PHYSICAL AGENTS
Theory and Practice

THIRD EDITION

PHYSICAL AGENTS
Theory and Practice
THIRD EDITION

BARBARA J. BEHRENS, PTA, MS
Coordinator, Physical Therapist Assistant
Program
Mercer County Community College
Trenton, NJ

HOLLY BEINERT, PT, MPT
Clinical Coordinator, Physical Therapist
Assistant Program
Mercer County Community College
Trenton, NJ

F.A. Davis Company • Philadelphia

F. A. Davis Company
1915 Arch Street
Philadelphia, PA 19103
www.fadavis.com

Copyright © 2014 by F. A. Davis Company

Printed in the United States of America

Last digit indicates print number: 10 9 8 7 6 5 4 3 2

Senior Acquisitions Editor: Melissa Duffield
Manager of Content Development: George W. Lang
Developmental Editor: Robin Levin Richman
Art and Design Manager: Carolyn O'Brien

As new scientific information becomes available through basic and clinical research, recommended treatments and drug therapies undergo changes. The author(s) and publisher have done everything possible to make this book accurate, up to date, and in accord with accepted standards at the time of publication. The author(s), editors, and publisher are not responsible for errors or omissions or for consequences from application of the book, and make no warranty, expressed or implied, in regard to the contents of the book. Any practice described in this book should be applied by the reader in accordance with professional standards of care used in regard to the unique circumstances that may apply in each situation. The reader is advised always to check product information (package inserts) for changes and new information regarding dose and contraindications before administering any drug. Caution is especially urged when using new or infrequently ordered drugs.

Library of Congress Cataloging-in-Publication Data

Physical agents : theory and practice / [edited by] Barbara J. Behrens, Holly Beinert. — Third edition.
      p. ; cm.
  Includes bibliographical references and index.
  ISBN 978-0-8036-3816-7
  I. Behrens, Barbara J., 1959- editor. II. Beinert, Holly, editor.
  [DNLM: 1. Physical Therapy Modalities. WB 460]
  RM700
  615.8'2—dc23
                    2014013175

Jo Ann Beine, PTA, MLS
Faculty
Physical therapy Assistant Program
Arapahoe Community College
Littleton, Colorado

Michelle Duncanson
Physiotherapist
Coordinator and Professor OTA & PTA program
Department of Health Studies
Niagara College
Welland, Ontario, Canada

Nancy Greenawald, EdS, MBA, BS PT
Program Coordinator
Physical Therapist Assistant Program
Montgomery College, Takoma Park-Silver Spring
   Campus
Takoma Park, Maryland

Heather MacKrell, PT, PhD
Program Director
Department of Health Sciences
Calhoun Community College
Tanner, Alabama

Amber L. Ward, OTR/L, BCPR, ATP
Occupational Therapy Coordinator, Adjunct Professor
Department of Neurology, Occupational Therapy
   Assistant Program
Carolinas Healthcare System, Cabarrus College of Health
   Sciences
Charlotte, North Carolina

Some clinicians greatly fear physical agents and others look to physical agents to help them to accomplish therapeutic treatment goals, knowing that it's all in how you use the agents. Throughout this text, concepts behind the physical agents are explained and then simple "why do you need to know" type activities are interspersed so that some of the fear factor can be reduced. There are examples of both theoretical and practical applications so the reader can consider and apply the concepts.

First, let's look at the chapter organization, followed by the special chapter features.

Chapter Organization

Each chapter includes many learning activities and features to help foster a greater understanding of the chapter's main objectives. Chapters begin with Learning Outcomes, Key Terms, and Chapter Outlines to help guide the reader through the content. Chapters end with a Summary, multiple-choice Self-Test Review Questions, Discussion Questions to promote further critical thinking, a Bibliography of suggested resources, list of cited References, and a Let's Find Out section with a variety of lab activities.

Special Features

A number of special features supplement the narrative and appear as appropriate:

- **Patient Perspective** provides a personal, unique story that reflects the content, followed by relevant questions.
- **Why Do I Need to Know About...?** connects concepts to clinical applications.
- **Let's Think About It** appears as appropriate, to focus attention on specific issues that the reader should consider.

- **Check It Out** is a lab activity (no equipment) that includes precautions, contraindications, and the rationales for both.
- **Before You Begin...** is a brief description of safety considerations to be taken prior to therapeutic interventions.
- **Case Studies** for application is a real-life scenario, which may appear at the end of the chapter before the Let's Find Out feature.
- **Let's Find Out** is a longer lab activity with equipment, and also includes precautions, contraindications, and rationales for both.

As noted, each of the lab activities (Check It Out and Let's Find Out) includes the contraindications and precautions for the physical agent as well as the rationales for its use. Clinical decision-making opportunities start with decisions regarding indications for modalities, which are just as important as the contraindications, and their individual rationale statements. Patient scenarios enable the student/learner ample opportunities to engage in thought provoking exercises focused on each of the physical agent modalities while learning about new techniques and gaining confidence in their ability to accomplish treatment goals.

The ability to provide a sound physiological rationale for what one is doing with a physical agent and then accomplish a therapeutic treatment goal with that physical agent is both an art and a science. The tools within the text have been written with the ultimate goal in mind that with one, the other can be accomplished. It just takes a willingness to understand and practice rather than fear of the unknown. There is so much that we can do if we just apply what we already know rather than fear it! We hope that you will be able to impart that to your students/learners and patients.

—*Barbara J. Behrens, PTA, MS*

I've heard that the third time is the charm, well here goes! The third edition of this text is a real charm and a marriage of many things, including:

- The minds and ideas from Holly Beinert and me as we collaborated on what to do with various topics that needed to be included or needed to be elaborated on a bit more.
- The lab manual and the text, but updated to include more pedagogic materials and, we hope, make them more useful and relevant.
- The blending of years of student/learner experiences and suggestions for what we should do in "the next edition of the book."
- The:
  - "I've always wanted to include that. . . " version
  - "I wish I could put that in there. . ." version
  - And oh, "I forgot to thank. . ." version

I couldn't do any of what I do without a firm foundation of support around me and that includes those who give of themselves, sometimes without even knowing it:

- The foundation of support that I mentioned. . . .
- 17 years of Mercer PTA Program alumni have provided themselves as awesome examples for photographic subjects, lab examples, patient scenarios, and the periodic exam question to ponder.
- An incredibly supportive set of faculty members from the PTA program at Mercer, who have lent their clinical expertise, patience, laughter, and editorial skills along the way in the development of innumerable lab and lecture activities for physical agents. Thank you Holly Beinert, Jessica Sliker, and Kristen Collins!
- Robin Levin Richman, who kindly nudged when deadlines were approaching.

- Lisa Thompson whose ability to edit and "see the big picture" among the drivel will never cease to amaze me.
- Melissa Duffield who encouraged Holly and I to give birth to a "third child."
- Kate M. who patiently revisited the art and photography for us so that what we envisioned and what you see are one and the same!
- George for his ability to organize the FAD team into high gear.
- T., who alerts me to the morning light after a long night of revisions!
- Everyone around me who "tolerated the process well" as I worked on the third edition.
- The following contributors to the second edition of this book: Ute H. Breese, Med, PT, OCS; Elizabeth Buchanan, PT; Joy Cohn, PT, CLT-LANA; Cheryl Gillespie, PT, DPT, MA; Burke Gurney, PT, PhD; Stacie Lynn Larkin, PT, Med, ACCE; Ethne Nussbaum, PT, PhD, Peter C. Panus, PT, PhD; Russell Stowers, PTA, MS; and Kristin von Nieda, DPT, Med.

—Barbara J. Behrens, PTA, MS

I would like to extend a very large thank you to the PTA alumni who so graciously gave their time during the photoshoot for this third edition, especially Jessica Sliker, Kristen Collins, Diana Diaz, and the PTA Class of 2013. Thank you to Barbara Behrens for inviting me along this journey and trusting me with a project so close to her heart. I would also like to thank my family, Paul, Betsy, Neil, and Sean, for their everlasting love and support. Lastly, I thank Jackson Ryan Alexander, who provides daily doses of happiness, laughter, and love, without which success is not possible.

—Holly Beinert, PT, MPT

TABLE OF CONTENTS

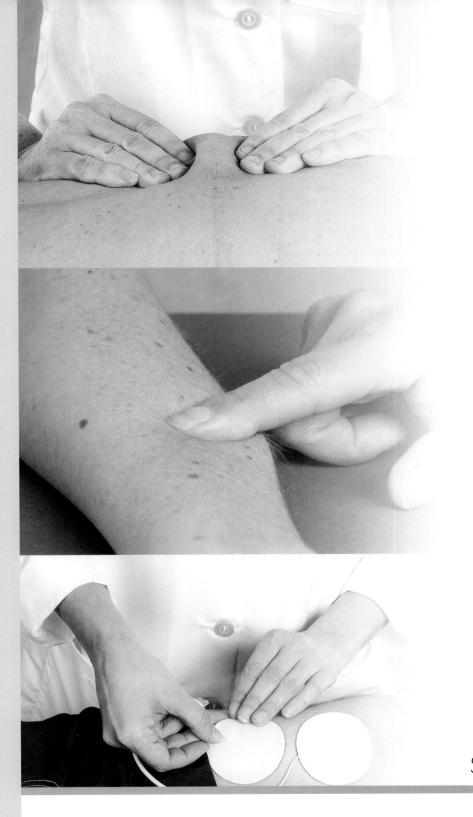

The Concept of Adjunctive Therapies

CHAPTER 1

Evidence-Based Practice With Physical Agents

Holly C. Beinert, PT, MPT

Learning Outcomes

Following the successful completion of this chapter, the learner will be able to:

- Define evidence-based physical therapy practice.
- Outline the five-step process of evidence-based practice (EBP) implementation.
- Discuss the benefits of EBP.
- Discuss the barriers to EBP and approaches for reducing them in clinical education and clinical practice.

Key Terms

Bias
Clinical expertise
Evidence-based practice
Exclusion criteria
Experimental design

Hierarchy of evidence
Inclusion criteria
Nonexperimental design
Peer-reviewed journals
Quasi-experimental design

Research design
Research subjects
Systematic review
Variables

Chapter Outline

Defining Evidence-Based Practice
Arguments for Using Evidence-Based Practice
The Five-Step Process for Implementing Evidence-Based
   Practice
    Ask
    Acquire

    Appraise
    Apply
    Assess
Sources of Evidence
Evidence in Action

"Knowledge is power" —*Sir Francis Bacon*

Patient Perspective

"Do you have to go to school to learn how to do this?

Evidence-based practice (EBP) is the use of the best current evidence to assist clinicians and their patients in the clinical decision-making process. All health care providers are obligated to provide current and accurate information regarding treatment options, so that the patient is able to provide truly informed consent. This textbook provides foundational information regarding the use of physical agents as a treatment intervention. Research will continue to expand and add to the knowledge base of those who incorporate the principles of EBP into their careers, making them more effective health care providers than those who rely solely on a textbook.

Defining Evidence-Based Practice

EBP is an approach to clinical decision making that integrates best research evidence, clinical expertise, and patient values.[1] Sackett, the first medical doctor to document the process of **evidence-based practice,** and colleagues define it as "conscientious, explicit, and judicious use of current best evidence in making decisions about the care of individual patients."[2] According to Physical Therapist Assistant (PTA) Pete Levine, "Being evidence based is a state of mind."[3] It requires that the Physical Therapist (PT) and PTA stay up to date with clinically relevant research and then implement the findings to provide improved quality of patient care. Once the evidence has been gathered and analyzed, clinical expertise is necessary to determine if the evidence applies to a particular patient, and if so, how.[1] Research evidence does not replace clinical expertise. Once the therapist decides to implement current research data into patient care, **clinical expertise,** or the proficiency of clinical skills and abilities, is required to do it safely and effectively.[2,4] Lastly, the patient's unique presentation, values, and goals must be taken into account when the therapist is making clinical decisions.

Arguments for Using Evidence-Based Practice

The number one reason for getting on board with EBP is that it benefits the patient. According to Iles and Davidson, "The appropriate use of evidence about the effectiveness of various treatment strategies should result in clinicians selecting techniques known to be effective, and ultimately lead to improved patient outcomes."[5] This is supported by the American Physical Therapy Association's *Vision 2020* statement, in which it states that PTs and PTAs will render evidence-based services (Box 1-1).[6] Incorporating EBP will increase the credibility of the physical therapy profession within the health care industry. Lastly, changes in health care structure and reimbursement provide motivation for justification of services for reimbursement, as well as a greater need to provide the best outcomes possible in the most efficient manner. Insurance companies have already begun to deny reimbursement for PT services that are not supported by evidence. Depending on the setting, reimbursement may be determined by the diagnosis and not the length of stay or number of physical therapy interventions

---

BOX 1-1 | American Physical Therapy Association's *Vision 2020 statement*[6]

The following is the APTA *Vision 2020 Statement*:

"Guided by integrity, life-long learning, and a commitment to comprehensive and accessible health programs for all people, physical therapists and physical therapist assistants will render evidence-based services throughout the continuum of care and improve quality of life for society."

provided. Therefore, providing physical therapy interventions that help patients to meet their goals in a shorter period of time benefits both patients and the facility.

The Five-Step Process for Implementing Evidence-Based Practice

According to Sackett et al (2000) and Del Mar et al (2004), the five steps of EBP are (1) asking an answerable clinical question, (2) acquiring the best available evidence, (3) appraising the evidence, (4) applying the evidence to clinical practice, and (5) assessing the process.[7,8]

ASK

Asking an answerable clinical question requires the clinician to recognize when there is a gap in his or her clinical knowledge. The clinician then needs to be able to form a structured question that defines the problem, the intervention, and the outcomes of interest.[5]

To connect the clinical process of implementing EBP to everyday life, we will follow an example of this process that is not related to physical therapy. Imagine that you have just moved into your first apartment. As a housewarming gift, your friends bought you a houseplant called an African violet. They didn't know that you have never taken care of a houseplant before. You immediately recognize that there is a gap in your knowledge because you do not know how to keep this plant alive. You create the following question in your head: "How do I keep an indoor African violet plant alive?"

ACQUIRE

This step requires that the clinician have access to journals or databases in order to acquire the best available evidence.[9] Investing in database memberships can play a very important role in providing access to quality articles. Conducting free searches using resources such as the local library system, PubMed, PEDro, Medline, and Google Scholar is also a possibility.

To find an answer to your question regarding taking care of your houseplant, where would you go? Let's say that you asked your friend because she has a lot of plants. Unfortunately, your friend has never owned nor cared for an African violet, but she does advise you to provide it with lots of sunlight. Your next step leads you to the experts who have cared for African violets. You go to the library and search in the archives of *The Plant Journal* and the *Journal of the American Society for Horticultural Science*. Lastly, you make a trip to your local hardware and garden store to talk with one of the associates. You are doing a lot of work to gather answers.

APPRAISE

After articles have been gathered, the clinician must be able to critically appraise the evidence to determine its clinical importance.[5] It is important to read more than just the abstract and conclusion. You must familiarize yourself with interpreting research data. The reader must be cognizant of subject selection and management, measurement reliability and validity, research validity, and study credibility, to name a few.

Entire textbooks and continuing education courses have been devoted to the topic of how to conduct a proper analysis of research. This section covers some of the foundational and basic information pertaining to the appraisal of evidence quality. Further self-directed learning is recommended.

LET'S THINK ABOUT IT...

Self-directed learning is the process by which the individual takes responsibility for furthering his knowledge regarding a specific topic and takes it upon himself to conduct research on that topic. The *February 2009 Project Information Literacy Progress Report* states that students frequently conduct "everyday life research," defined as the ongoing information-seeking strategies for solving problems that may arise in daily life (e.g., health and wellness, finance and commerce, news, domestic, career, and spiritual).[9] Students in the survey reported that everyday life research differed from educational course-related research in that it is personal, is curiosity driven, and has no deadlines.[9]

Following are questions that you need to ask:

1. Where would you go to find the most reliable information about purchasing a new car? Would you trust this source more or less than the car salesman? Why?
2. What would you do if you needed to find out how to make your own modeling clay before your nephew arrives in an hour?
3. Do you consider reading research articles to improve the quality of patient care personally important or is it work related? Is there a deadline? Is it driven by curiosity?

Research Design

Research design is the plan for conducting a research study.[10] Some research designs are stronger than others and in an effort to make selecting the best current research easier, the Centre for Evidence-Based Medicine in Oxford, England, created a **hierarchy of evidence,** which ranks research designs based on their ability to minimize bias.[11] **Bias** is a systematic deviation from the truth owing to uncontrolled influences in the study.[10] Even in research designs that minimize bias, clinicians should not rely on the conclusions of research studies to make decisions regarding patient care without first critically appraising the study to determine whether or not the conclusion is supported by the data presented.[12]

In an **experimental design,** researchers place the subjects into two or more groups and keep all variables the same except for the one they are testing. The group not receiving the test intervention is called a *control group* and the researchers measure the results so that they can compare the two groups. An example would be a study designed to determine if the addition of moist heat prior to stretching increases passive range of motion (ROM). The researchers may have two groups, both of which receive the same stretches. Only one of the groups would receive moist heat prior to the stretching. Passive ROM would then be measured in both groups to determine if there is a difference. **Variables** are characteristics that can vary from group to group. When a study aims to test cause-and-effect relationships, the variable that is controlled by the researchers is called the independent variable. In the example above, the addition of moist heat is the independent variable. The variable that is measured is called the dependent variable. Therefore, in the above example, passive ROM is the dependent variable.

While similar in many ways to an experimental design, a **quasi-experimental** design lacks random subject assignment. While the validity of quasi-experimental designs tends to be weaker than that of experimental designs, they are often used when researchers have difficulty obtaining sufficient numbers of subjects to form groups.[10] There are many different types of quasi-experimental designs. One of the most commonly used quasi-experimental designs includes testing two groups of subjects prior to and after an intervention. However, it is important to remember that the two groups were not randomly assigned; therefore, there may be additional differences between the two groups aside from the intervention provided. An example would be a study designed to determine the effects of biofeedback on balance control and coordination in two groups of pediatric patients with the rare Joubert syndrome. Because the condition is so rare, the researchers may be able to find only two clinics in the country that treat children with this diagnosis. If the researchers were to provide biofeedback only to children in one of those clinics, it would not be a random assignment. Can you think of additional differences that these groups of subjects may have that were not controlled?

In **nonexperimental designs,** researchers observe and collect data without manipulating the subjects. These are also referred to as observational studies.[10]

A **systematic review** is often conducted by trained reviewers who gather many studies regarding a specific research question, creating a thorough research paper incorporating the findings of many researchers.[10]

Subjects

Research subjects are the people from whom data will be collected in an effort to answer the research question. **Inclusion criteria** define the characteristics the subjects must possess in order to be included in the study.[10] For example, if researchers were trying to determine the effectiveness of cervical mechanical traction in reducing pain in patients with mechanical neck disorders, it would make sense that all subjects have a mechanical neck disorder. **Exclusion criteria** define characteristics that will make subjects ineligible to participate in the study because they are considered variables that may interfere with the study outcome.[10] To continue with the same example, subjects with mechanical neck disorders may be excluded from the study if they have had recent cervical surgery, have signs and symptoms of an upper motor neuron lesion, or are currently taking steroidal medication.

The number of subjects included in a study will have an impact on the strength of the study as well. Imagine that two separate studies attempted to answer the question regarding the effectiveness of cervical mechanical traction in reducing pain in patients with mechanical neck disorders. In the first study, 75% of the subjects showed decreased pain with cervical mechanical traction and in the second study only 25% of the subjects showed decreased pain following the same intervention. When you read further, you notice that the first study had only four subjects, so three of the four subjects had decreased pain. The second study had 100 subjects and only 25 of them demonstrated pain relief. Which results might be due to chance? Which is more mathematically meaningful?

Statistics

Statistics are tools that researchers use to understand and evaluate the data that they collect from the studies that they do with their subjects. Each statistical test has a specific purpose, indications for use, methods for their application, and performance limitations. Further learning about the many statistical tests is the only way to be able to consider whether the researcher utilized the appropriate test for her study, and whether it was used correctly. Table 1-1 defines the most common statistical terms.

You have gathered potential solutions to keeping your African violet alive. Your neighbor takes care of many houseplants and although she has never owned an African violet, she tells you to give the plant lots of sunlight. The associate at the hardware store brought you to the aisle containing plant food products. The back of the bag you chose indicates that the product will meet the unique needs of all indoor plants. Lastly, you read information from *The Plant Journal* and the American Society for Horticultural Science. These two sources indicate that the leaves of the African violet should not get wet. Therefore, placing the plant in a dish and watering from the bottom is a good idea. They also informed you to take the flowers off of the plant when it flowers, to rotate the plant in the sun, and to water it only when it is dry. Which of these sources is most objective?

APPLY

Once the clinical importance has been determined, the clinician must integrate the evidence with clinical expertise and patient values.[5]

Initiating change in your clinical practice can be quite difficult; however, working in a supportive environment with other clinicians who hold EBP in high esteem will foster practice growth.

Now it is time to go home and apply your newfound knowledge. You have decided that the advice on the plant food product is not objective because the company that makes it has a monetary stake in your decision to use its product. You place the plant in the sun, water it carefully so that you do not get the leaves wet, and wait for it to flower.

TABLE 1-1 | Statistical Terminology Defined[10]

Mean	The sum of the data points divided by the number of scores. Also known as the average
Median	The middle score in a data set
Mode	The score that occurs most frequently in a data set
Negative Predictive Value	The proportion of subjects with a negative test result who do not have the condition of interest
p Value	The probability that a statistical finding occurred owing to chance
Positive Predictive Value	The proportion of subjects with a positive test result who have the condition of interest
Power	The probability that a statistical test will detect, if it is present, a relationship between two or more variables or a difference between two or more groups
Reliability	The extent to which repeated measurements agree with one another
Sensitivity	The proportion of subjects with the condition of interest that have a positive test result
Specificity	The proportion of subjects without the condition of interest who have a negative test result
Standard Deviation	The average absolute distance of scores from the mean score of a data set
Validity	The degree to which a study appropriately answers the question being asked. Also, the degree to which a measurement tool captures what it is intended to measure

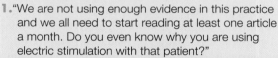

LET'S THINK ABOUT IT...

How does a clinician initiate this type of discussion with coworkers? Compare the two following approaches. Which is more likely to get your coworkers on board with EBP?

1. "We are not using enough evidence in this practice and we all need to start reading at least one article a month. Do you even know why you are using electric stimulation with that patient?"
2. "I read a really interesting article this weekend, which showed that 10 sessions of ultrasound used at 1 MHz, 1 W/cm², 100% for 5 minutes in patients with knee osteoarthritis decrease pain, improve functional outcomes, and help the 50-m walk time. I'm really excited to use this with Mr. Smith for the next 10 visits to see if we can get the same results. Here is a copy of the article if you are interested."

ASSESS

Lastly, the clinician is required to assess the steps that he/she took, as well as the effectiveness of the treatment outcome. The clinician must identify ways to improve effective patient care.[5]

One year later, your African violet is alive and well. You have a new neighbor and you decide to bring her an African violet as a welcome gift. She asks you how to take care of it and you know exactly what to tell her, where you got your information, and how successful you have been with implementing it.

Table 1-2 outlines the five steps of EBP. The first column summarizes the steps taken to answer the question "How do I keep an indoor African violet plant alive?" The second column shows the five steps as they apply to a clinical question regarding effective use of low-level laser therapy and the third column has been left blank, so that you can fill it in based on one of the two case studies outlined at the end of the chapter.

Sources of Evidence

Information regarding physical therapy can come from many sources. Often that first source we turn to is the opinion of other clinicians who may have more experience than we do. This may include instructors, authors of textbooks and articles, and co-workers. We can also rely on our own clinical experience to help guide us in the decision-making process with our current patients. Lastly, we can look toward **peer-reviewed journals.** These journals have panels of experts on various topics who then evaluate research studies for credibility and relevance prior to publishing it in the journal in an effort to publish only high-quality research.[10]

Evidence in Action

Implementing evidence-based medicine into daily practice is not without challenge. Staying current with the evidence requires a commitment to learning, and clinicians are encouraged to set aside time each week to locate and read journal articles.[5] Creating a journal club at work promotes

TABLE 1-2 | Steps for Implementing EBP

		AFRICAN VIOLET EXAMPLE	PHYSICAL AGENT EXAMPLE[14]	YOUR OWN
1	Ask	"How do I keep an indoor African violet plant alive?"	Does current research support the use of low-level laser therapy for knee osteoarthritis?	
2	Acquire	A. Neighbor who has never cared for an African violet B. *The Plant Journal* C. The American Society for Horticultural Science D. Sales associate at local plant shop	Alfredo, P., Bjordal, J., Dreyer, S., Ferreira, Zaguetti, G., Ovanessian, V., & Marques, A. (2012). Efficacy of low level laser therapy associated with exercises in knee osteoarthritis: A randomized double-blind study. *Clinical Rehabilitation* 26(6), 523–533. doi:10.1177/0269215511425962	
3	Appraise	You appraise the source's experience and level of bias.	While reading the article, you note that the subjects included all had osteoarthritis, were between 50 and 75 years of age, were male and female, and had pain and limited function for at least 3 months. You note that the subjects were placed into one of two groups randomly and that the therapists who measured and treated the subjects were both blinded. The p values indicate statistically significant improvement in the laser group over the non-laser group for pain relief and functional improvement.	
4	Apply	You place the plant in the sun, water it carefully so you do not get the leaves wet, and wait for it to flower.	Because your patient is a 60-year-old man who has had pain and limited function for 7 months and has no contraindications for low-level laser therapy, you decide to include low-level laser therapy three times a week for the first 3 weeks using the parameters included in the study.	
5	Assess	Is the plant still alive 1 month later? One year later?	Provide assessment and documentation of ROM, pain levels, strength, and functional status as compared with the findings of the initial examination and evaluation.	

encouragement of and support for the implementation of EBP. Clinicians can take turns presenting clinically relevant research articles to peers, managing discussions, and assisting in the application of the evidence into clinical practice. Clinicians who are seeking employment can ask potential employers how they promote EBP in their clinics, whether a journal club is in place or would be welcomed, and whether they offer access to databases and journals for their employees. In addition to the time required, lack of access to evidence has also been cited as a barrier to EBP.[5] Employers may provide access to various peer-reviewed journals and databases. Clinicians may also choose to subscribe to resources on their own.

Successful implementation of EBP requires the commitment and participation of each practicing clinician, as well as support from management and leaders. Clinicians are encouraged to follow the five steps for implementing EBP, discuss the findings with colleagues and patients alike, and explain to their patients why each physical therapy intervention was chosen. Managers and leaders can foster learning activities by creating and supporting journal clubs,

providing access to journals and time to stay current, as well as providing incentives for employees.[13]

Providing accurate, thorough, and clinically meaningful documentation is a vital component to EBP. When we provide good clinical documentation, it allows us to analyse patient outcomes to determine if the chosen interventions are effective in meeting the physical therapy goals. The final step, assessment, allows us to better navigate the many options available to us as clinicians.

Summary

Being an evidence-based clinician is an ongoing process that requires a strong commitment to patient outcomes and professional growth. When health care providers make treatment choices based on sound evidence, it fosters self-confidence and patient confidence. Understanding why you are choosing a modality and which parameters to use will maximize your patient outcomes and effectiveness as a health care provider.

Review Questions

1. Which of the following is not typically used in EBP?
   a. Best current research evidence
   b. Clinical expertise
   c. Patient goals and values
   d. What your coworkers do

2. The use of EBP in clinical decision-making skills benefits whom?
   a. The patient
   b. The clinician
   c. The profession
   d. All of the above

3. Which of the following is the first step in implementing EBP?
   a. Asking a clinical question
   b. Acquiring data
   c. Appraising the data
   d. Applying the data

4. Which of the following research designs has at least two groups, with one of them being a control group?
   a. Case study
   b. Experimental
   c. Quasi-experimental
   d. Nonexperimental

5. Which of the following best defines "research subject"?
   a. The person collecting the data
   b. The person analyzing the data
   c. The person from whom data are being collected
   d. The person excluded from the study

Patients' Frequently Asked Questions

1. Why am I doing this?
2. Is this going to work?
3. What do you know about this?

CASE STUDY 1

You are on your final clinical affiliation in a busy outpatient facility and you have two clinical instructors. The facility specializes in treating the upper quadrant and you see many patients being treated for their shoulders. After 3 weeks in the clinic, you realize that one of your clinical instructors performs ultrasound with regular ultrasound gel. The other clinical instructor calls the patients' doctors to request a prescription for a gel containing fluocinonide so that she can do phonophoresis. You ask each clinician for his or her clinical rationale for choosing between ultrasound and phonophoresis. Neither clinician provides a strong response. The first clinician states, "That's how I've always done it" and the other states, "I think the medicine helps." The following week, you start working with a patient who has shoulder pain. You do not know which gel (regular ultrasound gel or gel containing fluocinonide) is likely to produce better results. Therefore, you decide to do a literature review to answer the following question: "Which intervention is more effective in reducing shoulder pain: ultrasound or phonophoresis?" You decide to utilize your school library's online database this weekend to conduct your research.

1. What keywords will you enter into the database search engine?
2. What factors do you consider important when considering if the evidence is relevant to your patient?
3. Once you determine the type of gel most likely to be effective for your patient, how will you present your decision to the patient and your clinical instructors?
4. Lastly, how will you measure the effectiveness of your decision?

CASE STUDY 2

You have just started your first job as a licensed clinician and one of your first patients has Bell's palsy. You have been working on initiation, facilitation, movement control, and relaxation of the facial muscles using proprioceptive neuromuscular facilitation (PNF) principles and techniques. During today's treatment session the patient tells you that he had neuromuscular electric stimulation (NMES) on his thigh years ago after tearing his anterior cruciate ligament. He is wondering if the same thing can be used on his face. You decide to do a literature review to answer the following question: "Is neuromuscular electric stimulation effective in treating Bell's palsy?" You decide to utilize the American Physical Therapy Association's (APTA) online database, Hooked on Evidence to conduct your research.

1. What keywords will you enter into the database search engine?

2. What factors do you consider important when determining if the evidence is relevant to your patient?

3. Once you determine if NMES is best suited for your patient, how will you present your decision to him?

4. Lastly, how will you measure the effectiveness of your decision?

5. Choose one of these two case studies and fill in the third column of Table 1-2, indicating the steps you would take to implement EBP.

DISCUSSION QUESTIONS

1. How would you explain the importance of EBP to a clinical instructor who has limited clinical experience with this concept?

2. Imagine that your family doctor prescribed a blood pressure medication for a female family member in her late 20s. When asked what the current literature states regarding the use of this medication in young women, the doctor cannot answer the question. The family decides to get a second opinion and when asked the same question, the second doctor is able to reference two articles regarding the effectiveness of the medication versus other nonmedicinal interventions as well as the side effects in women during their childbearing years. How has the use of EBP influenced your confidence in the doctor and the treatment intervention?

3. Might knowing the funding source of a research trial affect your interpretation of the results?

4. Two randomized controlled trials are identical in setup except for the number of subjects. The first trial tested 20 subjects and the second trial tested 500 subjects. Which trial is stronger? Why?

5. If a research article uses only male subjects, can you conclude that the results would be the same for women? Would it depend on what is being tested?

REFERENCES

1. Mellion, LR: Evidence-based research. Advance for Physical Therapy & Rehab Medicine 13(3): 6, 2012.
2. Sackett, DL, Rosenberg, WM, Gray, JA, Haynes, RB, Richardson, SW: Evidence based medicine: What it is and what it isn't. British Medical Journal 312: 71–72, 1996.
3. Levine, P: An evidence-based state of mind. Advance for Physical Therapy & Rehab Medicine, Web content, 2010.
4. Higgs, J, Jones, M, Loftus S, Christensen, N: Clinical Reasoning in Health Professions, 3rd ed. Butterworth Heinemann, Oxford, England, 2008.
5. Iles, R, Davidson, M: Evidence based practice: A survey of physiotherapists' current practice. Physiotherapy Research International 11:93–103, 2006.
6. Vision Statement for Physical Therapy. American Physical Therapy Association, Vision 2020, http://www.apta.org/vision2020/
7. Sackett, DL, Straus, SE, Richardson, SW, Rosenberg, W, Haynes, BR: Evidence-Based Medicine. Churchill Livingstone, London, 2000.
8. Del Mar, C, Glasziou, P, Mayer, D: Teaching evidence based medicine. British Medical Journal 329: 989–990, 2004.
9. Head, AJ, Eisenberg, MB: Finding Context: What Today's College Students Say about Conducting Research in the Digital Age. University of Washington, Project Information Literacy Report, February 2009.
10. Jewell, DV: Guide to Evidence-Based Physical Therapist Practice, 2nd ed. Jones & Bartlett Learning, Sudbury, MA, 2011.
11. Levels of Evidence. Centre for Evidence-Based Medicine: Oxford website. Available at: http://www.cebm.net. Accessed June 16, 2012.
12. Feise, R. Is cervical traction effective for patients with mechanical neck conditions? Journal of the American Chiropractic Association, 2009.
13. Schreiber, J, Stern, P, Marchetti G, Provident, I: Strategies to promote evidence-based practice in pediatric physical therapy: A formative evaluation pilot project. Physical Therapy 89(9): 918–933, 2009.
14. Alfredo, PP, Bjordal, JM, Dreyer, SH, et al: Efficacy of low level laser therapy associated with exercises in knee osteoarthritis: A randomized double-blind study. Clinical Rehabilitation 26(6): 523–533, 2011.

2

Tissue Response to Injury

Holly C. Beinert, PT, MPT | *Barbara J. Behrens, PTA, MS*
Stacie Larkin, PT, MEd

Learning Outcomes

Following the successful completion of this chapter, the learner will be able to:

- Define pain.
- Describe the factors that affect an individual's perception of pain.
- Define acute and chronic pain.
- Define analgesia and anesthesia, and differentiate between them.
- Explain the gate control theory of pain; provide examples of the use of physical agents based on this theory.
- Define endogenous opiates, listing events that can trigger the release of these substances.
- Describe therapeutic interventions for a patient in acute pain, including methods of encouraging active patient participation in the recovery process.
- Describe the team approach to the treatment of patients with chronic pain.
- Discuss analgesic and anti-inflammatory medications and their impact on therapeutic interventions.
- Describe key events that occur in the three stages of wound healing.
- Identify precautions for handling wounds during each of the three stages.
- Describe appropriate therapeutic treatment interventions for wounds in each of the three stages.
- Define the following terms that are commonly used in the clinical setting to describe symptoms related to tissue responses:
  - pain
  - altered sensation
  - edema (swelling)
  - loss of function
- Describe the common concepts for the theory of pain transmission and perception and explain it in terms that a patient would understand.
- Describe the similarities and differences between the endogenous opiates in terms that a patient would understand.
- Discuss the impact of the psychological component on pain perception by comparing his or her findings and experiences with those of classmates in a guided class discussion.
- Discuss a classic theory of pain transmission and how it can be applied to pain-relieving techniques.
- Differentiate between the key events in the three stages of wound healing by describing each of those key events and what triggers them.
- Describe the necessary precautions in handling wounds during each of the stages of healing.

Key Terms

Acute pain
Analgesia
Anesthesia
Chronic pain
Dermatome
Dorsal horn

Edema
Endogenous
Erythema
Inflammation
Ischemia
Myotome

Narcotic
Nociceptor
Pain
Proliferation
Remodeling
Scleratome

Chapter Outline

> *"Behind every beautiful thing, there's some kind of pain."* —Bob Dylan

Patient Perspective

"I keep hearing the phrase 'no pain, no gain'; is that really necessary?"

Pain perception is one of the most common reasons or symptoms that causes an individual to seek the assistance of a medical or allied health professional. It can be a sign of physical, physiological, or psychological dysfunction. This explains why there are so many different pain assessment instruments developed to measure it.[2] Depending on the individual, pain may be thought of as the body's warning system or the body's way of letting the individual know that something is wrong. Without the sensation of pain, additional tissue damage or injury may occur. Pain may, however, have numerous adverse effects, resulting in symptoms such as muscle guarding that over time can lead to weakness, decreased range of motion, fatigue, insomnia, increased irritability, anxiety, depression, decreased appetite, sexual dysfunction, and emotional distress.[3-6] Although an individual seeks assistance to relieve his or her pain, it must be remembered that pain management is only one aspect of the complete care of the patient geared toward improving function and reducing disability. Depending on the additional rehabilitation needs of the individual, several therapeutic interventions may be used.

Definitions

Pain is defined as "an unpleasant sensory and emotional experience associated with actual or potential tissue damage, or described in terms of such damage" (Box 2-1).[7] This definition avoids tying pain to just a physical stimulus and instead emphasizes that our willingness to call something painful can be influenced by other factors. These factors include our focus of attention, level of anxiety, degree of suggestibility, level of arousal, degree of fatigue, previous emotional and psychological experience, and cultural mores.[3,4,8,73] In other words, although a sensation may start as a physical or chemically mediated stimulus to a **nociceptor** (pain receptor), our willingness to call the sensation painful or to respond to the painful stimulus is variable depending on past learning and current circumstances and is purely subjective. Only the individual experiencing the "pain" knows the true quality of that sensation and the personal meaning of that sensation. One aspect of a therapeutic intervention for a patient experiencing pain involves controlling the perception and/or sensation of pain. Providing the patient with a way to manage his or her level of discomfort can ultimately lead to improved function.

The body's response to trauma is a complex interaction of sensory, motivational, and cognitive processes that determine a sequence of behavior that characterizes pain (Fig. 2-1).[1,6] On a systemic level, the sympathetic component of the autonomic nervous system responds to the perceived threat by a "fight-or-flight" reaction. This reaction involves numerous body systems and typically includes increased heart rate and sweating, expansion of the bronchioles (small airways), dilation of the pupils, shunting of blood from the skin and digestive tract to the muscles and brain, decreased peristalsis, and contraction of the sphincters (Fig. 2-2).[9]

Initially, when experiencing pain resulting from trauma, the person will try to withdraw from the stimulus. Muscle guarding occurs as the body's way to immobilize the injured area and prevent further damage (Fig. 2-3). This reaction of the muscles requires a high level of metabolic activity at the same time as it compresses the blood vessels. The compromised circulation is often inadequate to supply metabolic needs, leading to **ischemia,** local anemia due to

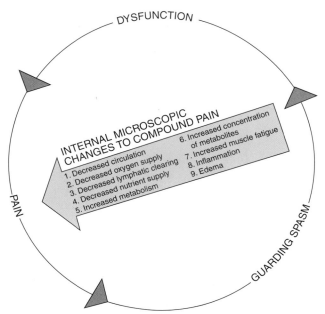

FIGURE 2-1 Primary pain cycle and associated internal changes.
(From Mannheimer, JS, and Lampe, GN, eds. Clinical Transcutaneous Electrical Nerve Stimulation. FA Davis, Philadelphia, 1984, p 10, with permission.)

mechanical obstruction of the blood supply.[76] This ischemia becomes a new source of pain. In addition, the compromised circulation impedes the removal of the metabolic wastes, many of which sensitize nociceptors, resulting in further enhancement of pain.

Edema is the accumulation of excess watery fluid in cells, tissues, or serous cavities.[76] Edema resulting from injury causes disruption of the capillaries and lymphatics, with an increase in capillary permeability as a result of compression from muscle guarding. This further compounds the problems of nutrient supply and waste removal, thereby causing additional pain perception and subsequent additional muscle guarding. Thus, a vicious circle of pain, muscle guarding, and pain can evolve. Finally, **endogenous** pain-producing substances are those that are produced within the body. Examples are potassium, serotonin (5-hydroxytryptamine [5-HT]), bradykinin, histamine, prostaglandins, leukotrienes, and substance P, which are commonly released into the injured area (Box 2-2).[6,10]

These substances can directly activate nociceptors, or they may act alone or in combination to sensitize nociceptors to other agents. For example, histamine excites polymodal nociceptors, bradykinin increases the synthesis and release of prostaglandins from nearby cells, and prostaglandin E produces hyperalgesia and sensitizes nociceptors.[6] The body responds to trauma by an acute inflammatory response. The symptoms associated with the **inflammation** are a warning to the individual, indicating tissue damage. Inflammation is a complex of cytological and chemical reactions that occur in response to injury.[76] The symptoms experienced are the cardinal signs of inflammation: pain, heat, **erythema** (redness of the skin), edema, and loss of function.

BOX 2-1 | The Terminology of Pain Perception

The use of appropriate terminology is helpful when discussing pain management.

- *Analgesia:* The absence of pain or noxious stimulation; the absence of the sensibility to pain; or the relief of pain without a loss of consciousness.
- *Anesthesia:* A loss of sensation, usually by damage to a nerve or receptor, that is, numbness; or the loss of the ability to feel pain caused by the administration of drugs or medical interventions.

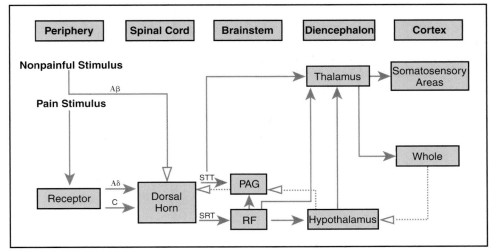

FIGURE 2-2 Schematic representation of ascending and descending connections responsible for pain sensation. Ascending pathways are represented by solid lines. Pain stimulus triggers a response in the peripheral sensory receptors. Stimulus is sent to the spinal cord via the A-delta (Aδ) and C fibers and then to the brainstem (PAG = periaqueductal gray matter and RF = reticular formation) via two tracts (STT = spinothalamic tract and SRT = spinoreticulothalamic pathway). Information is relayed to the thalamus and hypothalamus and then on to the somatosensory areas and other areas of the cortex. Descending, inhibitory pathways are represented by dashed lines. Descending modulation of pain perception is thought to block pain signal transmission in the dorsal horn of the spinal cord. Nonpainful sensory stimulus (transmitted via A-beta [Aβ]) is also thought to block pain signal transmission in the dorsal horn.[10,21]

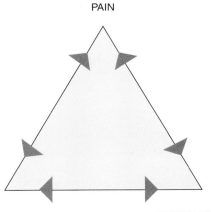

FIGURE 2-3 The pain triangle depicts an interrelationship between each of the points of the triangle. Pain perception has the ability to increase muscle guarding, which could then cause a decrease in circulation and impair the healing process. Conversely, treatment interventions that address pain in addition to its cause and the dysfunction itself will help to break the cycle, increasing circulation by decreasing protective muscle guarding.

BEFORE YOU BEGIN

Remember that on a local level, the body reacts to injury in three primary ways:

1. Muscle guarding
2. Edema formation
3. Release of endogenous pain chemical mediators

BOX 2-2 | Pain-Producing Substances Triggered by Injury

Injury triggers the release of the following endogenous pain-producing substances into the injured area:[6,10]

- Potassium
- Serotonin (5-HT)
- Bradykinin
- Histamine
- Prostaglandins
- Leukotrienes
- Substance P

ACUTE AND CHRONIC PAIN

Pain can be classified as acute or chronic.[6,11-13] **Acute pain** is most often the result of infection, injury, or internal disease. It is predictable in characteristics, easily localized by the patient, relatively easy to diagnose and treat, and often readily relieved. **Chronic pain,** however, may or may not relate to an actual physical injury and may persist well beyond the presence of obvious physical findings to support it. The longer the pain persists, the more likely it is to be referred away from the site of the actual cause or lesion.[11] The pain associated with an injury can also result in decreased function of the injured body part. Range of motion may be limited as a result of increased pain with motion due to the added stress at the site of injury. Also, muscle contraction produces pain because of the "tension" created at the injury site by the contraction. Pain may cause protective muscle guarding, which further increases pain perception. The end result is the pain-muscle guarding cycle.[10] The prolonged protective guarding of a muscle can lead to ischemia of the tissue because of compression of the blood vessels. The ischemia can also further sensitize already irritated nociceptors and increase pain perception. The combination of the prolonged painful event and resultant muscle guarding may lead to an inability to use the body part without pain.

Chronic pain is pain that lasts longer than 3 months[1] and leads to a long-term loss of function, as well as imposing many psychosocial stresses on the patient and his or her friends and family. The mechanism by which acute pain is similar to or different from chronic pain is not fully understood. The extent to which pain is perceived and responded to may be a function of the influences of biological, psychosocial, behavioral, neurohormonal, and neurochemical factors.[1–3,11–15] There are reasons postulated for this that are not yet completely understood. Various mechanisms have been proposed to account for chronic pain. The most commonly described mechanisms are as follows:[6,10,13]

- *Mechanical:* Clinical examples of mechanical irritation include entrapment syndromes such as carpal tunnel syndrome.
- *Chemical:* Chemical irritation in the injured area occurs as the body releases various substances in reaction to trauma, inflammation, or ischemia. These substances increase the sensitivity of the nociceptor,[6] enhance each other's action, and facilitate the release of prostaglandin E. A positive-feedback loop of pain causes inflammation and more pain results.
- *Regeneration:* As nerves are regenerating following surgery or trauma, there can be a period of marked increase in discharges from the peripheral nerve fibers that transmit pain signals (A-delta and C fibers).[6,13]
- *Reflexes:* Motor reflexes that normally act to protect tissue from acute pain can persist and produce changes associated with chronic pain such as muscle guarding. This can result in ischemia and nerve compression. Overactivity of sympathetic reflexes can result in vasoconstriction, ischemia, and trophic changes.
- *Inhibitory failure:* Inhibitory failure involves a breakdown in the usual response of the central nervous system (CNS).[6] In response to significant pain, the CNS normally releases chemicals called endogenous opiates. These chemicals exert control at the first relay of incoming injury signals in the **dorsal horn** of the spinal cord and decrease or block the transmission of further pain signals. "The dorsal horn of the spinal cord acts like a computer that processes the incoming sensory signals, rearranging and modulating them before sending them on to the next higher level."[21] Some examples of this inhibitory failure are thalamic pain, pain associated with brain or spinal cord injury, and pain associated with demyelinating diseases such as multiple sclerosis.

WHY DO I NEED TO KNOW ABOUT...
CARDINAL SIGNS OF INFLAMMATION

Pain
The resultant pain perception is due to the stimulation of the pain receptors and free nerve endings of A-delta and C fibers by the chemicals present at the site and the mechanical pressure of the edema.

Increased Tissue Temperature
Increased tissue temperature and erythema are the result of the vasodilation of the blood vessels, allowing more blood to pass through the area and increasing metabolic rate.

Erythema
Vascular changes occur with an inflammatory response that allows fluid and cells to exude from the blood vessels that promote phagocytosis, fibroblastic activity, and the beginning of the formation of new capillary beds.

Edema
The fluid exudate in the extravascular space accumulates due to the increased permeability and vasodilation of blood vessels.

Loss of Function
This is the ultimate result of sensitization of pain receptors, tissue damage, fluid retention impeding range of motion, and an active unchecked inflammatory response.

The transition from acute to chronic pain has not been well defined. If pain meets the following three criteria, however, it is usually termed chronic pain[6]:

1. The cause is uncertain or not correctable.
2. Medical treatments have been ineffective.
3. Pain has persisted for longer than 3 months.

Chronic pain is often treated by a team approach with a heavy emphasis on psychological support, behavior modification techniques, and guidance.[11,16–21] The team can include a coordinating physician and/or nurse practitioner, a psychologist, a physical therapist, an occupational therapist, a social worker, and a vocational rehabilitation counselor. Recreational therapists, dietitians, biofeedback technicians, and other health care providers also play roles on some teams. The team attempts to empower the patient and his or her family through education. Physical therapy treatment intervention emphasizes active management of the pain[17] through the proper use of activity alternating with rest, body mechanics, posture education, stretching, strengthening, cardiovascular conditioning,[16] relaxation techniques, work conditioning or hardening, and home use of physical agents such as heat, ice, and transcutaneous electrical nerve stimulation (TENS).[17] Manual techniques and physical agents are kept to a minimum but may include joint or soft tissue mobilization techniques, ultrasound, and electrical stimulation. Other members of the team deal with drug dependency, stress management, assertiveness training, behavioral modification, family therapy, and vocational counseling as needed.

Psychological Implications

On a psychological level, the individual reacts to the on-going misery and stress of chronic pain, the failure of adequate pain relief, changes in role and social status, and financial hardship. Many people experience depression in the face of these problems. Patients with chronic pain may also engage in pain behavior and pain games as maladaptive behavioral responses to their situation (Fig. 2-4).[5,6]

MEDICAL MANAGEMENT AFTER PAINFUL INSULT TO SOFT TISSUES

Medical management often involves the use of prescription or over-the-counter analgesic medications to help alleviate acute symptoms associated with pain. **Analgesia** is a state in which painful stimuli have been reduced.[76] Therefore, analgesic medications are characterized by a reduced response to painful stimuli. It is hoped that their use will decrease the potential for progression into a chronic condition and the associated difficulties

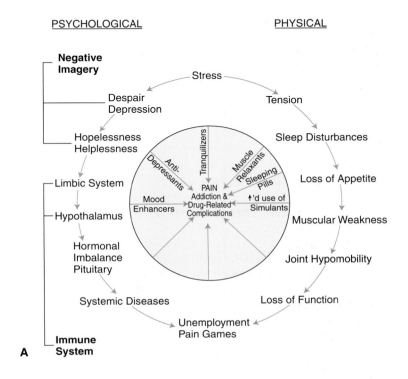

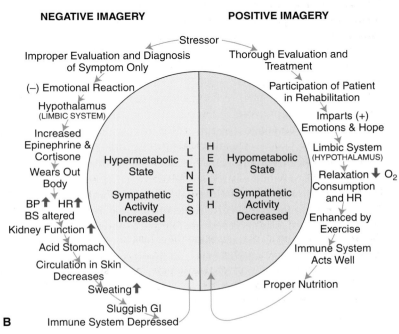

FIGURE 2-4 Chronic pain cycle.
(A) Psychological and physical impact.
(B) Psychological feelings or attitudes toward illness.
(Adapted from Mannheimer, JS, and Lampe, GN, eds. Clinical Transcutaneous Electrical Nerve Stimulation. FA Davis, Philadelphia, 1984, pp 12–13, with permission.)

previously described. Medications used to relieve pain are referred to as analgesics, which may be of two classifications: non-narcotics and **narcotics.**

Narcotics include any drug derived from opium or opium-like compounds with analgesic effects associated with both mood and behavior changes and the potential for dependence.[76] Narcotic analgesics include codeine and morphine. Examples of non-narcotic drugs are aspirin and nonsteroidal anti-inflammatory drugs (NSAIDs). Each class of drug affects the body in different ways to alter the painful experience. Non-narcotic pain medications selectively affect the hypothalamus of the brain. In addition, the synthesis of prostaglandins is inhibited and bradykinin is prevented from stimulating pain receptors at the site of injury. NSAIDs interrupt the inflammatory response by making cell membranes less permeable and by inhibiting prostaglandin synthesis. Narcotic analgesics are used to alleviate severe pain. The mechanism of action affects the CNS to decrease anxiety and the response to pain. The drugs do not affect the peripheral nerves and receptors, so the pain stimulus is still present. In effect, the patient does not respond to the stimulus because of the depression of the CNS.[6]

The adverse effects of this group of medications include gastrointestinal irritation, toxicity, mental confusion, drowsiness, and hypersensitivity. Narcotic analgesics, in addition to the adverse effects previously mentioned, can produce tolerance and physical addiction to the drug. In some cases, the use of electrical stimulation for pain control and continuous low-level heat therapy has decreased the need for the use of analgesic medications.[18,21]

Electrical stimulation is believed to produce analgesic effects through stimulation of the peripheral and central nervous systems. Electrical stimulation devices are available for use in the clinic and as portable models (see Chapters 13 and 15) that the patient can use at appropriate times during the day as needed. The portable units are generally the size of a "beeper" and run on rechargeable batteries. The portability of the electrical stimulators allows the patient greater autonomy in his or her own care and the option for use of extended periods of stimulation. When the unit and electrodes are used appropriately, side effects are minimal. There is a chance for a chemical burn at the stimulation site, hypersensitivity reactions to the stimulation, or allergic reactions to the adhesives used to hold an electrode in place.[7,8] These are minimal in comparison with the adverse reactions that may result from ingested medications.

It is important to differentiate between the terms *analgesia* and **anesthesia.** While analgesia refers to reduced pain, anesthesia refers to a loss of sensation, not necessarily the sensation of pain, resulting from neurological depression or dysfunction.[76]

Patient Perspective

Remember that your patient is the only individual who can actually quantify what he or she is feeling. The answers you provide to the questions below can have a positive or an adverse effect on the results of the therapeutic intervention for a given patient. Fear is often linked with pain, despite the fact that a patient might not express it.

Patients' Frequently Asked Questions

1. How can such a small area hurt so much?
2. Why is it that some people don't seem to "suffer" as much with pain?
3. Why does someone who is having a "heart attack" feel pain down his or her left arm?
4. Why does "swelling" happen?
5. Why does healing take so long to happen with some people and not with others?

REFERRED PAIN

Pain arising from deep body structures but felt at another, distant site is called referred pain.[19,21,23,24] It is considered an error in the localization of pain.[23,24] Mechanisms that cause the referral of pain are based on the convergence of cutaneous (skin) and visceral (internal organ) afferent nerve fibers within the spinal cord. Areas of skin that are innervated by a particular nerve root are referred to as **dermatomes.** Areas of bone that are innervated by a specific nerve root are known as **sclerotomes,** and **myotomes** are the areas of muscle innervated by a nerve root.

These areas may overlie each other, complicating the diagnostic process. Referred pain may be an indicator of the spinal segment in which there is a problem.[23] Pain in the L5 dermatome (buttock, leg, and foot) could arise from irritation around the L5 nerve root, the L5 disc, any facet involvement of L4 to L5, any muscle supplied by the L5 nerve root, or any visceral structure having L5 innervation.[23] Another common example of referred pain is the pain associated with angina (ischemia of the heart) and with myocardial infarction (heart attack). An individual experiencing these conditions may feel pain radiating down the arm in the T1 and T2 dermatomes.[21,25] Pain is felt here because the pain fibers innervating the heart arise from the T1 to T5 nerve roots (Fig. 2-5).

Not all referred pain follows a segmental (spinal nerve) pattern. Pain referred from an active trigger point follows a predictable and characteristic pattern for the muscle that is harboring the trigger point. These trigger points are defined by their referred pain pattern.[25] It is important to

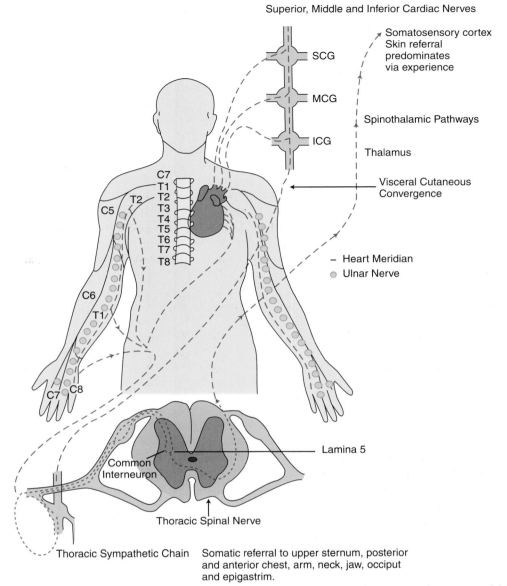

FIGURE 2-5 Diagram of dermatomes. When someone is experiencing a "heart attack," pain can be perceived throughout the left upper extremity, which corresponds to the overlap of dermatome, myotome, and scleratome.
(Adapted from Mannheimer, JS, and Lampe, GN, eds. Clinical Transcutaneous Electrical Nerve Stimulation. FA Davis, Philadelphia, 1984, p 109.)

be aware of common referral patterns to identify the anatomical source of pain correctly and treat it appropriately.[20] Also, because pain that is perceived by the patient appears to arise from the area of referral and not the deeper, more distant structures, it is important to be able to explain to the patient why you may not be treating him "where it hurts" but rather that you are treating the source of the pain. Failure to educate the patient regarding the pain pattern and source may feed into feelings of helplessness and of not being heard. The patient has informed you that his "leg hurts," but you seem to ignore him and instead treat his back. The perception of the patient may be that you are not listening or that you do not care about his or her recovery. Patient education can make a substantial difference in improving your rapport with your patient and enhance overall treatment effectiveness.

Pain Assessment

Pain is a subjective experience, and as such it is difficult to measure. It is essential, however, to have some means of monitoring an individual's perception of pain at any given time to monitor response to treatment and activity. The McGill Pain Questionnaire (MPQ),[20,24,26] visual analog scales (VASs),[3] and numeric pain-rating scales (NPRSs)[3,27] are some pain assessment tools commonly used in the assessment of pain perception (see Chapter 3).

MCGILL PAIN QUESTIONNAIRE

The MPQ is made up of several parts and attempts to measure the patient's perception of pain. Body diagrams for pain location and word descriptors for pain quality are included. The patient's description of pain intensity and the pattern of pain related to activity compose the remainder of the questionnaire. The advantages of using the MPQ include collecting quantitative and qualitative information regarding pain and providing information on the effects of different treatments and activities on pain perception.

VISUAL ANALOG SCALES

Although not as sensitive as the MPQ, the VAS is a quick means by which patients can rate pain.[3,6] The patient is given a piece of paper marked with a line that is 10 cm long. At one end is written, "the worst pain I ever felt," and at the other, "no pain at all." The patient is asked to mark the line at the point corresponding to the intensity of pain felt at that moment. Records can be kept by measuring the position of the marks on the scale from treatment to treatment. The numeric pain-rating scale (NPRS) is a variation of the VAS. The patient is asked to rate his or her pain "on a scale of 0 to 10, 0 being no pain and 10 being the worst pain imaginable." This information is then recorded in the patient's chart. Further description of pain assessment is detailed in Chapter 3.

Pain Perception

The mechanisms of pain perception are not completely understood,[6] although some pieces of the puzzle are better identified and understood than others. Pain signals must be picked up by sensory receptors in the periphery and the signals must be transmitted to the brain for us to perceive pain. This is not a simple stimulus-response situation.[6,10] Many factors modify the signal before and after it reaches the brain.[6,28–32] The following is a brief review of the neural mechanisms of pain perception.

PAIN RECEPTORS

Specialized receptors called nociceptors signal actual or potential tissue damage.[6,9,21] The receptors in the skin are understood better than the receptors found in the viscera and cardiac and skeletal muscle.[6] The nociceptors are actually three distinct types of free nerve endings that respond to different stimulus modalities (Table 2-1). The nociceptors do not normally respond to sensory stimuli in nondamaging ranges. For example, high-threshold mechanoreceptors (HTMs) do not usually respond to light touch. The sensitivity of HTMs increases following mild injury, however, causing the surrounding tissue to become more sensitive to pressure. Polymodal nociceptors become increasingly sensitive following repeated heat or chemical activation,[30–32] possibly accounting for the hyperalgia experienced in injured skin. Pain sensation is elicited by a noxious stimulus that is the result of excitation of the various sensory receptors and free nerve endings of the skin and internal structures. The nerve fiber types that are the mediators of pain impulses in the CNS are the A-delta and C fibers. A-delta fibers transmit discriminative touch stimuli from the skin. A-delta fibers are sensitive to crude touch, pain, and temperature. C fibers are the afferent fibers coming from pain receptors.[9]

PAIN FIBER TYPES AND CENTRAL PATHWAYS

Once a pain receptor is stimulated, the nerve fiber transmits a signal to the dorsal horn of the spinal cord. A few ascending and descending fibers branch off to form Lissauer's tract and communicate with neighboring spinal segments. The main fiber continues in the dorsal horn to make connections with neurons of lamina I, II, III, IV, and V. Lamina III is also known as the *substantia gelatinosa*. Synaptic connections are then made with neurons, giving rise to the lateral spinothalamic tract. These neurons cross over to the opposite side of the spinal cord at the ventral white commissure (Fig. 2-6). The fibers of the lateral spinothalamic tract ascend the spinal cord and enter the brainstem, where some fibers send branches to the reticular formation. Other fibers continue to the thalamus, where they form synapses with neurons that ascend to the primary and secondary somatosensory cortex. The fibers that have been projected to the reticular formation then synapse with other fibers that relay pain information to the thalamus, hypothalamus, and

TABLE 2-1 | Types of Nociceptors

TYPE	RESPONDS TO	FIBER CONNECTION	SENSATION	SPEED OF CONDUCTION
High-threshold mechanoreceptor	Strong mechanical stimulation	A-delta	Sharp "pricking" Well localized	Fast
Mechanothermal nociceptor	Strong mechanical stimulation Noxious heat	A-delta	Sharp "pricking" Well localized	Fast
Polymodal nociceptor	Strong mechanical stimulation Noxious heat Irritant chemicals	C	Dull Aching Burning Poorly localized	Slow

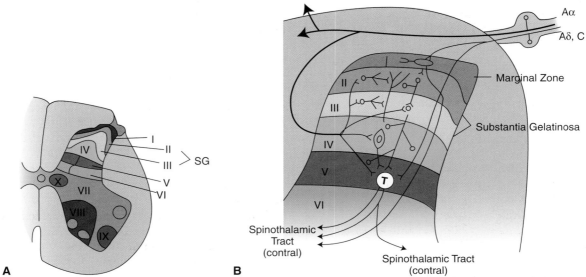

FIGURE 2-6 Spinal cord dorsal horn illustration with crossover of information. The main fiber continues in the dorsal horn to make connections with neurons of lamina I, II, III, IV, and V. Lamina III is also known as the substantia gelatinosa. Synaptic connections are then made with neurons, giving rise to the lateral spinothalamic tract. These neurons cross over to the opposite side of the spinal cord at the ventral white commissure. The fibers of the lateral spinothalamic tract ascend the spinal cord and enter the brainstem, where some fibers send branches to the reticular formation. Other fibers continue to the thalamus, where they form synapses with neurons that ascend to the primary and secondary somatosensory cortexes. The fibers that have been projected to the reticular formation then synapse with other fibers that relay pain information to the thalamus, hypothalamus, and limbic system. The end result of all these connections is the perception of pain.[1,9]
(Adapted from Manheimer, JS, and Lampe, GN, eds. Clinical Transcutaneous Electrical Nerve Stimulation. FA Davis, Philadelphia, 1984, p 45. Originally adapted from Heavner, JE: Jamming spinal sensory input: Effects of anesthetic and analgesic drugs in the spinal cord dorsal horn. Pain 1:239, 1975.)

limbic system. The end result of all these connections is the perception of pain.[1,9]

PERIPHERAL FIBERS

Each type of nociceptor is attached to one of two distinct types of primary afferent (sensory) neurons: small myelinated A-delta fibers and small unmyelinated C fibers. The A-delta fibers conduct impulses at a rate faster than the C fibers. Stimulation of A-delta fibers evokes a sharp and pricking pain sensation that is well localized and of short duration (sometimes referred to as "first pain"[23]). Stimulation of C fibers produces a longer-lasting burning sensation, which is dull and poorly localized (sometimes referred to as "second pain"[23]).

DORSAL ROOT GANGLIA

The cell bodies of the A-delta and C fibers, together with those of the larger sensory fibers (A-β), are found in the dorsal root ganglia at the various levels of the spinal cord. Primary afferent (sensory) signals are transmitted from these ganglia by axonal processes to specific areas of the spinal cord.

DORSAL HORN OF THE SPINAL CORD

A-delta and C fibers carrying pain signals travel through the lateral division of the dorsal root. They may then ascend several spinal segments before entering the spinal gray matter. "The dorsal horn of the spinal cord acts like a computer that processes the incoming sensory signals, rearranging and modulating them before sending them on to the next higher level."[21] Many factors influence which signals are emphasized and which are ignored.

Within the dorsal horn, A-delta and C fibers communicate with several different types of neurons in different layers of the gray matter.[24] These include nociceptive-specific neurons that receive input only from A-delta and C fibers (pain fibers) and wide-dynamic-range neurons that receive input from A-delta mechanoreceptive (nonpainful) fibers as well as from A-delta and C fibers. Nociceptive-specific neurons assist in discrimination of the specific type of pain, that is, thermal, mechanical, or chemical, but do not localize the pain sensation well. The wide-dynamic-range cells contribute to the localization of burning or pricking pain as well as the discrimination between touch and noxious pinching. These cells receive input from both the viscera and the skin. It is thought that this convergence of noxious stimuli may be the basis for referred pain, because the brain may be unable to discriminate between a visceral and a cutaneous source of stimuli. Wide-dynamic-range cells are also called T (transmission) cells and form the basis for the gate control theory (Fig. 2-7).[20,24]

PAIN PATHWAYS
Ascending

For an individual to be aware of pain, the noxious input to the dorsal horn of the spinal cord must travel to the brain. Several ascending tracts are responsible for the transmission of pain signals.[9] The axons of most of the transmission

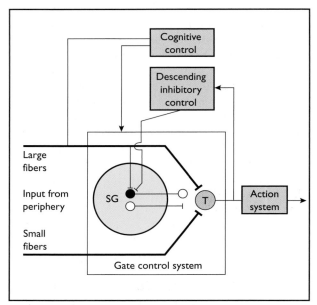

FIGURE 2-7 The gate control theory. The new model includes excitatory (open circle) and inhibitory (shaded circle) links from the substantia gelatinosa (SG) to the transmission (T) cells, as well as descending inhibitory control from brainstem systems. The round knob at the end of the inhibitory link implies that its actions may be presynaptic, postsynaptic, or both. All connections are excitatory, except the inhibitory link for the SG to T cell.
(From Bonica,[6] p 10, with permission.)

cells cross over and ascend via the spinothalamic tract. This tract transmits the pain signal to the thalamus. The thalamus acts as a general relay station for sensory information and has precise projections to the portion of the brain called the somatosensory cortex.[9] Once the signal reaches the cortex, it is perceived as a sharp, discriminative, and relatively localized sensation.[9] The second pathway is called the spinoreticulothalamic pathway. As the name implies, signals travel from the spine to the reticular formation of the brainstem and to the thalamus. Signals are also thought to connect to nuclei in the periaqueductal gray area of the midbrain and to areas of the limbic system. The information that this pathway conveys is perceived as diffuse, poorly localized somatic and visceral pain (Fig. 2-8).[9,33]

Descending

The descending control system for the modulation of pain is not completely understood. There is evidence that naturally occurring substances called endogenous opiates exist that inhibit the perception of pain.[6,10] Examples include methionine enkephalin (met-enkephalin), beta-endorphin (β-endorphin), serotonin, dynorphin,[34,35] and dopamine. They work via various mechanisms and are effective for different lengths of time. Release of endogenous opiates is stimulated by systemic pain, intense exercise, laughter, relaxation, meditation, acupuncture, and electrical stimulation.[6]

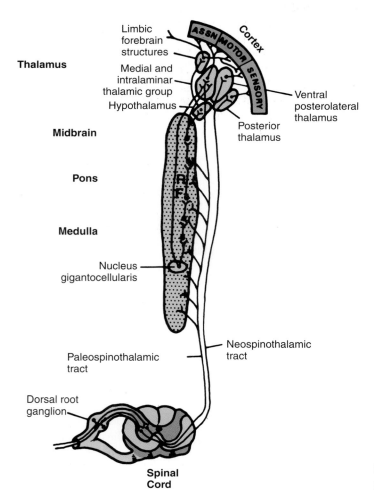

FIGURE 2-8 Generalized conceptualization of projections from pain pathways traversing the neuraxis.

Pain Theories

A number of theories have been proposed to explain the nature of pain and how it is perceived. The gate control theory is considered by some the most complete model of pain.[24] The reader should be aware, however, that knowledge of the nature of pain and the mechanisms of its perception continues to expand.

GATE CONTROL THEORY

The gate control theory was proposed in 1965 by Melzack and Wall and was modified in 1975 and 1982 (Fig. 2-9).[20,26,24] They stated that sensory mechanisms alone failed to account for the fact that nerve lesions do not always cause pain. Instead, they proposed a more complex interaction of peripheral and central mechanisms. Injury activates small-diameter myelinated afferent nerve fibers (A-delta fibers) and small-diameter unmyelinated afferent fibers (C fibers). These nerve impulses excite central transmission cells (T cells) that were proposed to be in the substantia gelatinosa of the dorsal horn of the spinal cord. These T cells receive a convergence of excitatory and inhibitory influences, some from nociceptors and some from other sensory nerve endings. Whether further transmission occurs and the pain signal is sent on to higher centers to be perceived by the individual depends on the summation of inhibitory and excitatory influences. In addition, Melzack and Wall proposed that descending control from the brainstem and cortex also strongly influenced the excitability of the transmission cells. They stated that "psychological factors such as past experience, attention, and emotion influence pain response and perception by acting on the gate control system."[27]

ENDOGENOUS OPIATES

In the years since 1965, much has been learned about pain control mechanisms. The accuracy of the original statement by Melzack and Wall that facilitation and inhibition occur and influence the perception of pain is clear; where and how this facilitation and inhibition occur are not clear. A new class of neurotransmitters called endogenous opiates[6,10] has been discovered. These naturally occurring "pain killers," including enkephalins, endorphins, serotonin, and dopamine, operate in different parts of the nervous system and are effective for varying lengths of time. They may partially account for the "descending control mechanisms" referred to by Melzack and Wall. Enkephalins, which are short-acting endogenous opiates that operate at the spinal cord level, are now thought to "block the gate" by interfering with A-delta and C fiber signal transmission to T cells. They have a very short half-life, meaning that they are effective while actually present in the tissue and for only a short time afterward. Nonpainful sensory stimulus is effective in triggering the release of enkephalins.

Endorphins are another class of endogenous opiates. They act in several different areas of the nervous system (including the dorsal horn) to inhibit pain signal transmission or to decrease the amount of chemical irritants present in the system.[6,10] The half-life of these neurotransmitters is 4 hours. The release of endorphins is stimulated by a variety of factors, including intense pain, intense exercise, acupuncture, laughter, meditation, and relaxation.

Serotonin (5-HT) and dopamine are also capable of influencing pain perception; however, the mechanisms of their actions are not well understood. Serotonin is released from platelets and activates the primary afferent pain fibers,[6,35,36] which would seem to increase the number of pain signals. However, serotonin is also involved in the descending (brain to spinal cord) system that inhibits signals from peripheral nociceptors.[37] Serotonin is a necessary link in the analgesic system.[35–37] Dopamine, a neurotransmitter well known for its role in influencing movement through basal ganglion functioning, may also be used by the body to synthesize morphine and codeine.[30] More continues to be learned regarding these substances and the roles they play in the human body.

Clinical Versus Experimental Pain

Experimental pain is pain that is induced to study physiological, psychological, emotional, and behavioral responses to stimuli. Subjects are often healthy volunteers who are

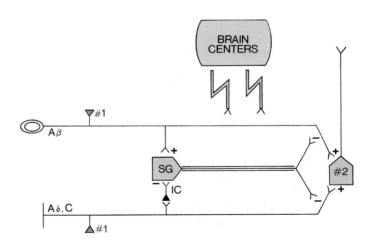

FIGURE 2-9 Gate control theory.
(From Michlovitz, SL: Thermal Agents in Rehabilitation, ed 3. FA Davis, Philadelphia, 1996, p 45.)

aware of the controlled nature of the study or patients with pain who are submitting to induced pain to have their responses or pain tolerance measured. Although experiments with pain have greatly expanded our knowledge of the responses to such stimuli, the controlled nature of the stimulus and the situation may very well bias subjects' responses. Care should be taken in extrapolating experimental results to clinical situations. As Wall stated, "In the real world outside the laboratory, the variation in the relationship between pain and injury occupies all portions between injury with no pain and pain with no injury."[38]

Pain Management

PAIN AS A SYMPTOM OF DYSFUNCTION

A general shift across disciplines has occurred from pain relief to pain management.[74] Rehabilitation typically focuses on pain that is caused by physical dysfunction or is the result of disease. Pain is usually a symptom of dysfunction. The underlying dysfunction or problem, as well as the symptom of pain, should be treated. A complete approach to working with a patient experiencing pain should include the following:[39,40]

1. Gathering background information, including mechanism of injury (if applicable), prior medical problems, work background, recreational activity, health habits, and sleep patterns.
2. Assessment of pain location, temporal aspects, quantity, and quality. Pain assessment forms, including pain-rating scales, should be part of routine documentation.
3. Physical examination, including range-of-motion measurements, volume and girth assessments (if applicable), strength assessments, postural evaluation, joint alignment and mobility, soft tissue examination, and functional ability.

The intervention plan that results from this evaluation should prioritize, then address, all pertinent problems. Effective initial therapeutic treatment intervention with pain-relieving modalities or medications prescribed by a physician is important to minimize the pain-dysfunction-guarding cycle (see Fig. 2-3) and can be critical to the success of the plan; however, limiting the treatment of pain to medication or physical modalities such as ice massage, hot packs, ultrasound, and/or soft tissue massage is seldom effective in addressing all of the underlying causes of pain and restoring lost function.

Frequently, poor posture and body mechanics, decreased flexibility, and an overall decline in fitness are contributing factors to the dysfunction causing pain.[39] Common examples include the patient with a severe forward head and rounded shoulders who complains of neck pain or shoulder pain due to tendinopathy and the truck driver with shortened hamstring muscles who complains of low back pain. If these patients are only treated symptomatically with pain-relieving modalities and the issues related to posture, overuse, and muscle length are not addressed, there is a high likelihood that they will either achieve poor control of their pain or become "revolving-door patients" who return on a frequent basis with the same or related pain complaints.

It is also important that the psychological and emotional aspects of the patient's pain problem not be ignored.[75] Positive reinforcement of pain behavior may increase the likelihood of an acute pain problem becoming a chronic pain problem.[14,16] Involvement in decision making and treatment activities by the patient is important to foster a sense of personal responsibility over dependency. If properly administered, even the physical modalities may include education and active involvement on the part of the patient. For example, instruction in proper body mechanics, positions of rest, the appropriate use of heat, and relaxation techniques including deep breathing and visualization can all be part of an effective home program.

THERAPEUTIC INTERVENTION—CLINICAL DECISION MAKING

The form that treatment takes, the timing with which it is administered, and the attitude of the health care professional toward the patient and his or her problem are all critical to the successful treatment of pain. The importance of correcting dysfunction as a means of treating pain was previously discussed. The various tools that can be used as therapeutic treatment interventions to provide analgesia are briefly reviewed next. They are discussed in greater depth in subsequent chapters of this text.

Thermal Agents

Thermal agents include the following:

- Superficial heating agents such as hot packs, paraffin, fluidotherapy, infrared lamps, and warm whirlpool baths (>98.6°F)[41,42]
- Deep-heating agents such as ultrasound and shortwave diathermy
- Cold agents such as cold packs, ice massage, ice towels, and cold baths

The decision of which thermal modality to use should include consideration of several factors, most notably goal of treatment, stage of healing of the injury, depth of the target tissue, patient tolerance and preference, and ease of application (especially for home use).

Electrotherapeutic Devices

Transcutaneous electrical nerve stimulation (TENS) is an application of electrotherapy specifically designed for pain managment.[43-45] TENS units are small, portable, battery-powered pulsed stimulators. The stimulus parameters used with these devices are based on the theories of pain perception. Two of the more commonly used protocols are sensory-level (conventional or high-rate) TENS, which is set at 75 to 100 pulses per second (pps), a short pulse duration, and sensory paresthesia level of intensity[38] to "block the gate," and low-rate TENS, which is set at a low rate (1 to 4 pps), a moderate duration, and a motor threshold level of intensity to stimulate the release of endorphins.[38]

Electrical stimulation as a treatment intervention and form of pain management is discussed in more detail in Chapter 14.

Biofeedback is another electrotherapeutic device modality that is frequently used in the management of pain. Biofeedback is used to monitor various functions in the body, including muscle activity, skin temperature, skin conductance, heart rate, respiratory rate, blood pressure, and brain waves. The information picked up by the biofeedback unit in the form of electrical potentials is then translated into an audio and/or a visual signal that the patient can relate to activity of the body. The idea is to bring physiological functioning that normally occurs below our level of awareness to our conscious attention so that we can learn to control various body systems. A common application in physical therapy is the monitoring of muscle function[46] to enhance muscle activity in a weak muscle or to promote relaxation in a tense muscle.

Tissue Repair

A predictable sequence of reactions of the body occurs from injury through the completion of healing. There are both physical and psychological factors that may influence the phases of this sequence. Estimates of the length of each phase vary,[47,48] but it is generally agreed that they overlap.[48,49] Certainly factors such as the size of the insult or wound, the presence of cardiovascular and pulmonary system diseases, infection and immunosuppressive disorders, and the administration of immunosuppressant drugs influence the course of recovery.

The goals of this next section are to (1) describe the normal response to tissue trauma, (2) discuss factors that affect wound healing, and (3) introduce ways in which physical agents and electrotherapy can be used to influence tissue healing.

TISSUE RESPONSE TO TRAUMA: INFLAMMATION AND REPAIR

The body responds to injury of vascularized tissue with a series of events, collectively called inflammation and repair.[47] Vascular, cellular, hormonal, and immune system responses occur to minimize tissue damage and restore function. Scar tissue replaces damaged tissue that cannot regenerate. Although scar tissue may restore a certain structural integrity to the tissue, it is not as strong as the original tissue (maximal tensile strength of scar tissue is between 70% and 80% of normal tissue[50,51]), is poorly vascularized, may disrupt organ functioning, may restrict movement (especially if it occurs near a joint), and may be disfiguring.

Inflammation (Days 1 to 10)

The initial phase of healing is described as the inflammatory, or "self-defense," response. This normal process, which is a prerequisite to healing, does have uncomfortable and sometimes distressing symptoms, including the "cardinal signs of inflammation": redness, heat, swelling, and pain. In addition, there is typically a loss of function.[49] These signs are the result of complex interactions of the vascular, hemostatic, cellular, and immune systems. (Refer to the Why Do I Need to Know About... feature at the beginning of the chapter.)

Immediately following injury, changes in severed vessels occur as the body attempts to wall off the wound from the external environment.[49] Platelets aggregate, blood coagulation is initiated, severed lymph channels are sealed off, and arterioles constrict. These brief but important compensatory mechanisms serve to protect the individual from excessive blood loss and increased exposure to bacterial contamination.

Within a few minutes of injury, vasodilation of the injured vessels occurs, resulting in increased blood flow, redness, and heat. Noninjured vessels dilate in response to chemicals such as histamine and prostaglandins released from injured tissues.[48] An increase in the hydrostatic pressure also occurs within the vessels. At the same time, the capillaries and venules become more permeable (because of chemicals called bradykinins and histamine), allowing the release of cells, macromolecules, and fluid from the vascular system into the interstitial spaces. Lymph vessels that normally clear osmotically active particles from this area are unable to keep up with the demand. Edema occurs as fluid moves in to the interstitium to restore the balance of osmotic pressures.

The makeup of the edema fluid changes as the stages of inflammation progress and with the magnitude of injury. Initially the fluid is a clear, watery substance called transudate. As more cells and plasma proteins enter the interstitial space, the edema fluid becomes viscous and cloudy and is called exudate. If the exudate contains large numbers of leukocytes (white blood cells), it is called pus.[49]

For healing to commence, the wound must be decontaminated (through phagocytosis) and a new blood supply must be established (revascularization).[50] Phagocytosis is carried out first by polymorphonuclear leukocytes. In a few days, another type of phagocyte called a macrophage appears. These cells remain in the wound until all signs of inflammation are gone. Macrophages attack and engulf bacteria and dispose of necrotic tissue in the wound. They have been called the "director cells" of repair because, by emitting certain chemical signals, macrophages recruit fibroblasts to form scar tissue. The number of fibroblasts relates to the amount of scar tissue. If there are not enough macrophages or they cannot function well enough because of a lack of oxygen, there will be no signal to stimulate the fibroblasts, and a chronic wound results.

Another important component of healing is the release of growth factors. Growth factors stimulate the production of many of the necessary components of the tissue extracellular matrix. These growth factors are referred to as cytokines. Growth factor beta-1 stimulates collagen production.[52] Fibroblasts are also intricately involved in wound healing and scarring. Fibroblast growth factors (FGFs) appear to be a key component during the beginning of cellular **proliferation** (or growth), differentiation, migration, and matrix deposition phases of wound healing.[53,54] Hepatocyte growth factor (HGF) is involved in antifibrotic activities, assisting in the prevention of excessive fibrous deposition of healing tissues.[55] There are also osteogenic growth factors involved in the enhancement of bone repair. Gene therapy for recombinant osteogenic growth factor is now available and has the potential for use in nonunion fractures and the enhancement of bone repair (Box 2-3).[55]

As this phase comes to a close, chemicals are released from blood vessels to dissolve clots. The lymphatic channels open to assist in reducing wound edema.[50]

Proliferative Phase (Days 3 to 20)

Revascularization and rebuilding of the tissue occur in the proliferative phase. Revascularization is thought to be triggered by the macrophages through the release of growth factors ("director cells" of the inflammation phase). Intact blood vessels at the edges of the wound develop small buds and sprouts that grow into the wound area. These outgrowths eventually come in contact with and join other arteriolar or venular buds and form a functioning capillary loop. These loops are what create the bright pink color seen throughout healing wounds. They are extremely fragile when first formed and can be easily disrupted. Immobilization or protected movement is important to prevent bleeding. Vigorous heating at this time may also cause increased bleeding and is contraindicated.

Rebuilding of the structure of the wound occurs through resurfacing with epithelial tissue and restrengthening with connective tissue. This phase is extremely active and is highly dependent on the oxygenation of the tissue. Hypoxic wounds build poor-quality scars. Fibroblasts, which form scar tissue, respond to changes in the electrical potential at the wound (chemotactic influence) and migrate into the inflamed area along fibrin strands.

Three processes occur simultaneously to close the wound and are outlined in Table 2-2. The process of wound contraction deserves special mention. The purpose of this process is to decrease the open area that the skin must ultimately cover. It occurs through action of the myofibroblasts located at the edge of the wound. This is a normal part of the healing process, starting around day 4 postinjury and continuing to days 14 through 21. Depending on the location of the wound, the results of this contraction process may or may not restrict movement. For example, the contraction of a large scar in the hand may cause functional problems, whereas the contraction of a large scar on the buttocks may not. Wound contraction is one of many different forces that may lead to a contracture and subsequent loss of passive motion.

Remodeling or Maturation Phase (Day 9 Onward)

The long-term goal of wound healing is the return of function. During the final phase of healing, **remodeling** (the process of reshaping and reorganizing) of the scar tissue occurs. Ideally, there should be a balance between the formation of new collagen and the breakdown of old collagen. As long as the scar looks "rosier" than normal, remodeling is under way;[56] this process may continue for years. The desired outcome is a scar that is pale, flat, and pliable. Abnormal scars form when more collagen is produced than is reabsorbed. Overproduction of collagen can result in a hypertrophic scar or keloid scar (Fig. 2-10). These scars appear red, raised, and rigid.

During remodeling, randomly oriented collagen fibers are replaced with fibers that are oriented both linearly and laterally. Through processes that are not fully understood, the scar takes on some of the characteristics of the structure it is replacing: repaired ligamentous tissue will

---

BOX 2-3 | Growth Factors (Cytokines) Involved in Tissue Repair

Growth factor beta:	*for collagen production*
Fibroblast growth factors:	*for cellular proliferation*
	differentiation
	migration
	matrix deposition phases
	of wound healing
Hepatocyte growth factor	*for antifibrotic activity*
	prevents excessive
	fibrous depositions
Osteogenic growth factors	*for bone repair*

TABLE 2-2 | Three Stages of the Proliferative Phase of Healing

STAGES OF PROLIFERATIVE PHASE	CHANGES WITHIN THE WOUND
Epithelization (granulation)	Wound is filled in with granulating tissue, from the edges in and from structures such as hair shafts and sweat glands out Epithelial cells seek out a moist, oxygen-rich environment Epithelial cells can only cover 2 cm of open wound
Wound contraction	Myofibroblasts pull the entire wound together Occurs from 4 to 14–21 days
Collagen production	Wound tensile strength is dependent on cross-linking Weak electrostatic forces hold edges together

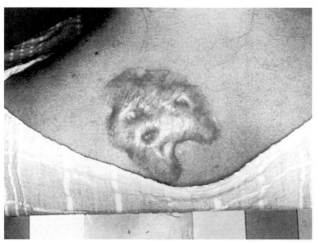

FIGURE 2-10 A keloid of the left posterior scapula area that is the result of thermal injury to the back. This thermal injury occurred as the result of carbon dioxide laser treatment of a decorative tattoo.
(Courtesy of David B. Afelberg, MD, Palo Alto, CA, as shown in Reed and Zarro,[47] p 11.)

ultimately have a different structure than the repaired joint capsule only millimeters away. Two theories have been proposed to explain how collagen realigns appropriately. The induction theory hypothesizes that scar tissue tries to mimic the characteristics of the tissue it is healing. The tension theory hypothesizes that the collagen fibers that lay down during remodeling respond to internal and external stresses that are placed on the wound and align accordingly. The application of dynamic splints, serial casting, continuous passive motion (CPM) machines, neuromuscular electrical stimulation (NMES), scar massage, and positional stretching techniques to wounds or scars to increase flexibility and range of motion is based on this theory. NMES is detailed in Chapter 13.

DELAYS IN WOUND HEALING

Delayed closure of a wound simply means that a wound is taking longer than expected to heal.[56] There are two types of delayed closure. The first is intentionally created by the medical staff when a choice is made to not suture a wound closed (healing by first intention) but rather to leave it open to granulate and reepithelialize on its own (healing by second intention). Reasons for promoting healing by second intention include dirt in the wound, infection, and excessive drainage. The second type of delayed closure is not deliberate and involves many factors affecting the conservative treatment of a wound. It is important to consider whether the delay is caused by (1) a factor related to the patient's general physical or mental condition or (2) an iatrogenic factor, such as the way the wound is physically managed and treatments, including drugs and therapies (Box 2-4).[52,56] Factors that can be changed should be addressed (Tables 2-2, 2-3, and 2-4).

BOX 2-4 | Factors That Increase the Likelihood of a Wound Becoming Chronic

- Medications such as certain nonsteroidal anti-inflammatory drugs, steroids, and immunosuppressive drugs used for transplant patients
- Comorbidities such as acquired immunodeficiency syndrome (AIDS), diabetes, cancer, and peripheral vascular disease[56]
- Cellular toxicity of commonly used antimicrobial agents such as povidone-iodine (e.g., Betadine; Becton Dickinson Acute Care, Franklin Lakes, NJ), hydrogen peroxide, and acetic acid
- Radiation therapy
- Chemotherapy
- Malnutrition

TABLE 2-3 | Effect of Local Factors on the Promotion or Impairment of Wound Healing

LOCAL FACTORS	PROMOTION OF WOUND HEALING	IMPAIRMENT OF WOUND HEALING
Surgical technique	Close approximation of wound edges	Excessive tension Devitalized tissue
Blood supply	Patent	Atherosclerosis Venous stasis Tissue ischemia
Infection	None	Bacteria Mycobacteria Fungi or yeast
Medications	Some topical antibiotics (e.g., mupirocin [Bactroban])	Topical steroids Many systemic and topical antibiotics Antineoplastic drugs Hemostatic agents (aluminum chloride or Monsel's solution)

Continued

TABLE 2-3 | Effect of Local Factors on the Promotion or Impairment of Wound Healing — cont'd

LOCAL FACTORS	PROMOTION OF WOUND HEALING	IMPAIRMENT OF WOUND HEALING
Trauma	None	Chronic trauma Foreign body Factitial trauma
Microenvironment	Occlusive dressings	Dry dressings Photo-aged skin Radiation injury
Ulcer type		Pressure ulcers Tumor (Marjolin's ulcer) Neuropathic ulcers (malperforans ulcers)

Source: From Daly, p 41, with permission.[50]

TABLE 2-4 | Effect of Systemic Factors on the Promotion or Impairment of Wound Healing

SYSTEMIC FACTORS	PROMOTION OF WOUND HEALING	IMPAIRMENT OF WOUND HEALING
Nutrition	No deficiencies	Deficiency of protein, calories, vitamins (especially A and C), trace metals (especially zinc and copper)
Age	Young	Advanced chronic illness (hepatic, renal, hematopoietic, cardiovascular, autoimmune, carcinoma)
Illness	None	Endocrine disease (e.g., diabetes mellitus, Cushing's disease) Systemic vascular disorders (periarteritis nodosa, vasculitis, granulomatosis, atherosclerosis) Connective tissue disease (e.g., Ehlers-Danlos syndrome)
Systemic medications		Corticosteroids, aspirin, heparin, coumadin, penicillamine, nicotine, phenylbutazone, and other NSAIDs; antineoplastic agents

Source: From Daly, p 41, with permission.[50]

An important area beyond the scope of this chapter is wound coverage with dressings. The traditional concept of promoting wound healing by "airing" the wound has given way to an understanding of the importance of maintaining a moist environment at the wound bed. Semiocclusive or occlusive dressings are now used to promote reepithelization, avoid the formation of a crust (scab or eschar), decrease bacterial exposure, and decrease the secondary trauma of frequent dressing changes.[56–58]

Chronic wounds are wounds that are not healing despite conservative or surgical treatment.[56] This does not mean that healing is impossible but that intervention will be needed to improve the chances of successful wound closure. Some of the factors that are likely to increase the chance of chronicity of a wound are summarized in Box 2-4. Age is also a factor in wound healing. The neonate may have a modified response because of the immaturity of organ system functioning. Children have a greater capacity for tissue repair than adults but lack the reserves necessary to counteract any significant trauma. This is shown by "an easily upset electrolyte balance, sudden elevation or lowering of body temperature, and rapid spread of infection."[59] Older adults undergo the same healing process as young adults but do so more slowly. They are, however, "more susceptible to wound healing problems due to the interactions of body systems, environmental stresses, and disease with an aging process that takes place over many years."[60] Aging leads to decreased efficiency in many body systems, including the cardiovascular, pulmonary, immune, and integumentary systems.[60] This decrease in efficiency affects healing. It is important to remember, however, that there is more variability in the older population than in any other age group: what may be true for a fragile, debilitated 60-year-old with diabetes mellitus may not be true for a healthy, robust 80-year-old (Table 2-5, Box 2-5)

PHYSICAL THERAPY INTERVENTIONS FOR SOFT TISSUE HEALING

Physical agents play a vital role in the management of soft tissue injuries (for both closed and open wounds). For closed wounds, including sprains and strains, physical therapy management initially involves rest, ice, compression,

TABLE 2-5 | The Effects of Aging on the Healing Response[53,56]

PHASES OF HEALING	EFFECTS OF AGING
Inflammatory, "self-defense" phase	• ↓ 'd and disrupted vascular supplies → ↓ 'd clearance of metabolites, bacteria, and foreign materials • ↓ 'd supply of nutrients • ↓ 'd inflammatory response • → ↑ 'd likelihood of "chronic wounds" • ↓ 'd rate of wound capillary growth
Proliferative phase	• ↓ 'd metabolic response • ↓ 'd migration and proliferation of cells • Delayed maturation of cells • Delayed wound contraction
Remodeling phase	• Delayed collagen remodeling • ↑ 'd tertiary cross-linking of collagen → less flexible and weaker scars

BOX 2-5 | Factors That Influence Wound Healing

- Balance is critical to the success of the healing process.
- If there is no inflammatory response, there is no healing.
- If there is too little inflammatory response, healing is slow.
- If there is too much inflammatory response, healing is prolonged and excessive scar tissue forms.

Other Factors
- Virulence of the bacteria
- Presence of foreign objects
- Presence of necrotic tissue
- Poor oxygen supply
- Dehydration
- Certain vitamin deficiencies (vitamin C, vitamin E,[70] vitamin D[71])
- Lack of protein[70]
- Irradiated tissues[72]
- Immunosuppression

and elevation (RICE) of the affected part. As the inflammatory stage resolves, other therapeutic interventions can be applied, including ultrasound, hot packs, whirlpool, shortwave diathermy, and electrical stimulation, to further promote healing, increase soft tissue extensibility, and decrease any pain that may be present. Range-of-motion exercises, strengthening exercises, and functional activities are added

as the soft tissue heals and is better able to tolerate these forces.

If the trauma includes an open wound, therapy may include the following:

- Hydrotherapy (whirlpool or now, more commonly, pulsatile lavage with suction) to cleanse and débride the wound
- Electrical stimulation to promote wound healing[56,61-65]
- Vacuum-assisted closure (VAC) to assist with the closure of acute, subacute, and chronic wounds[66]
- Pulsed ultrasound to promote wound healing during the proliferative and remodeling phases[66-68]
- Hyperbaric oxygen chambers to promote healing of chronic wounds[66,69]
- Ultraviolet-C radiation (UVC) for the treatment of infected wounds[56]
- Early controlled mobilization of the injured part, including management of bracing with adjustable locks and exercise to prevent contractures and minimize muscle atrophy
- Positioning programs to protect healing tissue and avoid the development of pressure sores or contractures
- Design of seating systems (if applicable) to prevent the development of pressure sores and provide optimal mobility
- Advising staff, patients, or family members in the selection of pressure-relieving devices (specialty beds, mattresses, and seat cushions)
- Patient and family education in appropriate home activities

Summary

This chapter has dealt with the topics of pain and wound healing. It is important to be aware that knowledge of pain perception, pain management mechanisms, and wound healing continues to expand rapidly. To provide the most effective therapeutic treatment interventions for patients, health care providers must be ready to modify choices as new information and interventions become available.

Pain is a frequent concern for patients involved in rehabilitation. Skillful management of the physical, physiological, and psychological aspects of the patient with pain is a responsibility of all members of the rehabilitation team. An understanding of pain mechanisms will lead to appropriate choices of treatment interventions and approaches.

Wound healing progresses through a series of predictable stages, each of which may require different handling. Wound closure may be intentionally delayed if there is debris in the wound, infection, or excessive drainage. Errors in wound management, as well as factors relating to the patient's underlying physical and mental condition, may lead to the development of chronic wounds. The rehabilitation team may be involved in numerous aspects of wound care, ranging from débridement to the prevention of secondary complications to optimization of mobility during the patient's recovery.

Review Questions

1. Which of the following terms is defined as "an unpleasant sensory and emotional experience"?
   a. Analgesia
   b. Pain
   c. Anesthesia
   d. Inflammation

2. Pain, heat, erythema, edema, and loss of function are signs of which of the following?
   a. Inflammation
   b. Chronic pain
   c. Wound healing
   d. Ischemia

3. Chronic pain is pain that lasts longer than which of the following?
   a. 1 month
   b. 2 months
   c. 3 months
   d. 4 months

4. Which of the following best describes the two main categories that an analgesic drug may fall into?
   a. Legal and illegal
   b. Narcotics and non-narcotics
   c. Aspirin and NSAIDs
   d. Toxic and non-toxic

5. Melzack and Wall proposed the gate control theory of pain perception. Which of the following is a psychological factor that they feel may influence pain response and perception?
   a. Culture
   b. Past experience
   c. Gender
   d. Age

CASE STUDY

Phil is a 40-year-old Federal Express driver who has been referred to physical therapy subsequent to intermittent pain, weakness, and cramping in his dominant left hand thumb. Extension and abduction of the thumb reproduce his pain. There are no fractures, and he describes the onset of the pain as gradual. The hand is edematous with exquisite tenderness over the anatomical "snuff box."

- What could potentially cause his pain to be intermittent?

- At 40, would you expect this injury to heal as quickly as if Phil were 20? Why or why not?
- Because this is Phil's dominant hand, how does the *Pain Triangle* fit into his recovery?

DISCUSSION QUESTIONS

1. If a patient asked you to explain the nature of pain, how would you explain why some people seem to feel more discomfort than others? What terminology would you use to ensure that your explanation is easily understood by the patient?

2. How would the psychological implications of pain perception influence your approach to a patient with chronic pain? Would this approach change in any way if this were an acute pain syndrome rather than a chronic pain syndrome?

3. If the patient asked you why he or she is feeling pain in an amputated limb or pain that travels down an arm or a leg, how would you explain it? Be careful to use terminology that a patient would understand.

4. How would you explain the inflammation and tissue repair process to a patient? Be careful to use terminology that the patient would understand. Your explanation should address the significance and necessity of the process.

5. Prepare an explanation for a patient that would discuss the importance of proper nutrition and wound care to promote tissue healing. Your explanation should include the rationale for keeping the wound moist as opposed to the patient's expressed desire to "let the wound dry."

REFERENCES

1. Loeser, JD, and Melzack R: Pain: An overview. Lancet 353:1607–1609, 1999.
2. Turk, DC, and Melzack, R: Handbook of Pain Assessment, ed 3. Guilford Press, New York, 2010.
3. Tyrer, SR (ed): Psychology, Psychiatry and Chronic Pain. Butterworth Heinemann, Oxford, 1992.
4. Sternbach, R: Psychology of Pain, ed 2. Raven Press, New York, 1986.
5. France, RD, and Krishnan, KRR: Chronic Pain. American Psychiatric Press, Washington, DC, 1988.
6. Bonica, JJ: The Management of Pain, Vols 1 and 2, ed 2. Lea & Febiger, Malvern, PA, 1990.
7. Merskey, HM: Pain terms. Pain 3(suppl):S215–S221, 1986.
8. Kwako, J, and Shealy, CN: Psychological consideration in the management of pain. In Mannheimer, JS, and Lampe, GN (eds): Clinical Transcutaneous Electrical Nerve Stimulation. FA Davis, Philadelphia, 1984, p 29.
9. Gilman, S, and Newman, SW: Manter & Gatz's Essentials of Clinical Neuroanatomy and Neurophysiology, ed 10. FA Davis, Philadelphia, 2003.
10. Kandel, ER, Schwartz, JH, and Jessell, TM: Principles of Neural Science, ed 4. Elsevier, New York, 2000.
11. Sternbach, RA: Acute versus chronic pain. In Wall, PD, and Melzack, R: Textbook of Pain, ed 4. Churchill Livingstone, New York, 1999, p 173.
12. Bowsher, D: Acute and chronic pain and assessment. In Wells, PE, Frampton, V, and Bowsher, D (eds): Pain Management in Physiotherapy. Butterworth Heinemann, Oxford, 1996.
13. Tandon, OP, Malhotra, V, Tandon, S, and D'Silva, I: Neurophysiology of pain: Insight to orofacial pain. Ind J Physiol Pharmacol 47:247–269, 2003.
14. Brookoff, D: Chronic pain: 1. A new disease? Hosp Pract (Off Ed) 35:Jul 15, 2000.
15. Aronoff, GM: Evaluation and Treatment of Chronic Pain. Williams & Wilkins, Baltimore, 1992.
16. Sculco, AD, Paup, DC, Fernhall, B, and Sculco, MJ: Effects of aerobic exercise on low back pain patients in treatment. Spine J 1:95–101, 2001.
17. Barr, RB: Physical modalities in chronic pain management. Nurs Clin North Am 38:477–494, 2003.
18. Nadler, SF, Steiner, DJ, Erasala, GN, Hengehold, DA, Abein, SB, and Weingand, KW: Continuous low-level heatwrap therapy for treating acute nonspecific low back pain. Arch Phys Med Rehabil 84:329–334, 2003.
19. Graven-Nielsen, T, and Arendt-Nielsen, L: Induction and assessment of muscle pain, referred pain, and muscular hyperalgesia. Curr Pain Headache Rep 7:443–451, 2003.
20. Melzack, R, and Wall, PD: Pain mechanisms: A new theory. Science 150:971, 1965.
21. Bowsher, D: Central pain mechanisms. In Wells, PE, Frampton, V, and Bowsher, D (eds): Pain Management in Physiotherapy. Butterworth Heinemann, Oxford, 1996.
22. Nadler, SF, Steiner, DJ, Erasala, GN, Hengehold, DA, Abein, SB, and Weingand, KW: Overnight use of continuous low-level heatwrap therapy for relief of low back pain. Arch Phys Med Rehabil 84:335–342, 2003.
23. Bowsher, D: A note on the distinction between first and second pain. In Mathews, B, and Hill, RG (eds): Anatomical and Physiological Aspects of Trigeminal Pain. Excerpta Medica, Amsterdam, 1982.
24. Melzack, R: Pain: Past, present and future. Can J Exp Psych 47:615–629, 1993.
25. Travell, JG, and Simmons, DG: Myofascial Pain and Dysfunction: The Trigger Point Manual. Williams & Wilkins, Baltimore, 1983.
26. Melzack, R: The McGill Pain Questionnaire: Major properties and scoring methods. Pain 1:277, 1975.
27. Wall, PD: On the relation of injury to pain. Pain 6:253, 1979.
28. Melzack, R, and Wall, PD: Pain mechanisms: A new theory. Science 150:971, 1965.
29. Cepeda, MS, Africano, JM, Polo, R, Alcala, R, and Carr, DB: Agreement between percentage reductions calculated from numeric rating scores of pain intensity and those reported by patients with acute or cancer pain. Pain 106:439–442, 2003.
30. Loomis, CW, et al: Monomaine and opioid interactions in spinal analgesia and tolerance. Pharmacol Biochem Behav 26:445, 1987.
31. Roberts, MH: Involvement of serotonin in nociceptive pathways. Drug Des Deliv 4:77, 1989.
32. Matsubara, K, et al: Increased urinary morphine, codeine and tetrahydropapaveroline in parkinsonian patient undergoing L-3,4-dihydroxyphenylalanine therapy: A possible biosynthetic pathway of morphine from L-3,4-dihydroxyphenylalanine in humans. J Pharmacol Exp Ther 260:974, 1992.
33. Takeuchi, Y, and Toda, K: Subtypes of nociceptive units in the rat temporomandibular joint. Brain Res Bull 61:603–608, 2003.
34. Jansen, AS, Farkas, E, MacSams, J, and Loewy, AD: Local connections between the columns of the periaqueductal gray matter: A case for intrinsic neuromodulation. Brain Res 784: 329–336, 1998.
35. Gardell, LR, Ibrahim, M, Wang, R, Ossipov, MH, Malan, TP, Porreca, F, et al: Mouse strains that lack spinal dynorphin upregulation after peripheral nerve injury do not develop neuropathic pain. Neuroscience 123:43–52, 2004.
36. Witta, J, Palkovits, M, Rosenberger, J, and Cox, BM: Distribution of nociceptin/orphanin FQ in adult human brain. Brain Res 997:24–29, 2004.
37. Miranda, HF, Lemus, I, and Pinardi, G: Effect of the inhibition of serotonin biosynthesis on the antinociception induced by non-steroidal anti-inflammatory drugs. Brain Res Bull 61:417–425, 2003.
38. Melzack, R, and Wall, PD: The Challenge of Pain. Basic Books, New York, 1983.
39. Magee, DJ: Orthopedic Physical Assessment, ed 5. WB Saunders, Philadelphia, 2007.
40. Saunders, HD: Orthopedic Physical Therapy: Evaluation, Treatment, and Prevention of Musculoskeletal Disorders. Educational Opportunities, Edina, MN, 1985.
41. Ceylan, Y, Hizmetli, S, and Lilig, Y: The effects of infrared laser and medical treatments on pain and serotonin degradation products in patients with myofascial pain syndrome. A controlled trial. Rheumatol Int 24:260–263, 2004. Epub 2003 Nov 20.
42. Walsh, MT: Hydrotherapy: The use of water as a therapeutic agent. In Michlovitz, SL (ed): Thermal Agents in Rehabilitation, ed 3. FA Davis, Philadelphia, 1996.
43. Chesterton, LS, Foster, NE, Wright, CC, Baxter, GD, and Barlas, P: Effects of TENS frequency, intensity and stimulation site parameter manipulation on pressure pain thresholds in healthy human subjects. Pain 106:73–80, 2003.
44. Sluka, KA, and Qalsh, D: Transcutaneous electrical nerve stimulation: Basic science mechanisms and clinical effectiveness. J Pain 4:109–121, 2003.
45. Rakel, B, and Frantz, R: Effectiveness of transcutaneous electrical nerve stimulation on postoperative pain with movement. J Pain 4:455–464, 2003.
46. Colborne, GR, Olney, SJ, and Griffin, MP: Feedback of ankle joint angle and soleus electromyography in the rehabilitation of hemiplegic gait. Arch Phys Med Rehabil 74:1100–1106, 1993.
47. Reed, B, and Zarro, V: Inflammation and repair and the use of thermal agents. In Michlovitz, SL (ed): Thermal Agents in Rehabilitation, ed 3. FA Davis, Philadelphia, 1996.
48. Hardy, MA: The biology of scar formation. Phys Ther 69:1014, 1989.
49. Kloth, LC, and McCulloch, JM: The inflammatory response to wounding. In Kloth, LC, and McCulloch, JM (eds): Wound Healing: Alternatives in Management, ed 3. FA Davis, Philadelphia, 2002.
50. Daly, TJ: The repair phase of wound healing: Re-epithelialization and contraction. In Kloth, LC, and McCulloch, JM (eds): Wound Healing: Alternatives in Management, ed 3. FA Davis, Philadelphia, 2002.
51. Cooper, DM: Optimizing wound healing. Nurs Clin North Am 25:165, 1990.
52. Alaish, SM, Yager, DR, Diegelmann, RF, and Cohen, IK: Hyaluronic acid metabolism in keloid fibroblasts. J Pediatr Surg 30:949–952, 1995.
53. Cool, SM, Snyman, CP, Nurcombe, V, and Forwood, M: Temporal expression of fibroblast growth factor receptors during primary ligament repair. Knee Surg Sports Traumatol Arthrosc 2:490–496, 2004. Epub 2003 Dec 23.
54. Hirano, S, Bless, DM, Massey, RJ, Hartig, GK, and Ford, CN: Morphological and functional changes of human vocal fold fibroblasts with hepatocyte growth factor. Ann Otol Rhinol Laryngol 112:1026–1033, 2003.
55. Baltzer, AW, and Lieberman, JR: Regional gene therapy to enhance bone repair. Gene Ther 11:344–350, 2004.
56. Feedar, JA, and Kloth, LC: Conservative management of chronic wounds. In Kloth, LC, and McCulloch, JM (eds): Wound Healing: Alternatives in Management, ed 3. FA Davis, Philadelphia, 2002.
57. Hollinworth, H: Wound care: Pathway to success. Nursing Times 88:66, 1992.
58. Bayley, EW: Wound healing in the patient with burns. Nurs Clin North Am 25:205, 1990.
59. Garvin, G: Wound healing in pediatrics. Nurs Clin North Am 25:181, 1990.
60. Jones, PL, and Millman, A: Wound healing and the aged patient. Nurs Clin North Am 25:263–273, 1990.
61. Kloth, LC: How to use electrical stimulation for wound healing. Nursing 32:17, 2002.
62. Kloth, LC: Electrical stimulation in tissue repair. In Kloth, LC, and McCulloch, JM (eds): Wound Healing: Alternatives in Management, ed 3. FA Davis, Philadelphia, 2002.
63. Feedar, JA, Kloth, LC, and Gentzkow, GD: Chronic dermal ulcer healing enhanced with monophasic pulsed electrical stimulation. Phys Ther 71:639, 1991.
64. Akai, M, and Hayashi, K: Effect of electrical stimulation on musculoskeletal systems: A meta-analysis of controlled clinical trials. Bioelectromagnetics 23:132–143, 2002.
65. Houghton, PE, Kincaid, CB, Lovell, M, Campbell, KE, Keast, DH, Woodbury, MG, et al: Effect of electrical stimulation on chronic leg ulcer size and appearance. Phys Ther 83:17–28, 2003.

66. Hess, CL, Howard, MA, and Attinger, CE: A review of mechanical adjuncts in wound healing: Hydrotherapy, ultrasound, negative pressure therapy, hyperbaric oxygen, and electrostimulation. Ann Plast Surg 51:210–218, 2003.

67. Ziskin, MC, McDiarmid, T, and Michlovitz, SL: Therapeutic ultrasound. In Michlovitz, SL (ed): Thermal Agents in Rehabilitation, ed 3. FA Davis, Philadelphia, 1996.

68. Kloth, LC, and Niezgoda, JA: Ultrasound for Would Débridement and Healing. In McCulloch, JM, and Kloth LC (eds): Wound Healing: Evidence Based Management, ed 4. FA Davis, Philadelphia, 2010

69. Niezgoda, JA, and Kindwall, EP: Oxygen therapy—management of the hypoxic wound. In McCulloch, JM, and Kloth LC (eds): Wound Healing: Evidence Based Management, ed 4. FA Davis, Philadelphia, 2010.

70. MacKay, D, and Miller, AL: Nutritional support for wound healing. Altern Med Rev 8:359–377, 2003.

71. Passeri, G, Pini, G, Troiano, L, Vescovini, R, Sansoni, P, Passeri, M, et al: Low vitamin D status, high bone turnover, and bone fractures in centenarians. J Clin Endocrinol Metab 88:5109–5115, 2003.

72. Payne, WG, Walusimbi, MS, Blue, ML, Mosielly, G, Wright, TE, and Robson, MC: Radiated groin wounds: Pitfalls in reconstruction. Am Surg 69:994–997, 2003.

73. Coghill, RC, McHaffie, JG, and Yen, YF: Neural correlates of interindividual differences in the subjective experience of pain. Proc Natl Acad Sci U S A. 100: 8538–8542, 2003.

74. American Society of Anesthesiologists Task Force on Chronic Pain Management: Practice guidelines for chronic pain management. Anesthesiology 112:810–833, 2010.

75. Mallen, CD, Peat, G, Thomas, E, et al: Prognostic factors for musculoskeletal pain in primary care: A systematic review. Br J Gen Pract 57:655–661, 2007.

76. Stedman's Concise Medical Dictionary for the Health Professions, ed. 4. Lippincott Williams & Wilkins, New York, 2001.

LET'S FIND OUT

Lab Activity: Tissue Response to Injury
These lab activities provide students/learners with the opportunity to review tissue response concepts that may have been presented previously in other courses.

Pain

1. Look up the definition of pain in three dictionaries and develop a composite definition that encompasses all of them.

   Source/Definition:

   _____

   _____

   Source/Definition:

   _____

   _____

   Source/Definition:

   _____

   _____

   Composite Definition: _____

   _____

   _____

   _____

2. How much of the definition was based on psychological factors and how much on physical factors?

   Psychological Factors: _____

   _____

   Physical Factors: _____

   _____

3. How could this potentially be useful information for you as a clinician?

   _____

   _____

   _____

   _____

4. Look up and write down the definitions of analgesia, anesthesia, and paresthesia.

   Analgesia:

   _____

   Anesthesia: _____

   _____

   Paresthesia: _____

   _____

5. What is the difference between the three?

_____

_____

- Which would be a symptom of more concern?

_____

_____

- Why?

_____

_____

Edema

1. Review your definitions for edema or look it up again and write it below.

_____

_____

_____

2. Based on the definition that you have written, how would edema potentially limit function?

_____

_____

_____

3. What would you consider to be a reliable indicator of the amount of edema present? Why?

_____

_____

_____

_____

Pain Transmission

1. Review your text and describe why sensory input to an intact peripheral nerve is capable of providing pain relief in the same location on the opposite side of the body.

_____

_____

_____

_____

Endogenous Opiates

1. What are the differences between enkephalin and beta-endorphin?

_____

_____

_____

_____

2. If it is possible to stimulate the liberation of one or both of the listed endogenous opiates, which would be more difficult to stimulate?

_____

_____

_____

_____

3. What pharmacological agents potentially inhibit the liberation of the longer-lasting endogenous opiates?

_____

_____

_____

_____

Psychology and Pain

1. Interview three people of different ethnic groups and generations to find out how they would describe the pain associated with each of the following stimuli:

	First Person	Second Person	Third Person
A severe sunburn			
Overexposure to sub-freezing temperatures			
Hitting a thumb with a hammer			
An extremity that "falls asleep"			

2. Compare the sensation descriptions that you have solicited. Are there any differences in reported responses that surprised you? Why or why not?

_____

_____

_____

_____

3. What practical knowledge could you gain from this activity?

_____

_____

_____

_____

4. Providing sensory stimulation to an area will decrease the perception of painful stimuli in that area.

- What response from your interviewees supports this theory?

_____

_____

_____

- What is the name of this theory, first described in 1965 by Melzack and Wall?

_____

_____

_____

- How can this information be applied practically today?

_____

_____

Stages of Wound Healing

1. What are the three stages of wound/tissue healing, and approximately how long does each stage last?

First: _____

_____

_____

Second: _____

_____

_____

Third: _____

_____

_____

2. What is the primary purpose for each of the stages, and what is the indicator for whether or not that stage of healing is occurring?

Stage	Purpose	Indicator
First		
Second		
Third		

Precautions in Handling Wounds in Each Stage

1. Each of the stages of wound/tissue healing involves a significant number of activities. Wound/tissue healing is vulnerable to potential setbacks that could delay the healing process. Review your texts for examples of precautions that may adversely affect this process.

First: _____

_____

_____

Second: _____

_____

_____

Third: _____

_____

_____

Lab Questions

1. What have you learned from the activities in this lab exercise about tissue responses to injury?
2. Do all patients respond the same way to the same types of stimuli? Why or why not?
3. What types of factors tend to influence the way that a patient responds to "painful stimuli"?
4. How will the responses that you noted from your classmates influence your expectations for patient responses in the future?

CHAPTER 3

Patient Responses to Therapeutic Interventions

Barbara J. Behrens, PTA, MS | Stacie Larkin, PT, MS

Learning Outcomes

Following the completion of this chapter, the student/learner will be able to:

- Describe the potential patient responses to therapeutic treatment interventions.
- Outline examination techniques for pain assessment, the presence of edema, muscle guarding, range-of-motion deficits associated with edema, and muscle strength.
- Select appropriate assessment tests and measurements to determine the effectiveness of a treatment intervention with a physical agent.
- Describe and identify expected responses to the application of superficial heat.
- Provide the rationale for skin assessment before and after the application of physical agents to the skin by demonstrating the techniques on a classmate.
- Differentiate between normal and abnormal responses to heat observed in a controlled activity with classmates.
- Document observations of skin appearance of a classmate in terms that would be appropriate for a patient record.

Key Terms

Assessment
Blanching
Capillary refill
Edema
Erythema
Evaluation

Examination
Girth
Intervention
Melanin
Mottling
Muscle guarding

Muscle spasm
Muscle tone
Palpation
Pigmentation
Visual analog scale
Volumeter

Patient Perspective

"Is this really supposed to make my knee so red?"

The importance of assessing a patient's response to treatment cannot be overstated. It is critical in determining the success of any treatment intervention with a patient. This chapter focuses on the clinician's role in assessing the patient's response to interventions with physical agents. The purpose of these observations is to ensure safety in administration of treatment, monitor patient progress, and adjust dosage when necessary.

Examination, Evaluation, and Intervention

For consistency's sake, the definitions given for examination, evaluation, and intervention are those that can be found in the American Physical Therapy Association's *Guide to Physical Therapist Practice*, second edition (2003):

Examination: "The process of obtaining a history, performing relevant systems reviews, and selecting and administering specific tests and measures"

Evaluation: "A dynamic process in which the physical therapist makes clinical judgments based on data gathered during the examination"

Intervention: "Purposeful and skilled interaction of the physical therapist with the patient/client . . . using various physical therapy methods and techniques to produce changes in the condition that are consistent with the diagnosis and prognosis"

After a thorough initial examination and evaluation, a plan of care is created by the physical therapist that includes anticipated goals and expected outcomes. Physical agents and mechanical modalities are most commonly used for the goals of:

- Decreasing pain
- Reducing soft tissue/joint edema and inflammation
- Increasing blood flow and enhancing delivery of nutrients to tissue
- Promoting muscle relaxation
- Increasing the extensibility of connective tissue
- Increasing muscle strength

Skin (Integument) Assessment

Assessment of the skin's (integument) characteristics, including color, continuity, and temperature, is necessary when determining the condition of the soft tissue being treated. Skin pigmentation or color is based on the amounts of **melanin** and hemoglobin that are present. Melanin is a substance that gives skin and hair their color and may also be referred to as a pigment. Temperature of the skin surface indicates the current state of the tissue. Elevated skin temperatures indicate either inflammation in the area or possibly infection or a burn. Decreased skin temperatures may indicate vascular compromise. One should also inspect for any wounds, blisters, or rashes, as they will also affect the decision of which interventions are most appropriate and safe to use.

SKIN PIGMENTATION OR COLOR

Pigmentation of human skin is determined by the presence of a biochemical compound known as *melanin*. Persons with darker skin tones have a greater amount of melanin. Fairer-skinned individuals will appear to respond differently to the increases in subcutaneous circulation than will individuals with olive or black skin tones, and changes in blood flow will be more obvious compared with an individual with darker skin. The skin of fair-skinned patients will appear pink or red after prolonged exposure to the sun or heat. This coloration is readily visible due to the decreased levels of melanin. Both darker-skinned and lighter-skinned individuals respond to prolonged exposure to the sun or heat; however, the changes in skin pigmentation and in local circulation will be different and might be less apparent in some than in others. This is one of the reasons it is important to enlist a patient's responses when asking about his or her experiences with exposure to the sun or heat. In most instances, the patient will be able to tell from his or her own skin whether any changes have occurred in response to heat. It's also why it is important for students to work with classmates who have different skin types from their own and observe their classmates' responses.

Patients who have areas of skin that have been continually exposed to severe weather conditions, and have marked weathering of their skin, will also respond less noticeably to changes in local circulation. Skin coloration may vary because of the day-to-day elements, including temperatures, to which the skin is exposed. Skin texture will also vary depending on the forces it encounters. Scars in the treatment area make the skin respond in a particular way to physical, mechanical, or electrotherapeutic treatment interventions. For example, where there is scar tissue, there is altered circulation and the response to thermal agents will thus be different. Clinicians must become cautious observers of the skin and surrounding tissues they are treating, noting subtle changes when they occur.

Uniformity of skin coloration and pigmentation provides information regarding the local circulation and the potential sensitivity of the skin to thermal agents. Skin that is pale or bluish in appearance may indicate a decrease in blood flow to that area (for example, frostbite). Skin that is pink or red may indicate an increase in blood flow to that area (for example, a thermal burn or an acute injury). It is important to be sure that the modality chosen for a given patient takes into consideration the current status of the tissue being treated. Heating agents are commonly applied to promote circulation, which will enhance the nutrient base for tissue healing. However, use of a heating agent would not be indicated if the skin is already red, inflamed, and warm when palpated, as this would only increase the blood flow to the area.

The presence of scars must also be observed and taken into consideration when choosing a modality. Immature scar tissue, which when pink, is well vascularized. When immature scars are exposed to heat, they will turn bright red in response. Mature scar tissue, which is often pale in appearance, is not as well vascularized as is noninjured or repaired tissue and will likely retain a lighter appearance regardless of being heated or cooled. Sensation may also be impaired around the scar. For these reasons, the presence of a scar and skin pigmentation or coloration in the treatment area are important to note and to monitor closely during the application of any thermal agent. Failure to note the presence of a scar in the treatment area and whether or not the patient has sensation and uniform circulation in and around that scar may result in patient injury that could easily have been prevented.

CIRCULATORY IRREGULARITIES

Because circulatory changes can be noted to some degree by appearance, it is important for the clinician to observe and identify various skin types and their responses to local changes in circulation. One simple test for circulatory impairment is known as the capillary refill test, or blanching. **Blanching** of the skin is the term used to describe the response to applied pressure on the surface of the skin. Those with intact or unimpaired circulation will have a temporary change in pigmentation when pressure is applied, and as the capillary beds refill with blood the original pigmentation will return. **Capillary refill** is the return of the pre-pressure pigmentation and it should occur in less than 3 seconds.[1] Areas where arterial circulation is impaired may not respond by blanching when pressure is applied; they may remain unchanged, or the return to pre-pressure pigmentation make take longer than 3 seconds, indicating that the underlying tissue has impaired circulatory function. Mature scar tissue is another example where blanching may not be observed. Mature scar may remain pale when pressure is applied to it. This may indicate that the patient will have an increased sensitivity to heat or cold. The application of pressure to the skin is a simple activity that provides quick information regarding the ability of the capillary beds and arterioles to respond to this form of stimuli (Fig. 3-1).

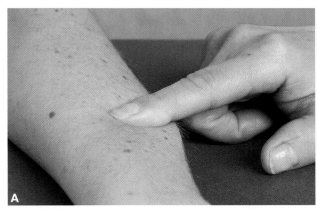

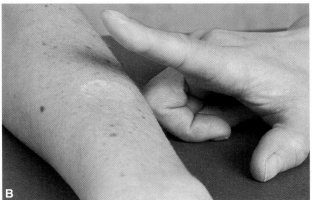

FIGURE 3-1 Capillary refill. **(A)** Before; **(B)** after.

appearing blanched. Wherever the thermal agent was applied should have the same pigmentation throughout. There should not be inconsistencies. Mottling is one of the types of inconsistencies that could be observed. If mottling occurs, the application time and/or intensity of the thermal agent should be decreased during the next application (Fig. 3-2).

SKIN SURFACE TEMPERATURE

As with the observation of the pigmentation of the skin, the surface temperature of the skin can provide information regarding the circulatory status of the underlying tissue. The simple act of touching, or **palpating,** the treatment area prior to treating with thermal agents can provide a wealth of information helpful to clinicians. Warmth may indicate inflammation of the underlying tissues, whereas coolness may indicate poor circulation. Surface temperature of the skin should change in response to environmental influences. If the temperature of the room is cool but the skin temperature feels warm, this could indicate that there is an underlying inflammatory process taking place in the palpated area. At a minimum, it would require that the clinician palpate an uninvolved area to determine whether or not areas outside of the treatment area also feel warm when palpated.

CHECK IT OUT 3-1

ACTIVITY: CAPILLARY REFILL

- Observe the skin in an area that you want to "investigate."
- Press on the skin in that area with your thumb.
- Observe what happens to the skin directly under your thumb once you release the pressure.
- How long does it take for the appearance of the skin to return to the pre-pressure appearance?
- Try it again on someone with a different skin type and try it over a scar.
- Were there any differences in what you saw? Why or why not?

MOTTLING OF THE SKIN

Spotty patches of erythema that occur after the application of thermal agents is referred to as **mottling** of the skin. It may be indicative of overheating or overcooling of the skin. It may also be indicative of repeated or prolonged use of superficial thermal agents. *Mottling should be considered a warning sign of potential inability of the tissue to respond appropriately and adequately to the thermal agent.* In other words, rather than seeing a uniform erythema throughout the treatment area, what is observed is splotchy with areas that are various colors, with some indicating an erythema and others almost

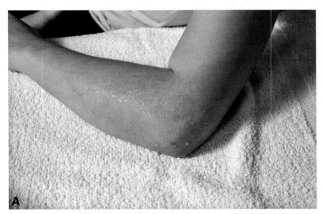

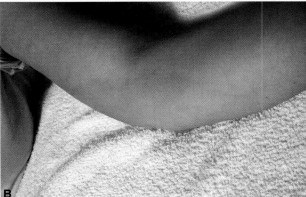

FIGURE 3-2 **(A, B)** The extremity exhibits signs of uneven erythema with white patches, indicating excessive exposure to a thermal agent. The condition is referred to as mottling of the skin.

The application of heat will cause local vasodilation, an increase in the surface temperature of the skin, accompanied by **erythema,** a redness of the skin, and possibly perspiration depending upon the modality selected. The application of cold will cause a decrease in the surface temperature of the skin accompanied by a reflex vasodilation erythema (after about 8 minutes of application time). These responses can be detected via observation of the pigmentation or color changes of the skin and via **palpation,** which involves physically touching the patient to feel the surface temperature of the skin.

BEFORE YOU BEGIN

OBSERVATIONS

If there are any alterations in the appearance or temperature of the skin, these areas are prone to a different response to thermal agents. Watch these areas more closely!

Skin temperature as perceived via palpation, pigmentation, or color and overall integrity provide the clinician with valuable information regarding the patient's response or his/her potential response to the application of a thermal agent. This information will help determine whether a given intervention is appropriate and safe to perform. If a clinician fails to visually inspect the treated area before and after treatment interventions with physical agents, then the safety and efficacy of the treatment cannot be assured. However, if it is a routine aspect of patient care to visually inspect the area pre- and post-treatment, then that is one more way to assure patient safety and the potential efficacy of the intervention used.

Pain Assessment

Pain represents the most difficult complaint to quantify and objectively document. Pain assessment encompasses a variety of techniques used to quantify and measure the impact it has on the patient's ability to perform functional activities. There may be a strong psychological component to the expression of pain. The patient is the only individual who can describe the intensity of his or her experience. Due to these complexities, many researchers and clinicians have attempted to compile an objective set of baseline measures to reflect the experience of pain. Pain scales have been used in an attempt to quickly measure the level or quantity of discomfort a patient is experiencing.

PAIN SCALES: VISUAL ANALOG AND NUMERIC PAIN RATING

Visual analog scales (VASs) involve the use of a 10-cm line drawn on a piece of paper, with a beginning and an end anchor identified by word descriptors like "no pain" and "pain as bad as it can be," respectively. Patients are asked to place a mark on the line indicating their level of discomfort (Fig. 3-3). The clinician then measures the distance in centimeters from the start of the line and records

1.   Please mark on the scale how much pain you have.

Visual Analog Scale

No Pain ——————— Pain as Bad as It Could Be

2.   Where is your pain?

On the drawings below, please mark the areas where you feel pain. Put E if external, or I if internal, near the areas that you mark. Put EI if both external and internal.

FIGURE 3-3 **(1)** Visual analog scale. Patients are to indicate the level of pain they are experiencing by marking on the 10-cm line. The distance from the start point of the line is measured and recorded for future assessment comparisons. **(2)** Anatomical pain drawings.
(Parts 1 and 2, excerpted from of the McGill Pain Questionnaire, Courtesy of R. Melzack.)

the measurement. After treatment, the patient is given a new, unmarked 10-cm line and asked to reassess the level of discomfort and to mark the new line (Fig. 3-4). The clinician then measures the distance to the new mark and again records the length of the line in centimeters. For each assessment, the patient is given a clean, new line to indicate his or her level of discomfort so that past responses do not influence how the patient rates his or her current pain level. If the results of the line measurements are recorded regularly, then it will be possible for the clinician to actually chart the patient's progress. This may assist the clinician in determining whether the selected treatment interventions have been appropriate and effective for relieving the patient's pain according to the patient's reported responses.

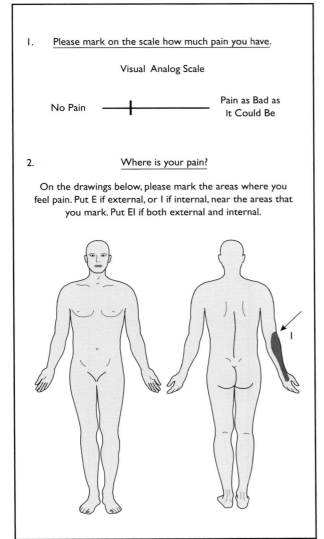

1.   Please mark on the scale how much pain you have.

Visual Analog Scale

No Pain ———————|——————— Pain as Bad as
                                                          It Could Be

2.   Where is your pain?

On the drawings below, please mark the areas where you feel pain. Put E if external, or I if internal, near the areas that you mark. Put EI if both external and internal.

FIGURE 3-4 Drawing of a 10-cm line that a patient has used, indicating the level of discomfort. The beginning of the line has the descriptor "no pain" and the end of the line has the descriptor "pain as bad as it can be."
(Parts 1 and 2, excerpted from the McGill Pain Questionnaire, Courtesy of R. Melzack.)

A similar assessment may be done with numbers from 0 to 10 marked along a 10-cm line, and thus is a numeric pain-rating scale (NPRS). A change of 3 points on the NPRS or a change of 28 mm on the VAS is needed for it to be considered a detectable change.[2] The drawback with marking the numbers is that the patient has a reference point to refer to, which may influence how he or she marks the line. Clinically, however, it is the NPRS that is most commonly used, as it is very quick to use.

FACTORS THAT INFLUENCE PAIN RATINGS

Use of either the VAS or the NPRS involves assessment of the level of discomfort before and after treatment to determine whether the treatment had any effect on the patient's pain. The type of questions asked of the patient is important, and clinicians must be careful to encourage the patient to respond not to the presence of pain, but rather to the presence of whatever sensation or symptom is the greatest. Optimally, a clinician would ask the patient to rate his or her discomfort and, after treatment, let the clinician know just what he or she is feeling. The questions should not reinforce the perception of pain by using the word "pain" in the question.[3,4] Rather than asking a patient, "Are you still in pain?" or "Do you still hurt?" instead ask, "What are you feeling now?" to find out about the primary complaint the patient is experiencing.

Patients who are not motivated to recover may skew their responses and invalidate their subjective responses to treatment. The patient may also attempt to control the "recovery time" by assigning an arbitrary number to his or her "acceptable" level of pain to be able to return to work. He or she may decide that he is willing to discontinue therapy only when his pain, as he reports it, returns to a level of 3. If using the unmarked line, he or she may arbitrarily decide that his assessment of pain must be one-third the distance from the starting point. This decision may be made by the patient before he will be satisfied that he can return to work. This is another reason pain ratings are just one factor in pain assessment. Pain scales are simple, quick, subjective measures for a pain complaint. They are not flawless, however, and should not be used as the sole source for pain assessment.

PAIN INVENTORIES

Inventories for pain assessment represent another tool for quantifying and documenting the subjective complaints of pain. The McGill-Melzack Pain Questionnaire[5,6] was formulated in an attempt to create an instrument that would be universally applicable for many cultures and diagnoses, and for multiple levels of cognitive understanding. Patients who reported that they were experiencing pain and had been diagnosed with a painful condition were surveyed to describe their pain with whatever words they could use to adequately capture their individual experience. The patient reactions or expressions were categorized as affective, emotional, behavioral responses to the painful experience. Participants in the survey were then asked to rank-order the phrases or words that were offered from least annoying to worst experience. Many translations took place so that the information could be used with a patient from virtually any culture. A standardized version of the test was formulated and a methodology for grading or interpreting it was also developed. Individual categories of descriptors are graded according to their ranking within the category. Thus, if there are four words in a category, the first word listed is ranked as the least bothersome, and the fourth word as the most annoying and potentially serious.

Some of the descriptors include words such as "sharp" or "dull," which will assist the clinician in assessing the ease of localization of the discomfort. As discussed in Chapter 2, pain receptors can be A-delta fibers, transmitting fast "pain or injury," or they can be C fibers, which are responsible for the transmission of the "pain of suffering" or a difficult-to-identify or -localize aching sensation. The McGill-Melzack Pain Questionnaire records information about and evaluative components of the patient's pain experience and is quite comprehensive (Fig. 3-5).[5,6]

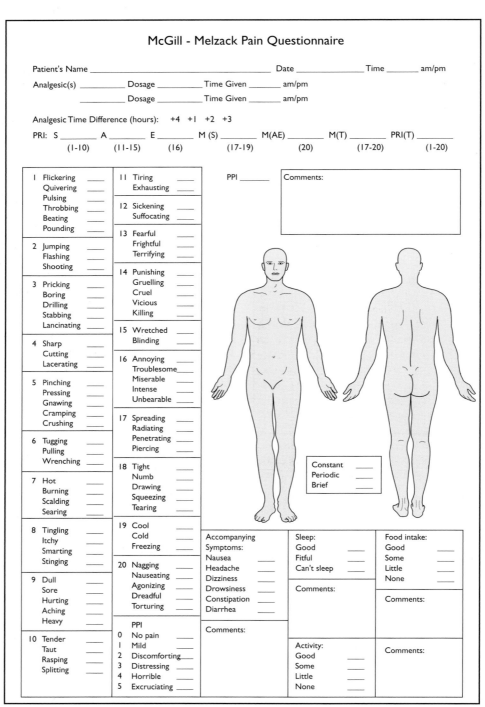

FIGURE 3-5 The McGill-Melzack Pain Questionnaire.
(Courtesy of R. Melzack.)

CHECK IT OUT 3-2

ACTIVITY: SENSATION

Localize the treatment/testing area and without showing your patient/partner what you are doing, ask him/her to tell you whether or not he/she feels something and if so, where and what it feels like.

- You can use a pencil point for sharp and the eraser end for dull "probing/touching" in the treatment/target area.
- A cold or warm hand can be used to help determine the patient/partner's ability to distinguish temperature.
- Be careful *not* to ask "Do you feel THIS?" or "Did that feel sharp?" These are leading questions!

ANATOMICAL PAIN DRAWINGS

Line drawings of the anatomy allow the patient to locate just where he or she is experiencing discomfort. If a patient is instructed to fill in the areas that correspond to the pain, the completed drawing guides the clinician to the primary area(s) of discomfort. This type of information can be extremely important if radiating pain is present, because it may indicate the original source. It also acts as a road map for clinicians working with patients who are experiencing multiple areas of involvement, because the patient is instructed to "color in" the worst area first. Caution should be observed when interpreting these drawings if the clinician is unable to solicit responses directly from the patient. Some patients may have difficulty recognizing a particular part of the body on the line drawing. This would be another reason the drawing should be completed in the presence of a clinician who is able to answer questions as they arise. Technology has introduced computer animation to pain drawing and pain drawing analysis, which may lead to further refinement of the data obtained.[7-12]

Word inventories, not anatomical drawings, should be completed by patients while they are comfortably positioned and relaxed, possibly while they are waiting to be seen by the clinician. The anatomical pain drawings, however, should be completed in the presence of a clinician so that any sequencing can be noted. Although the information obtained in these inventories is useful, it is by no means complete and should be accompanied by other performance-related assessments.

PRESSURE ALGOMETERS OR DOLORIMETERS

Objective tools have been developed to help determine tissue sensitivity in the form of strain gauges; however, their use clinically is not widespread. *Dolor* in Spanish means "pain," so a dolorimeter is a meter that measures pain with a force transducer, that is, something that measures the amount of pressure that can be applied before a patient reports that he feels discomfort. Most of the determinations that are made are based on the experience of the clinician. Strain gauges are calibrated to detect the amount of applied pressure administered to a patient. They then can objectively quantify just how much force was exerted on the surface of the skin before the patient complained of discomfort.

These devices are referred to as dolorimeters or pressure algometers (Box 3-1).[13-17]

OTHER MEANS TO ASSESS PAIN

Facial expression can be another way of assessing a patient's subjective complaint of pain. Facial musculature, particularly in the forehead and around the eyes, will contract in response to pain perception. A patient may not verbally express discomfort because of his or her cultural background but will appear to be in pain. After treatment, the patient appears more comfortable, despite other objective responses indicating that there has been no change in the level of discomfort that he or she is experiencing. This is truly an interpretation but may provide the clinician with additional information regarding the patient's pain (Fig. 3-6).

Pain Intensity Scales

A wide variety of instruments have been developed for the assessment of pain in various patient populations. Some of these instruments utilize the observations of the clinician if the patient is nonverbal, a child, an infant, or a cognitively impaired adult. Several examples have been provided that are used by the NIH Clinical Center to measure pain intensity and patient responses to treatment interventions. Examples of other tools can be found in Appendix: Pain Assessment Tool Kit (see pages 51–52).

The ability to perform a functional activity or perform a certain range of motion can also provide information regarding a patient's current level of pain. Rather than focusing on the patient's pain through pain scales as a means to determine progress, it becomes even more important to focus treatment goals on returning the patient to his or her

---

BOX 3-1 | Pain Assessment

1. Pain is only quantifiable by the individual *when* they are experiencing it.
2. Diagrams work well for some patients to describe their pain; they do not work for all patients.
3. Some patients may not objectively assess their discomfort.
4. Some patients may be motivated not to report that they feel better. This is why you need to assess more than just their subjective response to a treatment intervention.

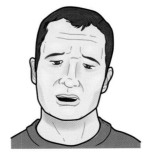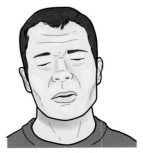

FIGURE 3-6 Facial expression can indicate whether an individual is experiencing pain.

prior functional level. Range-of-motion (ROM) measurements taken before and after a treatment intervention can provide clear objective data regarding the patient's ability or willingness to move. When ROM is limited, the cause of that limitation needs to be identified. Pain secondary to muscle guarding, joint restriction, nerve impingement, and edema are some possibilities. **Muscle guarding** is the protective response of muscles after injury whereby the muscle length remains shortened to limit function. It is a temporary symptom that should resolve as the primary symptoms and insult resolve, but it can often be referred to by patients as a "**muscle spasm**" (see later in this chapter). After treatment for these impairments, it is necessary to reassess the patient's ROM to see if a change has occurred in the quantity and the quality of the motion. Pain should also be assessed to see if the increase in ROM results with a decrease in pain, as one would expect. If there was no change in pain, yet gains were made in ROM, this is still considered a positive outcome as functional gains have been made.

Another means to determine whether progress is being made is to assess the frequency, dosage, and types of pain medication a patient is taking. When a patient reports a decrease in use of pain medications or stops taking a more potent prescription medication for pain management and is not managing his or her discomfort with an over-the-counter pain medication, this is valuable information that indicates a positive change in the patient's pain level.

WHEN PATIENTS ARE NOT IMPROVING AS EXPECTED

Most patients who seek assistance in the management of pain have legitimate complaints. However, there are occasions when the potential for secondary gain, or the potential of a legal battle, may influence a patient's response to treatment. When a patient is not progressing as anticipated, it is important to reevaluate and determine whether any change has occurred or if any new problems have arisen. Working with patients who are influenced by outside sources to prolong the course of treatment may be particularly frustrating. Resources such as *The Guide to Physical Therapist Practice*, revised second edition (2003), can provide the therapist with the general range of therapy visits needed to achieve the anticipated goals and expected outcomes for a given diagnostic classification. When therapy progress is happening slowly or not at all, the physical therapist must reexamine the patient to evaluate progress, modify the treatment plan, or possibly consider discontinuation of therapy if it is no longer providing any benefit to the patient.

Edema Assessment

Edema, or swelling, is an abnormal increase in the amount of interstitial fluid. It may be diffuse throughout the area or localized to the injury site. When swelling is contained within a joint capsule, it is referred to as joint effusion. Edema in small quantities is a normal response to trauma, and it is necessary for the repair process of tissue healing. Prolonged and/or massive edema can interrupt repair by impeding the diffusion of nutrients to cells or perhaps by leading to tissue fibrosis. To accurately assess the quantity of edema present in an area, there are several options available, depending on the location of the edema. The options include:

- Circumferential or **girth** measurements
- Volumetric water displacement
- Joint mobility
- Functional performance

CIRCUMFERENTIAL OR GIRTH MEASUREMENTS

Using a tape measure can be one of the quickest, easiest, and most accurate ways to assess the presence of edema. For consistency of measurement, the following factors must be adhered to:

1. Use a tape measure that does not stretch.
2. Measure with the same tape measure each time.
3. The same therapist should record the measurements each time.
4. Measurements are most accurate and comparable when taken at the same time of day.
5. Use bony landmarks as reference points for measurement.
6. Use the same measurement technique each time you measure.
7. Remember to use the same unit of measurement each time a measurement is taken (centimeters or inches).

If these factors are adhered to, then there will be a reasonable degree of accuracy and reliability of the measurements (Fig. 3-7). Further details regarding circumferential measurement are provided in Chapter 8.

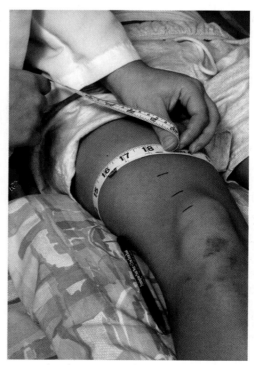

FIGURE 3-7 The clinician is performing circumferential girth measurements using a tape measure. She is using bony landmarks as reference points and areas distal and proximal to them that have been marked.

BEFORE YOU BEGIN

EDEMA ASSESSMENT

- Make sure that you use the same measurement tools each time.
- Make sure that it's assessed at the same time each time it is assessed and that whoever is doing the assessment is familiar with the measurement tools that are being used.

WHY DO I NEED TO KNOW ABOUT...

SKIN SURFACE TEMPERATURE

Consider the following before treatment:

1. If the skin of the area being treated is warm and red in appearance (compared with the surrounding area), then inflammation or infection may be present. This would be a contraindication for the use of heating agents.
2. If the skin of the area being treated is cooler and paler (compared with the surrounding area), then circulation may be compromised. Vascular insufficiency is a contraindication for all heating and cooling agents.
3. If there is scar in the treatment area, then be sure sensation has been tested and that it is intact. This is important when using modalities where you are dependent on the patient's response to guide the intensity and duration of treatment.

VOLUMETRIC WATER DISPLACEMENT

When edema is confined to distal extremities, volumetric measurements may be considered practical and accurate. A **volumeter** is a device that measures water displacement to record the volume that a distal extremity occupies when submerged in water. If an edematous extremity is placed in a known volume of water and the displaced water is measured, then the volume of that part of the extremity can be determined (Fig. 3-8). Subsequent

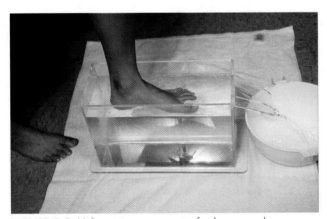

FIGURE 3-8 Volumetric assessment of edema can be performed using a volumeter and water displacement. The patient places the edematous extremity into the water, and the displaced water is measured to determine the volume of the edema.

measurements will reveal the status of the edema and whether the volume of displaced water increases, decreases, or remains unchanged. Some critical factors for accuracy of this form of measurement include the following:

1. The time of day for subsequent measurements should be the same as the initial time of measurement. Variations in the time of day may lead to variations in measurements because patients may retain fluids at different times during the day or in response to medication schedules.
2. The same temperature of water must be used for each measurement. Water changes density at different temperatures, which could potentially make readings inaccurate.
3. The unit of measurement must remain constant (ounces or milliliters of water).

Hand and foot volumeters are commercially available in Plexiglas (Volumetrics Limited, Idyllwild, CA). Commercial devices have known values for accuracy.

There can be several disadvantages to volumetric measurements if they are used as the sole source of assessment of edema. This form of assessment looks at total volume of the part immersed but does not account for individual areas of excessive edema relative to the diffuse edema. It does not enable the clinician to document precisely *where* the edema is located, simply that *there is edema*. It is not as practical to use for the assessment of an entire extremity, as would be circumferential measurements. Despite the disadvantages, it can be a useful and time-efficient form of edema assessment for the foot and ankle or hand.

Clinicians are cautioned that comparisons with the uninvolved upper extremity might not yield reliable data because hand dominance plays a significant role in the size of one's hand. Volumetric assessment of edema is most beneficial for assessing the presence of edema in a specific distal extremity when it is compared with that same specific distal extremity upon subsequent visits after receiving treatment interventions. Any attempt to compare one's left to right hand could potentially yield a difference when there is no pathology present. In addition, if one's nondominant hand is involved and then compared volumetrically with an injured dominant hand, the volumes may appear to be the same. Hence comparisons between left and right are not typically beneficial.

FUNCTIONAL PERFORMANCE LIMITED BY EDEMA

A patient's ability to perform activities of daily living (ADLs) may be impaired by the presence of edema. Limitations in movement caused by an increase in edema may inhibit the patient's ability to get dressed or don a garment. Putting on socks or stockings may be very difficult if there is a significant quantity of edema in the lower extremity. These specific activities can also be a means to assess progress toward functional goals.

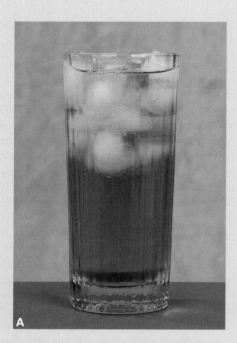

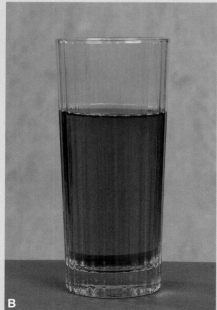

FIGURE 3-9 Glass of iced tea. **(A)** ice; **(B)** no ice.

WHAT SHOULD BE MONITORED FOR EDEMA MANAGEMENT?

Assessment of edema will take into account all of the elements that apply to the individual patient. If the possibility of volumetric and circumferential measurements is feasible, then monitor both. To be considered valid, the form of assessment must be kept consistent for a given patient. If a patient had an acute ankle sprain and the initial evaluation used volumetric measurements for edema, then any reassessment of the edema must also use volumetric measurements. Likewise, if the initial evaluation used circumferential measurements, then subsequent assessments of edema must include circumferential measurements.

Soft Tissue Assessment

Muscle guarding can inhibit or delay a patient's recovery. Two components of the assessment of soft tissue are palpation of muscle tone and observation of posture. Each of these assessments helps to outline a clearer picture of the patient's overall condition and how it is affecting them.

MUSCLE GUARDING

Muscle guarding is a clinician's term for what a patient refers to as a "muscle spasm." Muscle guarding is a protective response in a muscle that results from pain or fear of movement. Terminology is important especially when referring to motor responses of muscles. Unfortunately, patients tend to confuse the term "spasm" with "spasticity" despite the fact that these are quite different. Spasticity is a type of motor response that is mediated or controlled by a higher mechanism in the brain or spinal cord and not a peripheral nerve or local area of involvement. Muscle guarding occurs to protect the area from further trauma by contracting the surrounding muscles and providing an "exoskeleton." It is an indication of the degree of motor unit firing present in a muscle that exists to protect the area. This is one of the reasons that it can be measured using electromyographic (EMG) monitoring equipment. Prolonged muscle guarding can result in a shortening of the underlying tissue and a feeling of "hardening" so that the muscle now feels harder than the surrounding tissue. The actual number of sarcomeres, which are the units of contraction in the muscle, may decrease due to the prolonged immobility and shortened position of the muscle.[18]

When patients report that they "feel a muscle spasm" it is important for clinicians to differentiate between a localized response and a centrally mediated response and help patients to understand what is happening and why. Muscle guarding is particularly sensitive to stress and anxiety, especially if the guarding is present in the paraspinal musculature. If patients are anxious about what is occurring and do not understand the treatment interventions that are taking place or the anticipated outcomes, muscle guarding could potentially increase. Some thermal agents are used to help reduce or eliminate perceived increases in muscle guarding. It is important to palpate the area before and after applying a therapeutic intervention to determine whether the treatment technique produced any changes in the muscle tone. Palpation of the treatment area before and after a treatment intervention is also a way to validate the outcome of the chosen approach. If the clinician examines the area via palpation before the initiation of treatment and fails to reexamine the area after the application, it is difficult to determine whether change occurred as a result of the selected intervention (Fig. 3-10).

MUSCLE TONE

Muscle tone refers to the resistance of the muscle to passive stretch or elongation, or how "tight" it feels. When a muscle guards, it assumes a shortened state to help protect the area from further injury. Its tone may therefore be increased protectively, causing it to feel harder than uninvolved tissue when palpated. Ease in reaching the determination that a muscle is guarding comes with experience in palpating a multitude of soft tissue injuries on a wide variety of patients. Muscle tightness and its causes are difficult to assess objectively without an external source of measurement such as a surface EMG reading of the electrical activity taking place within the muscle. In other words, an EMG reading could supply a measurement of the number of sarcomeres that were actually firing to contract the muscle and produce the current state of the muscle.

Tissue tone assessment relies heavily on the experience of the clinician monitoring it. In many acute conditions, the patient will experience some degree of tenderness in the injured soft tissue. Tissue tone changes may or may not be one of the first palpable signs of injury. If muscle guarding is present, then it will typically occur in both the agonist and the antagonistic muscle groups crossing or surrounding the injured area to protect the area from further trauma. When both the agonist and antagonist co-contract, motion in the involved area is limited, leaving less chance for injury to occur. Palpation comparison of the involved with the uninvolved side will provide further insight concerning the level of discomfort or tightness that the patient is experiencing.

POSTURAL ASSESSMENT

Postural changes are likely to be observed in patients who are experiencing pain and muscle guarding. Postural changes can be observed throughout the body but this is especially noticeable when the injured area involves the cervical postural muscles. For example, patients who have been involved in automobile accidents in which they have been hit from behind and injured their cervical spine, who have had a whiplash or cervical strain, exhibit different sitting/standing postures than do individuals who have not experienced this type of trauma. In this situation, the cervical muscles guard in both anterior and posterior regions supporting the head and limit all mobility of the head. This may visually look as if they have a stiff neck, avoiding any active cervical movements. If the cervical muscles are not assessed and treated, a forward head posture may result, wherein the head is displaced anteriorly on the cervical spine due to the increased muscle tone or guarding in the upper posterior cervical musculature. Ultimately, this type of muscle guarding in the cervical spine results in an increased cervical lordosis (Fig. 3-11).[19]

Range-of-Motion (ROM) Assessment

As with other forms of assessment, the measurement of joint ROM can provide an objective measure of the available movement within a given joint. It is important to look at both the quantity of motion available and the quality of that motion. In the case of muscle guarding, an agonist muscle may limit the antagonistic direction of joint ROM. The presence of edema can also impede joint movement, resulting in

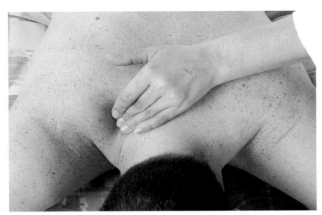

FIGURE 3-10 This clinician is palpating the area to be treated before the application of any physical agent. The same approach will be repeated after the administration of a therapeutic intervention to assist the clinician in determining whether a soft tissue change occurred.

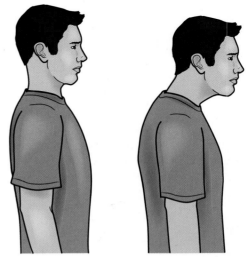

FIGURE 3-11 (A) Normal cervical posture and (B) forward head posture.

a decrease in ROM. The simple assessment of ROM must be a part of every peripheral joint assessment and reassessment to determine whether progress had been made with a particular treatment intervention. Measurements of available joint ROM with a goniometer can provide additional objective baseline information with which to make a comparison after therapeutic treatment interventions.

Muscle Strength Assessments

Muscle strength assessment can be accomplished either manually or with the use of sophisticated equipment to record force or torque production. A manual muscle test (MMT) assesses the strength of specific muscles or gross muscle actions. MMTs are performed when the area to be tested is stabilized and both active and passive ROM measurements have been assessed and recorded in the patient's chart. Manual resistance is then applied as the patient attempts the requested motion either in a position in which they are not moving against gravity or they are asked to move against resistance. The patient is provided with verbal instructions to resist the movement or force being applied to the area. The patient's response to the resistance is graded from trace to normal depending on the patient's position, completed ROM, and ability to perform against resistance when applied.

More reproducible testing of muscle performance may involve the use of a commercially manufactured dynamometer that measures the force applied at a given speed of motion. This is referred to as isokinetic force testing. "Iso" refers to the speed, which can be set to a fixed number, and "kinetic" refers to the fact that motion takes place. This type of equipment provides for proximal stabilization when resistance is applied to the distal extent of the tested extremity. One advantage of this type of device is that the patient will experience resistance only if he or she meets the preset speed of the resistance arm. In other words, if the patient is unable to contract quickly enough to "catch up" with the resistance arm, the patient will not experience any resistance. This means that if a patient experiences pain with a resisted contraction, he will not injure himself further with an isokinetic device. If the patient does not "push," there is nothing to push against. This is quite different from the use of free weights to assess muscle strength, wherein the patient may be able to lift the weight but not let it down without injury. Isokinetic dynamometers provide a torque or force reading to indicate the maximal level of torque exerted by the muscle. Subsequent tests will reveal increases in torque output if a patient is progressing and all testing factors are kept constant, such as test position, speed, and stabilization. The term **assessment** has been used throughout this section and it refers to a continuation of the primary assessment, in which the physical therapist or physical therapist assistant reassesses changes in the patient's condition, and performs appropriate physical examinations.

Patient Perspective

Remember that your patient is curious about all of the assessments, tests, and measurements that clinicians take and record. Your patient may want to know what the test results mean and why you are taking the time to record the information. Also, the word "test" may increase anxiety and therefore increase muscle guarding, which may have a negative impact on the results of your assessments or testing. Keeping the patient informed about what you are doing and why you are doing it will most often decrease the anxiety that your patient might be feeling. This also means that you need to consider the terminology that you are using and be sure to keep things simple. Although you understand medical terminology, do not assume that your patient will understand it. Terms as simple as "edema" can be lost on a patient.

The following questions are commonly asked by patients during or after an assessment. Your challenge is not in answering them as much as it is in the words that you choose to use to answer them.

Patients' Frequently Asked Questions

1. Why are you taking so many different types of measurements?
2. What do all of the numbers mean?
3. Why is the treatment area "red" after treatment; does that mean something "bad" has happened?
4. Why can't I bend my elbow as much when it's my shoulder [or hand] that is injured?
5. What is the difference between that water tank and a tape measure for swelling?
6. Why does "the injured area" feel hot after I exercise?
7. Why doesn't the pain relief that I get in therapy last longer after the first visit?
8. What difference does poor posture make on neck or back problems?
9. Why is it so hard to get dressed in the morning, but after I have been up for a while, I seem to be able to move more easily?

Summary

This chapter has presented many areas in which specific tests and measures can provide valuable information regarding the condition of a patient. It is important to gather information from multiple sources to help provide the clearest picture of the condition and progress that a patient is making. Without objective measures, the subjective complaints of the patient cannot be substantiated. The future of the profession of physical therapy rests on our ability to accurately quantify and qualify what we do for our patients. Capturing that information from a variety of sources is critical.

Review Questions

1. Skin types with the greatest amounts of melanin will appear_____ relative to those skin types with a lower amount of melanin present.
   a. Lighter
   b. Darker
   c. Softer and more pliable
   d. Tougher and scarred

2. The presence of a scar in the treatment area that is about to be treated with a thermal agent is only a factor if:
   a. The scar is mature and well vascularized
   b. The scar is immature and not well vascularized
   c. The scar tissue lacks sensation and vascularization
   d. The scar is unremarkable

3. Blanching is another term used to describe which of the following normal phenomenon?
   a. The response of arterioles to pressure
   b. The appearance of fair-skinned individuals after exposure to heat
   c. Capillary refill after pressure to the area is released
   d. An indication that excessive heat or cold has been applied

4. The patient you are working with this afternoon has a palpable difference in skin temperature between the involved and uninvolved sides, with the involved side noticeably warmer than the uninvolved side. What could this potentially indicate if that area on that side also had an erythema?
   a. Nothing in particular; you do not have enough information
   b. That one side has an active process taking place
   c. That the involved side is actively inflamed
   d. That heat would potentially be indicated for this patient

5. A patient another clinician worked with yesterday is on your schedule for today. You were informed that the patient was involved in a motor vehicle accident (MVA) and that an attorney has been engaged to attempt to gain a large sum of money for the patient in a court case. Which of the following pain scales would be the most objective for you to use to attempt to gather data regarding the patient's progress?
   a. Visual analog scale
   b. Numeric pain-rating scale
   c. The McGill-Melzack Pain Questionnaire
   d. All of the above are objective and equally reliable as long as they are administered correctly

6. If you decided to use anatomical pain drawings as part of a pain assessment for a patient, which of the following would be the most important for you as a clinician to remember to do to assure that no information was lost?
   a. Place the patient's name on the form prior to giving it to him or her
   b. Collect the form from the patient after it has been completed
   c. Place the form in the patient's chart after it has been completed
   d. Watch the patient complete the form

7. Which of the following statements most accurately describes the response of muscles that have been subjected to a soft tissue injury whereby they temporarily protect the area and limit ROM?
   a. Sprain
   b. Strain
   c. Muscle spasm
   d. Muscle guarding

8. One of the patients you were working with last week was initially evaluated via volumeter for the presence of edema in her nondominant left hand. Today is her fourth session and you have been asked to reassess the presence of edema. Which of the following scenarios is most likely and why?
   a. You use a volumeter again and compare left with right and there is no difference between the two hands. She has not improved.
   b. You use a volumeter again and determine that the volume displaced today is less than it was on the first visit. She has improved.
   c. You use a tape measure today to reassess her edema because it is negligible. She appears to have improved.
   d. You determine that you will not have enough time for edema assessment today but base her improvement status on function rather than on anything else. She can now make a fist, so she is functional.

9. Which of the following methods could be used to help accurately determine the degree of muscle tone above and beyond normal that a patient was experiencing?
   a. A sarcomere measurement system
   b. An electrical conductivity measurement
   c. An EMG reading
   d. A dolorimeter

10. Other than an MMT, what can be used to objectively and accurately test the strength of muscles?
    a. ROM measurements
    b. An EMG reading
    c. A dolorimeter
    d. Isokinetic testing equipment

CASE STUDY

Richard is a 55-year-old retired truck driver who has been referred to physical therapy for treatment to relieve pain and stiffness in his right knee. Radiographs revealed arthritic changes in both knees. He had a medial meniscectomy in the right knee 2 years ago. His recent complaints of pain and stiffness are related to his present leisure and work activities. Richard is an avid golfer and country-western dancer and often acts as a chauffeur.

- What types of assessments would be important for this patient?

- What symptoms would you need to monitor, and what would you use to do that?
- Describe how you would approach Richard to determine the degree of discomfort that he is experiencing and when.

DISCUSSION QUESTIONS

1. Describe at least two pain assessments that evaluate the quality of a patient's pain experience.

2. Describe at least two pain assessments that attempt to quantify a patient's pain experience.

3. What are the components of edema assessment?

4. Which assessment tool(s) would provide data for the determination of multiple symptoms, for example, edema and muscle guarding? How is this possible?

BIBLIOGRAPHY

The Guide to Physical Therapist Practice, published by the American Physical Therapy Association, is the most comprehensive and well-organized source of information for the clinician; it deals with signs and symptoms and what to do with the information.

American Physical Therapy Association: A Normative Model of Physical Therapist Assistant Education: Version 2007. American Physical Therapy Association, Alexandria, VA, 2007.

American Physical Therapy Association: Guide to Physical Therapist Practice, ed 2. American Physical Therapy Association, Alexandria, VA, 2003.

REFERENCES

1. McCulloch, JM, and Kloth, LC: Wound Healing—Evidence Based Management, ed 4. FA Davis, Philadelphia, 2010, p 96.
2. Finch, E, Brooks, D, Stratford, P, and Mayo, N: Physical Rehabilitation Outcome Measures, ed 2. Lippincott, Williams, and Wilkins, Philadelphia, 2002, pp 180 and 244.
3. Warfield, CA (ed): Manual of Pain Management, ed 2. JB Lippincott, Philadelphia, 2002, pp 20–23.
4. Loeser, JD, and Melzack, R: Pain: An overview. Lancet 353:1607–1609, 1999.
5. Melzack, R: McGill Pain Questionnaire (1975). In Turk, DC, and Melzack, R (eds): Handbook of Pain Assessment. Guilford Press, New York, 1992, pp 154–161, 165–166.
6. Melzack, R: Short form McGill Pain Questionnaire (1987). In Turk, DC, and Melzack, R (eds): Handbook of Pain Assessment. Guilford Press, New York, 1992, pp 161–163.
7. Lowe, NK, Walker, SN, and MacCallum, RC: Confirming the theoretical structure of the McGill Pain Questionnaire in acute clinical pain. Pain 46:52, 1991.
8. Holroyd, KA, et al: A multi-center evaluation of the McGill Pain Questionnaire: Results from more than 1700 chronic pain patients. Pain 48:301, 1992.
9. Mann, HN, et al: Initial-impression diagnosis using low-back pain patient pain drawings. Spine 18:41, 1993.
10. Swantson, M, et al: Pain assessment with interactive computer animation. Pain 53:347, 1993.
11. North, RB, et al: Automated "pain drawing: Analysis by computer-controlled, patient interactive neurological stimulation system. Pain 50:51, 1992.
12. Toomey, TC, et al: Relationship of pain drawing scores to ratings of pain description and function. Clin J Pain 7:269, 1993.
13. Fischer, AA: Clinical use of tissue compliance meter for documentation of soft tissue pathology. Clin J Pain 3:23, 1987.
14. Fischer, AA: Pressure threshold measurement for diagnosis of myofacial pain and evaluation of treatment results. Clin J Pain 2:207, 1987.
15. Atkins, CJ, et al: An electronic method for measuring joint tenderness in rheumatoid arthritis. Arthritis Rheum 35:407, 1992.
16. Bryan, AS, Klenerman, L, and Bowsher, D: The diagnosis of reflex sympathetic dystrophy using an algometer. Bone Joint Surg (Br) 73:644, 1991.
17. Cott, A, et al: Interrater reliability of the tender point criterion for fibromyalgia, Rheumatology 19:1955, 1992.
18. Soderberg, GL: Skeletal muscle function. In Currier, DP, and Nelson, RM (eds): Dynamics of Human Biologic Tissues. FA Davis, Philadelphia, 1992, pp 92–93.
19. Calliet, R: Neck and Arm Pain, ed 3. FA Davis, Philadelphia, 1991, pp 74–75.

Appendix: Pain Assessment Tool Kit

NIH PAIN INVENTORY SAMPLES OF PAIN INTENSITY SCALES

Researchers at the NIH Clinical Center use a variety of pain intensity scales to help them in determining whether or not their patients are responding to the treatment interventions that they are utilizing. The variety of pain scales provides opportunities for patients and caregivers to monitor pain. These examples can be applied for infants, children, adults, and those who are cognitively impaired or nonverbal. It's not a "one size fits all" formula when attempting to quantify pain. More information about pain intensity scales can be obtained through the NIH Clinical Center.

WONG-BAKER FACES

The Wong-Baker FACES Pain Rating Scale combines pictures and numbers to allow the user to rate his/her pain by matching it to a facial expression. Children over the age of 3 are capable of understanding and using this scale, as are adults who might not be English speakers. The faces used in the scale range from a happy, smiling face to a sad, clearly very upset and crying face. Each face also has a numeric rating with 0 representing "no hurt" and 10 representing "hurts worst." There is a total of six faces.

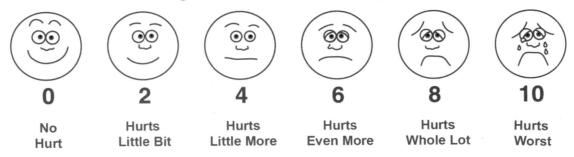

Wong-Baker FACES® Pain Rating Scale

0	2	4	6	8	10
No Hurt	Hurts Little Bit	Hurts Little More	Hurts Even More	Hurts Whole Lot	Hurts Worst

©1983 Wong-Baker FACES® Foundation. Visit us at www.wongbakerFACES.org.
Used with permission. Originally published in Whaley & Wong's Nursing Care of Infants and Children. ©Elsevier Inc.

COMFORT SCALE

Other populations including children, cognitively impaired adults, adults whose cognition is temporarily impaired by medication or illness, the learning disabled, and sedated patients in an ICU or operating room setting can still have their pain rated via an objective tool. The COMFORT Scale is a pain scale that may be used by a health care provider when a person cannot describe or rate his/her own pain. The COMFORT Scale provides a pain rating between 9 and 45.

CRIES PAIN SCALE

Neonatal patients have special needs and therefore they have their own special pain scale. The CRIES Pain Scale was designed for that population and setting. The CRIES pain scale is an observer-rated assessment tool. This assessment is performed by a health care provider. The CRIES tool assesses crying, oxygenation, vital signs, facial expression, and sleeplessness, which are all signs that a neonate is potentially in pain. The CRIES Pain Scale is generally used for infants 6 months of age and younger.

	DATE/TIME						
Crying - Characteristic cry of pain is high-pitched 0 – No cry or cry that is not high-pitched 1 – Cry high-pitched but baby is easily consolable 2 – Cry high-pitched but baby is inconsolable							
Requires O$_2$ for SaO$_2$ <95% - Babies experiencing pain manifest decreased oxygenation. Consider other causes of hypoxemia, (e.g., oversedation, atelectasis, pneumothorax) 0 – No oxygen required 1 – <30% oxygen required 2 – >30% oxygen required							
Increased vital signs (BP* and HR*) - Take BP last as this may awaken child, making other assessments difficult 0 – Both HR and BP unchanged or less than baseline 1 – HR or BP increased but increase in <20% of baseline 2 – HR or BP is increased >20% over baseline							
Expression - The facial expression most often associated with pain is a grimace. A grimace may be characterized by brow lowering, eyes squeezed shut, deepening naso-labial furrow, or open lips and mouth 0 – No grimace present 1 – Grimace alone is present 2 – Grimace and non-cry vocalization grunt are present							
Sleepless - Scored based upon the infant's state during the hour preceding this recorded score 0 – Child has been continuously asleep 1 – Child has awakened at frequent intervals 2 – Child has been awake constantly							
TOTAL SCORE							

FLACC SCALE   CHECKLIST OF NONVERBAL INDICATORS

LET'S FIND OUT

Lab Activity: Superficial Heat

This lab activity was designed to emphasize the importance of observational skills for patient responses to therapeutic interventions and to lay the foundation for problem-solving. Throughout the lab activity, students/learners will be provided with a guide for the application of a commonly utilized thermal agent and some assessment techniques that would be appropriate to note as patient responses both prior to and after the application of the thermal agent.

Equipment That You Will Need

towels   minute timer
hot packs   thermometer

Precautions and Why

Precaution	Why?
Past experience with the agent	It is always helpful to solicit this information from a patient. It will guide you in determining whether a previous attempt with this intervention was successful or not and whether any adverse responses were experienced. It will also help to establish a rapport with the patient with regard to his/her expectations for an intervention.
Open wounds	Fresh granulated tissue is too fragile for the application of many physical agents; however, proximal application techniques may enhance circulation to healing areas.
Peripheral vascular disease	If there is a diagnosed difficulty with circulation to the lower extremity, a proximal application technique of a thermal agent may exacerbate lower extremity discomfort.
Advanced age	Older patients may have less adipose or connective tissue to insulate them against extremes of heat or cold. This may make them more susceptible to burns. In addition, their superficial layer of skin is often thinner and more fragile.
Pregnancy	Application of heat or cold directly over a pregnant uterus is contraindicated; however, application to other areas of the body is not contraindicated.
Impaired cognitive ability	If a patient is unable to communicate discomfort, application of heat or cold would be contraindicated; however, if he/she has cognitive limitations but is able to provide this information and the skin blanches appropriately, the intervention may be undertaken with caution.
Metastases	Application of heat or cold directly over a metastasis is contraindicated because it could potentially increase circulation to the area. However, if the malignancy is terminal and the patient has found heat or cold to be beneficial as a palliative treatment, it may be applied with caution. Special care should be taken to ensure that nerve roots to distally related areas are *not* treated with heat, because they may increase circulation to the metastasized area
Anticoagulant medications	The patient may experience hyperemia easily and be unable to regulate his or her temperature effectively.

Contraindications and Why

Contraindication	Heat	Why?
Unreliable patient responses	X	The patient may burn without warning.
Metastasis in the treatment area	X	An increase in circulation may enhance the spread of the malignancy.
Absence of sensation in the treatment area	X	The patient may burn without warning.
Frostbite in the treatment area	X	The patient may have an inability to adapt to sudden temperature changes, and application of heat or cold may be extremely painful.
Peripheral vascular disease distal to the treatment area	X	Heat may produce a local increase in circulation, which would exacerbate patient discomfort rather than relieve it.
Acute inflammation	X	Heat could exacerbate the inflammatory response, causing further bleeding and potentially inducing shock.
Deep vein thrombosis	X	Heat would exacerbate the inflammatory response in an area that cannot accommodate circulatory changes. A clot could potentially dislodge and travel to the heart, lungs, or brain.
Acute hemorrhage	X	Heat would exacerbate the inflammatory response and increase discomfort.
Fever	X	Heat would exacerbate the inflammatory response and increase discomfort.
Over a pregnant uterus during the first trimester	X	There is no indication for this application. Studies have not been performed to show the effects on the fetus to determine whether or not it would be detrimental.

Observation of Skin Types and Responses to the Application of Superficial Heat

Select two classmates (patients) who have different skin types and list them below. Record your observations of their knees in terms of skin type, location of any visible scars (noting the age and condition of each), and ability to differentiate among heat, cold, light touch, dull touch, sharp touch, and pain.

Classmate/Patient	Scar (location, age, condition)	Sensation (heat, cold, sharp, dull, pain)

A. Position both patients so that each is supine with his or her knees supported in about 10 to 20 degrees of flexion by placing a towel roll, pillow, or bolster underneath his or her knees (Fig. 3-12).

B. Remove two standard size hot packs from the Hydrocollator unit. Wrap one hot pack in towelling so that there are four layers of towel between the hot pack and the patient (Fig. 3-13). Wrap the second hot pack in towelling so that there are six layers between the patient and the hot pack. *(Use only towels, not commercial covers, for this exercise.)*

C. Record the following information while the hot packs are on the patients' knees.

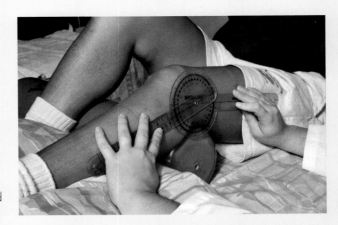

FIGURE 3-12 Patient is positioned so that the knee is in approximately 20° of knee flexion, after the skin has been inspected for scars and sensation.

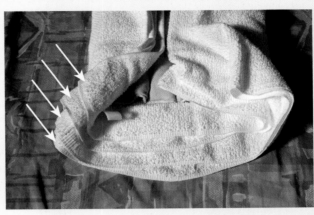

FIGURE 3-13 Standard size hot pack has been removed from the Hydrocollator unit and placed on two towels that have been folded in half, providing four layers of towel between the patient and the pack.

Patient 1 (4 layers)	After 3 Minutes	After 6 Minutes	After 9 Minutes	After 12 Minutes
Appearance of treatment area under the pack				
Patient report of "how it feels" under the pack				

Patient 2 (6 layers)	After 3 Minutes	After 6 Minutes	After 9 Minutes	After 12 Minutes
Appearance of treatment area under the pack				
Patient report of "how it feels" under the pack				

Patient's Observations Regarding His or Her Heated Knee

D. Ask the patients to get up and walk around. Observe their gait, and ask each to describe how the treated knee feels as he or she walks on it.

	Patient 1 (4 Layers)	Patient 2 (6 Layers)
How does the heated knee feel? (tight, loose, etc.)		
Is there symmetry in the gait?		
Were there any differences between the perceptions of the two patients?		

E. How would you describe what you observed in the patient's knee after the hot pack had been applied for 6 minutes?

- Was there any uniformity in what you observed? _____
- Why or why not? _____
- Patient 1 (4 layers): _____
- Patient 2 (6 layers): _____

F. If the patient had any scars, did the scar tissue respond the same way as the nonscarred or uninvolved tissue?

Patient 1 (4 layers): _____

Patient 2 (6 layers): _____

G. How would the presence of a scar in the treatment area potentially affect your treatment?

_____

_____

_____

_____

H. Remove the hot packs from the patients and observe the knees again, recording any differences in appearance and sensation from that which you observed before the hot pack application. Place the hot packs in the Hydrocollator unit for reuse.

During the application of the thermal agents, did you find that the patient ever neglected to tell you that the sensation was too strong, resulting in an adverse response? If yes, what would you do in the future to prevent this from occurring?

_____

_____

_____

_____

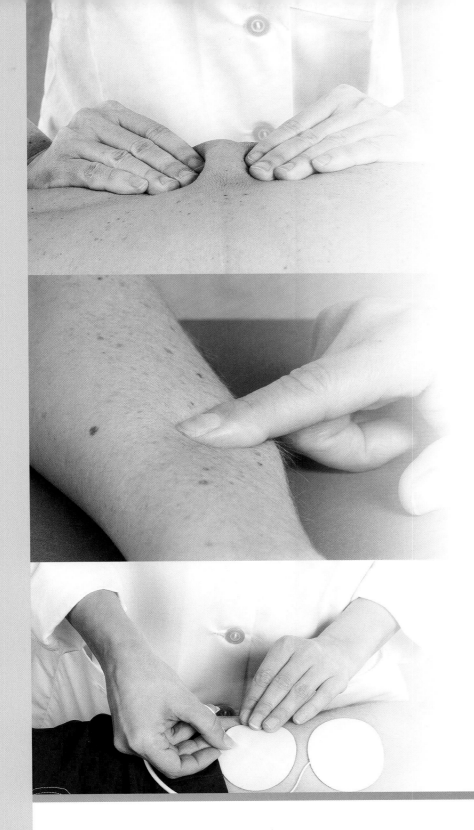

Thermal and Mechanical Agents

CHAPTER *4*

Therapeutic Heat and Cold

Barbara J. Behrens, PTA, MS | Susan Michlovitz, PT, PhD CHT Kristin von Nieda, DPT, MEd

Learning Outcomes

Following the successful completion of this chapter, the learner will be able to:

- Describe the different types of heating and cooling agents commonly utilized as therapeutic treatment interventions in the clinical environment.
- Discuss the application techniques for heating and cooling agents commonly utilized as therapeutic treatment interventions in the clinical environment.
- Differentiate between the possible choices of heating and cooling agents commonly utilized as therapeutic treatment interventions in the clinical environment.
- Discuss the clinical decision making involved in using heating or cooling agents commonly utilized as therapeutic treatment interventions in the clinical environment to optimize therapeutic benefit.
- Describe safety considerations for the use of heating and cooling agents commonly utilized as therapeutic treatment interventions in the clinical environment.
- Describe the normal sensations perceived in response to the application of a variety of thermal agents through having the agents applied to them by a classmate and recording the sensations. The thermal agents for this exercise include:
  - Hydrocollator packs
  - Paraffin
  - Fluidotherapy
  - Shortwave diathermy
  - Cryotherapy
- Identify practical application techniques and challenges for thermal agents by participating in problem-solving activities in guided lab activities using physical agents.
- Integrate the problem-solving process into the application of therapeutic cold for a patient by practicing the techniques with a classmate, discussing outcomes, and soliciting feedback.
- Integrate the problem-solving process into the application of therapeutic heat for a patient by practicing the techniques with a classmate, discussing outcomes, and soliciting feedback.

Key Terms

Afferent neurons
Alpha motor neuron
Axon reflex
Clonus
Cold vasodilation
Conduction
Convection
Conversion
Counterirritation
Cryotherapy
Efferent neurons

Erythema
Evaporation
Fluidotherapy
Homeostasis
Hot pack
Hydrocollator pack
Hyperemia
Hypothalamus
Mechanoreceptors
Metabolic rate
Muscle guarding

Muscle spindle
Nerve conduction velocity (NCV)
Paraffin bath
Perfusion
Peripheral vascular disease (PVD)
Radiation
Raynaud's disease
Specific heat
Subcutaneous tissue
Thermal conductivity

Chapter Outline

Temperature Regulation
Physical Mechanisms of Heat Exchange
    Conduction
    Convection
    Radiation
    Conversion
    Evaporation
Therapeutic Heat
    Physiological Effects of Heat
    Intervention Goals
    Heat and Exercise
Methods of Heat Application
    Superficial Heating Agents
    Intervention Considerations

Cryotherapy
    Physiological Effects of Cold
    Intervention Goals
    Methods of Cold Application
    Intervention Guidelines
    Safety Considerations with the Application of Cold
        Treatment Interventions
    Clinical Decision Making: Heat or Cold?
Documentation

"By three methods we may learn wisdom: First, by reflection, which is noblest; second, by imitation, which is easiest; and third by experience, which is the bitterest." —Confucius

Patient Perspective

"I've heard that you should use heat and I've also heard that you should use ice to relieve pain. Which one works better or does it really matter?"

Heating and cooling agents are age-old remedies for pain control. Each has a role during the phases of tissue healing and recovery and with disorders such as arthritis that lead to muscle ache and joint stiffness. This chapter provides the background for developing problem-solving skills for appropriate and safe clinical application of heating and cooling agents. Knowledge of the body's physiological responses to heat and cold in combination with therapeutic treatment goals that have been set for each patient provides the basis for decisions regarding the use, method of application, and intervention duration of these agents. Prior experience with each of these agents must also be taken into consideration as it may affect the decision-making process and, ultimately, selection of the agents utilized.

Temperature Regulation

Our bodies must maintain optimal temperature ranges to be capable of working properly to sustain life and function. There are several temperature regulatory systems in place that help to maintain a relatively stable body temperature or help restore that temperature if fluctuations occur. **Homeostasis,** which is a stable state or state of equilibrium wherein body systems operate more efficiently, is maintained through the interaction of local and central neural mechanisms. Sensory receptors in the skin, muscles, and joints respond to changes in temperature. Sufficient intensity of and exposure to the stimulus are needed for activation of the temperature-regulating center in the **hypothalamus** within the brain. The hypothalamus acts as the "body's thermostat" to maintain a normal range of human body temperature from 36°C to 38°C (96.5°F to 99.5°F). When sensory information reaches the hypothalamus, the information is integrated and interpreted along with information on the temperature of the blood circulating through the hypothalamus. This results in the activation of temperature-regulating mechanisms, including the following:[1]

- Changes in circulation (e.g., vasodilation or vasoconstriction of blood vessels)
- Shivering, to maintain heat
- Sweating, to lose heat

Several mechanisms come into play for the body to lose heat, which are identified in Table 4-1. Knowledge of basic neuroanatomy and neural transmission is necessary to understand temperature regulation in the body. Neural transmission is a function of first-, second-, and third-order afferent and efferent neurons or nerve fibers. **Afferent neurons** conduct sensory information from the periphery to the spinal cord and brain. **Efferent neurons** conduct motor information from the brain to the periphery. First-order neurons transmit information from thermal receptors or free nerve endings and terminate in the dorsal horn of the spinal cord. Second-order neurons transmit information along ascending or descending tracts of the white matter of the spinal cord and terminate in the thalamus. Third-order neurons transmit ascending sensory and descending motor information between the thalamus and the cerebral cortex. For example, if one steps on a nail there is a withdrawal response from the nail. The sensory afferent input to the cerebral cortex stimulates an efferent response resulting in a motor effect (Fig. 4-1). Chapter 1 of this text provides detailed information about the neurophysiology of pain.

| TABLE 4-1 | Pathways of Heat Loss |
PATHWAY	MECHANISM
Skin (major pathway)	• Radiation and conduction—heat is lost from the body to cooler air or objects. • Convection—air currents move warm air away from the skin. • Sweating—excess body heat evaporates sweat on the skin surface.
Respiratory tract (secondary pathway)	• Evaporation—body heat evaporates water from the respiratory mucosa, and water vapor is exhaled.
Urinary tract (minor pathway)	• Urination—urine is at body temperature when eliminated.
Digestive tract (minor pathway)	• Defecation—feces are at body temperature when eliminated.

From Scanlon, VC, and Sanders, T: Essentials of Anatomy and Physiology, ed 6. FA Davis, 2011, Philadelphia, p 379.

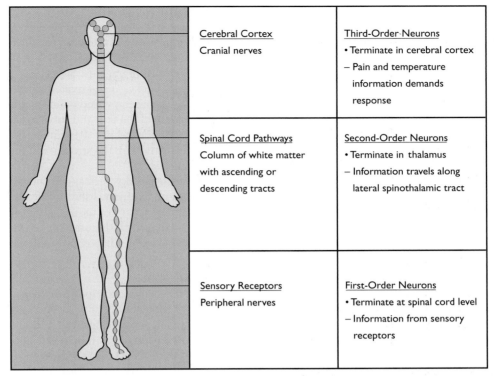

	Cerebral Cortex
	Cranial nerves
		Third-Order Neurons
		• Terminate in cerebral cortex
		– Pain and temperature
		  information demands
		  response

	Spinal Cord Pathways Column of white matter with ascending or descending tracts	Second-Order Neurons • Terminate in thalamus – Information travels along lateral spinothalamic tract
	Sensory Receptors Peripheral nerves	First-Order Neurons • Terminate at spinal cord level – Information from sensory receptors

FIGURE 4-1 First-, second-, and third-order neuron transmission pathways for sensation perception.

Physical Mechanisms of Heat Exchange

The means by which therapeutic heat or cold is delivered to the target tissue is attributed to the following physical mechanisms: conduction, convection, radiation, conversion, and evaporation, which will be discussed in further detail. The extent of temperature change results from several of the following factors:

● Temperature difference between the thermal agent and the tissue area being treated
● Time of exposure to the thermal agent
● Thermal conductivity of the tissue area being treated
● Intensity of the thermal agent

Adipose tissue, skeletal muscle, bone, and blood have different levels of **thermal conductivity.** Essentially, this means that just as the tissue types differ, they do not conduct temperature changes in the same way either. Adipose tissue acts as insulation to underlying tissues, thus limiting the degree of temperature change in deeper tissues. Blood and muscle, which contain relatively high water contents, readily absorb and conduct thermal energy or temperature changes.

CONDUCTION

Thermal loss or gain through direct contact between materials with different temperatures is referred to as **conduction.** Heat absorbed by the body when using a hot pack is an example of heat exchange by conduction. When cold packs are applied to the skin, heat is lost from the skin via conduction.

CONVECTION

Convection is exemplified by the transference of thermal energy to a body by the movement of air, matter, or liquid around or past the body. An example of convective heat is a hot-air furnace or a convection oven. These devices circulate warmed air around a room, and the temperature of the contents changes. A freezer works in much the same way; however, the cold air around the objects within the contained environment become cooled rather than heated. A clinical example is the use of **Fluidotherapy,** whereby warm air is circulated through a bed of fine-grained cellulose particles. The movement of the warm cellulose particles around a body part results in a temperature change of the skin and underlying subcutaneous tissue that have been submersed within the media.

RADIATION

Radiation or radiant energy transfers heat through air from a warmer source to a cooler source. Examples of radiant heat include the glowing coals of an open fire or the heating element on an electric stove. A therapeutic example is an infrared heat lamp. The infrared element in the lamp does not come in contact with the tissue. This form of thermal transfer is highly directional. When radiant heat is generated from the lamp, only those body areas in the immediate vicinity of the lamp receive direct heating effects. (*The infrared lamp, though, is not in common use in clinical practice.*)

CONVERSION

Conversion refers to the temperature changes that result from energy being transformed from one form into another, such as the conversion from mechanical or electrical energy into heat energy. A clinical example is continuous-wave or uninterrupted therapeutic ultrasound, in which sound waves (mechanical energy) are transformed to heat (thermal energy) as they are absorbed by the tissue. Ultrasound is addressed in detail in Chapter 5.

EVAPORATION

Evaporation is defined as the transformation from a liquid state to a gas state. This transformation requires an energy exchange. Heat is given off when liquids transform into gases. Sweating results from heat production within the body. Cooling occurs as the perspiration evaporates from the surface of the skin. Vapocoolant sprays cause the cooling of the skin via evaporation. Some physicians use ethylchloride, which is a vapocoolant spray used to "freeze" the skin prior to administering some forms of injections. The use of ethylchloride must be handled with extreme caution since it numbs the area, which may be appropriate for the task a physician is performing but not for day-to-day activities.

LET'S THINK ABOUT IT...

Respiration plays a key role in the evaporative process and also in maintaining proper pH levels. If you've ever been in a closed environment, for example a car, where you were actively engaged in an activity that produced significant increases in your respiration, you probably noticed that the windows fogged up. Your body was attempting to cool itself via the mechanism of evaporation. Both your respiratory and musculoskeletal systems were also participating in the process. Your body temperature was most likely elevated due to the activity. . . .

Therapeutic Heat

Several heat agents are available for heat application to tissues. Generally, two categories are described: superficial and deep heating agents. Superficial heating agents, such as hot packs, air-activated heat wraps, warm whirlpool, Fluidotherapy, and paraffin, primarily increase the temperature of the skin and **subcutaneous tissue** with less of an effect on deeper structures. See Figure 4-2 for further clarification on the structure of the skin and subcutaneous tissues.

Deep heating agents, such as continuous uninterrupted ultrasound and continuous shortwave diathermy, can increase the temperature of tissues at depths of 3 to 5 cm. Shortwave diathermy is discussed in Chapter 10 and ultrasound is addressed in Chapter 5.

PHYSIOLOGICAL EFFECTS OF HEAT

Physiological changes in response to heat application vary according to the intensity of the agent, the duration of application, and the area being treated. Therapeutic levels of heating are categorized as mild and vigorous. Heating is considered mild when tissue temperatures are less than 40°C (104°F), and vigorous heating occurs when tissue temperature reaches 40°C to 45°C (104°F to 111.2°F).[2] At these temperatures, **hyperemia** or **erythema** is noted. An erythema is redness of the skin, caused by an increase in the blood flow in the capillaries (hyperemia) in the lower layers of the skin. Temperature increases greater than 45°C (111.2°F) have the potential to result in thermal pain and irreversible tissue damage.[3,4]

Elevating the tissue temperature results in an increase in blood flow to the area, which is attributable in part to the vasodilatory response in surface blood vessels.[5] The increase in blood flow removes heat from the area, whereas blood that is relatively cooler flows into the area,

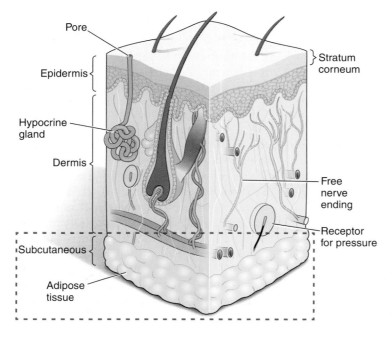

FIGURE 4-2 Subcutaneous tissue lies beneath the dermis and is a thick layer of connective tissue and adipose (fatty tissue). The adipose acts as insulation that assists in insulating the body to maintain a stable temperature. It also stores energy gained from ingested foods from the digestive system. Subcutaneous tissue also acts as a shock absorber, helping to protect the underlying tissues from injury.

thus preventing excessive heat accumulation. Conversely, therapeutic heating levels may not be reached because the increased blood flow may not allow for adequate heat build up in the area. Heat accumulation is affected by the intensity and duration of the stimulus, as well as the rate of heat absorption by the tissue. If therapeutic heating levels are reached with local application, reflex heating in other areas of the body may also occur. Local heat application has both direct and indirect heating effects. For example, when heat was applied to the low back area, an increase in subcutaneous blood flow and vasodilation to the distal extremities was reported.[1,5,6]

An older technique involved trying to increase circulation to the extremities of someone with **peripheral vascular disease (PVD)** via the indirect effect. Patients with PVD have restricted blood flow to the lower extremities and may have difficulty tolerating heat locally that could cause a distal response. This is not commonly used in contemporary practice. However, the effect should be recognized for those patients who do have comorbidities where a distal effect may be undesirable.

The application of superficial heating agents generally does not allow for increases in muscle temperatures, unless those structures are themselves superficial or the conductive heat agent is left on for 30 minutes or longer. Increased temperature in the muscles and tendons of the hand and foot may occur with the use of superficial heating agents, because insulation from adipose tissue is not prevalent in these areas.

Changes in **metabolic rate** in association with changes in tissue temperature have been reported. An increase in tissue temperature correlates with an increase in metabolic rate.[1] An increase in metabolic rate may be used advantageously to facilitate tissue healing. Conversely, in the face of acute inflammation, heat may exacerbate the inflammatory process owing to the increase in metabolic rate and internal heat production. In that case, cold, which slows metabolic rate, can thus reduce potential tissue damage.

LET'S THINK ABOUT IT...

If you are going to work with a patient in the clinic today, one of the first things that can be done to help assess whether or not there is an acute inflammatory process in the treatment area is to palpate the area. If it is already warm or hot, then there is already significant metabolic activity taking place there. The application of more heat would potentially make that worse and cause tissue damage.

Heat may have a beneficial role in wound healing based on the increase in blood flow. The increase in blood flow improves perfusion of the wound and peri-wound tissue. Improved **perfusion** essentially means that there is improved blood flow in the wound and through the vessels that supply the surrounding area. This results in an increase in oxygen tension of the wound, and the increase in oxygen allows for greater clearing of bacteria from the wound site.[7] Increasing tissue temperature to therapeutic levels ($40°C$ to $45°C$; $104°F$ to $111.2°F$)[2] can facilitate the release of oxygen from the blood's hemoglobin, thus improving tissue nutrition.

INTERVENTION GOALS

Based on the physiological effects of therapeutic heat, intervention goals are easy to identify. Therapeutic heating agents are used as adjunctive intervention techniques for achieving functional goals. This means that the therapeutic heat is not the only treatment intervention provided for the patient, but it is used in addition to other techniques to facilitate the accomplishment of the treatment goals.

Heat contributes to the alleviation of pain and to pain management, which may allow increased functional activity or improved range of motion (ROM). The increase in motion may in turn lead to improvement in activities of daily living (ADLs). When heat is used for reduction of muscle guarding, it may lead to pain reduction and further improvement in mobility. By affecting the visco-elastic properties of tendon and muscle with the use of heat, tissue extensibility is enhanced, potentially allowing for return of lost motion.

Each of the therapeutic goals—pain reduction, pain management, reduction of muscle guarding, and increased tissue extensibility—is addressed in relationship to specific thermal agents. It is important to recognize the connection between these therapeutic goals and the overall functional goals of each patient. Therapeutic goals are broad based, but each patient is an individual whose personal goals must be considered with each treatment intervention. Although there are sound physiological rationales behind each of the following therapeutic goals that can potentially be accomplished with each of the thermal agents, if the patient does not understand, accept, or believe in what the clinician is attempting to accomplish, then the stated goal will be more difficult to attain.

Pain Reduction and Management

The use of superficial heat for the alleviation or management of pain is well recognized, but the mechanism by which heat produces analgesia is not fully understood. Several mechanisms have been proposed to explain pain relief in response to therapeutic heat.

In 1965 Melzack and Wall[8] proposed the *gate control theory of pain*, in which a spinal "gating" mechanism was responsible for pain mediation (see Chapter 2). Small A-delta fibers and C fibers are primary afferents that transmit pain impulses from free nerve endings or nociceptors to the spinal cord. When therapeutic heat is used, the thermal stimuli provide input to the spinal gating mechanism, which in effect overrides the painful stimuli. When there is greater non-noxious input (heat) than noxious input (pain), the "gate" is in a relatively closed position, thus inhibiting transmission of pain to second-order neurons or ascending tracts. Although the model was proposed almost 50 years ago, there are still aspects of that model that have stood the test of time. The theory proposed by Melzack and Wall serves as a good conceptual framework to discuss the application of physical agents (Fig. 4-3).

No Stimulation

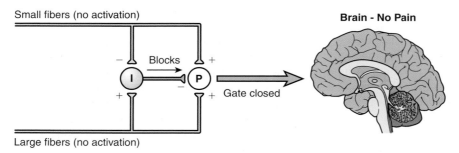

Non-Pain Stimulation

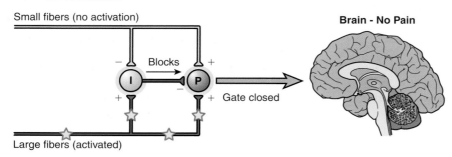

Painful Stimulation

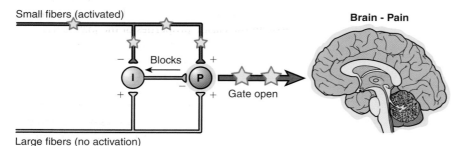

FIGURE 4-3 Schematic representation of the gate control theory of pain.

Gammon and Starr[9] postulated that thermal stimuli (heat or cold) produced **counterirritation.** Pain was not as readily perceived because the thermal input countered painful stimuli. This may explain why a common response to initial injury is rubbing or pressure, both of which could be considered counterirritants. This sensory response of rubbing, pressure being applied to an area that is uncomfortable, has also been postulated as being a form of **mechanoreceptive** input or sensory information to the spinal cord as a part of Melzack and Wall's gate control theory. That form of sensory information travels at a much faster speed than pain information and is theorized to literally close the "gate" at the dorsal horn preventing anything other than sensory information from ascending to the brain. This is also why the location for the sensory input is important for successful pain relief.

Heat has also been shown to elevate the pain threshold[9,10] and increase **nerve conduction velocity (NCV).**[11] The ability of a nerve to carry an impulse from point A to point B can be timed and measured in meters per second.

There are known values for the speed at which impulses travel along normal peripheral nerves, normal NCVs. An elevated pain threshold may delay the onset and perception of pain. Clinical relevance associated with the change in nerve conduction velocity has not been demonstrated.

Reduction of Muscle Guarding

Muscle guarding is a protective response in muscle that results in a sustained isotonic muscle contraction for both the agonists and antagonists that surround the injured area to help provide a virtual exoskeleton of muscle until healing takes place. It may occur in response to: (1) trauma, as a protective mechanism to guard against the potential pain and further injury or pain associated with joint movement. or (2) a painful stimulus that activates or perpetuates the pain-spasm-pain cycle.[12]

Heat has been used to relieve muscle guarding[13,14] and to increase tissue flexiblity.[15] When muscle temperature is sufficiently elevated, as can be seen with the use of deep heating agents, the firing rate of the **muscle spindle** afferents (type II) is decreased, whereas that of the Golgi tendon organs (type Ib) is increased.[16] Muscle spindles are sensitive to stretch in the muscle. The resultant decrease in alpha motor neuron activity leads to a decrease in tonic muscle activity. In other words, there is a decrease in muscle guarding resulting from decreased stimuli to the muscle (Fig. 4-4).

The reduction in muscle guarding as the direct result of elevated muscle temperature does not explain the reduction seen with the use of superficial heating agents. This muscle relaxation may be explained by an indirect reduction in muscle spindle firing as a direct result of elevating skin temperature. The increase in skin temperature causes a decrease in gamma efferent activity, thus altering stretch on the muscle spindle and producing a decrease in the firing rate and an overall decrease in **alpha motor neuron** activity.[17] Alpha motor neurons are large lower motor neurons of the brainstem and spinal cord. They innervate skeletal muscles over which we also have voluntary control. Heat application has a direct effect on pain and muscle guarding (spasm) such that the pain-spasm-pain cycle[13] can be interrupted by influencing pain as well as the muscle guarding. A reduction in pain can lead to a reduction in guarding or spasm, thus further reducing pain.

Tissue Extensibility

Shortening of connective tissue may result from injury or immobilization. The visco-elastic properties of muscle, tendon, and ligaments are affected.[18] The use of heat has been shown to decrease viscosity and increase the elastic properties of connective tissue, specifically muscle, tendon, and joint capsule.[2] However, a sufficient load must also be applied to produce residual elongation of the tissue over a long time.[17] The temperature range needed for residual length changes is 40°C to 45°C (104°F to 111.2°F).[2]

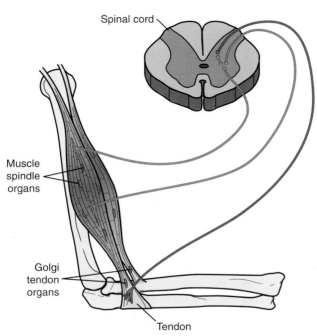

FIGURE 4-4 Golgi tendon organ (GTO) and muscle spindle.

Spinal cord

Muscle spindle organs

Golgi tendon organs

Tendon

Furthermore, the potential for irritation and tissue damage is lessened when heat is applied *during* the stretching procedure.

Residual elongation of connective tissue is dependent on a sufficient increase in tissue temperature, the timing of the application, and the type of stretch applied. The stretch is best applied during heat application, if possible, or immediately after removal of the heat source. A low-load prolonged stretch was reported as preferable to a high-load brief stretch because it resulted in less tissue damage and greater increases in ROM.[18–21]

CHECK IT OUT 4-1

- Apply heat in a neutral joint position and stretch immediately after the removal of the heat.
- Apply heat at the patient's end ROM in a stretched but supported position using gravity to assist in the stretch if possible.
- Think about the best position for every patient *prior* to applying heat rather than just applying heat the same way for every patient every day.

Patients diagnosed with arthritis who have pain and limited motion associated with joint stiffness may benefit from the use of therapeutic heat. The direct effect of heat is an increase in the elastic properties of the joint capsule,[22] and the reduction of associated pain may also contribute to a resultant increase in ROM.

HEAT AND EXERCISE

A greater increase in blood flow is reported with heat and exercise than with either heat or exercise alone.[23] An initial decrease in isometric muscle strength was seen during the first 30 minutes after deep heat application, and subsequent increase in strength was measured during the next 2.5 hours.[24] Endurance was shown to decrease after heat applications.[25,26] These findings are of particular interest because muscle performance may be altered in response to heat. The clinical implications of the relationship between the use of heat and exercise are important considerations for planning and implementing exercise programs and for evaluating patient performance. To assess progress or limitations in strength and endurance accurately, measurements should be taken consistently either before or after exercise. If an initial measurement is taken before exercise and a subsequent measurement is taken after exercise, comparison of the results may lead to erroneous conclusions about the patient's performance and the efficacy of the intervention.

BEFORE YOU BEGIN

Make sure you know the goal of the treatment intervention. If the patient has muscle guarding, you may wish to position to reduce "stretch" on muscle. If heat is being used to increase ROM, you may position with joint at or near the end range of available motion.

Methods of Heat Application

SUPERFICIAL HEATING AGENTS

Heat from superficial heating agents generally penetrates to depths of less than 2 cm from the surface of the skin. Subcutaneous tissue that is well vascularized reaches its maximum temperature increase within 8 to 10 minutes of application.[27-29] Skin and subcutaneous tissue temperatures increase 5°C to 6°C (41°F to 42.8°F) after 6 minutes and are maintained up to 30 minutes after application. An intervention duration of 15 to 30 minutes is necessary for an increase in muscle temperature of 1°C (33.8°F) at depths up to 3 cm.[27,28,30] Temperature of a joint capsule in the foot increased 9°C (48.2°F), in response to 20 minutes of heat exposure at 47.8°C (118°F).[31] It is therefore possible to heat joint structures using superficial heating agents when these structures are closer to the skin surface. Therefore, in this instance heat should be applied for 15 to 30 minutes for maximal benefit.

Hydrocollator Packs

The commercial **Hydrocollator pack**, or **hot pack**, is one of the most common ways to deliver superficial moist heat. Generally, hot packs contain a hydrophilic substance, such as silica gel or betonite, encased in channelled canvas covers. They are stored in thermostatically controlled units that are filled with water at a temperature range of 71°C to 79°C (159.8°F to 174.2°F).[2] Frequent use, low water levels, and faulty thermostats can affect the temperature of the hot packs, so it is important to check the water level (replenishing water levels frequently) and temperature to ensure optimal heat delivery so that therapeutic heat levels are achieved. The hot packs should be checked for ruptures in the canvas or for mold formation, which can weaken the canvas and allow leakage. When a hot pack leaks, it should be discarded and replaced with a new one.

The temperature of the hot pack itself is regulated by the length of time it is stored and the temperature of the water in which it is stored. After a hot pack has been used, a period of 20 to 30 minutes is needed for the hot pack to reach the temperature of the water in the storage unit. This is an important consideration if hot packs are frequently used in a busy clinical setting.

Before application to the patient, the hot pack is covered with six to eight layers of towelling that insulates the hot pack from heat loss and protects the patient from potential burn. Commercial terrycloth covers are also available and are equivalent to two to four layers of towelling (Fig. 4-5).

Thermal energy is conducted from hot packs to the skin surface, and heat is absorbed superficially. The resultant change in temperature depends on the thermal conductivity and the size of the area being treated, the temperature of the hot pack, the size of the hot pack, and the duration of the application.

Hot packs are manufactured in several sizes and shapes to better match the body part to which they are applied.

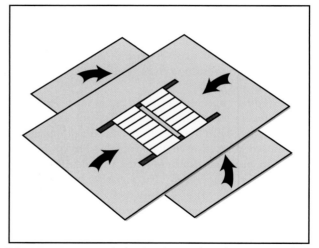

FIGURE 4-5 Hot pack that has been placed on two towels, folded in half to provide eight layers of towelling.

The standard size of 10 × 12 inches is suitable for treating medium size flat surface areas. The oversize pack is approximately twice the size of the standard pack and is suited for larger flat surface areas. Cervical packs are designed to fit the contours of the neck and are also appropriate for use around peripheral joints (Fig. 4-6). Size and shape are important because the mechanism of heat transfer is conduction, so optimal contact with the skin surface ensures optimal heat absorption. The weight of the hot packs also helps to maintain contact with the body surface. Weight of the pack increases with the size and is a consideration when deciding to use this form of superficial heat. Patients may not tolerate the weight of the pack during treatment.

LET'S THINK ABOUT IT...

There are many sizes and shapes of hot packs to allow for better contouring and therefore conduction of the thermal energy of the hot pack. Try them and see what size or shape works best in the following areas of the body and describe your patient positioning techniques, filling in the information in Table 4-2.

Preparing the patient for treatment includes proper positioning and draping of the patient, visual inspection of the area to be treated, and assessment of the patient's ability to report sensory changes. The area to be treated must be accessible and free of clothing and jewelry to ensure even heating.

- Select and prepare the hot pack with the appropriate layers of towelling.
- Make sure the patient is in a comfortable position, and that any muscles being treated are in an unloaded and resting position, and apply the hot pack.
- Instruct the patient in what to expect to experience from the heat, and ask him or her to report any

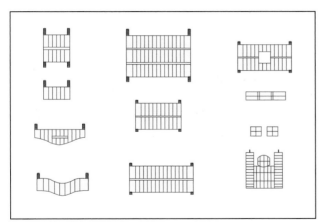

FIGURE 4-6 Variety of hot packs that are available. Variation in sizes allows for the selection of the appropriate size pack to fit the treatment area. Left column (*top to bottom*): standard size, half size, cervical packs. Middle column (*top to bottom*): oversize, spinal sizes. Right column (*top to bottom*): knee or shoulder pack, obstetric size, others.

TABLE 4-2	Choosing Hot Pack Shapes and Sizes
HOT PACK SHAPE/SIZE	**POSITIONING**
Shoulder	
Hip	
Knee	
Cervical spine	

abnormal or unusual sensations such as overheating or burning.

- Monitor the initial response to intervention during the first 5 to 10 minutes by asking the patient for feedback and by visually inspecting the skin, emphasizing that the sensation of heat should be warm, not hot. The old adage of "the hotter, the better" must be dispelled.

- If necessary, adjust the layers of towelling by adding more towelling to reduce heat delivery or removing towelling to increase heat delivery. Maximum skin temperature change is achieved within the first 10 minutes of hot pack application and maintained for approximately an additional 10 minutes. Therefore, the application time is typically 20 minutes.

- Observe the skin again after the hot pack is removed and assess the patient's response to the intervention.

Commercial hot packs are also available for home use. In addition to packs, there are reusable, microwavable products that deliver heat in a similar manner to Hydrocollator packs. Detailed instruction to patients and care providers regarding safe and appropriate use is essential,

and a demonstration on use is recommended. Use of superficial heating agents at home, as part of an established home program, may be beneficial to the patient in maintaining ROM, managing pain, and alleviating joint stiffness. Refer to Table 4-3 for a quick summary of the pros and cons of hot packs.

Paraffin

Paraffin is another superficial heating agent in which conduction is the method of heat transfer. **Paraffin baths** contain a mixture of paraffin wax and mineral oil, which are combined to lower the melting point and the specific heat in comparison to water.[2] In other words, since **specific heat** is the amount of heat per unit mass required to raise the temperature by one degree Celsius, the addition of mineral oil to the wax makes it possible for the melting temperature of the wax to be lower than it normally would be and thus tolerable to immerse one's hand into for treatment. Paraffin is stored in double-walled, thermostatically controlled, stainless steel tanks, and temperatures are maintained in the range of 47.0°C to 54.4°C (117°F to 130°F). The low specific heat of paraffin allows patients to tolerate the higher temperatures. Also, moist heat tends to be perceived as comfortable by the majority of patients.

Paraffin is best suited for distal extremity joints, such as the wrist, hand, and foot, because of the primary methods of application: "dip and wrap" and "dip and immerse." The former is far more popular, more practical, and safer than the latter. The dip-and-wrap method involves dipping and removing the body part from the paraffin bath for 8 to 10 repetitions. A solid glove is formed that serves to insulate the body part against heat loss. It is common to place a plastic bag over the glove and to wrap a towel around the extremity to further assist in heat retention. The wrapped extremity is then positioned in elevation to minimize edema formation (Figs. 4-7 and 4-8). Intervention duration is 15 to 20 minutes, after which time the glove is removed. If the patient wants to squeeze the paraffin after removal until the clinician is ready to work with the patient, this should be encouraged if not contraindicated. The temperature of the treated part is highest at that point in time and the activity could prove beneficial to the patient. The used wax may then be discarded or returned to the unit to be reused.

TABLE 4-3	Pros and Cons of Hydrocollator Packs	
PROS	**CONS**
Inexpensive	Heavy
Readily available	May not conform to all areas of the body
Slow, progressive heat delivery	Great source of burns owing to clinician negligence!

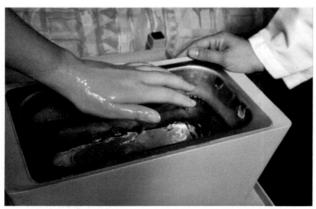

FIGURE 4-7 Paraffin unit with an application of paraffin to the hand.

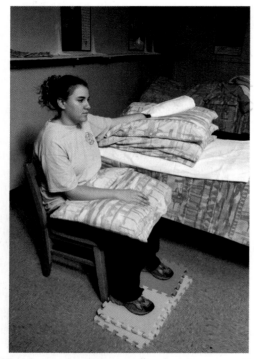

FIGURE 4-8 Hand with the paraffin glove is wrapped in a towel and positioned in an elevated position.

The dip-and-immerse method is similar to the above method in that the patient is asked to dip and re-immerse the body part, allowing the glove to form. Rather than wrapping the hand or foot, the part is re-immersed and left in the paraffin bath for the duration of the intervention. This method is more effective in raising tissue temperature but places the patient at greater risk for burn. This method also does not allow for elevation of the body part being treated and an increase in edema may result. As with any therapeutic heat application, careful monitoring of the patient during and after intervention is essential to safe practice. For reasons of practicality and safety, other techniques of heat should be selected rather than the paraffin dip and immerse.

Before intervention, the patient should be instructed to remove clothing and jewelry from the area and to thoroughly wash and dry the area to be treated. The skin must be visually inspected and sensation and heat tolerance assessed. The patient should be instructed in what to expect during the paraffin application and to report any abnormal sensations. Care should be taken by the patient to avoid touching the sides or bottom of the unit to minimize the risk of skin burn.

Paraffin has advantages over Hydrocollator packs in that it conforms to the body part and may provide more evenly distributed and intense heat. However, the higher temperatures may not be as easily tolerated. The temperature of the unit must be checked prior to having the patient immerse his or her hand into the unit. If it is warmer than 47°C to 54°C (117°F to 130°F) then it should be unplugged and uncovered for a few minutes until the temperature returns to a lower and safe level. Other than that, there is no way of adjusting the level of heat delivery to the patient, as is the case with hot packs. Home units are available but are more expensive than commercial hot packs. For in-clinic use, the paraffin "glove" should be disposed when removed from the patient's hand or foot. If only one person is using the paraffin, such as in the case of home use, the paraffin can be returned to the bath after each use. If too much sediment builds up in the unit, then the paraffin wax should be disposed and replaced. Refer to Table 4-4 for a summary of the pros and cons of paraffin and the Let's Find Out paraffin lab activities later in this chapter.

Fluidotherapy

Fluidotherapy allows stimulation of both thermoreceptors and mechanoreceptors and therefore can serve for the simultaneous uses of enhancing motion while reducing pain and hypersensitivity. Fluidotherapy units contain particles of natural cellulose enclosed in a cabinet, through which dry, warm air is circulated. The method of heat exchange that occurs with Fluidotherapy is convection. The units are thermostatically controlled, and specific temperatures, which can be set by the clinician, vary between 38.8°C and 47.8°C (102°F and 118°F). Lower temperatures are recommended for patients

TABLE 4-4	Pros and Cons of Paraffin	
PROS	**CONS**
Inexpensive	Unable to see the area being treated
Completely conforms to the treatment area	Patient is unable to move during treatment
Patient can purchase for home use	Only exposed to heat with first dip and then insulated from further heating by paraffin Only applicable to hands and feet

with more acute conditions who might be more prone to the development of edema. The turbulence level has a separate control. The moving suspended particles create a medium similar to that of a liquid and stretching and exercise can be performed during this form of heat application.

Fluidotherapy units have been manufactured to accommodate the distal upper extremity (Fig. 4-9) and the distal lower extremity (Fig. 4-10). Fluidotherapy can be utilized clinically for pain relief, tissue healing, and increasing ROM. It is also indicated to promote desensitization of hypersensitive tissues. The effects of Fluidotherapy are the result of the combination of heat and the movement of the natural cellulose particles.

WHY DO I NEED TO KNOW ABOUT...
STATUS OF CIRCULATION AND SKIN INTEGRITY

If there is impaired (e.g., reduced) circulation, heat cannot dissipate from the area and one risks the possibility of burning the patient. If there is an open area of skin, paraffin can potentially penetrate into that area and cause an irritation or a burn.

Unlike paraffin and Hydrocollator packs, there is no loss of heat over time when Fluidotherapy is administered. The temperature is selected and maintained for the duration of the treatment intervention when using Fluidotherapy owing to its thermostat, which the other heating options do not have available. The constant temperature may result in greater heating, and elevated temperatures in joint capsules of the hand and foot have been reported.[32] Unlike paraffin and a hot pack, Fluidotherapy allows movement of the extremity during heat application.

Preparation for Fluidotherapy interventions is similar to that for paraffin intervention. The area to be treated needs to be thoroughly washed and dried, and jewelry and clothing need to be removed from the area. Sensation and heat tolerance must be assessed, and the skin carefully inspected. Open lesions must be covered and sealed with

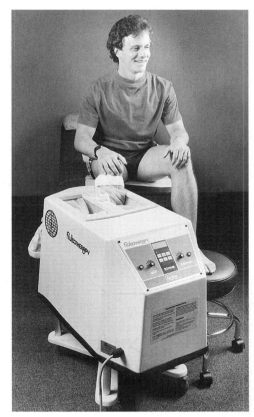

FIGURE 4-10 Fluidotherapy for the foot and ankle.
(From Michlovitz, SL: Biophysical principles of heating and superficial heat agents. In Michlovitz, SL, (ed): Thermal Agents in Rehabilitation, ed 2. FA Davis, Philadelphia, 1990, p 99, with permission.)

an airtight barrier before the start of the intervention to prevent the cellulose particles from entering the wound. The barrier contributes to the creation of a moist wound environment and potential autolytic debridement where the wound sheds unwanted tissue from itself.

Fluidotherapy has been reported to be safe when used in the presence of splints, bandages, tape, metal implants, plastic joint replacements, and artificial tendons.[32] Splints that are designed to apply a stretch to joints can be applied before intervention in the Fluidotherapy unit so that the stretch can be applied during the heat application to the joint. Exercise equipment, such as small balls, can also be used by patients during the intervention. A quick summary of the pros and cons of Fluidotherapy is provided in Table 4-5.

Air-Activated Heat Wraps

Continuous low-level heat can be delivered via air-activated heat wraps. These heat wraps are comfortable and provide a low-profile, low-level heat source that can be worn during activity and sleep for up to 8 hours at a time. These wearable heat wraps maintain a temperature of approximately 40°C (104°F) and elevate tissue temperature. They can be purchased inexpensively at pharmacy chain stores, and worn safely by the patient during ADLs and work and during sleep.

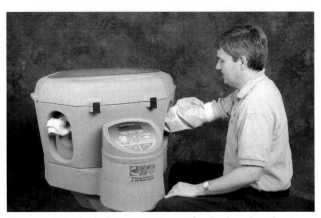

FIGURE 4-9 Fluidotherapy treatment for the hand and wrist.
(From Michlovitz, SL, and Nolan, TP (eds): Modalities for Therapeutic Intervention, ed 4. FA Davis, Philadelphia, 2005, with permission.)

TABLE 4-5 | Pros and Cons of Fluidotherapy

PROS	CONS
Easy to set up for patients	Expensive
Little to no maintenance of the units themselves	Patients with chronic obstructive pulmonary disease (COPD) may not be able to tolerate the dry environment around the unit
Thermostatically controlled temperature throughout the treatment time	
Applicable for hands, upper extremities, and lower extremities	
Patients are encouraged to move during treatment owing to the medium itself	
Ability to control turbulence of the medium during treatment	
Turbulence can be used to treat patients with sensitivity issues for desensitization in the hands or feet	

These wraps are available in different sizes and shapes to accommodate body size and contour (Figs. 4-11 and 4-12). Applying low-level heat over a long time (e.g., hours) has been the concept of the use of electric heating pads. With an electric heating pad, the patient must be at the site of an electrical outlet. Also, some of the pads may

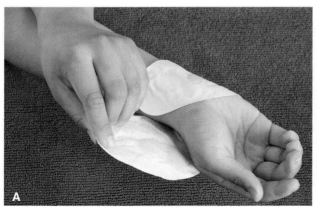

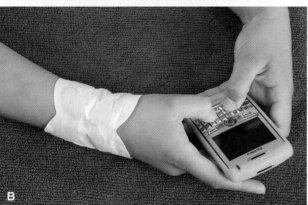

FIGURE 4-11 Air-activated heat wrap (Thermacare, Procter & Gamble, Cincinnati, OH) **(a)** applied to the wrist and **(b)** worn during activity.
(From Michlovitz, SL, and Nolan, TP (eds): Modalities for Therapeutic Intervention, ed 4. Philadelphia: FA Davis, 2005, with permission.)

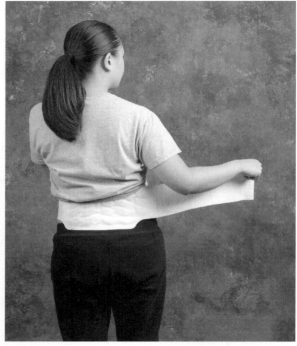

FIGURE 4-12 Air-activated heat wrap (Thermacare, Procter & Gamble, Cincinnati, Ohio) being applied to the low back.
(From Michlovitz, SL, and Nolan, TP (eds): Modalities for Therapeutic Intervention, ed 4. Philadelphia: FA Davis, 2005, with permission.)

heat up enough to produce superficial burns, particularly if the person falls asleep while the electric heating pad is plugged in and turned on. Studies have been done that show these air-activated heat wraps are effective in controlling pain, improving muscle flexibility, and improving function in patients with acute and chronic low back pain.[14,15] In addition, pain levels are improved, stiffness is reduced, and hand grip strength is increased when wearing these wraps on the wrist in those with tendinitis, arthritis, and symptoms consistent with carpal tunnel syndrome.[33]

INTERVENTION CONSIDERATIONS

The selection of the appropriate heating agent is based on the size and location of the area to be treated, the depth of tissue targeted for intervention, the intervention goals, and the contraindications and precautions associated with the intervention and the heating agent. Table 4-6 lists the contraindications and precautions for superficial heating agents. For example, use of a hot pack is appropriate as a treatment intervention for a patient with low back pain if the goals of the intervention are to decrease pain and muscle guarding. Diathermy may also be appropriate, especially if deeper muscles are to be heated. However, diathermy would not be considered appropriate if the patient had low back pain after a surgical procedure for the spine in which a metal rod was used as a fixation device. Diathermy is covered in Chapter 10

The treatment intervention and the response to the intervention must be carefully monitored, regardless of the thermal heating agent used. Before the intervention the patient's cognitive status, and ability to communicate must also be determined, and the area must be carefully inspected to assess the patient's sensation, and heat tolerance. Deficits in any of these areas will require more careful monitoring during the treatment intervention.

Cryotherapy

Cryo means "cold or freezing," and **cryotherapy** refers to the practice of using cold to achieve therapeutic goals. Cooling agents, such as cold packs, a cool whirlpool, and ice massage, are used in the management of pain and edema and are effective in decreasing muscle guarding and muscle guarding or spasm that is controlled by central mechanisms. The primary methods of this form of thermal exchange, or in this case heat abstraction or cooling, are conduction and convection.

PHYSIOLOGICAL EFFECTS OF COLD

When cold is applied to the surface of the skin, the initial response is vasoconstriction of superficial blood vessels. If skin temperature is sufficiently lowered, the cooler temperature stimulates free nerve endings, which in turn causes reflex vasoconstriction. Local blood flow is also decreased. However, when a sufficient amount of cooled blood flows through the general circulation, the hypothalamus may be stimulated, resulting in further reflex vasoconstriction. The vasoconstriction and the resultant reduction in blood flow are a means for the body to retain heat by restricting the volume of cooled blood in systemic circulation. Shivering

TABLE 4-6 | Contraindications to and Precautions for the Use of Superficial Heating Agents and Diathermy

GENERAL CONTRAINDICATIONS FOR HEATING AGENTS	RATIONALE
Acute inflammation	Local heat application may exacerbate the inflammatory response.
Existing fever	Heat application may further elevate body temperature.
Malignancies	The increased blood flow that results from localized heat application may promote a metastasis.
Acute hemorrhage	Hemorrhage may be prolonged if heat is applied after an acute injury.
Peripheral vascular disease (PVD)	Heat increases metabolic demands and a patient with PVD has a diminished capacity to meet the increase in metabolic demands of heated tissue.
Radiation (x-ray therapy)	Tissue that is devitalized by x-ray therapy should not be heated.
SPECIFIC CONTRAINDICATIONS FOR DIATHERMY*	
Metal implants or any metal within the treatment area (snaps, zippers, hair pins)	Metal will alter the flow of electromagnetic energy and may result in a burn.
Cardiac pacemakers	Pacemaker function may be altered.
PRECAUTIONS FOR THE USE OF HEAT	
During menses	May have an increase in blood flow if heat is applied to the low back.
In the presence of sensory deficit	There is an increased potential for a burn; need to be monitored closely.
During pregnancy	The effect on the fetus has not been established; heat application to peripheral joints may be given with caution.

*Diathermy equipment should not be operated within close proximity to cardiac pacemakers or other equipment that may be adversely affected by electromagnetic radiation (traction, electrical stimulation equipment).

is also a heat-retaining mechanism and may result if a large area of the body is exposed to cooler temperatures.

Vasodilation has been reported to occur in response to extended exposure to cold.[34,35] Lewis[35] postulated that cycles of vasodilation followed periods of vasoconstriction to increase the flow of relatively warmer blood to the body areas affected by cold. He termed this phenomenon the "hunting response" and proposed that it occurred as a result of an **axon reflex**. Axon reflex is the term used to describe the phenomenon where a peripheral nerve is stimulated and carries that impulse along the nerve fiber away from the cell body until it reaches a branching, where it is diverted to an end organ without entering the cell body. It does not involve a complete reflex arc. That is why it is referred to as an axon reflex and not a true reflex.

Cold vasodilation was also reported to occur without the cycling component and was attributed to local responses in deeper tissues.[36] Responses have included the following:

- Skin vessels were shown to maximally constrict at 15°C (59°F) followed by vasodilation at temperatures below 15°C (59°F), reaching maximal vasodilation at 0°C (32°F),[36] and
- Cold-induced vascular responses, to which the prevention of local tissue injury is ascribed.[34,37,38] The hunting response is described as cycles of vasoconstriction-vasodilation lasting approximately 12 to 30 minutes during cold exposure.[39-47] Vasodilation occurs before the vasoconstrictive phase of the hunting response, and changes in sensation accompany the cycles. Cold vasodilation was also reported to occur without the cycling component and was attributed to local responses in deeper tissues.[37]

Tissue temperature changes in response to cold applications have been reported at depths of 1 to 4 cm,[48] depending on the temperature gradient and the duration of the exposure. More intense cold and longer durations result in greater decreases in tissue temperature. The presence of adipose tissue also affects the depth of cold penetration because it acts as insulation. It may not be possible to lower temperatures of deeper structures if the intensity of the cooling agent and the duration of the application are not adequate, and if the area of the body being treated has low conductivity. However, cooling of muscles and joints is possible when these structures are located more superficially without the presence of excessive adipose tissue. For tissue temperature changes at greater depths to be noted, longer application times are needed.

Decreases in tissue temperature to 10°C (50°F) or below may result in thermal damage to tissues.[48] Thermal damage may trigger an inflammatory response and result in an increase in edema. This may account, in part, for somewhat conflicting results in animal studies of the effect of cryotherapy on post-traumatic edema.[49-52]

The visco-elastic properties of tissue are also affected by cold application. Just as heat increases elasticity and decreases viscosity, cold has the opposite effect. Tissues that are cooled may not respond as favorably to length changes, and ROM measures after cold application may not be accurate.

Therapeutic cold reduces the metabolic rate and slows the production of metabolites, resulting in less metabolically generated heat production. The reduction in the metabolic rate also decreases the oxygen demand for tissues, such that tissues can accommodate the decreased blood flow.

INTERVENTION GOALS

Knowledge of the physiological effects of cold helps to identify the benefits of the use of therapeutic cold as an adjunctive treatment intervention in physical therapy. The rationale for using cold is similar to that of the use of therapeutic heat. Addressing impairments, such as edema, pain, muscle guarding, and abnormal muscle tone, helps in attaining meaningful therapeutic goals related to mobility and function (Table 4-7).

Edema Reduction

Cold is commonly used in the management of acute inflammation. Vascular responses to cold affect cell wall permeability, thus inhibiting fluid accumulation in the interstitium. In a study of microcirculatory changes in response to cold, Smith and colleagues[54] suggested that the amount of interstitial fluid is controlled by an increase in the reabsorption rate. They reported that there was an increase in the diameter of venules, but no change in arteriolar diameter in response to cold.

The decrease in blood flow associated with vasoconstriction and the decrease in metabolic rate with cold application may result in less accumulation of metabolites and chemical irritants in the injured area. The presence of chemical irritants may themselves trigger an inflammatory and pain response. By minimizing the presence of these irritants, a decrease in the rate of the inflammatory response *may* be possible. The lack of pain in the injured area then helps promote mobility, which in turn can facilitate an increase in blood flow and a reduction in edema.

Cold applications in combination with compression have been reported to be more effective than compression alone for the management of edema. Basur and associates[55] compared the use of cold and compression with the use of compression alone in the management of acute ankle sprains. They reported that edema was better controlled when using combined cold and compression rather than compression alone. Levy and Marmar[56] reported similar

TABLE 4-7	Treatment Goals for Therapeutic Cold	
INDICATION	**RATIONALE**
Pain reduction	A-beta and C fiber stimulation
Muscle guarding reduction	Decreased muscle spindle activity
Inflammation reduction	Decreased vascular responses
Hemorrhage containment	Decreased by minimizing effects of active bleeding

findings in their study of the postoperative management of patients with total knee arthroplasties. In addition to improved edema control with cold and compression, they also reported less pain and a greater increase in ROM. The intensity and duration of cold application appear to influence the effect on edema. More intense cold applied for longer durations may have an adverse effect. Therefore, less intense cold applied for durations of 20 to 30 minutes is recommended. To maximize edema reduction, concomitant compression is also advised. A recent review concluded that more evidence is needed to determine whether cold positively affects the consequences of acute soft tissue injury.[56]

Pain Reduction

Cryotherapy is commonly used to decrease pain. The proposed mechanisms by which cold influences pain are similar to those for heat. Cooling agents applied to the skin surface may elevate the pain threshold. Cold is also a counterirritant and may lessen pain sensation by stimulating thermal receptors.

Pain associated with edema and inflammation is both directly and indirectly mediated with cryotherapy. Analgesia is a direct effect of therapeutic cold. Further pain reduction may result from the decrease in chemical irritant response to the decrease in metabolic rate. There may be a decrease in stimulation of mechanoreceptors in the area of injury as edema is reduced. The decrease in pain promotes an increase in mobility, which has been associated with an earlier return to function.

Reduction of Muscle Guarding

Muscle guarding is a local reaction to injury, in which a tonic contraction is sustained in an attempt to guard or protect the tissue from further injury. It is also a component of the pain-spasm-pain cycle, and as such may be reflexively affected by a decrease in pain. Muscle tightness may be reduced following cryotherapy if sufficient analgesia is induced to allow stretch of the muscle. However, there are some patients who have an aversion to cryotherapy who will not permit a clinician to apply it to them regardless of what they are told.

Reduction of Muscle Spasticity

Spasticity is differentiated from muscle spasm in that it is associated with increased resistance to passive stretch, an increase in deep tendon reflexes (DTRs), and clonus. **Clonus** is defined as the spasmodic alteration of contractions between antagonist muscle groups because of a hyperactive stretch reflex from an upper motor neuron lesion. Several studies indicate that spasticity can be reduced by cryotherapy.[57-62] Cold application temporarily decreases the amplitude of DTRs. The reduction may be a result of direct cooling of the muscle and can be attributed to stimulation of skin receptors.

Miglietta[60] investigated the effects of cold on sustained ankle clonus and reported that clonus was either decreased or eliminated after cold whirlpool at 18.3°C (65°F) for 15 minutes. The changes were maintained for several hours.

The decrease in spasticity associated with cryotherapy may have a positive effect on mobility and may allow an increased level of participation in a therapy program. Since the reduction in spasticity can be sustained for several hours, the exercise or activity should be initiated within that time frame. This becomes especially important when establishing a home program and instructing the patient, family members, and other care providers in carrying out the exercise program.

BEFORE YOU BEGIN
- Ask the patient if he or she has a known hypersensitivity to cold.
- You may choose not to use cold because you do not want to cause an adverse response.

METHODS OF COLD APPLICATION
Ice Massage
Ice massage is the application of ice directly onto the skin surface. Because it is an intense cold application, it is usually applied to small areas, such as a localized area on a muscle belly or trigger point. To cover an area 10 cm by 15 cm, a period of 5 to 10 minutes is needed.[63] However, numbness will be achieved more efficiently if the size of the area is smaller. Larger treatment areas attempted with an ice massage will allow for the area to re-warm as soon as the ice is moved off of the area. The treatment intervention time for ice massage can also be determined by the amount of time needed to numb the area. It is important to explain to patients that before numbness or analgesia occurs, the patient will experience stages of cold, burning, and aching. This discussion is necessary for the patient to understand that these sensations are normal responses, so that the patient may better tolerate the intervention. The ability to produce numbness depends on the size of the area treated. Smaller areas are recommended because the intensity and localization of the cold application do not allow for effective local temperature regulation, and tissue cooling is achieved.

Paper or Styrofoam cups can be filled with water and placed in a freezer. The use of paper or Styrofoam cups provides insulation to the therapist handling the ice cup. The skin surface to be treated must be exposed and the surrounding area draped with a towel to absorb the water as the ice melts. Refer to the Let's Find Out—Ice Massage: Lab Activities later in this chapter.

Cold Packs
Cold packs are a simple and effective method for cooling tissue. There are commercially available cold packs, as well as cold packs that can easily be made at home or in the clinic. Cold packs represent a means of delivering very cold temperatures to the treatment intervention area and are considered a good choice as a cold intervention. Commercial cold packs contain a semi-gelled substance, covered in durable plastic. They are manufactured in sizes similar to those of Hydrocollator packs. Cold packs are stored in freezer units and remain cold for up to 10 minutes after removal from the cooling unit. They may be applied either directly to the skin (if used by only one

person) or can be used with a wet or dry interface, depending on the desired intensity of the cold application. This form of cold pack conforms to irregular surface areas, but maintaining a constant cold temperature is problematic. Commercial cold packs are reusable and self-contained.

Ice packs can be made using a plastic bag or towel and crushed ice or ice cubes. The use of crushed ice allows for better conformity when applying the ice pack to the body part. The pack can be applied directly to the surface of the skin or it may be applied using a wet or dry towel as an interface. Keep in mind that the use of a terrycloth towel adds an air-space between the ice pack and the patient and air does not conduct cold. An Ace wrap or second towel may be used to secure the cold or ice pack and to absorb water as the ice melts. Ice packs can be easily made at home and are inexpensive.

Patients must be positioned and draped appropriately for the duration of the ice application keeping in mind the goals for the treatment intervention. This includes the need for support and elevation of the part being treated as well as consideration for neutral or unloaded positions where muscles do not have to work during the application of the ice pack. The average treatment intervention time for a cold or ice pack application is 10 to 15 minutes.

Cold or Ice Baths

Immersion in water that contains partially melted ice cubes is primarily used for distal extremities or larger body parts. Immersion of the body part allows complete conformity of the cooling agent to the skin. Therapeutic temperature ranges for cold baths are between 13°C and 18°C (55.4°F and 64.4°F) and lower temperatures within this range are tolerated for shorter durations. This method of cryotherapy is easily applied in the home setting; however, the patient is in a dependent position, which is not optimal.

Controlled Cold Units

Controlled cold units that apply simultaneous compression are available as portable home model units and can be effective in controlling postoperative pain and edema. One of these units is pictured in Figure 4-13. Different sleeves and cuffs are available for different parts of the body or areas of an extremity. Care must be taken to assure that the patient is cautious and follows the instructions supplied by the manufacturer of the units and does not use the unit more than indicated by his or her physician, as injury could potentially result.

INTERVENTION GUIDELINES

Patient preparation and proper positioning are primary considerations for any method of cold application.

- The treatment intervention must be explained prior to its initiation.
- Patients must be encouraged to ask questions, and clinicians must stress the importance of their verbalizing their response to the intervention.

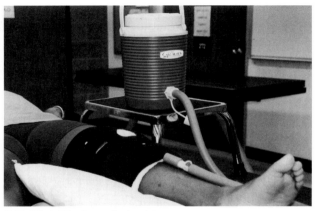

FIGURE 4-13 Controlled cold unit.
(From Michlovitz, SL, and Nolan, TP (eds): Modalities for Therapeutic Intervention, ed 4. FA Davis, Philadelphia, 2005, with permission.)

- Patient positioning is important and must consider body mechanics principles for both the patient and clinicians who will be interacting with the patient.
  - Support for the area being treated
  - Alignment of the area, relaxed, neutral or stretch, depending upon the treatment goals
- Clothing and jewelry need to be removed from the treatment area so that the area can easily be assessed and visualized.
- Visual inspection includes an assessment of skin integrity and appearance and tissue response before, during, and after cryotherapy interventions.
- The patient's subjective response must be checked periodically throughout the duration of the intervention.

SAFETY CONSIDERATIONS WITH THE APPLICATION OF COLD TREATMENT INTERVENTIONS

Precautions

Cryotherapy should be used with caution on patients with thermoregulatory problems, sensory deficits, hypersensitivity to cold, and impaired circulation. If cryotherapy is to be used, careful monitoring is essential. Appropriate adjustments of the treatment parameters may be necessary to decrease stress to body systems. For example, if a patient reports an abnormal level of discomfort in response to ice massage, perhaps a method involving less intense cold could be substituted. Cold should not be applied directly over an area of compromised circulation.

Cold applications can cause a transient increase in blood pressure.[64,65] Careful monitoring of blood pressure should be performed before, during, and after cold application if the patient is hypertensive. Intervention should be discontinued if an excessive elevation in blood pressure occurs. A quick summary of the pros and cons of the various forms of cryotherapy that have been discussed is presented in Table 4-8.

Contraindications

Cryotherapy is contraindicated for patients with particular cold sensitivities. One adverse response is known as cold urticaria, which may include both local and systemic

TABLE 4-8 | Pros and Cons of Various Forms of Cryotherapy Application Techniques

	EXPENSE		AVAILABILITY		RELATIVE SAFETY		CLINICIAN TIME		POSITIONING	
	Pro	Con	Pro	Con	Pro	Con	Pro	Con	Pro	Con
Ice massage	X				X			X	X	
Ice bath	X		X		X		X			X
Cold packs	X		X		X		X		X	
Controlled cold and compression units		X	X?		X	X	X		?	?

reactions. The local response is a skin rash, usually occurring as an allergic reaction that is marked by itching and small pale or red swellings, and often lasts for a few days. It may also be characterized by wheals, or raised, reddened areas, that appear in direct response to a local cold application.[66,67] The systemic response may include facial flushing, a drop in blood pressure, an increase in heart rate, and syncope.[68]

Patients with cryoglobulinemia, a rare blood disease in which specific blood proteins (cryoglobulins) form a gel when exposed to cold, are at risk for developing ischemia or gangrene because of the abnormal blood protein. This condition is seen in patients with multiple myeloma, chronic liver disease, and several rheumatic diseases.[69]

Patients with **Raynaud's disease** exhibit cycles of pallor, cyanosis, bright red coloration or rubor, and normal coloration in the hands and feet in response to cold. Numbness, tingling, or burning may also occur. These sensations are similar to the normal stages of sensation experienced with cold, so it is important to pay attention to visual cues as well as subjective responses from the patient.

Paroxysmal cold hemoglobinuria is characterized by the sudden presence of blood in the urine. It can result from either local or systemic exposure to cold. It may not be possible to observe this response in the clinic, but a complete and thorough patient history will help in identifying those individuals at risk.

CLINICAL DECISION MAKING: HEAT OR COLD?

Responses to both therapeutic heat application and cryotherapy may be similar. Both heat and cold are effective pain management techniques and both are beneficial in reducing muscle guarding. Some guidelines apply when making recommendations for the use of heat or cold. The benefits of cold in the management of acute injuries are well documented. For painful conditions associated with acute injuries, cryotherapy is the intervention of choice. Neither heat nor cold provides lasting benefit in the management of chronic pain,[70] but heat may aid in promoting relaxation and could be recommended for home use. Either heat or cold could be used for relief of joint stiffness. Heat enhances

the visco-elastic properties of connective tissue and may result in increased motion and decreased pain. Although cold has the opposite effect on connective tissue, it may provide greater pain relief for a given patient. An increase in motion may result, because pain no longer limits the motion.

For pain associated with muscle guarding, either heat or cold may be effective. If a patient has received heat interventions and there is no documented change in the pain level or in ROM, then a trial of therapeutic cold may be indicated.

Acute injuries are treated with cold because the rate of the inflammation is reduced. Heat is contraindicated for acute injuries because it may exacerbate the inflammatory process. However, an increase in blood flow may promote the reabsorption of exudates and may be appropriate in the management of chronic edema and inflammation.

Precautions and contraindications may guide the intervention choice when the intervention goal could be achieved with either heat or cold. Patient tolerance of the thermal agent should not be discounted. If either heat or cold produces discomfort, and if the intervention goal can be achieved with heat or cold, then patient preference may be the primary determinant.

Documentation

The goals of documentation are to provide an accurate and complete description of the intervention and the patient's response to intervention. Documentation should include all the necessary parameters and components so that the intervention could be easily reproduced by another clinician. Documentation of the use of any thermal agent should include a description of the type of agent used, the method of application, the area treated, and the position of the patient. For example, report that a cervical hot pack was applied to a patient's shoulder using eight layers of towelling. Also, report the position of the patient and the involved extremity if it was supported in a particular position.

Documentation of the patient's response to intervention is important because it provides a means for evaluating the effectiveness of the intervention and the patient's readiness to progress in the intervention plan. Both subjective and objective responses should be documented. Subjective statements by the patient regarding pain and activity levels are indications of how effective the use of thermal agents is for pain management. Pain levels can be better quantified by using a visual analog scale or verbal rating scale. Objective measures are essential in determining intervention efficacy. Girth and volume measures should be reported to reflect changes in edema and can be used to determine whether changes have been maintained over time. The same is true for goniometric measurements, which are useful in assessing changes in ROM in response to intervention. Improvement in function is the ultimate therapeutic goal. Although the use of heat or cold may not have a direct effect on function, the functional status of the patient reflects the overall effectiveness of the intervention plan.

Summary

Throughout this chapter, the safe and effective clinical application techniques for a variety of thermal agents have been presented. The goals of the heat or cold intervention, mechanisms of thermal exchange, patient positioning, general health, and the age of the patient all play an important part in the clinical decision making involved in the selection and use of thermal agents. Every patient is an individual with a specific set of symptoms and previous or co-existing medical conditions. Clinicians must fully understand not only the benefits of thermal agent application, but also the potential adverse effects that they may cause.

Review Questions

1. When sensory information reaches the brain, the information is integrated and interpreted along with information about the temperature of the blood circulating through the hypothalamus. Which of the following mechanisms regulates temperature?
   a. Vasodilation or vasoconstriction of blood vessels
   b. Shivering, to maintain heat
   c. Sweating, to lose heat
   d. All of the above are examples of temperature regulation

2. Elevating the tissue temperature results in an increase in blood flow to the area, attributable in part to the vasodilatory response in surface blood vessels. What mechanism normally prevents excessive heat accumulation?
   a. The decreased blood flow removes heat from the area, and blood that is relatively cooler from the circulatory system flows into the area
   b. The increased blood flow removes heat from the area, and blood that is relatively cooler from the circulatory system flows into the area
   c. The increased blood flow moves heat into the area, and blood that is relatively warmer from the circulatory system flows into the area
   d. The increased blood flow removes heat from the area, and blood that is relatively warmer from the circulatory system flows into the area

3. According to Melzack and Wall's gate control theory of pain, how does the application of therapeutic heat reduce the perception of pain?
   a. The theory has not been proved; therefore, it doesn't reduce pain perception
   b. Thermal stimuli inhibit nociceptor input to the spinal cord and open the gate in the spinal cord
   c. Thermal stimuli override painful stimuli and inhibit pain transmission
   d. Thermal stimuli override sensory input and open the gate in the spinal cord

4. Hydrocollator packs, or hot packs, are one of the most commonly applied forms of superficial moist heat in the clinical environment. After a 20-minute application of a hot pack on a patient, how long will it take for the pack to reach the temperature of the water in the storage unit?
   a. 20–30 minutes
   b. 30–40 minutes
   c. 60 minutes
   d. 5–10 minutes

5. Cold is commonly used in the management of acute inflammation and edema. Which of the following interventions has been the most successful in controlling pain and edema in the management of acute ankle sprains?
   a. Cold
   b. Compression
   c. No difference has been identified between the use of cold or compression separately or together
   d. Cold and compression

6. Muscle guarding is a protective mechanism to protect against potential pain and further injury or pain associated with joint movement. Heat application to relieve muscle guarding accomplishes all *but which* of the following?
   a. Increase in pain perception
   b. Muscle relaxation
   c. Increase in ROM
   d. Reduction of pain

CASE STUDY

Diagnosis: Ankle fracture with loss of ROM of the ankle in all planes.

Henry is a 45-year-old van driver who has been referred to physical therapy for treatment to relieve pain and stiffness in his left ankle. He has a healed bimalleollar fracture of the ankle. He is 8 weeks post-fracture, he has had surgery to reduce the fracture, and he has been out of his cast for 2 days. He is permitted weight-bearing to tolerance and is using crutches for ambulation. The primary goal of the physical therapy treatment intervention is to reduce pain and stiffness prior to using techniques to restore ROM.

1. What thermal agent(s) could you use to reduce pain and stiffness?

   Response: If swelling in the ankle were under control, the other options would include Fluidotherapy or warm whirlpool. The advantage to using either Fluidotherapy or whirlpool is that exercise can be performed during heat application. Moist heat packs are another option.

2. How would you carry out this intervention? What patient position would you use? What would be the duration of the application?

   Response: Fluidotherapy could be applied between 106°F and 108°F (41°C and 42°C), or whirlpool at about 102°F (39°C), with the foot and ankle immersed in the cellulose medium or water, respectively. The agitation for either modality would provide a desensitization and pain control. Henry would be positioned supine with his leg elevated on a pillow. Moist heat could be applied for 15 to 20 minutes; then ROM exercises would follow. (The physical therapist may determine that between heat and ROM exercises, joint mobilization techniques on Henry's ankle should be performed.)

3. Can you give an example of a situation in which heat would be contraindicated?

   Response: Is circulation intact? Does he have a dorsal pedis pulse? Does he have any comorbidities such as diabetes or PVD that may impede circulation and prevent dissipation of heat? You do not want to risk a burn as a result of heat application.

4. How would you determine whether heat was appropriate in accomplishing the intervention goal?

   Response: In part, you could determine whether pain and stiffness were relieved before exercise (self-reported by the patient).

DISCUSSION QUESTIONS

1. When would ice or cryotherapy be contraindicated and heat be indicated?

2. When would heat be contraindicated and cryotherapy potentially be indicated?

3. How would you explain the sensations that a patient should expect to feel during an application of superficial heat?

4. How would you explain the sensations that a patient should feel during cryotherapy?

REFERENCES

1. Scanlon, VC, and Sanders T: Essentials of Anatomy and Physiology, ed 4. FA Davis, Philadelphia, 2003, pp 376–379.
2. Lehmann, JF, and de Lateur, BJ: Therapeutic heat. In Lehman, JF (ed): Therapeutic Heat and Cold, ed 4. Williams and Wilkins, Baltimore, 1990.
3. Moritz, AR, and Henriques, FC, Jr: Studies in thermal injury. II. The relative importance of time and surface temperature in causation of cutaneous burns. Am J Pathol 23:695, 1947.
4. Henriques, FC, Jr: Studies in thermal injury. V. The predictability and the significance of thermally induced rate processes leading to irreversible epidermal injury. Am J Pathol 23:489, 1947.
5. Abramson, DI, et al: Changes in blood flow, oxygen uptake and tissue temperatures produced by the topical application of wet heat. Arch Phys Med Rehabil 42:305, 1961.
6. Abramson, DI, et al: Indirect vasodilation in thermotherapy. Arch Phys Med Rehabil 46:412–420, 1965.
7. Rabkin, JM, and Hunt, TK: Local heat increases blood flow and oxygen tension in wounds. Arch Surg 122:221, 1987.
8. Melzack, R, and Wall, PD: Pain mechanisms: A new theory. Science 150:971, 1965.
9. Gammon, GD, and Starr, I: Studies on the relief of pain by counter imitation. J Clin Invest 20:13, 1941.
10. Benson, TB, and Copp EP: The effects of therapeutic forms of heat and ice on the pain threshold of the normal shoulder. Rheumatol Rehabil 13:101, 1974.
11. Coseutino, AB, et al: Ultrasound effects on electroneuromyographic measures in sensory fibers in the median nerve. Phys Ther 63:1789, 1983.
12. DeVries, H: Quantitative electromyographic investigation of the spasms theory of muscle pain. Am J Phys Med 45:119, 1966.
13. Harris, R: Physical methods in the management of rheumatoid arthritis. Med Clin North Am 52:707, 1968.
14. Nadler, SF, Steiner, DJ, Erasala, GN, et al: Continuous low-level heat wrap provides more efficacy than ibuprofen and acetaminophen for acute low back pain. Spine 27(10):1012, 2002.
15. Nadler, SF, Steiner, DJ, Petty, SR, et al: Overnight use of continuous low-level heat wrap therapy for relief of low back pain. Arch Phys Med Rehabil 84:335–342, 2003.
16. Mense, S: Effects of temperature on the discharges of muscle spindles and tendon organs. Pflugers Arch 374:159, 1978.
17. LeBann, MM: Collagen tissue: Implications of its response to stress in vitro. Arch Phys Med Rehabil 47:345, 1966.
18. Enneking, WF, and Horowitz, M: The intra-articular effects of immobilization on the human knee. J Bone Joint Surg (AM) 5:973, 1972.
19. Kottke, FJ, Pauley, DL, and Ptok RA: The rationale for prolonged stretching for correction of shortening of connective tissues. Arch Phys Med Rehabil 47:345, 1966.
20. Warren, GC, Lehmann, JF, and Koblanski, JN: Heat and stretch procedures: An evaluation using rat tail tendon. Arch Phys Med Rehabil 57:122, 1976.
21. Light, KE, et al: Low-load prolonged stretch vs high-load brief stretch in treating knee contractures. Phys Ther 664:330, 1984.

22. Backlund, L, and Tiselius, P: Objective measurement of joint stiffness in rheumatoid arthritis. Acta Rheum Scand 13:275, 1967.
23. Greenberg, RS: The effects of hot packs and exercise on local blood flow. Phys Ther 52:273, 1972.
24. Chastain, PB: The effect of deep heat on isometric strength. Phys Ther 58:543, 1978.
25. Edwards, HT, et al: Effect of temperature on muscle energy metabolism and endurance during successive isometric contractions, sustained to fatigue of the quadriceps muscle in man. J Phys 220:335, 1972.
26. Wickstrom, R, and Polk, C: Effect of whirlpool on the strength endurance of the quadriceps muscle in trained male adolescents. Am J Phys Med 40:91, 1961.
27. Abramson, DI, et al: Changes in blood flow, oxygen uptake and tissue temperatures produced by the topical application of wet heat. Arch Phys Med Rehabil 42:305, 1961.
28. Greenberg, RS: The effects of hot packs and exercise on local blood flow. Phys Ther 52:273, 1972.
29. Lehmann, JF, et al: Temperature distributions in the human thigh produced by infrared, hot packs and microwave applications. Arch Phys Med Rehabil 47:291, 1966.
30. Whyte, HM, and Reader, SB: Effectiveness of different forms of heating. Ann Rheum Dis 10:449, 1951.
31. Borrell, RM, et al: Comparison of in vivo temperatures produced by hydrotherapy, paraffin wax treatment and Fluidotherapy. Phys Ther 60:1273, 1980.
32. Borrell, RM, et al: Fluidotherapy: Evaluation of a new heat modality. Arch Phys Med Rehabil 58:69, 1977.
34. Michlovitz, S, Hun, L, Erasala, GN, Henehold, DA, and Weingand, KW: Continuous low-level heat wrap therapy is effective in treating wrist pain. Arch Phys Med Rehabil 85:1409, 2004.
35. Lewis, T: Observations upon the reactions of the vessels of the human skin to cold. Heart 15:177, 1930.
36. Fox, RH, and Whyatt, HT: Cold-induced vasodilatation in various areas of the body surface in man. J Physiol 162:289, 1962.
37. Downey, JA: Physiologic effects of heat and cold. J Am Phys Ther Assoc 44:713, 1964.
38. Clarke, RSJ, Hellon, RF, and Lind, AR: Vascular reactions of the human forearm to cold. Clin Sci 17:165, 1958.
39. Clarke, RSJ, and Hellon, RF: Hyperemia following sustained and rhythmic exercise in the human forearm at various temperatures. J Physiol 145:447, 1959.
40. Behnke, R: Cold therapy. Athletic Train 9:178, 1974.
41. Behnke, R: Cryotherapy and vasodilation. Athletic Train 8:106, 1973.
42. Grant, AE: Massage with ice (cryokinetics) in the treatment of painful conditions of the musculoskeletal system. Arch Phys Med Rehabil 45:233, 1964.
43. Hayden, C: Cryokinetics in an early treatment program. J Am Phys Ther Assoc 44:11, 1964.
44. Knight, KL, Aquino, J, Johannes, SM, and Urbano, CD: Reexamination of Lewis cold induced vasodilation in the finger and the ankle. Athletic Train 15:248–250, 1980.
45. Moore, R, Nicolette, R, and Behnke, R: The therapeutic use of cold (cryotherapy) in the care of athletic injuries. Athletic Train 2:6, 1967.
46. Moore, R: Uses of cold therapy in the rehabilitation of athletes, recent advances, Proceedings of the 19th American Medical Association National Conference on the Medical Aspects of Sports. San Francisco, June 1977.
47. Murphy, AJ: The physiological effects of cold application. Phys Ther Rev 40: 1112, 1960.
48. Olson, JE, and Stravino, U: A review of cryotherapy. Phys Ther 52:840, 1972.
49. Michlovitz, SL: Cryotherapy. In Michlovitz, SL (ed): Thermal Agents in Rehabilitation, ed 2. FA Davis, Philadelphia, 1990.
50. Matsen, FA, Questad, K, and Matsen, AL: The effect of local cooling on post fracture swelling. Clin Orthop 109:201, 1975.
51. Jezdinsky, J, Marek, J, and Ochonsky, P: Effects of local cold and heat therapy on traumatic oedema of the rat hind paw. I: Effects of cooling on the course of traumatic oedema. Acta Universitatis Palackianae Olomucensis Facultatis Medicae 66:185, 1973.
52. Marek, J, Jezdinsky, J, and Ochonsky, P: Effects of local cold and heat therapy on traumatic oedema of the rat hind paw. II: Effects of various kinds of compresses on the course of traumatic oedema. Acta Universitatis Palackinanae Olomucensis Facultatis Medicae 66:203, 1973.
53. McMaster, WC, and Liddle, S: Cryotherapy influence on post traumatic limb edema. Clin Orthop 150:283, 1980.
54. Smith, TL, et al: New skeletal muscle model for the longitudinal study of alterations in microcirculation following contusion and cryotherapy. Microsurgery 14:487, 1993.
55. Basur, R, Shephard, E, and Mouzos, G: A cooling method in the treatment of ankle sprains. Practitioner 216:708, 1976.
56. Levy, AS, and Marmar, E: The role of cold compression dressings in the postoperative treatment of total knee arthroplasty. Clin Orthop Rel Res 297: 174, 1993.
57. Bleakley, C, McDonough, S, and MacAuley, D: The use of ice in the treatment of acute soft-tissue injury: A systematic review of randomized controlled trials. Am J Sports Med 32(1):251, 2004.
58. Knuttsson, E, and Mattssan, E: Effects of local cooling on monosynaptic reflexes in man. Scand J Rehabil Med 1:126, 1969.
59. Newton, M, and Lehmkuhl, D: Muscle spindle response to body heating and localized muscle cooling: Implications for relief of spasticity. Phys Ther 45:91, 1965.
60. Miglietta, O: Electromyographic characteristics of clonus and influence of cold. Arch Phys Med Rehabil 45:508, 1964.
61. Miglietta, O: Action of cold on spasticity. Am J Phys Med 52:198, 1973.
62. Eldred, E, Lindsley, DF, and Buchwald, JS: The effect of cooling on mammalian muscle spindles. Exp Neurol 2:144, 1960.
63. Hartvikksen, K: Ice therapy in spasticity. Acta Neurol Scand 38:79, 1962.
64. Waylonis, GW: The physiologic effect of ice massage. Arch Phys Med Rehabil 48:37, 1967.
65. Boyer, JT, Fraser, JRE, and Doyle, AE: The haemodynamic effects of cold immersion. Clin Sci 19:539, 1980.
66. Claus-Walker, J, et al: Physiological responses to cold stress in healthy subjects and in subjects with cervical cord injuries. Arch Phys Med Rehabil 55:485, 1974.
67. Austin, KD: Diseases of immediate type hypersensitivity. In Isselbacher, KJ, et al (eds): Harrison's Principles of Internal Medicine, ed 9. McGraw-Hill, New York, 1980.
68. Nadler, SF, Prybicien, M, Malanga, GA, and Sicher, D: Complications from therapeutic modalities: Results of a national survey of athletic trainers. Arch Phys Med Rehabil 84(6):849–853, 2003.
69. Horton, BT, Brown, GE, and Roth, GM: Hypersensitiveness to cold with local and systemic manifestations of a histamine-like character: Its amenability to treatment. JAMA 107:1263, 1936.
70. Schumacher, HR (ed): Cryoglobulinemia. In Primer on Rheumatic Diseases, ed 9. Arthritis Foundation, Atlanta, GA, 1988, p 82.

LET'S FIND OUT

Lab Activity: Thermal Agents
Hydrocollator (hot) packs

Equipment

Towels	Paraffin unit
Plastic bags	Ice cubes
Fluidotherapy	Ice packs
Thermometer	Pillows and pillow cases
Basin	Hydrocollator packs (various sizes)
Gowns	Shortwave diathermy
Minute timer	Ice bath

Before you begin, we need to first address the precautions and contraindications for the application of hot packs and other thermal agents. It's important to know what they are, but perhaps it is even more important to understand *why* each is either a precaution or a contraindication.

Precautions and Why

Precautions	Why
Over wounds	New granulation tissue is sensitive to heat and pressure and may not be able to withstand heat application. However, heat may enhance the circulation to the area once the wound is closed. Skin sensation must be intact to administer heat.
During pregnancy	Heat may be beneficial; however, it should not be applied over a pregnant uterus as it may increase the circulation to the fetus and the effects of this have not been studied.
With patients who are of advanced age	If the patient has intact sensation and is reliable, then the application of heat may be indicated. However, if the patient has fragile skin that does not blanche during depression, he or she may not be able to adapt to the increased temperature from heat.
During menses	Heat applied to the lower back of a female during menses may increase her flow. If she is prepared for this, then the application might be indicated depending upon the signs and symptoms of the physical therapy diagnosis.
Impaired cognitive ability of the patient	If a patient is able to communicate hot and pain in some meaningful way, then the patient may have heat applied. However, these patients should be monitored closely.
Previous experience with the physical agent	If a patient has had a poor response to the application of a thermal agent, he or she may be less receptive to trying it again. However, it is important that the clinician educate the patient and explain the potential benefits or risks of any modality before it is applied.

Contraindications and Why

Contraindications	Why
	Hydrocollator packs, paraffin, Fluidotherapy
Pregnancy *(during the first trimester)*	Not directly over a pregnant uterus as it may increase the circulation to the fetus and this has not been studied for safety with human subjects.
Undressed or infected wounds	The infection must be cultured and treated first. The wound must be covered to prevent cross-contamination.
Presence of a pacemaker	If the pacemaker is a demand pacemaker, then the application is a precaution. Heat received by patients with *non-demand* pacemakers may cause undue stress on the cardiac musculature.
Metastasis	Heat application directly over or proximal to a metastasis will increase the circulation to the area and may enhance the disease progression.
Existing fever	Heat to an area actively involved in the inflammatory process will result in an increase in the circulation to that area and potentially increase edema.
Acute inflammation	Heat to an area actively involved in the inflammatory process will result in an increase in the circulation to that area and potentially increase edema.
Acute hemorrhage	Heat to an area actively involved in the inflammatory process will result in an increase in the circulation to that area and potentially increase edema.
Peripheral vascular disease	Heat applied to an area with compromised ability to maintain homeostasis may result in increased pain perception and other complications.
Lack of sensation in the treatment area	The safety of heat applications relies on the ability of the patient to report changes in sensation to prevent a burn.

Application Techniques and Challenges

Select three classmates/patients to have hot packs applied to their lower back. You will be positioning them differently to compare the conduction of thermal energy from the hot pack to each of the patients. As with all treatments, inspect the area and note the presence of scars, edema, muscle guarding, or impairments in sensation. *Remember, scars may not conduct heat as uniformly as unscarred areas.*

Prone

1. Position one patient prone with a pillow underneath his/her abdomen and ankles to reduce lordosis and permit treatment in a neutral spine position (Fig. 4-14).

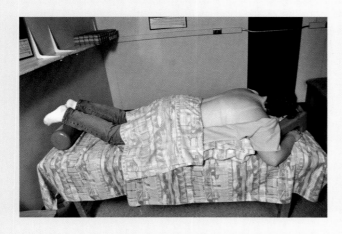

FIGURE 4-14 Patient positioning for application of lumbar hot packs. The sheet is draping the lumbar area in preparation for the application of heat.

2. Remove a standard size hot pack and place it in a commercial cover. Place a folded towel over the treatment area, and place the hot pack on top of the folded towel. Drape your patient.

How does the patient describe what he or she feels under the hot pack?

Initially _____

After 5 minutes _____

After 8 minutes _____

After 10 minuets _____

Does your patient ever report that the hot pack is getting too warm? If yes, after how long and what did you do?

_____

_____

_____

_____

Supine

1. Position your patient so that he or she is supine, with a pillow underneath the head and knees for support. The clothing should be removed in the treatment area so that it will not be in the way of the hot pack.

2. Remove a standard size hot pack and place it in a commercial cover. Place a folded towel on top of the cover and ask your patient to lift him- or herself up so that you can place the hot pack underneath him or her.

How does the patient describe what he or she feels on the back?

Initially _____

After 5 minutes _____

After 8 minutes _____

After 10 minutes _____

Does your patient ever report that the hot pack is getting too warm? If yes, after how long and what did you do?

_____

_____

_____

_____

Side-Lying

1. Position your patient so that he or she is side-lying. You will need to ensure that the hot pack is in good contact with the lumbar spine. It is important that the patient is well supported in neutral and is comfortable. (A wall or strap may work well.) *Describe the position that you decided upon, and indicate the rationale for your choices.*

_____

_____

_____

2. Remove a standard size hot pack and place it in a commercial cover. Place a folded towel over the treatment area, and place the hot pack on the folded towel. Secure the hot pack in place.

How does the patient describe what he or she feels on the back?

Initially _____

After 5 minutes _____

After 8 minutes _____

After 10 minutes _____

Does your patient ever report that the hot pack is getting too warm? If yes, after how long and what did you do?

_____

_____

_____

_____

Hydrocollator Application Questions

Remove the hot packs from your patients after 15 minutes, and reassess the treatment area. Leave a layer of towelling on the treatment area while you return the hot pack to the Hydrocollator unit. *(This will keep some of the heat and moisture from evaporating from the patient's skin.)*

	Prone	Supine	Side-Lying
1. Subjectively, which patient initially felt the most comfortable?			
2. Were all three patients still comfortable after 10 minutes? If no, who was not, and what is your explanation for this?			
3. How long did it take for the heat from the hot pack to plateau with each of the patients?			
4. Which position was the easiest for you to add towel layers for the patient if you needed to?			
5. Which patient had the greatest amount of erythema post–hot pack removal? Why?			
6. Which patient had the least amount of erythema post–hot pack removal? Why?			
7. When would each of the positions that you tried be indicated?			
8. How long post–hot pack removal did it take for the appearance of the treated area to return to its pre-treatment appearance/coloring?			
9. What is the temperature of the water within the Hydrocollator unit? (Was the water level in the Hydrocollator unit sufficient to cover the hot packs completely, and what difference if any would the water level within the Hydrocollator unit make?)			
Temperature?			
Water Level?			

Paraffin Dip Method

Application Techniques and Challenges

Select a classmate/patient to have paraffin applied to his or her hand. You should inspect and wash his or her hand, recording any observations you make. *Remember that scars or areas of decreased sensation are areas to be cautious of, owing to the lack of uniformity of patient response to sensation in that area.* Paraffin can be applied in several different methods. For this exercise, you will be using the dip method and making some notations regarding the patient's responses.

1. What is the temperature of the paraffin unit that you will be utilizing?
2. Ask your patient to dip his or her hand and wrist into the paraffin unit, remove it, and let the paraffin harden. (Fig. 4-15). Then instruct them to re-dip for 8 to 10 layers of paraffin (Fig. 4-16).
3. Wrap the dipped hand in plastic wrap (Figs. 4-17 and Fig. 4-18) and then in a towel (Figs. 4-19 through 4-21).

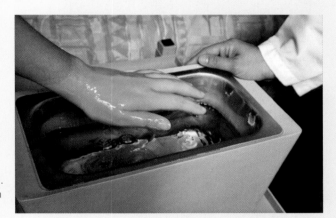

FIGURE 4-15 Dip method of paraffin application. After the first dip, the patient lets the wax harden before re-immersing for subsequent dips.

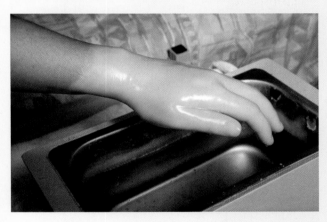

FIGURE 4-16 Dip method of paraffin application. The left distal upper extremity after several dips.

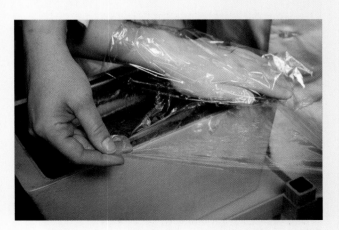

FIGURE 4-17 Dip method of paraffin application. Plastic wrap is wrapped around the paraffin-dipped hand.

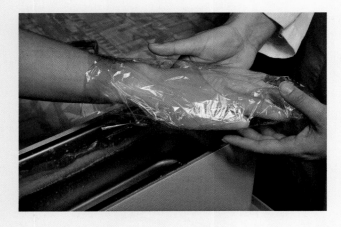

FIGURE 4-18 Dip method of paraffin application. Plastic wrap is secured around the paraffin-dipped hand.

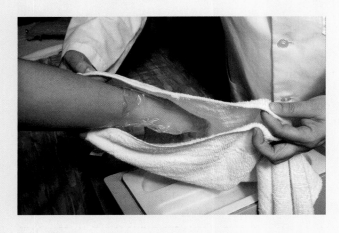

FIGURE 4-19 Dip method of paraffin application. Plastic-wrapped hand is inserted into a folded towel.

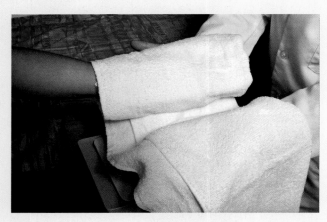

FIGURE 4-20 Dip method of paraffin application. Towel is wrapped around the paraffin-dipped hand.

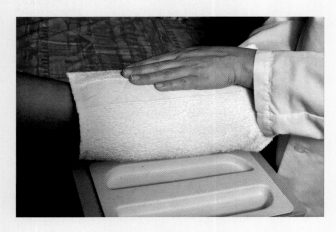

FIGURE 4-21 Dip method of paraffin application. Towel is secured around the paraffin-dipped hand.

4. Position your patient for a 15-minute treatment time, making sure that the dipped hand is supported and elevated above the heart.

	Initially	After 3 Minutes	After 6 Minutes	After 9 Minutes	After 12 Minutes
How does the paraffin feel to your patient?					
Ask your patient to describe how his/her hand feels after the paraffin is removed.					
Reassess your patient, then document your observations.					

The paraffin that you remove may either be "manipulated" in the patient's hand until it cools or immediately removed and then the hand reassessed. Some facilities will require that the paraffin be disposed of after patient use, whereas other facilities may return the paraffin to the unit for re-melting. Make sure that you have asked for and are familiar with the facility policy prior to terminating any treatment with paraffin.

Paraffin Application Questions

1. Describe the appearance of the treated hand after removal from the paraffin. Is there a difference and why would or why wouldn't you expect to see one? _____

2. What types of patient diagnoses would potentially be indicated for the dip method of paraffin application and why? _____

3. What would you do if prior to immersing your patient into the paraffin unit, you noted that the temperature was 140°F (45.8°C)? _____

Ice Massage

Application Technique and Challenges

Wrap an ice cube in a paper towel, or use a prepared "ice pop" for the ice massage (Fig.4-22).

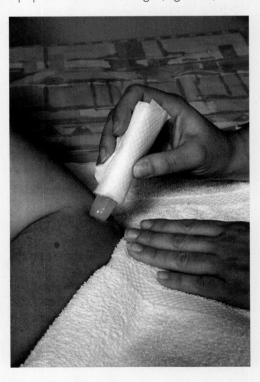

FIGURE 4-22 Ice massage to the lateral epicondyle with an "ice pop" wrapped in a paper towel.

Record the following observations:

Ice Massage	After 3 minutes	After 6 minutes	After 9 minutes
Skin appearance:			
Patient's report of how it feels:			

1. How long did it take for your patient to report numbness?
2. How large was the area affected by the treatment for the ice massage?

Patient Scenarios

Keep the following questions in mind while reading through each of the eight patient scenarios:

1. Would therapeutic heat or cryotherapy potentially be indicated?
2. When would cryotherapy be contraindicated?
3. If heat or cryotherapy is indicated, what would your treatment goal(s) be?
4. If heat or cryotherapy is indicated, *how* should what you selected be applied to the patient?
5. What if any positioning considerations are there for the patient?
6. How will you describe what the patient should expect from the treatment intervention selected?
7. How will you assess whether or not your selection was appropriate in accomplishing your treatment goal(s)?
8. What application technique(s) would you employ (if there are more than one option, describe each)?
9. When would heat be contraindicated?
10. What precautions there are for the patient described?
11. What additional information if any, would you need to know prior to applying therapeutic heat to the patient described?
12. Would therapeutic heat or cryotherapy potentially be indicated?
13. When would cryotherapy be contraindicated?
14. If heat or cryotherapy is indicated, what would your treatment goal(s) be?
15. If heat or cryotherapy is indicated, *how* should what you selected be applied to the patient?
16. What if any positioning considerations are there for the patient?
17. How will you describe what the patient should expect from the treatment intervention selected?
18. How will you assess whether or not your selection was appropriate in accomplishing your treatment goal(s)?
19. What application technique(s) would you employ (if there are more than one option, describe each)?
20. When would heat be contraindicated?
21. What precautions there are for the patient described in the following scenarios?

   A. John has been referred to the physical therapy department for an injury to his left ankle that was the result of a dispute that took place during a hockey game. He is a professional hockey player who has the goalie position. He was playing in the championship game last evening when another player collided with him on the ice. His left ankle is now edematous, particularly anterior to the lateral malleolus. He has acute tenderness in this area as well. The posterior aspect of the ankle has a large hematoma on both the medial and lateral aspects. There were no fractures noted by the physician who x-rayed the ankle last night. John's chief complaints are pain with palpation and pain with weight-bearing, as well as an inability to don his skates owing to the edema. John has no significant past medical history. He has previously encountered numerous fractures, sprains, strains, and lacerations during his career.

   B. Marylou is a gymnast who has been referred to the physical therapy department for an injury that she sustained to her cervical spine when she fell from the balance beam during practice this afternoon. She complains of stiffness and pain with movements in all directions in the cervical spine. There were no fractures apparent upon x-ray.

C. Betty is an older woman who has been referred to the physical therapy department because of pain and stiffness in her osteoarthritic hands. She has had an acute exacerbation of her arthritis after canning fresh fruits and vegetables from her garden. She lives and earns her livelihood on a farm and has rarely seen a medical professional in her lifetime. Betty has diabetes and has lost two toes to frostbite. There is no other significant medical history that Betty or anyone in her family knows of and she is very anxious to return to her farm to get back to work.

D. George is a perpetual "weekend warrior" who plays softball, soccer, and an occasional touch football game. He has been doing this with his friends since he graduated from college in 1990. He has been referred to the physical therapy department for an injury to his right knee. He slipped on the grass during a game of "ultimate Frisbee" and felt a sharp pain in the medial aspect of his right knee. There were no fractures identified upon x-ray. He is scheduled for a magnetic resonance imaging (MRI) scan of the knee next week. George complains of instability, pain, and swelling in the knee. He has a history of hypertension, which is being managed by medication, but no other complicating medical history.

E. Richard is a 55-year-old retired truck driver who has been referred to physical therapy for treatment to relieve pain and stiffness in his right knee. X-rays revealed arthritic changes in both knees. He had a medial meniscectomy in the right knee 2 years ago. His recent complaints of pain and stiffness are related to his present leisure and work activities. Richard is an avid golfer and country-western dancer and often acts as a chauffeur.

F. Charlotte is a 50-year-old secretary who has been referred to physical therapy for treatment to relieve symptoms associated with the automobile accident 3 weeks ago in which she was involved. She was driving to work and was struck from behind by another vehicle, sustaining cervical and lumbar sprains and strains. She is having difficulty maintaining an upright posture because of severe headaches, back pain, and intermittent paresthesias in her dominant right hand. She is a frail woman, and taught aerobics classes five nights a week but is unable to teach at all now. There were no fractures, and she is otherwise healthy.

G. Mike is a 37-year-old carpenter who has been referred to physical therapy subsequent to a fall that took place while he was working. He fell from the second story scaffolding of a house. In an attempt to break his fall, he reached for a nearby ladder and landed on a cement slab floor. His chief complaints are of pain with internal rotation, abduction, and horizontal adduction of the right shoulder. He has marked muscle guarding in the paraspinal musculature bilaterally throughout the lumbar spine. He also re-injured his left ankle, which he sprained approximately seven times before. As an independent contractor, he is anxious to resume work as quickly as possible to keep the project on schedule. Other than the injuries noted he has no significant medical history. His prior experiences with physical therapy yielded unsuccessful results with ultrasound.

H. Jimmy is a 67-year-old retired factory worker who has been referred to physical therapy to help relieve chronic arthritic joint stiffness and pain in his hands. He is diabetic and has had an amputation below the knee on his right leg. He ambulates with a prosthesis and no assistive device. He is an active man who is now frustrated by his inability to work on his sailboat. He cannot tie the lines without pain, and he feels that they are insecure.

CHAPTER 5

Therapeutic Ultrasound and Phonophoresis

Barbara J. Behrens, PTA, MS | Ethne L. Nussbaum, PT, PhD
Peter C. Panus, PT, PhD

Learning Outcomes

Following the successful completion of this chapter, the learner will be able to:

- Define the parameters and terminology to describe therapeutic ultrasound.
- Discuss the effects of varying the parameters of therapeutic ultrasound.
- Describe the clinical applications of therapeutic ultrasound.
- Discuss the theory and rationale for the application of therapeutic ultrasound.
- Discuss the clinical decision-making process for determining treatment parameters when using therapeutic ultrasound.
- Outline current clinical and research trends in the utilization of therapeutic ultrasound.
- Describe safety factors in the use of therapeutic ultrasound including contraindications, precautions, and equipment considerations.
- Discuss the clinical decision-making process and procedures for phonophoresis.

Key Terms

Absorb
Acoustics
Attenuation
Beam nonuniformity ratio (BNR)
Biophysical effects
Cavitation
Couplant
Dosage
Duty factor
Eddy currents

Effective radiating area (ERA)
Frequency
Heterogeneous
Intensity
Longitudinal wave
Megahertz (MHz)
Parameters
Penetration
Phonophoresis
Pitch

Power
Rarefaction
Reflection
Refraction
Standing wave
Transverse wave
Ultrasound
Vacuum
Vibration

"It's not what you look at that matters,
it's what you see." —Henry David Thoreau

Patient Perspective

"Ultrasound, isn't that what they used to take a picture of my baby when I was pregnant?"

Ultrasound is one of the most commonly used physical agent modalities in many outpatient facilities and it is probably one of the least understood by clinicians. That does not have to be the case since it has been in use for many years and is based on fairly simple physical principles that are applied to the human body. Ultrasound relies on the application of sound waves to accomplish a therapeutic treatment goal. Sound has physical properties that are well defined and understood. They form the basic foundation for the use of and our understanding of this modality. The same principles that modify sound can be used to modify the effects of ultrasound, which means that there will be several different terms that will be covered throughout this chapter that will need to be understood. Please keep in mind that with all terminology there are synonyms, so examples will be provided to help solidify how things relate to each other. The science of sound is often referred to as an acoustic branch of science, so one of the first terms referred to will be the acoustical aspects of sound.

Acoustic principles have been used for detection since early in the twentieth century. **Acoustics** is a term

Continued

that is used when discussing the sound and how it is created and measured, and the mechanical waves that can be produced in gases, liquids, and solids including **vibration**. During the development of underwater detection apparates in the 1920s, acoustical principles were used to detect the location of submarines. Sound waves were sent out, and as they returned to the sender "ping" qualities would enable the sender to locate structures underwater, including enemy submarines (Fig. 5-1). Today this form of underwater detection is used to locate schools of fish for deep-sea fishermen. In the 1920s it was also observed that extremely high-pressure waves were damaging to

living tissues. As early as the 1930s, low intensities of therapeutic ultrasound were used for the first time in physical medicine to treat soft tissue conditions with mild heating. Today therapeutic ultrasound is a commonly used modality in therapy clinics, applied for its deep heating ability. However, therapeutic forms of ultrasound that are available in the twenty-first century are capable of many more applications than providing just deep heating. Some of the research that is discussed in this chapter outlines the potential benefits of ultrasound for nonthermal applications.

Physical Principles

Sound is produced by the vibration of a medium. If a column of air is vibrated, the human ear may be able to perceive the disturbance dependent upon the **frequency** at which it is vibrated. However, owing to the high frequency at which ultrasound is operating, the vibration causes a frequency or pitch that is too high for the human ear to perceive; its frequency is beyond audible sound, hence the term *ultrasound*. **Pitch** is a term commonly associated with music and it refers to the perceived frequency of sound or what you hear. The human ear is capable of interpreting vibrations at frequencies up to 20,000 cycles per second (cps) but ultrasound causes events at a much higher frequency, in the 1 million to 3 million cps range.

A sound wave exerts pressure on the medium it travels through, alternately compressing, or "squeezing," and then releasing pressure on the particles of the medium. During the release phase, which is referred to as **rarefaction,** molecules are spread out more than during the compression phase (Fig. 5-2). Sound can be transmitted through liquid,

gas, or solid media, but not through a vacuum. A **vacuum** is a space where all gas, air, or matter has been removed, which is why sound cannot travel through it. There is nothing to transmit it.

Beating a drum is an example of transmitting a sound wave through air. We hear the disturbance of the air particles because the frequency or pitch of the sound is within our audible range of 30 up to 20,000 cps. Therapeutic ultrasound is typically applied at either 1 million cps (**megahertz**) or 3 MHz.

Sound is a form of energy that is transmitted as a wave. There are a number of principles from wave theory that are valid for sound and ultrasound. A principle common to all wave formation is that matter in a wave does not itself travel; only the wave energy is transmitted. Each vibrating particle collides with and displaces its nearest neighbor, transferring momentum in a chain reaction. A desk ornament, sometimes called Newton's Cradle, illustrates some principles of this type of energy transfer. Newton's Cradle consists of a frame with five metal balls suspended on thin rods from a horizontal bar so that they touch each other at rest. If one lifts and releases the first ball, the mobile will be set in motion. When the first ball swings back into place it bumps into the next ball, which in turn bumps into the one after it. In this way, the energy is transferred from ball to ball. Because the last ball is unopposed, it swings out into space. However, when it drops back into line, a new cycle is set in motion (Fig. 5-3). The model will continue to oscillate until it runs out of energy and the balls then come to rest. And how does this relate to ultrasound in the body?

Waves can travel through media in three modes: as longitudinal, transverse, and standing waves. When the particles of a medium are compressed and decompressed in the direction that a wave travels, it is termed a **longitudinal wave.** When particle movement is at right angles to the direction of travel, it is termed a *shear* or **transverse wave.** Shear waves propagate or start more readily in solids, and longitudinal waves in liquids and gases. Note that a wave traveling on the surface of water is a shear wave, which means that it is an exception to the rule. Sound travels in a longitudinal mode in human tissues. However, a shear wave may be propagated when a pressure wave reaches

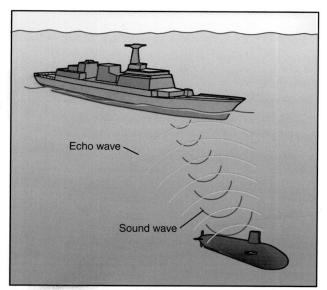

Echo wave

Sound wave

FIGURE 5-1 How sonar works.

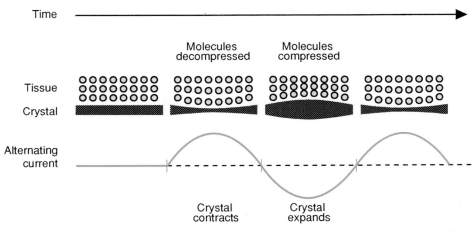

FIGURE 5-2 Schematic diagram showing the effect of a changing electrical field on crystal size and the effect of changing pressure on tissue molecules in the sound field.

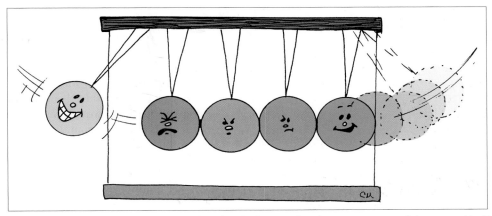

FIGURE 5-3 Newton's Cradle desk mobile. Movement of the first ball is translated into movement of the second ball just as compression force applied to soft tissues would be transferred to the underlying soft tissues during the application of ultrasound. Energy is lost as the distance from the source is increased and a rebound effect occurs, which can result in a cancellation of energy, or implosion.

bone, at which point the wave is transmitted along the periosteum, the outer covering of the bone.

If the source of a wave is kept stationary opposite a boundary and the path of the incident and reflected waves coincide, the resultant energy along the path is the algebraic sum of the two waves. In other words, since sound travels in sine waves you would be adding the sine waves together. If the waves are also exactly in phase so that the high and low peaks of the inbound wave reinforce the high and low peaks of the returning wave, very intense peaks and lows of **power** result and the position if the wave is stationary (Fig. 5-4).

This is called a **standing wave.** To prevent the formation of standing waves during a treatment intervention with ultrasound, the transducer must be continuously moved.

THERAPEUTIC ULTRASOUND

With therapeutic ultrasound, the wave transmitted to the tissues cannot be perceived as audible sound by either the patient or the clinician. However, if sufficient energy is delivered to the tissues, the patient will experience a sensation of mild warmth. Two characteristics of audible sound, pitch and volume, describe (or quantify) the frequency and power of sound. Both of these characteristics are important variables or **parameters** in therapeutic ultrasound that can be altered by the clinician administering the treatment.

Another important parameter in ultrasound is whether it is delivered in a continuous or an interrupted mode. The interrupted mode is more commonly referred to as pulsed ultrasound. The role of these and other parameters and the effects of ultrasound are discussed later in this chapter and in Box 5-1.

CHARACTERISTICS OF ULTRASOUND EMISSION AND RELEVANCE TO INTERVENTION OUTCOME

Characteristics discussed in this section include the following: frequency, pulsed- as opposed to continuous-wave delivery, absorption and **penetration, attenuation,** reflection and refraction, power, **intensity** and **dosage,** and beam profile. Understanding the clinical implications of these factors will assist the clinician in providing effective and safe applications using ultrasound (Table 5-1).

Constructive

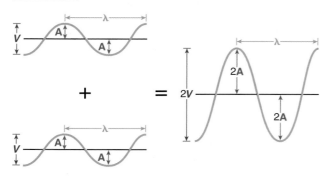

Properties of waves

λ Wave length – distance from crest to crest
V Frequency – number of crest passages per unit time
A Amptitude – distance from level of crest to level of trough

Destructive

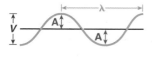

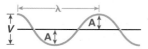

FIGURE 5-4 When sine waves have the same wavelength and are "in phase," they supplement each other and create a standing wave.

FREQUENCY

Frequency describes the number of events that take place within a set time frame. In sound waves, frequency refers to the number of completed wave cycles that pass a fixed point in 1 second. The higher the frequency is, the greater

TABLE 5-1 | Sound Terminology

SOUND		ULTRASOUND PARAMETERS
Pitch	Frequency	3 MHz to 1 MHz
Volume	Power	Watts (W)
Temporal quality	Mode of energy delivery	Continuous wave or pulsed wave

the number of cycles per second; conversely, a lower frequency means fewer cycles per second. Previously, the concept of pitch was mentioned in relation to the frequency of sound. Higher pitch sounds have higher frequency than lower pitch sounds. High-frequency sound waves vibrate air molecules more rapidly and thus expend their energy sooner, which means over a shorter distance, than do lower-frequency sounds (Fig. 5-5).

In contrast, lower-pitch sounds vibrate air molecules more slowly, thus expending their energy more slowly, and consequently have a greater capacity to travel distances than do higher-frequency waves. Consider the pitch of the sounds you would most likely hear if your neighbors were having a noisy party—would they be higher- or lower-pitch sounds? It is often the pounding of the bass speaker that alerts uninvited neighbors to the fact that someone is hosting a party. The fact that bass tones or lower-frequency sound waves travel a greater distance than higher-frequency sound waves is a physical characteristic of sound that will apply in determining whether to use a 1-MHz

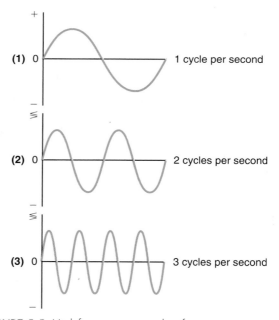

FIGURE 5-5 High-frequency versus low-frequency sine wave comparison. The author uses a slinky and stretches it to show how many more "rings/inch" there will be if it is only stretched about 2 feet versus 4 feet. The "rings" are closer together in the same space at a higher frequency.

(1 million cycles per second) or a 3-MHz sound wave for ultrasound therapy. The decision should depend on whether the target tissue lies in deep 2.5 cm (1 MHz) or superficial 1.5 cm (3 MHz) tissue layers.

PULSED OR CONTINUOUS ULTRASOUND

Continuous ultrasound refers to an uninterrupted flow of sound waves. Pulsed ultrasound is produced by intermittently interrupting the supply of electrical energy to the ultrasound head, which causes the acoustical energy, or sound waves, to be discontinuous or pulsed. The effects of ultrasound depend partly on duration of application; hence, there is a different effect when the output of the device is pulsed. If we continue the analogy to music, pulsed ultrasound would be similar to a musical note that is played repeatedly rather than held (Fig. 5-6.)

BEFORE YOU BEGIN

PARAMETER SELECTION QUESTION

1. Is the tissue I am treating superficial (use 3 MHz) or deep (use 1 MHz)?

Operational Definitions
Superficial: something that can be easily palpated, 1 to 3 cm deep
Deep: 3 to 5 cm deep within the tissue

The percentage of "on" time of ultrasound output is known as the **duty factor,** which can be expressed as a percentage or as a ratio. Clearly, when output is continuous, the duty factor is 100%; the output must have an "off" time for it to be considered pulsed. For example, if an ultrasound unit was programmed to have equalled "on" and "off" periods, this would mean that there would be output for half the time. The duty factor could be expressed as either 50% or a ratio of 1:1. Commonly used duty factors are shown in Table 5-2.

TABLE 5-2 | Common Duty Factors for Ultrasound

Continuous	Duty factor	100%
1:1 Ratio	Duty factor	50%
1:4 Ratio	Duty factor	20%

The intensity registered on an ultrasound unit during delivery of pulsed ultrasound indicates the intensity delivered *during* each pulse (i.e., the "on" period). It is a measure of the amplitude, strength or "intensity" of the sound wave during each pulse. This should be made clear in documentation by using the term "temporal peak intensity," or sometimes just (I_{SATP}) to describe the intensity of pulsed ultrasound treatment. The average intensity delivered during pulsed ultrasound is not shown on the unit. Average intensity of a treatment would depend on the duration of the "off" periods: the lower the duty cycle, the longer the "off" periods and therefore the lower is the average intensity. "Temporal average intensity" is sometimes abbreviated as the term I_{SATA}.

Practice varies with respect to documentation of pulsed ultrasound. Some clinicians describe intensity delivered during the pulse (I_{SATP}), yet others describe intensity averaged over the "on" and "off" pulse periods (I_{SATA}). The manner of reporting in textbooks and journals is similarly confusing. Thus, it is important that clinicians understand when using pulsed ultrasound that the unit controls always refer to the intensity delivered during the pulse. Appropriately, it is becoming the norm in current literature to define the terminology used for pulsed ultrasound intensity. In this chapter, intensity of pulsed ultrasound indicates the intensity delivered during the pulse, which is the intensity registered on the ultrasound unit (W/cm²).

BEFORE YOU BEGIN

PARAMETER SELECTION QUESTIONS

1. Is the tissue I am treating superficial (use 3 MHz) or deep (use 1 MHz)?
2. Are the signs and symptoms:
   a. Suggestive of acute inflammation?
Answer: Use a 20% duty factor, i.e., a ratio of 1:4, when treating acute inflammation.
   b. Suggestive of a chronic condition? (There are very few of the five cardinal signs of inflammation remaining with the exception of pain.)
Answer: Use a 100% duty factor, continuous wave, to produce a thermal effect.

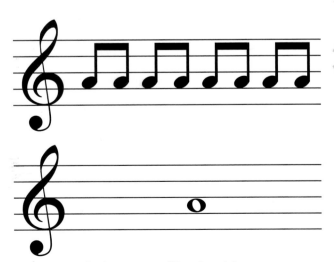

FIGURE 5-6 The first music staff has 8 eighth notes, representative of pulsed ultrasound. The second staff is followed by a whole note to be held for the entire measure, representative of continuous ultrasound. The pitch is the same for both, but one is *pulsed* and one is *continuous.*

When ultrasound is applied continuously (100% duty factor), the mechanical vibrations transmitted to the tissue molecules may cause heating of the underlying tissues. Thus, it is important to consider the underlying processes or metabolic state of the tissues when planning to use ultrasound. The five cardinal signs of acute inflammation are:

1. Pain
2. Erythema
3. Edema
4. Heat
5. Loss of function

If a heightened level of inflammatory activity were already present in the tissues, it would not be prudent to use continuous ultrasound because it could potentially make the condition worse by adding more heat to the area. A pulsed form of ultrasound, which would not likely generate additional heat in already hot tissues, might be more prudent. The relative acuteness of the patient's problem presents the second question that a clinician must consider when determining the parameters for ultrasound: Are the signs and symptoms suggestive of acute inflammation? Acute inflammation should be treated using a 20% duty factor and low intensity of ultrasound, delivered for periods of 10 to 20 minutes depending on the size of the treatment area and the transducer.

ABSORPTION AND PENETRATION

To **absorb** is to "take something in." **Penetrate** means to "enter into." "Penetration in ultrasound" is the term used to describe the distance from the sound source at which 50% of the original energy remains. As tissues absorb energy from a sound wave, a reduced amount of energy remains to be carried forward by the wave, which lessens its penetration; hence there is an inverse relationship between absorption and penetration. If energy penetrates deeply into the tissues, then it means it was not absorbed. If energy does not penetrate deeply, then the tissues have absorbed it (Fig. 5-7).

Energy from ultrasound is absorbed differently by different types of tissue depending on the compactness of the tissues. *Acoustic impedance* is the term that denotes the relative resistance of a medium to wave energy. The more dense or compact the molecules and the less compliant they are when squeezed, the greater their impedance or resistance. More work has to be done to transmit a wave against high impedance. Thus, it follows that over any given distance that a wave travels, when the medium is denser, a greater amount of energy is absorbed from the wave, and the distance decreases as that wave travels.

The density of a medium affects the distance that sounds travels. The rate of absorption of sound in air is relatively low because gas molecules are easily compressed; this explains the great distance that sound travels through air. In a dense medium such as brick, energy is rapidly consumed because the molecules resist compression. Unfortunately, there are few materials that completely absorb sound. However, the volume that you hear from your neighbor's party is not as high as the volume that you would hear if you were *at* your neighbor's party. Clearly, walls absorb some acoustical energy!

Human tissues represent a medium that is more dense than air but less dense than brick. Human tissues, however, are not a homogeneous medium, but consist of many layers and compartments of quite different densities. Each tissue layer transmits and absorbs ultrasound according to its specific acoustical properties. Fluid elements, such as blood and water, have the lowest impedance or resistance values and lowest acoustic absorption coefficients. This means that these elements are poor absorbers of ultrasound. Bone, the densest of all tissues, has the highest impedance value and highest acoustic absorption coefficient. This implies that bone is a good absorber of ultrasound. This is an important factor to consider when selecting the appropriate frequency of ultrasound, because the frequency controls the depth of penetration. In essence, this means that bone will absorb ultrasound easily, which may not be the desired effect. If a patient reports feeling a prickling sensation during a treatment with ultrasound, it may be that the periosteum, the outer highly innervated covering of bone, is absorbing the ultrasound, which means that the intensity of the ultrasound is too high.

REFLECTION AND REFRACTION

To reflect, according to *Webster's Dictionary*, is "to bend or cast back (as light, heat, or sound)." Sound waves may be partially reflected from boundaries or obstacles that they

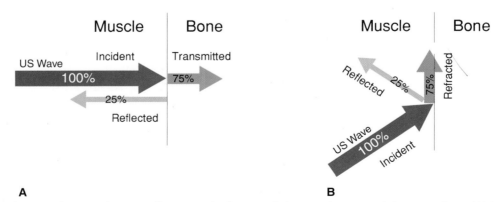

FIGURE 5-7 Schematic diagram showing reflection and refraction of ultrasound at a muscle-bone interface. (A) A wave arriving perpendicular to the boundary. (B) A wave arriving at an angle of 34° from the perpendicular.

encounter (see Fig. 5-7). The reflected portion of the wave continues to be subject to the effects of absorption, transmission, or further reflection on the original side of the boundary. The portion of the wave transmitted across the boundary is reduced in power as a result of **reflection.** Within biological tissues, such boundaries may be formed by any two **heterogeneous** tissue surfaces such as bone and nerve, muscle and adipose tissue, and many other examples.

In human tissues ultrasound repeatedly encounters boundaries. The acoustic properties of skin, fat, blood vessels, and muscle are similar. When ultrasound encounters boundaries between acoustically similar tissues, such as adipose and muscle, the amount of reflection is insignificant to treatment outcome. However, reflection increases in proportion to the difference in acoustic impedance of the two boundary materials. This means that when ultrasound encounters the boundaries in between bone and muscle, some of the acoustical energy is literally bounced back or reflected into the muscle and surrounding soft tissue and some is transmitted into the bone.

Because the impedance characteristics of metal and air are so different, the amount of reflection at a metal-air interface is about 99%, which means that the amount of ultrasound transmitted from a metal transducer to air is negligible. This is the reason for using a coupling medium between the transducer and the skin during ultrasound treatment. At a tissue-bone interface, about 25% of incident energy is reflected (see Fig. 5-7). If a wave meets a boundary at an angle, the reflected wave is directed away from the boundary on a new path that has the same angle but is a mirror image of the inward-bound wave.

The wave portion that is transmitted across a boundary is also subject to "bending" if the wave meets the boundary at an angle. This is known as **refraction.** As children, many of us played with a prism that split or refracted white light into the colors or wavelengths of the rainbow. The light was bent, that is, refracted at the glass-air interface because the prism walls were at an angle to the light source. Refraction is proportional to the difference in acoustic impedance of the boundary materials and to the incident angle of the wave. Refraction at boundaries formed by touching layers of skin, fat, blood, or muscle is very small. At tissue-air boundaries, however, because the impedance characteristics of tissue and air are so different, the transmitted wave changes direction by 90°. This means that the wave travels along the boundary of the original side instead of crossing it, which is known as total internal reflection. The clinical relevance is that ultrasound energy cannot be transmitted from the skin surface to air. For example, ultrasound applied to one surface of the hand would penetrate the tissue and at the opposite skin surface of the hand the beam would be bent back into the tissues where an additional amount of the remaining energy would be absorbed.

CAVITATION

Cavitation is the term for the stimulated behavior of micron-sized gas bubbles in the fluids in a sound field. These bubbles alternately shrink and expand as they lose and gain air during the compression and rarefaction phases of a sound wave, respectively. Cavitation can be potentially helpful or harmful to human tissues depending upon the type of cavitation. During *stable* cavitation the ebb and flow of gases causes small changes in bubble radius. It is thought that these effects may contribute to the increased cell membrane permeability that is observed following ultrasound application.

Cavitation activity increases as wave intensity increases. Under more intense pressure fluctuations, gas bubbles in an ultrasound field gradually increase in size, because they take in more air than they lose. During *unstable* cavitation, gas bubbles that have grown relatively large collapse violently under pressure. This event might have a parallel in the implosion of a building, which is a sight that most people find fascinating for a building but not for living tissues. To implode a building, explosive devices are set off in a highly orchestrated pattern so that the building loses its structural integrity and literally falls into itself. Although bubble collapse occurs on a microscopic scale in living tissue under the influence of ultrasound, it, too, can be highly destructive. However, a number of conditions must coexist for unstable cavitation to occur: ultrasound intensity must be high, the duration for bubble expansion must be relatively long, and there needs to be sufficient repetition of cycles for bubbles to reach a critical size. Frequency and cycle duration are inversely related; therefore, the duration for bubble growth is longer for lower-frequency waves. This explains why unstable cavitation occurs more readily at 1-MHz ultrasound rather than at 3 MHz.[1]

Unstable cavitation is more likely to occur during therapeutic ultrasound *when improper technique* is used, such as *not* moving the transducer during treatment, and may occur during pulsed or continuous modes of ultrasound.

BEAM QUALITIES

The importance of being aware of the characteristics of the beam of one's ultrasound device is often not fully appreciated. Two characteristics are of particular importance: the **beam nonuniformity ratio (BNR)** and the **effective radiating area (ERA)** (Figs. 5-8 and 5-9).

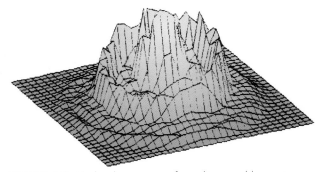

FIGURE 5-8 Hydrophone scan of an ultrasound beam in water showing uneven spatial distribution of energy. Characteristics: frequency 1 MHz; distance from transducer 0.5 cm; ERA 5.2 cm²; BRN 4.2.
(Courtesy of Excel Tech Ltd., Mississauga, Canada.)

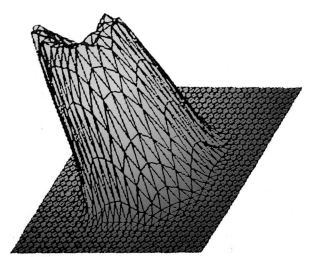

FIGURE 5-9 Hydrophone scan in water of an ultrasound beam of 1 MHz taken at a distance 10.0 cm from the transducer face.
(Courtesy of Excel Tech Ltd., Mississauga, Canada.)

Beam Nonuniformity Ratio

The BNR is the ratio of the peak power to the average power in the ultrasound beam measured in any cross-sectional plane. BNR is measured using an underwater microphone known as an acoustical hydrophone. The ultrasound applicator is mounted in a tank of degassed water, and the hydrophone moves over the surface of the applicator measuring the output intensity of the ultrasound head. A plot of the energy values is produced. BNR varies with distance from the transducer face. The BNR is measured at a fixed point at a distance of 0.5 cm from the transducer surface and it can be an indicator of the quality of the manufacturing process of the head. The result of the measurement is expressed in a ratio compared to one. (See Figs. 5-8 and 5-9.)

A beam ratio of 1:1 would mean that intensity would be unvarying over the entire cross-sectional area of the beam. However, this is not possible because of the physical phenomenon of wave interference, which occurs when waves meet in a medium. Acceptable BNRs for ultrasound devices in the United States are approximately 6:1 or lower. This means that as the transducer is moved over the skin, there is a "spot" in the tissues receiving ultrasound at an intensity of up to six times higher than the set dose (W/cm^2). This "hot spot" occurs whether the applicator is moved or held stationary. It is disturbing to find evidence in the literature that some devices operate with much higher BNR values than 6:1 because there is substantial evidence that very high doses of ultrasound can be hazardous to regenerating tissue.[2,3]

Effective Radiating Area (ERA)

The ERA (cm^2) describes the radiating area of the ultrasound applicator. This area is usually determined at a distance of 0.5 cm from the transducer face using the same underwater hydrophone mentioned previously. As a rule the ERA signifies the area of the beam that transmits

clinically effective radiation power (5% or more of the maximum intensity in that plane). By this rule, the very low-pressure area around the perimeter of the ultrasound beam is not considered to be part of the ERA. The ERA is less than the geometric area of the crystal that emits ultrasound. This is due to the fact that the crystal is housed inside of the head, making it impossible for the entire head to be part of the ERA. Accurate measurement of the transducer ERA is important because this value is incorporated into the intensity value registered on the device during ultrasound treatment (W/cm^2) (Fig. 5-10).

If the crystal is in some way defective and the actual ERA is not equal to the ERA measured at point of manufacture, then the registered dose is not an accurate reflection of the actual dose being received by the patient. The finding of discrepancies between actual and nominal ERA in supposedly functioning units is reported in the literature.[4,5] Furthermore, poor-quality crystals (those with high BNRs and low ERAs) are inefficient and are capable of operating with only a fraction of the surface area transmitting a sound wave. In the event of using a severely damaged crystal to deliver ultrasound, it would be hit and miss whether the target area actually received treatment.

To ensure that the intended dose of ultrasound can be delivered safely and reliably to the tissues, clinicians are encouraged to have the BNR and ERA of their ultrasound devices characterized on an annual basis, or more often if damage is suspected.

A short lab exercise at the end of this chapter, Let's Find Out: Testing the Transducer, has been developed to assist

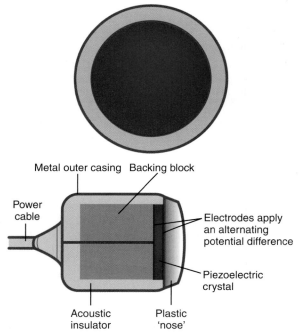

FIGURE 5-10 Comparison of (A) the transducer's effecting radiating area (ERA) with (B) the actual head of the transducer. (A) The darker area represents the crystal and the lighter outside area represents the housing for the head. (B) Side view of a transducer's construction and how the crystal is mounted inside the head itself.

in guiding one through determining whether or not there is acoustical output from transducers and viewing both the BNR and ERA of transducers.

BIOPHYSICAL EFFECTS

Biophysical effects refer to the physical effects on biological structures and processes. Therapeutic ultrasound can have significant or subtle biophysical effects on the underlying tissues, which will vary depending on whether the intensity delivered is high enough to cause heating of the tissues or whether heating is minimized or eliminated by using low-intensity and/or a pulsed-mode of delivery. The first two topic areas to be discussed in this section will be thermal and nonthermal ultrasound and their effects on the underlying tissues.

Thermal Ultrasound

Thermal ultrasound is the result of continuous ultrasound when it is administered in a treatment area that is no larger than twice the size of the transducer. The ultrasound beam does not itself transmit heat; however, heat is generated within the tissues as a result of increased molecular vibration due to absorption of ultrasound energy. Since the ultrasound is delivered in a continuous mode, which means that the duty factor is 100%, there is no "off" time, meaning that there is a constant flow of acoustical energy emanating from the transducer into the tissue below. Heat may be a result of *unstable* cavitation in the underlying tissues owing to the phenomenon of gas bubble "implosion" sending shock waves back through the tissues. This then releases energy that increases tissue temperature.

More heat is generated using ultrasound at a frequency of 3 MHz than at 1 MHz because more energy is delivered at the higher frequency. You can crudely mimic this effect by rubbing back and forth with a fingertip over a small area of your skin. Your skin will feel warmer where you were rubbing. Note that rubbing faster will produce greater heat. There is an inverse relationship between absorption and penetration, which means that when energy is absorbed, penetration is reduced. Thus, although heating is greater using 3-MHz ultrasound, the effect is more superficial when compared with 1-MHz ultrasound. Ultrasound at 3 MHz is too superficial for heating deeper lesions or structures that are not easily be palpated.

Energy from an ultrasound beam is also absorbed in proportion to the density of the tissue. Different tissues will therefore become heated in proportion to their density. Essentially, this means that the denser the tissue, the greater the absorption of ultrasound. This is the basis of the statement often seen in the literature that protein-rich structures selectively absorb ultrasound. It is probably more correct to state that ultrasound provides clinicians with an opportunity to deliver heat selectively to denser tissues, such as some forms of scar tissue, structures within the joint capsule, ligaments, and tendons.

General principles of heat transfer also apply to heating with ultrasound. This means that the temperature produced in the tissues will be the net effect of absorbed mechanical energy that is converted to heat and heat transfer to or from the tissues by conduction and convection. It was noted previously that ultrasound is rapidly absorbed by the periosteum, which becomes significantly heated. As a result, structures adjacent to bone gain additional heat in an ultrasound treatment by conduction of heat from the periosteum. Convection currents exist both within tissues via circulating blood and lymph, and external to tissues via circulating air or water acting on the skin. Clinically this means that, on the one hand, relatively dense, less vascular structures, such as branches of peripheral nerves, fresh scar tissue, the joint capsule itself, ligaments, tendons, and bone that rapidly absorb ultrasound and therefore heat well, also retain heat better than more vascular structures. Muscles, on the other hand, especially large, "red" postural muscles, have an abundant capillary network, with the result that they rapidly lose heat to adjacent cooler tissue through convection and conduction.

It is important to note that heating effectiveness of ultrasound is reduced if treatment is applied underwater. There are two reasons for this. First, some energy escapes from the skin surface to the water as a result of reflection. Second, some heat is transferred from the skin surface to the water by conduction. To compensate for that, the intensity of ultrasound should be increased by at least 50% when treatment is applied underwater. For example, if you typically apply ultrasound directly to the skin with gel coupling using an intensity of 1.0 W/cm², you would deliver 1.5 W/cm² to achieve similar thermal effects underwater.

Effects of tissue heating generally depend on the temperature produced rather than on the modality used to accomplish the temperature increase. Effects of ultrasound in the temperature range of 40°C to 45°C (104°F to 113°F) include reduced pain as a result of decreased nerve conduction velocity, increased metabolic rate, increased blood flow to assist in resolution of edema, enhanced immune system response, increased extensibility of soft tissue, and decreased viscosity of tissue fluids.[6] Temperatures above 45°C (113°F) are noxious (detrimental) to tissues and can cause irreversible tissue changes. However, pain is normally felt before dangerous temperatures are reached.

Nonthermal Ultrasound

Nonthermal ultrasound is most commonly associated with a pulsed mode of ultrasound, which means that the duty factor would be less than 100%. Lower duty factors represent longer "off" times and less potential for heat production. When heating effects of ultrasound are reduced, either by application of very low intensity or by using pulsed ultrasound, changes in cell function are noted. Mechanical vibration and acoustic streaming are possible mechanisms underlying the nonthermal changes.

MECHANICAL VIBRATION EFFECTS AND ACOUSTIC STREAMING

Cell membranes may become destabilized as a result of deformation and distortion. These are some of the forces cells are subjected to during ultrasound.[7] Radiation force is the proper term to describe this mechanism, but it is sometimes referred to by the slang term *micromassage*. Stable cavitation is also thought to contribute to these effects.[8] Cavitation produces **eddy currents** in the fluid surrounding a vibrating bubble. Eddy currents are interesting phenomena that can occur in fluids and gases. They are whirling currents of fluid (e.g., air or water) formed during turbulent flow such as what is created when the bubbles from unstable cavitation implode. Eddy currents turn back on themselves and eventually become detached from the main body of fluid, thereby opposing the main current flow. These small rotational current flows subject cell membranes and intracellular organelles in the vicinity of vibrating gas bubbles to additional rotational forces and stresses.[9] This fluid movement in a sound field is generally known as acoustic streaming, but in an ultrasound field in living tissue the scale of the events is microscopic, so it is sometimes called microstreaming.

To summarize the role of bubble activity (cavitation) in ultrasound mechanisms, it appears that gas bubbles are readily generated in an ultrasound field in living tissue, even at low intensities.[10] Bubble activity augments the mechanical effect of a pressure wave. The scale of cavitation depends on the ultrasound characteristics; the potential for bubble growth is limited when ultrasound is pulsed, the intensity is low, and the frequency is high. A higher frequency means that the cycle duration is shorter, so that the time for bubble growth is restricted. Pulsed ultrasound restricts the number of successive cycles for growth, which allows the bubble to regain its initial size during the "off" time. The likelihood of unstable cavitation during ultrasound is very low when using 3 MHz, 20% duty factor, and a low intensity. Unstable cavitation is a phenomenon, however, that must be considered in both thermal and nonthermal modes of ultrasound.

Patient Perspective

Remember that your patient does not understand what you are doing. It is important to explain ultrasound to him or her in terms that can easily be understood. Many patients are accustomed to feeling something with treatment interventions. This may or may not be the case with ultrasound. It is important for you to explain this before, during, and after your session with the patient.

Palpation of the area if appropriate, before and after treatment, can provide valuable information regarding soft tissue response to the treatment intervention as well as instil a more human touch to treatment.

Patients' Frequently Asked Questions

1. **Will I feel anything from this?**

Response: Therapeutic ultrasound is a treatment intervention in which the patient may not feel anything during the treatment itself with the exception of the transducer, which is the treatment head, moving over the surface of the skin. It is covered with a lotion or gel that helps to conduct the sound waves and sometimes might feel cool. If it feels uncomfortable in any way, patients must let the clinician know what they are feeling.

2. **Is this like what they use for babies?**

Response: Although they are both termed ultrasound, they are not the same. The ultrasound that is used during pregnancy is applied at a different frequency from that of the ultrasound used in physical therapy. Additionally, the techniques are different along with the purposes for the application. The ultrasound used during pregnancy is used to help provide an image of the developing child, which means that the information coming back to the sound head is what is most critical. This is in contrast to the ultrasound in physical therapy in which the energy that leaves the sound head is used as a treatment modality, not as an imaging technique.

3. **Would a dog be able to hear the ultrasound that is used in physical therapy?**

Response: No, the frequency range for dogs is between 67 and 45,000 Hz, which means that although they can hear a dog whistle and humans cannot, they would not be able to hear ultrasound at 1 million Hz.

4. **Why do you use that gel?**

Response: Since ultrasound is administered at such a high frequency, it does not travel through air. It needs something to transmit it, which is just what the gel or lotion does.

5. **Why do you move that "thing" on me during a treatment?**

Response: That "thing" is called a transducer and is delivering the ultrasound to the treatment area. It must be moved to prevent a buildup of too much energy in one place, which could potentially be damaging to the underlying tissues.

6. **If it is doing something, why don't I feel anything?**

Response: Ultrasound is a unique modality that works at deep tissue depths, which means that it is reaching into the soft tissue below the skin and affecting structures in a more subtle manner to increase circulation or promote the ability for structures to stretch.

7. **Is there a maximum number of treatments you can have with ultrasound? If yes, what is it?**

Response: Every treatment intervention that you receive in physical therapy is assessed to determine whether or not it was beneficial for you and your diagnosis and symptoms. If what we are doing is providing you with benefits that last and help us attaining your goals, then that approach will continue. However, if whatever is being used is not successful, then it will be discontinued.

Safety Considerations and Precautions in Applying Ultrasound

Precautions are common considerations that must be observed when working with patients to protect their safety. Some clinicians have held longstanding beliefs regarding ultrasound that may or may not be valid regarding potential precautions. It is important that the rationale behind these considerations be easily understood by anyone planning on administering ultrasound *prior* to any treatment application. Please refer to Box 5-2 for more detailed information.

Discomfort should not be experienced during treatment with ultrasound. Pain is usually a sign of too much periosteal heating, and treatment settings must be adjusted by decreasing intensity or moving the transducer more quickly. It is possible to cause a burn with ultrasound,[11] and this is the reason why some national radiation councils have regulated output limits for ultrasound.[12]

A stationary transducer technique is not safe for most clinical applications; there is a great risk of overheating at "hot spots" in the field and there is an added risk of standing wave formation. This caution especially applies when there are implanted materials in the tissues.[13,14] Metal reflects about 90% of incident ultrasound,[4] and therefore the chance of standing wave formation is increased. Plastic responds like periosteum and it absorbs a large percentage of ultrasound.[13,15] Generally, treatment over implanted materials is safe provided proper technique is used. It should be noted that a stationary transducer technique (20 minutes daily at intensity of 0.15 W/cm² I_{SATP}, pulsed 1:4) is used in treatment of fractures; however, the intensity is very low compared with most other clinical applications.

Skin integrity is not essential for ultrasound treatment, but direct contact with gel may be inappropriate over some skin lesions or in conditions such as dermatitis. A water-immersion technique can be used, provided infection control procedures are followed. Clinicians should protect themselves by wearing loose-fitting gloves when applying ultrasound underwater. A glove traps air, which reflects ultrasound, and thus prevents self-treatment at the same time as preventing the risk of cross-infection. The use of rubber gloves would further protect the clinician from unwanted sonation owing to the fact that rubber insulates against ultrasound transmission.

Transducer crystals are fragile and transducers should be handled with care. Intensity should be increased only when the transducer is in contact with a suitable medium, because a metal-air interface prevents transmission of the pressure wave. When energy cannot flow from the transducer, the metal cap itself becomes heated. Heat may affect the bonding of the crystal within the transducer. Repeated careless use of the transducer will eventually damage the crystal; hence, the potential rationale behind underwater application techniques. If the sound head that is available is too large to maintain contact with the treatment area, then an underwater technique might be a better choice for both the patient and the life of the transducer. Please note

BOX 5-2	Precautions for Using Therapeutic Ultrasound	
PRECAUTIONS	**WHY**
Open wounds	Sterile saline must fill the wound for transmission of the acoustical energy.
Impaired cognitive ability	The patient must be able to communicate any uncomfortable sensation under the transducer
Pregnancy	During the later stages of pregnancy there are no data to indicate that there would be any adverse effects as long as the treatment area does not include the abdomen, ankle,* or lower back (1 MHz).
Peripheral vascular disease	The presence of peripheral vascular disease is not a problem in itself; however, if the treatment area is involved, the patient's tissue may not be able to maintain homeostasis or respond to an increase in tissue temperature.
Advanced age	As long as the patient is alert and his or her sensation is intact, ultrasound should not cause any difficulties.
Previous experience with ultrasound	The patient may or may not have had a positive experience. It is important to elicit this from the patient, in addition to explaining the rationale for *this* application for *this* diagnosis.
Over joint or metal implants	Ultrasound may cause heterogeneous heating within the joint if a cementing medium was used. To avoid this, use 3-MHz ultrasound, which does not have sufficient depth to reach the internal aspects of joints. Metal implants tend to elevate in temperature faster than bone, but they also dissipate the heat faster, making them safe for ultrasound application.
Pain with pressure	Ultrasound involves the movement of a transducer along the surface of the skin. If this type of pressure is painful for a patient, an underwater technique with ultrasound can be employed.
Lack of sensation	Ultrasound may be administered in a thermal or a nonthermal mode. If administered in a thermal mode, the patient must be able to report pain as a potential adverse response.

*The superior medial aspect of the ankle referred to as SP-6 by acupuncturists is a popular point for labor induction via acupuncture or acupressure, and this area may be used to induce or encourage uterine contractions.

that heating effectiveness of ultrasound is decreased if treatment is applied underwater.

CONTRAINDICATIONS

Ultrasound is contraindicated over or close to the site of any abnormal growth. Ultrasound promotes cell proliferation and cell activity. Abnormal cell division occurs in many serious medical conditions, including cancer and tuberculosis, and in non-life-threatening diseases such as psoriasis. The clinician should be extraordinarily cautious in treating undiagnosed pain in patients with a past history of malignancy.[16] Tissue being treated with radiation therapy should not be treated with ultrasound.

Rapid cell division is also a feature of fetal development and, as yet, the effect of therapeutic ultrasound on the human fetus is unknown.[17,18] For safety's sake, ultrasound treatment should never be applied over the lower back or abdomen of a pregnant woman. It should be noted that diagnostic ultrasound, at 2.5 MHz, is used at significantly lower doses than therapeutic ultrasound (less than 0.1 W/cm^2).

The contraindication to treatment over epiphyseal plates in children has been passed on as part of the tradition of ultrasound. These plates give rise to new bone cells and also create another heterogeneous surface area. The original work that gave rise to concern was done on legs of anesthetized dogs at very low frequency (0.8 MHz) and high intensity (0.5–3.0 W/cm^2) using a stationary transducer. These characteristics would have caused high absorption and intense heating of bone. Subsequent work on animal bone by Dyson[19] and others[20] suggests that healing fractures in fact benefit from ultrasound at low doses. In view of the adverse treatment characteristics of the early work and advantages found in recent work, treatment over epiphyseal growth plates in children is not considered a contraindication at the present time. However, it is suggested that if this area is treated, it should be done with caution and only low treatment intensity should be used.

Treatment of the orbits of the eyes and directly over the gonads is contraindicated. Ultrasound should not be applied over the area of a thrombus.[21] Treatment of the calf after a deep vein thrombosis is also contraindicated: it is thought that ultrasound might dislodge a thrombus, which could have catastrophic consequences.

Pain and temperature awareness must be checked before treatment with continuous-mode ultrasound. Sensation must be intact to proceed with heating dosages owing to the possibility that ultrasound can cause a burn. If the patient is unable to accurately report that type of sensation, the administration of ultrasound would be considered unsafe for that patient.

Infection that is enclosed under tension, that is, abscesses, should not be treated with ultrasound. Infection with open drainage can be treated using very low pulsed dosages but should be discontinued if there are any signs of increased redness, heat, or pain.

Ultrasound vibration may interfere with operation of any implanted medical device, such as a pacemaker, and should be avoided directly over the device. Ultrasound should not be applied below the ribs directed toward the heart.[22]

Ultrasound should not be used when there is uncontrolled bleeding. It is ideal for enhancing resorption of fluid, but treatment should begin after bleeding has ceased or after replacement factor has been administered in conditions such as hemophilia. See Box 5-3 for a more detailed list of contraindications.

SECOND-ORDER EFFECTS OF NONTHERMAL ULTRASOUND

The primary site of ultrasound interaction is the cell membrane.[7] Destabilization of membranes leads to increased permeability, which allows various ions and molecules to diffuse into cells, where they precipitate a series of secondary events. Research on ultrasound has particularly focused on influx of calcium ions because calcium is a known second messenger for other cell functions, including protein synthesis. Histamine has also attracted interest because of its influence on circulation and stimulating effect on protein synthesis. Clinically, it has been demonstrated that ultrasound facilitates tissue repair, and researchers are exploring various events that could explain the clinical benefits.[23] Some of the observed effects are discussed later.

Histamine and other vasoactive substances are released from granules in mast cells and from circulating platelets during ultrasound.[24] The extent of mast cell degranulation is in proportion to the ultrasound intensity. It is important to keep treatment intensity low as there is some indication from animal research that high-intensity ultrasound could produce too much histamine, which could potentially prolong inflammation rather than producing the desired stimulus to healing. Prolonged inflammation can potentially occur with any heat treatment given during the acute inflammatory stage of an injury.

Increased plasma and cells for repair appear in the extravascular tissues following ultrasound. The result is an enhanced inflammatory response. Inflammation is an essential step in tissue repair because it brings cells that are normally in the circulation into the injury site. It is hypothesized that ultrasound may enhance the normal response. For example, monocytes arrive at the wound site and are turned into macrophages, which cleanse the wound. The macrophages also release growth factors that attract fibroblasts.

Phagocytic activity of macrophages is increased during ultrasound. Accompanying this is an increase in the concentration and activity of lysosomes. Lysosomes are the enzymes that break down foreign material. Clearing of tissue debris and bacteria is essential for tissue regeneration to begin.

Fibroblasts increase in number and show increased motility following ultrasound, a response that has been linked to macrophage release factors.[25] An increase in early fibroblast activity may provide a better basis for the subsequent step of fibroblast attachment and proliferation. Ultrasound also increases protein synthesis by fibroblasts. Protein synthesis is the basis of collagen production.

BOX 5-3 | Contraindications for Using Therapeutic Ultrasound

CONTRAINDICATIONS	WHY
Pregnancy	There is no physical therapy indication for application of ultrasound over a pregnant uterus, and there are no data to indicate what effect, if any, the therapeutic application of ultrasound would have on a fetus.
Abnormal growth (presumed malignant)	Thermal applications of ultrasound can potentially elevate tissue temperature, increase circulation to the area, and thus may enhance growth.
Metastasis	Thermal applications of ultrasound can potentially elevate tissue temperature, increase circulation to the area, and thus may enhance the growth or spread malignancy to other tissues.
Lack of sensation (thermal application)	If the patient is unable to report pain, he/she can easily burn with thermal applications of ultrasound.
Thrombus	The application of ultrasound directly over a thrombus may cause the clot to dislodge and move to the heart, lungs, or brain.
Pacemaker	There is no indication to apply ultrasound directly over a pacemaker. The potential for interference between the pacemaker and the ultrasound device exists.
Psoriasis	Ultrasound must be applied to the skin via an acoustical medium without airspace. Psoriatic skin may have too many irregularities to permit passage of the ultrasound into the patient.

Angiogenesis is enhanced following ultrasound.[25] This is the process of endothelial cell "budding" and formation of new blood vessels. The mechanism by which ultrasound stimulates this process is not clearly identified. It may be secondary to enhanced macrophage activity.

Capillary density is increased in ischemic tissue after repeated treatment with ultrasound. The effect, though, is only evident after repeated doses. The same effect has not been demonstrated in non-ischemic tissue.[26]

Ultrasound enhances wound contraction.[25] During wound contraction, healthy collagen fibers at the edge of the lesion exert a centralizing pull on the wound edges, which assists in closing the wound. Accelerated contraction is an advantage in tissue repair because less scar tissue is required to fill the wound gap. Ultrasound has been shown to increase myofibroblast activity, which may be the mechanism through which ultrasound enhances wound contraction.

In summary, the effects of ultrasound have been examined during different stages of tissue repair. Benefits have been demonstrated for various components of the inflammatory, proliferation, and maturation processes. Research is ongoing to identify the mechanisms and interactions that occur.

SEQUENCE OF ULTRASOUND IN A TREATMENT PLAN

Stimulation of tissue healing by pulsed ultrasound is a cascade of events triggered by the treatment and the benefit is not immediately evident. Pulsed ultrasound may be sequenced prior to any other activities in a treatment plan to take advantage of possible pain-relieving effects of the modality.[27-29]

One of the purposes of thermal treatment with ultrasound is to increase tissue temperature and subsequently tissue length; therefore, stretch must be imposed on the tissue immediately after ultrasound. Without proper sequencing, thermal doses of ultrasound are pointless. There are numerous methods of stretching tissues, and clinicians generally have individual approaches they prefer.[30] The important point is not how the stretch is achieved but that heated tissues should be stretched through the full available range of motion, without increasing pain levels. Independent or assisted exercise using static stretch techniques, mechanical devices, proprioceptive neuromuscular facilitation techniques, or end-of-range mobilization techniques are all appropriate methods of applying stretch.

Some research suggests that optimal results are achieved if the stretch is maintained until tissue temperature returns to baseline.[31-33] Based on studies that investigated the time it takes for human tissues to cool after heating with ultrasound,[34,35] full-range stretching activities should continue for a duration of 8 to 10 minutes post-ultrasound. Strengthening and other activities that do not fully stretch the shortened tissue should be postponed until after the cool-down period.

It is the practice of some clinicians to apply ice in combination with ultrasound. The reason for applying ice is not clear. Cooling changes the depth at which ultrasound is absorbed because attenuation increases as temperature decreases.[36] This means that the amplitude of the intensity decreases exponentially owing to the decrease in temperature caused by the ice application. Prior cooling with ice would result in more superficial absorption of ultrasound. In fact, ice and ultrasound appear to have contradictory effects. Ice causes vasoconstriction, decreases cell metabolism, and overall has an anti-inflammatory effect. Low-dose ultrasound is a pro-inflammatory agent. Ice effectively restricts bleeding and swelling in acute tissue trauma; low-dose ultrasound should be initiated 24 hours after injury to promote resolution of the edema and repair of tissue. Application of ice immediately before or after ultrasound would likely inhibit the beneficial effects of the ultrasound treatment.

The use of ice and thermal doses of ultrasound also appears to be contradictory.[37] Decreasing tissue temperature, and thereby increasing stiffness, prior to or after using ultrasound to heat the tissues in order to resolve the stiffness, appears to be indefensible! Moreover, there is no advantage to rapid cooling of tissues during or after stretch.[38] The application of any heating modality when sensory nerves have been numbed is a dangerous practice, and for this reason ice should not be applied before ultrasound.

The use of ice for pain control at the end of a treatment session that initially included thermal ultrasound may be seen clinically. There seems to be no conflict in this practice, as long as the ice application is of brief duration. Research shows that for an application of less than 8 minutes, the effect of ice is very superficial (less than a 1/2 inch or 1 to 2 cm).[39] Therefore, a 5-minute ice pack will relieve post-treatment pain without counteracting the benefit achieved from deep heating ultrasound, stretch, and exercise.[40]

ULTRASOUND TREATMENT PROCEDURES

A minimum amount of preparation is required for ultrasound treatment, which probably accounts for its high favor among clinicians. No discomfort is experienced during treatment with ultrasound, which no doubt explains why it is well accepted by patients.

Preparation for Treatment

Before uncovering the body part to be treated and positioning the patient, all jewelry and personal accessory items should be removed from the treatment area.

Treatment in a whirlpool, or in water that has been vigorously stirred, is not recommended because air interferes with ultrasound transmission. Air bubbles on the patient's skin should be gently smoothed away before underwater treatments administered using a basin of water.

Air bubbles are also trapped on the skin under gel: they are just less obvious and thus get overlooked. When skin is generously covered in hair, trapped air can be a problem. Ultrasound devices, with electronic coupling indicators, confirm this by switching off power. Transmission improves if air is removed by smoothing down hair with a wet cloth before applying the gel or if gel is applied to the transducer and not the patient.

Patient Education and Consent to Treat

Patient consent implies that the patient has been advised of the benefits and risks of the procedure, as well as the sensation he or she should experience during the procedure.

In the case of pulsed ultrasound, there should be no sensation other than the gliding of the transducer on the skin. When ultrasound is administered in a continuous mode, mild skin heating occurs, usually at doses above 0.8 W/cm².

Pain is a sign of excess periosteal heating. Patients should be instructed that the appropriate sensation is mild warmth and that excess heat, or pain, should be reported immediately.

For patient safety, and to ensure delivery of effective treatment, inability to report skin warmth should be an exclusion criterion for continuous-mode ultrasound. Potential to cooperate should be considered when patients are very young, very old, or have limited understanding.

Preparation of Equipment

The treatment space must be organized for safety, comfort, and access. Clinicians should be seated with back support or standing and positioned so that the tissues being treated and device controls are simultaneously visible and within easy reach.

Time and intensity controls should be at zero before the main power is switched on and returned to zero after treatment. A reminder is appropriate at this point that the clinician checks on the ultrasound unit that the intensity meter is set at W/cm² (not total watts).

Patient Position

Patient comfort is basic to treatment with any modality. Support is required for trunk and limbs, whether the patient is lying or sitting. Injured limbs need the additional support of pillows or rolled towels and should be positioned in elevation when there is edema, even though treatment periods are relatively short.

Specific positioning must be considered in addition to general principles. For example, the supraspinatus tendon lies partly under the acromion process. If the arm is passively extended, the humeral head rotates forward from underneath the acromion process, and the tendon can be reached where it inserts into the posterior aspect of the greater tubercle; in other positions, this tendon is not accessible. The patient can be seated in a high-backed chair with his or her arm resting on padding over the chair back to achieve the required position.

Technique

Acoustically conductive gel is applied to the transducer. There should be a 1- to 2-mm layer that would be sufficient to allow gliding of the sound head without creating a mess. The sound head is moved in overlapping circles or linear paths from the moment power is increased. Overlap ensures even distribution of energy to the treated tissue (recall that maximum intensity is distributed in the central one third of the ultrasound beam). The rate of transducer movement is slow, at a maximum of 3 to 4 cm/sec. If the transducer is "raced" over the skin, ultrasound effects may be reduced.

To ensure maximum penetration, the sound head should be parallel to the tissue surface, which means adjusting the angle of the sound head to the contours of the part being treated. In other words, the transducer is "pointed" toward the target tissue. This applies to treatment given in contact, when air gaps must not be allowed between the transducer and skin, and to water-immersion techniques, when treatment should be applied as close as possible to the skin.[1]

Adjustment of Parameters During Treatment

If a patient reports pain during a thermal mode treatment with ultrasound, the clinician must immediately lower the intensity. There are two options for proceeding: the treatment can be delivered at a lower intensity, provided the patient still feels skin warmth, or the intensity can be delivered at a higher frequency, which will result in less periosteal heating and should eliminate pain. If pain persists despite the use of one of these steps or the patient complains of increased pain associated with the condition, treatment should be terminated.

Repetition of Treatment

There is no limit to the number of ultrasound treatments that can safely be applied, but treatment should continue only if measurable and sustained benefits are noted.

Observation and Documentation of Ultrasound Treatment

Assessment after treatment and prior to the next treatment is essential to demonstrate to the patient, as well as to satisfy the clinician and any third-party payer, that ultrasound is effective for the patient's problem.

Some immediate benefits can be expected. Ultrasound has a soothing effect on pain, possibly from stimulation of mechanoreceptors in the skin acting via a gate control mechanism, or from the sedative effect of heat. Another possible immediate benefit is a change in the "feel" of tissue as a result of heating effects. Palpation will provide the surest sign of such improvement. An example is the softening of an unresolved hematoma after ultrasound. However, the feel of tissues is a subjective measure, and as such is difficult to document.[41]

Incomplete documentation makes it difficult to repeat successful treatment or to determine how to modify treatment. Good documentation includes details of the patient's position; the treatment area; the technique; the transducer size; the machine settings for frequency, duty factor or pulse ratio, intensity, and duration of treatment; and the nature and sequence of other activities.

Care of Therapeutic Ultrasound Equipment

BIOMEDICAL DEPARTMENT INSPECTION

Electrical safety checks should be left to technical experts who may be available through institutional biomedical departments or through manufacturers or distributors of equipment. Specialized equipment is required to measure the total power, spatial distribution of power (BNR), and ERA of the ultrasound beam to recalibrate machines. In view of the fact that displayed dosage tends to be unreliable, recalibration every 6 months is advisable.

CLINICAL MONITORING

Clinicians should watch for signs of damaged or worn equipment. When the metal face of a transducer is old, it becomes dull or ridged and may not transmit ultrasound adequately. Undue heating of the transducer is a sign that energy is being lost within the transducer instead of being transmitted to the patient. The most common damage is inflicted by dropping the head. A dent in the transducer casing is a sign that the crystal might be damaged.

A water displacement test can be performed to see if the unit is emitting any sort of pressure wave. The ultrasound applicator is held underwater with the transducer face angled upward but not parallel to the surface of the water. Tilting the face in this way will protect the crystal from a possible pressure wave being reflected from the water-air boundary back to the transducer face. Intensity is turned up to 1.0 W/cm². The beam should produce a cone-shaped displacement of water at the surface opposite the transducer face. The displacement should disappear as the intensity is reduced. Note that this simple test does not replace regular checks by qualified technicians. Another method for testing this is depicted in Figure 5-11.

The conductivity of gels and medicated topical agents for **phonophoresis** can be tested in a similar manner. The height and shape of the water displacement are compared, using the method noted earlier, with and without a layer of the **couplant** (1 to 2 mm) spread over the transducer face.

REVIEW OF ULTRASOUND BASICS

Further research is essential in the field of therapeutic ultrasound. Randomized controlled clinical trials are needed to confirm the promising findings of preclinical studies and uncontrolled human trials.

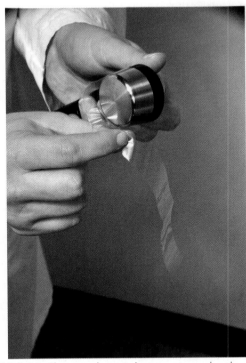

FIGURE 5-11 The transducer is being wrapped with a layer of cellophane tape. Once a "well" is created, then water can be added. Adjust the intensity to continuous and 1 W/cm². There should be movement of the water indicating that there is acoustical energy being emitted from the crystal. This simple exercise enables clinicians to test the transducer for output. It is recommended that this be performed frequently.

An understanding of the physical properties and physiological effects of ultrasound is fundamental for effective use of the modality. Distribution of energy in an ultrasound beam is dependent on frequency and beam characteristics. When the BNR is higher than 6, damaging "hot spots" might occur in the tissues. A moving head technique is required to distribute the points of maximum intensity evenly throughout the treated tissue. Absorption and penetration depend on frequency and the density of the tissue encountered.

Good clinical outcomes using ultrasound are achieved by careful treatment planning. Low-intensity pulsed ultrasound stimulates cellular activities that in turn trigger a chain of events leading to enhanced tissue repair. Benefit is obtained at dosages of about 1.0 W/cm^2 I$_{SATP}$ (20% duty cycle) for about 5 minutes per 5 cm^2 of treatment area (an area equal to the size of the transducer). Heating of tissue by ultrasound is for the treatment of chronic inflammatory conditions that restrict movement. Heating occurs with continuous-mode ultrasound using intensities between 0.8 and 1.5 W/cm^2 or higher. Tissue stretching should be performed immediately following heating. Appropriate timing is an important aspect of treatment.

Therapeutic Equipment

GENERATORS AND TRANSDUCERS

Therapeutic ultrasound machines generate a pressure wave by causing a crystal to vibrate. The crystal, which is made of natural quartz or a synthetic material, contracts and expands in response to an applied alternating electric current (refer to Fig. 5-1). The crystal is housed inside an applicator called a transducer, which is the term used to describe a device that converts energy from one form into another. Current is delivered to the crystal via an insulated cable. As the current alternates in phase, the crystal changes its shape from concave to convex. In effect, the crystal vibrates; hence, electrical energy is converted to mechanical energy.

The treatment surface of the transducer consists of a metal plate that acts as an interface between the vibrating crystal and the patient's tissues. Continuity between the crystal, metal plate, and tissues is essential for transmission of the pressure wave to the tissues. Reflection at a metal-air boundary is about 99%. Therefore, an air gap between the transducer face and skin will prevent the pressure wave from leaving the transducer. This results in heating of the transducer, which is potentially damaging to the crystal.[42] An acoustically conductive couplant, oil or water based, is normally used between the transducer face and skin to ensure continuity. Ultrasound units may feature a light-emitting diode (LED) on the transducer head or some other type of signal to warn the operator when skin contact is inadequate. When contact is poor, power is interrupted and the unit timer pauses until good contact is resumed. This type of feature has been developed in an attempt to assist the clinician in improving the application technique: special attention has to be given to keeping in contact with the contours of the limbs and joints.

It has been noted that ultrasound treatment is applied at different frequencies. In older machines, a separate transducer had to be purchased for each frequency. Some devices offer 1 or 3 MHz on the same transducer head. Transducers are not interchangeable on ultrasound devices; you should not attempt to fit one transducer to another unrelated ultrasound unit. Transducer crystals are delicate and can be damaged by being dropped. This is a problem for clinicians because it is difficult without sophisticated measuring equipment to check the integrity of a crystal.

Therapeutic transducers are available in a variety of sizes from 1 cm^2 to 10 cm^2, with 5 cm^2 the most frequently used. The appropriate size, however, should be selected according to the anatomic area to be treated. For example, a 5-cm^2 or 10-cm^2 applicator may be suitable for use around the knee, whereas a 1-cm^2 applicator may be more appropriate to access the web space between the thumb and first digit of the hand.

Ultrasound units are produced with various options. Flexibility is an advantage because setting ultrasound characteristics specific to the tissue condition will lead to better treatment outcomes. Options should be available for the following characteristics:

- Frequency (1 or 3 MHz)
- Transducer size (various ERAs/external dimensions)
- Continuous or pulsed modes (with several options for pulsed modes)
- Dosage (intensity) from 0.1 to 3.0 W/cm^2

Features should include

- Intensity display (analogue or digital type)
- Treatment timer
- Electronic contact monitor (LED on the transducer housing or head, or some type of alert signal on the console)

Intensity and Power of Ultrasound

The measured energy output of an ultrasound transducer should register on the device in two ways: as power and as intensity. Power, measured in Watts (W), refers to the electrical energy delivered to the crystal. Intensity, measured in Watts per square centimeter (W/cm^2), refers to the average power distributed over the ERA of the transducer. An intensity of 1 W/cm^2 would mean that 1 Watt of electrical energy was being delivered for each square centimeter of the ERA of the transducer. Intensity is the term used to describe clinical treatment.

BEFORE YOU BEGIN

PARAMETER SELECTION QUESTIONS

1. Is the tissue I am treating superficial (use 3 MHz) or deep (use 1 MHz)?
3. Are the signs and symptoms suggestive of acute inflammation?
   (Use a 20% duty factor, i.e., a ratio of 1:4, when treating acute inflammation.)
4. What is the transducer BNR? (Consider the potential for "hot spots" in the treatment field.)
5. What is the transducer ERA? (The treatment area should be approximately twice the size of the ERA of the transducer.)

The appropriate intensity of ultrasound to use in treatment is determined by the treatment goal—it depends on whether thermal or nonthermal effects are most wanted. Intensity of 3.0 W/cm² is often stated as the safe limit for treatment, based on the World Health Organization guidelines.[43] Lower intensities, however, are usually effective. A prudent approach to using any form of applied energy is to use the lowest dosage that achieves the desired effect.

In order to reproduce ultrasound treatment reliably and safely, it is important to document accurately and set treatment parameters correctly. It is critical for the reader to comprehend the difference between intensity (W/cm²) and power (W).

Using faulty equipment forces the clinician into errors that he or she cannot detect and can make the difference between effective and ineffective treatment. For example, if the efficiency of the crystal or its housing is impaired, the electrical signal is not converted to ultrasound energy and the patient does not receive the dose registered on the meter. A discrepancy of 20% between the registered dosage and actual output is the limit of acceptability.[4]

DOSAGE OF ULTRASOUND TREATMENT

Dosage incorporates the parameters previously discussed (frequency, intensity, and duty factor) as well as treatment time. Treatment time is based on the size of the treatment area relative to the ERA. The most recent evidence suggests that treatment time should be about 5 minutes per transducer ERA for treatments delivered in either pulsed or continuous mode. For example, for treatment of a 5-cm² area using a transducer with ERA of 5 cm², an effective treatment time would be approximately 5 minutes. For a treatment area of 10 cm², the treatment time using a transducer with ERA of 5 cm² would double (10 minutes). Areas larger than 10 cm² can be treated using pulsed ultrasound, but the time must be increased accordingly. With respect to thermal treatments, it is important to note that ultrasound does not produce clinically meaningful heating of deep tissues when the surface area treated exceeds 10 cm². Longer treatment times than 5 minutes per 5 cm² of surface area might be necessary to elevate deep tissue temperature if the patient is not capable of tolerating intensities greater than 1 W/cm². These examples are given as a starting point for the dosage of ultrasound.

Principles of Therapeutic Application

A HISTORICAL PERSPECTIVE

Ultrasound was used therapeutically as early as 1930 using devices that produced only continuous-mode output.[43] During that early period, it was thought that treatment benefit resulted entirely from heating effects. During the 1960s, although pulsed ultrasound was available, the common approach in rehabilitation was still to use continuous-wave output in the range of 0.5 to 1.5 W/cm². Then the development of focused ultrasound for medical diagnostics and continuing interest in ultrasound hyperthermia for treatment of cancer promoted intensive investigation into ultrasound effects. One finding of the early research was that ultrasound affected tissue growth using very low intensities. This knowledge, generated largely by medical biophysicists, filtered through to physical therapy literature in the early 1980s, leading to a gradual change in practice, in particular, a lowering of treatment dosage. The medical research also gave impetus to research activities led by physical therapists directed specifically toward therapeutic effects of ultrasound.

A Current Perspective: Research on Therapeutic Ultrasound

Research through the 1980s was most commonly conducted by scientists who were not themselves users of therapeutic ultrasound.[44-46] This trend has now been reversed. Also, the research in the early 1980s concentrated mainly on low-intensity pulsed ultrasound to promote tissue healing. However, current work also includes studies that evaluate heating dosages of ultrasound.

Heating Tissues with Continuous-Wave Ultrasound

The literature on heating of human tissues using ultrasound is limited because invasive procedures are required to measure temperature at depth.[48-50] Some researchers have used a pig (porcine) model to simulate heating in humans;[51,52] others have used tissue specimens.[53] Heating effectiveness has been examined using ultrasound intensity in the range of 0.5 to 3.0 W/cm². It has been demonstrated that tissue temperature can be increased to 40°C or higher using ultrasound, as measured by thermistors inserted at various tissue depths.[48] However, some investigators evaluated effectiveness of thermal dosages of ultrasound by measuring tissue extensibility rather than temperature.[48,49,54] The research demonstrates that tendon heats at a faster rate than muscle.[49] It appears that the duration (10 minutes) and area (10 cm²) of ultrasound are both critical factors in effective heating because increased tissue extensibility was not produced when duration was decreased or treatment area increased.[55,54] However, further research on tissue heating with ultrasound is essential. It is not the purpose here to review all of the literature; the reader is encouraged to consult the reference list provided at the end of the chapter for additional information.

Interestingly, the literature demonstrates that ultrasound does not effectively heat large muscle bellies such as those of gastrocnemius or quadriceps. The likely explanation for this finding is that muscles have low capacity to absorb ultrasound and an excellent blood supply that dissipates any heat generated by ultrasound. Other modalities should be considered for heating large muscles: shortwave preferentially heats vascular tissue and may be a more effective approach to muscle heating than ultrasound. In contrast, ultrasound is effective for heating skin and subcutaneous tissue or high-protein content tissue such as tendon and ligament. Structures adjacent to bone, including the deep muscle layer, are also effectively heated by ultrasound because of conduction of heat from the periosteum.

CLINICAL STUDIES USING ULTRASOUND AS A HEATING AGENT

There are a few controlled clinical studies that examine the effectiveness of ultrasound in chronic inflammatory connective tissue conditions, including lateral epicondylitis[48,52,57] and osteoarthritis.[57] The signs and symptoms of these conditions include soft tissue swelling, decreased range of movement, loss of strength, pain, and impaired function. The conditions have different etiologies but there are some common underlying problems, including chronic inflammatory changes, with fibrosis, tissue contracture, and possibly adhesion development.[52-55]

Clinically, there is no good rationale for using ultrasound as a sole treatment intervention for chronic conditions of the type noted earlier. When tissues are heated, the goal is usually to increase extensibility; thus, stretch must be applied and exercise through the range of motion must follow. What, then, can be learned from studies that treat chronic conditions with heating levels of ultrasound but without appropriate adjunctive treatment? Conversely, can ultrasound in combination with other treatment interventions be properly evaluated? A dilemma is apparent for the researcher and clinician. For the reader it is clear: the literature must be approached critically. We need to be able to justify what we do with physical agent modalities. At the same time we do not want to discard treatments based upon the negative findings of research when the research is problematic, the number of subjects in the study is small, and the treatment might yet be beneficial.

CLINICAL STUDIES USING ULTRASOUND TO FACILITATE TISSUE REPAIR

The difficulty in studying effects of ultrasound on human tissue wounds is obvious, with the result that most of the research has been carried out on experimental animal wounds. Animal studies often draw criticism because loose-skinned animals, typically rats and guinea pigs and, to a lesser extent, pigs, have skin that heals differently from human skin. While there are drawbacks to using animal models for ultrasound research valuable information has emerged, which can and should be extrapolated to clinical practice, albeit with discretion.

Animal studies have been used to demonstrate the effects of ultrasound on wound contraction,[31] rate of wound healing,[53-55,58,59] rate and quality of tendon healing,[30,60-62] formation of new blood vessels,[63] activity of the phagocyte system,[64] and the role of calcium ions.[65] Pulsed ultrasound delivered at intensities of approximately 1.0 W/cm² I_{SATP}, using a 20% duty cycle, consistently appeared to accelerate healing in a variety of experimental wound models, including open wounds, tendon repair, and tissue damage induced by trauma or drug infiltration.

There are a number of clinical studies that have looked at the healing effects of ultrasound on venous ulcers[66-69] and pressure ulcers.[70] Treatments using ultrasound in continuous mode did not produce benefit.[67] Some treatments using low-intensity pulsed ultrasound (20% duty cycle) at a dosage of 1.0 W/cm² I_{SATP} for 5 to 10 minutes were beneficial.[66,69] However, it should be noted that no benefit was seen when pulsed ultrasound was delivered at the same intensity (1.0 W/cm² I_{SATP}) but using a 10% duty cycle.[68] What is the optimal pulse ratio for stimulation of tissue healing? It has been shown that when the intensity is extremely high, even though the pulse is short (2 milliseconds), the occurrence of unstable cavitation is enhanced,[71] which may explain the lack of benefit using a 10% duty cycle.

More recent investigations have demonstrated that pulsed ultrasound (1.0 to 2.5 W/cm² I_{SATP}; 20% duty cycle) produced benefit when used in repetitive type of soft tissue injuries. In these studies, it is important to note the use of relatively long ultrasound duration (15 minutes) and increased treatment frequency (20 to 24 sessions over a 6-week period) compared with earlier studies.[51,52]

A new area of interest in ultrasound use has emerged, with the finding in large multicenter human trials that bone healing is enhanced with low-intensity ultrasound (0.15 W/cm² I_{SATP}, pulsed 1:4) applied for 20 minutes daily using a stationary transducer technique.[20,72]

In contrast with the facilitation of human tissue repair demonstrated by use of low-dose pulsed ultrasound, a study using high-intensity ultrasound to treat damaged tissues demonstrated a worsening of subjects' symptoms. Muscle inflammation and pain from delayed-onset muscle soreness (DOMS) were induced in human volunteers and then ultrasound was applied to the muscle at 1 MHz, 1.5 W/cm² for 5 minutes using a 10-cm² transducer size.[73] Compared with controls, the treatment increased subjects' symptoms of pain. The results of this work suggest that such high-intensity ultrasound can aggravate tissue injury during the acute phase. Important points for treatment that can be deduced from the research include the following:

- The area of tissue that can be realistically heated using ultrasound is an area equivalent to twice the size of the radiating area of the transducer, that is, 2 × ERA.
- Water-immersion techniques considerably diminish skin and tissue heating. To compensate, treatment intensity should be increased by 50% or until the patient reports feeling warmth on the skin.
- Using a frequency of 1 MHz, an intensity of 1.0 W/cm² and a stroking technique at a rate of 3 to 4 cm/sec, a change in temperature of 4° to 6°C can be expected in dense tissue close to bone.
- Therapeutic temperatures (40°C or 104°F) are achieved with 10 to 15 minutes of ultrasound treatment using intensities of 1 to 1.5 W/cm².[74,75]

Treatment techniques for the facilitation of tissue healing include the following:

- Pulsed ultrasound is most likely to improve tissue healing using low intensity of 1.0 to 2.5 W/cm² I_{SATP}, with a 20% duty cycle.
- Brief treatment duration, of about 2 minutes for each surface area equivalent to the ERA of the transducer, is sufficient to stimulate the healing process in chronic ulcers.

- Soft tissue injuries, such as strains, sprains, subacute hematomas, and so on, should be treated for up to 5 minutes per ERA of the transducer.
- Treatments should be repeated daily or every 48 hours to enhance healing.

RELIABILITY AND EFFICIENCY OF ULTRASOUND EQUIPMENT

A number of investigators have evaluated the accuracy of ultrasound equipment.[2,4,5] There appears to be agreement that equipment is not reliable and clinical units should be checked regularly. Researchers have found units with BNR values[2] and ERA characteristics[4] that do not agree with values reported by the manufacturer. The availability of suitable technology (since about 1980) and increasing awareness of the importance of accurate measurement of BNR and ERA have promoted this area of research.

TRANSMISSION PROPERTIES OF ULTRASOUND COUPLANTS

Some studies have compared transmission properties of ultrasound coupling media to determine their relative acoustic transmission efficiency.[11,74,75]

The medium used to compare coupling media is usually degassed water. The results show that acoustic conductivity differs among products. The properties required of a couplant are that it lubricates the skin, absorbs very little ultrasound, has sufficient viscosity not to "run off," has no odor, does not stain clothing, and is not susceptible to bubble formation. A sterile, semisolid, 3.3-mm-thick gel dressing called Geliperm (Geltech Sons Ltd., Newton Bark, Chester, England) apparently transmits 95% of incident ultrasound power.[76] Testing of this product was carried out underwater with the adhesive dressing applied directly to the transducer face. Although this product transmits well, it should be noted that it would be difficult to apply a dressing to skin without trapping air, which would significantly decrease its acoustic conductivity. The purpose of the dressing is to allow treatment directly over abrasions and wounds, using water or gel lubricant between the dressing and transducer. The authors who tested the product recommended using a syringe to fill shallow wounds with sterile saline before applying the dressing, to eliminate air gaps between the tissue and dressing. An adhesive transparent wound dressing available in North America (Opsite, Smith & Newphew, Inc., Lachne, Quebec, Canada) transmitted less than 10% of radiated ultrasound power when tested using similar procedures.[77]

PHONOPHORESIS

The suffix *phoresis* means movement or transmission in a medium and as we have already discussed in this chapter, *phono* applies to sound. When the two are put together as in phonophoresis, the meaning implies using sound waves to transmit or move something. Phonophoresis is the use of the mechanical properties of ultrasound's energy waves to deliver drugs through the skin (transcutaneously) for both local and systemic tissue sites. Ultrasonic energy has been documented to transcutaneously deliver a wide variety of agents from proteins to various substances that are either attracted to or repelled by water which are known as hydrophilic and hydrophobic drugs.[90-93] However, the mechanical energy parameters for many investigations reporting ultrasonic enhanced transcutaneous delivery are not within the 1 to 3 MHz frequency range currently available to clinicians within the United States. Additionally, when investigators examine these promising new ultrasonic parameters, less research is focusing on the frequencies that are clinically used.

As stated, phonophoresis is the practice of applying ultrasound through a medicated couplant. The mechanism by which phonophoresis may enhance uptake of drugs is not so simple. One theory is that ultrasound pressure drives the drug into the skin. An alternative theory is that heating of superficial tissue causes vasodilation of dermal capillaries, which speeds up the rate at which drugs are absorbed into the circulation. Another theory suggests that increased permeability of cell membranes enhances diffusion of the drug into the cell, which is the site of the chemical interactions. The studies on phonophoresis reflect all three theories.

The goal of some early studies[78,79] and some more recent work[80] was to determine the depth to which drugs were driven by ultrasound. Investigative procedures such as muscle sectioning in rabbits and joint aspirations in dogs were carried out as soon as 10 minutes after phonophoresis. Whereas drugs appeared in greater amounts at the depth of muscles, no benefit was found at the depth of the canine knee. It remains uncertain whether the drug needed more time to diffuse to greater depth or if in fact benefit is limited to the depth of muscle.

It is unclear from a review of the literature whether drugs that normally diffuse through the skin diffuse in greater amounts after ultrasound.[73,80,81] Early uncontrolled clinical trials[81-83] showed that patients with a variety of inflammatory conditions benefited from phonophoresis using hydrocortisone preparations; implying, as with the above in-depth studies, that the drug was successfully transmitted through skin by the ultrasound. However, in two recent controlled studies on epicondylitis,[84,85] hydrocortisone preparations of 10% and 1% were used without significant benefit compared with ultrasound alone. A topical nonsteroidal anti-inflammatory drug was rubbed on the skin in another study, and the same amount of drug was absorbed regardless of whether ultrasound was added.[86] In preliminary testing it was shown that less than 1% of ultrasound power was transmitted when 10% hydrocortisone acetate was mixed in gel and used as a couplant. Poor transmission qualities of some preparations may account for lack of benefit.[81]

The question of how much ultrasound is transmitted through phonophoretic preparations[75,87-89] was not examined until long after early clinical trials. A variety of topical creams, ointments, and gels were generally found to be less efficient than regular gels and water for transmission. For most products tested, transmission was better at a frequency of 1.5 MHz and 3 MHz than at 0.75 MHz, and there was no difference in transmission between intensities of 0.3 W/cm^2 and 1.0 W/cm^2.[87] Preparations tested at 1.5 W/cm^2 suggested that drug-containing media that transmitted 80% ultrasound power could be considered good media. There was a choice of corticosteroids, local anesthetics, and non-steroidal anti-inflammatory and salicylate drugs that met this criterion. The products tested included a variety of creams, ointments, gels, other media, and mixed media. Conflicting findings have been reported on some preparations.[88] Transmission through hydrocortisone cream has been reported as 47%.[89,90] Neither level is satisfactory and it makes it difficult to explain the earlier clinical successes of hydrocortisone phonophoresis.

The confusion in this field may be because of lack of uniformity in research methods. There are differences in the preparation of phonophoretic products, especially in concentration of active ingredients, in the type of base (gel, ointment, or cream), and in the dosage and number of ultrasound treatments. It seems that in preparation for phonophoretic treatment, a clinician should at the least perform a crude underwater test on the medicated product to see if it transmits any ultrasound.

Current experimental and clinical research evidence suggests that phonophoresis possesses the potential for transcutaneous delivery of anti-inflammatory pharmaceutics and potentially other medications. However, current evidence as to the pharmacokinetics of the depth of penetration and the clinical value of the pharmaceutics at these various tissue depths remains to be defined. The current discussion will present published investigations using phonophoretic parameters currently available to clinicians.

Parameters for Phonophoresis

As with transfer of the mechanical energy from the ultrasound transducer to the surface of the skin, the coupling gel used during phonophoresis should allow the transfer of the mechanical energy from the ultrasound transducer to the surface of the skin. Inclusion of a drug into the coupling gel should minimize the loss of the conductance of the mechanical energy. However, not all phonophoretic couplants are equal in the conductance of the mechanical energy.[94–97] There is a difference in couplant transmission of the mechanical energy that is independent of the drug.

Thus, clinicians should inquire about the phonophoretic gels used and how they were prepared. For example, whipping a drug into an acoustically conductive gel although normally effective for mixing purposes is *not* effective for acoustical gels as it adds air, which significantly decreases the ability of the medium to transmit ultrasound. Additionally, the drug being delivered should be stable in an ultrasonic field, and not provide additional resistance to the conduction of the mechanical wave in the coupling gel.

Phonophoresis has one clear advantage over iontophoresis, which is the ability to deliver both ionized and nonionized drugs.[90] As with iontophoresis, the stratum corneum has been proposed as the primary impediment to transcutaneous phonophoretic drug delivery.[91,98] Several phenomena have been proposed as responsible for phonophoretic enhancement of this form of drug delivery across the skin.[91,98,99] These phenomena include:

- Stable cavitation of gas bubbles within the stratum corneum
- Convective transport
- Thermal heating increasing the kinetic energy of the drug
- Mechanical stresses induced by the pressure variations of the wave

Additionally, this transport may occur either within the stratum corneum itself or through hair follicles and sweat glands as with iontophoresis. Iontophoresis is discussed in greater detail in Chapter 11.

There are a variety of types of transport systems that can occur within the tissues in the body. Transappendageal refers to transport via hair follicles or other appendages, transcellular transport, which occurs through the corneocytes in the outer layer of the skin, the stratum corneum, and intercellular transport, via the extracellular matrix. Mitragotri and co-investigators[99] examined these phenomena in vitro with clinically relevant frequencies, 1 to 3 MHz, and intensities, 0 to 2 W/cm^2. The conclusion from the investigation was that phonophoretic enhancement of transcutaneous drug delivery was the result of stable cavitation occurring intracellularly at the cell membrane of the corneocytes in the stratum structure. In this analogy, the **corneocytes** are the bricks (Fig. 5-12).

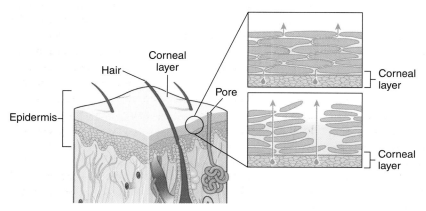

FIGURE 5-12 The corneocytes are the "bricks" in the brick-and-mortar-like construction of the epidermis. When the corneocytes are uniformly arranged, the passage of substances through the corneocyte layer cannot occur as easily as it can when there is a break in the surface. The presence of hair follicles and pores permit transappendageal transport to occur to facilitate absorption into deeper layers. However, transappendageal transport is *not* enhanced by phonophoresis.

Cavitation from ultrasound appears to disorder the structures of the stratum corneum enhancing the passive movement of drugs down a concentration gradient from the exterior skin surface to deeper layers. Additionally, this cavitation enhancement of transcutaneous drug transport occurs at 1 MHz and *not* 3 MHz. Thus, unlike iontophoretic transcutaneous transport, transcutaneous phonophoretic transport is not transappendageal.

Transcutaneous transport of all drugs may not be enhanced by phonophoresis and those that are enhanced by phonophoresis may not all be enhanced to the same extent. Mitragotri and co-investigators[99] proposed that the phonophoretic enhancement, compared with passive delivery, is directly proportional to the organic solubility of the drug, and inversely proportional to the passive permeability of the drug.

WHY DO I NEED TO KNOW ABOUT...
ACOUSTICAL PROPERTIES

If the drug was whipped to make a paste for application onto the skin, the drug may not pass through the skin. Whipping adds air and air is not acoustically conductive.

BEFORE YOU BEGIN
You *must* ask the patient if he or she has any allergies to medications and document his or her response in the patient's chart.

- Phonophoresis involves the delivery of a medication across the patient's skin.
- It is *not* sufficient to rely on anyone else or believe that anyone else has already asked the patient whether or not he or she is allergic to the medication that is about to be administered.
- Remember to check the acoustical capability of the drug by applying it to the surface of the transducer, surrounding the transducer with cellophane tape and adding water.
- If the surface of the water is disturbed when the intensity of the ultrasound is increased, then the drug is acoustically conductive. If not, it is not.

The comparison supported their conclusion that variations in previously reported phonophoretic enhancement for various drugs are the result of physicochemical differences in the agents being phonophoresed. Some drugs such as fluocinolone acetonide and dexamethasone are enhanced by phonophoresis (12-fold); other drugs such as indomethacin and hydrocortisone are also enhanced by phonophoresis but not to the same degree (3- to 5-fold); and some drugs such as lidocaine and salicylate are not enhanced by phonophoresis. Finally, one investigation reported enhanced back-diffusion of a drug into the phonophoretic gel when compared with passive application.[101] The drug was applied to the skin, then ultrasonic gel covered the drug and the area was sonated. See Table 5-3 for a summary of studies and medications delivered via phonophoresis and the indications for their use.

EXPERIMENTAL PHONOPHORESIS OF ANTI-INFLAMMATORY DRUGS

As previously discussed, the transcutaneous permeation of *all* anti-inflammatory drugs is not enhanced by phonophoresis. Thus, subsequent discussion focuses on those investigations using agents for which transcutaneous permeation is augmented by phonophoresis. The early phonophoretic investigations have been previously reviewed.[91] Several researchers documented cortisol delivery at intramuscular and deeper tissue levels.[101-103] However, those experimental parameters do not parallel the clinical use of the modality, and the relevance of these results in clinical practice is debatable. The phonophoretic delivery of several different nonsteroidal anti-inflammatory drugs (NSAIDs) has been examined. In vivo 1-MHz phonophoresis augmented the effects of indomethacin.[104-106] This augmentation was both intensity and time dependent, with higher intensity and longer times resulting in higher systemic blood drug levels. The phonophoretic enhancement also occurred with continuous and pulsed modes of ultrasound at 1 MHz. These investigations do not define whether the ultrasonic transducer was moved during the application. However, as a result of the epidermal histological appearance during 1 MHz at 0.75 W/cm^2 continuous ultrasound or 1.5 W/cm^2 1:2 pulsed ultrasound, the transducer may have remained stationary during the application. Finally, even after the phonophoretic application was terminated, the systemic blood drug levels continued to increase. This final pharmacokinetic information demonstrates that even after clinical phonophoretic application, the augmented drug delivery continued. A similar time- and intensity-dependent phonophoretic enhancement of flufenamic acid using an in vitro synthetic membrane has also been documented.[106,107] However, no phonophoretic enhancement of the NSAIDs, salicylate, or benzydamine have been observed.[109,110]

In humans, hydrocortisone was phonophoresed at 1 MHz continuously on the volar, palmar aspect at 1.0 W/cm^2 for 5 minutes.[111] No drug was detected in the proximal venous blood either during or up to 15 minutes post-phonophoresis. Finally, the maximal tissue depth for which 1-MHz phonophoresed hydrocortisone has an anti-inflammatory effect was also examined in the pig.[112] Hydrocortisone was phonophoresed with a continuous mode at 1.5 W/cm^2 for 5 minutes. No anti-inflammatory effect was observed for the phonophoresed hydrocortisone. In these investigations, a 10% (weight/volume) hydrocortisone concentration was used for phonophoresis. In contrast to hydrocortisone phonophoretic investigations, examination of dexamethasone phonophoresis has resulted in positive outcomes. In the previous investigation by Byl and colleagues in the pig,[112] dexamethasone phonophoresis, at parameters previously described for hydrocortisone, resulted in subcutaneous anti-inflammatory effects at the phonophoretic application site. However, no anti-inflammatory effects were observed in sub-muscular or sub-tendinous tissues underneath the application site.

TABLE 5-3 | Clinical Phonophoresis in Musculoskeletal Dysfunction

DYSFUNCTION	MHz	PARAMETERS W/cm^2	MIN	PHARMACOLOGICAL AGENT	Rx	OUTCOME
DOMS elbow flexors	1	1.5	5	0% TS (NSAID)	3	Mixed results[115]
Musculoskeletal dysfunction	1	2.0 max.	9	1% Hydrocort (Nonsteroidal anti-inflammatory drug)	8–10	Effectiveness
	1	2.0 max.	Maximum	10% Hydrocort	5–7	10% > 1%[117]
Musculoskeletal dysfunction	1	1.5	8	0.05% Lidex (Topical steroid)	9	Phono vs US; similar objective outcome[118]
Musculoskeletal tendonitis	3	1 (20% pulsed)	5	0.015% DexLido Glucocorticosteroid *Topical anesthetic	5	Phono vs US; similar objective & subjective Outcome[119]
TMJ dysfunction	1	0.8–1.5	15	1% Indo (nonsteroidal anti-inflammatory drug)	2	Subjective & objective improvements[116]

* Supply meaning of asterisk
Abbreviations: **Dex/Lido:** X% dexamethasone plus X% Lidocaine; **DOMS:** delay onset muscle soreness; **Hydrocort:** hydrocortisone; **Indo:** indomethacin; **Lidex:** fluocinonide; **Phono:** phonophoresis; **Rx:** number of treatments; **TMJ:** temporomandibular joint; **TS:** trolamine salicylate; **US:** ultrasound. The concentration of lidocaine in the coupling gel could not be determined from the methods.

Additionally, anti-inflammatory effects were observed at tissue sites distal to the phonophoresis, suggesting a systemic delivery of the dexamethasone. In humans, 1 MHz continuous mode phonophoresis at 1.5 W/cm^2 for 8 minutes was conducted on the volar, palmar surface, and proximal venous blood samples were collected at the cubital fossa.[113] These phonophoretic parameters were similar to those previously described for hydrocortisone.[111] Forty percent of the subjects receiving the dexamethasone phonophoresis demonstrated measurable, but not quantifiable, venous drug levels. In contrast, another human investigation examined 1 MHz continuous dexamethasone phonophoresis at 1.0 W/cm^2 for 10 minutes.[114] Phonophoresis was conducted on the volar, palmar surface, and proximal venous blood samples were collected at the cubital fossa. No measurable dexamethasone was detected in the proximal venous blood. With similar phonophoretic parameters, what may account for the differing pharmacokinetic results in the human dexamethasone phonophoretic investigations.

In the porcine (pig) investigation documenting subcutaneous anti-inflammatory effect following dexamethasone phonophoresis[112] and the human investigation measuring proximal venous dexamethasone post-phonophoresis,[113] the concentration of dexamethasone in the phonophoretic gel was 0.33%. In the pharmacokinetic human investigation that was unable to document measurable dexamethasone in the venous blood following phonophoresis, the concentration of drug in the phonophoretic gel was 0.017%.[114] The differences in the dexamethasone concentration in the phonophoretic gel may account for the differing results in the investigations examining dexamethasone phonophoresis.

As hypothesized,[91] phonophoresis enhancement of NSAIDs and SAIDs is selective, being in part dependent upon the chemical structure and hydrophobicity, or water-repelling, property of the agent. Additionally, optimal phonophoretic delivery of the agent is dependent upon the phonophoretic frequency and intensity, treatment duration, and mechanical transmitting properties of the coupling gel.

CLINICAL PHONOPHORESIS OF ANTI-INFLAMMATORY DRUGS

Stronger conclusions may be based on clinical investigations using control or alternative treatment groups. Therefore, only these clinical investigations will be currently reviewed. Several different investigations have examined the clinical benefit of phonophoresis with different anti-inflammatory drugs, and the results have been mixed. Both NSAIDs and SAIDs have been used in these clinical investigations, and the phonophoretic parameters and major outcome(s) are summarized in Table 5-3.

Decreases in pain perception of delayed-onset muscle soreness (DOMS) in elbow flexors by 10% trolamine salicylate phonophoresis was examined in a multi-control investigation.[115] There was no significant reduction of DOMS when compared with sham ultrasound or passive application of 10% trolamine salicylate. However, trolamine salicylate phonophoresis reduced the DOMS when compared with an equivalent treatment with ultrasound alone, as the ultrasound treatment increased the DOMS when compared with the sham ultrasound or passive hydrocortisone application. In contrast, phonophoresis of 1% indomethacin did reduce the subjective and objective complaints of pain in patients with temporomandibular joint (TMJ) dysfunction.[116] The patients receiving comparable ultrasound therapy as treatment for their TMJ dysfunction did not demonstrate a significant reduction in their dysfunction. These results suggest that the clinical improvement in the patients receiving the indomethacin phonophoresis was the result of the addition of the drug to the ultrasound therapy.

Similarly, a retrospective review compared 1% and 10% hydrocortisone phonophoresis in patients with various musculoskeletal dysfunctions.[117] Patients being treated with 10% hydrocortisone for their dysfunction required fewer treatments and demonstrated improved subjective assessment of the dysfunction with 10% hydrocortisone phonophoresis. In contrast, the use of 0.05% fluocinonide phonophoresis was compared with a similar duration of ultrasound in the treatment of various musculoskeletal dysfunctions.[118] Both groups demonstrated similar subjective and objective improvements in the various dysfunctions. The investigators concluded that the addition of the fluocinonide to the ultrasound treatment was not significantly beneficial. Finally, phonophoresis of dexamethasone with lidocaine in the treatment of tendonitis was compared with the use of a similar treatment of ultrasound alone.[119] As with the fluocinonide phonophoretic investigation,[118] no additional improvement was observed in either the subjective or objective outcomes when dexamethasone with lidocaine was added to the ultrasound treatment. Several conclusions concerning the success of these various clinical investigations may be made based on the potential for enhancement of transcutaneous drug permeation by phonophoresis[91] and the time required for optimal phonophoretic application:[97] first, the success of the indomethacin phonophoresis in comparison with the salicylate phonophoresis.[115,116] Theoretical constructs suggest that indomethacin would be enhanced by phonophoresis, whereas salicylate would not. Additionally, the phonophoretic application duration in the indomethacin investigation was three times as long as in the salicylate investigation. Based on previously discussed phonophoretic parameters, this additional time should enhance the transcutaneous permeation of the indomethacin compared with the salicylate.

In the investigations examining SAIDs,[117–119] the investigation documenting enhanced success with 10% compared with 1% hydrocortisone did not include an ultrasound-only treatment group.[117] This may explain the proposed success in this investigation compared with those documenting no difference between ultrasound and phonophoresis with an SAID.[118,119] Phonophoresis of dexamethasone would be predicted to have enhanced the delivery of the drug.[97] However, the clinical investigation demonstrated several experimental design deficiencies.[119] The phonophoretic treatment duration was just 5 minutes with pulsed (20% duty cycle) 3-MHz ultrasound. Both the short treatment duration and the 3-MHz frequency would not augment the transcutaneous transport of dexamethasone.[97] Additionally, the 0.015% dexamethasone concentration in the coupling gel may have been insufficient to provide an anti-inflammatory in the subcutaneous tissues. The final concentration of lidocaine in the coupling gel could not be determined from the methods. Finally, the authors assumed that the mechanical conduction efficiency of their coupling gel was similar to that of another steroid with efficient mechanical conduction. However, for the phonophoresis, dexamethasone tablets were crushed and mixed into the coupling gel. These crushed tablets may contain inert material, which potentially alter the mechanical conduction of the gel.

Finally, other cutaneous localized disorders may also be clinically treated with phonophoresis of anti-inflammatory drugs. A case study reported the use of phonophoresis in the treatment of cutaneous epitheloid granulomas that are associated with sarcoidosis.[120] Treatment of the nodules on the dorsal aspect of the hand with SAIDs had previously failed. Continuous mode hydrocortisone phonophoresis at 0.5 to 0.6 W/cm² for 5 minutes was used to treat the nodules. The phonophoretic frequency was not stated. Following a month of twice per week treatments, the nodules were markedly reduced. The anti-inflammatory effect of the hydrocortisone phonophoresis was concluded to be local, as nodules in other parts of the body were not reduced. These clinical results suggest that phonophoresis of anti-inflammatory drugs may be of clinical benefit in other cutaneous conditions such as hypertrophic scarring, keloid formation, or psoriasis.

PHONOPHORESIS AND PHONOPHORETIC PRODUCTS: INDICATIONS FOR TREATMENT

Apart from ultrasound, there are other modalities to stimulate tissue healing, such as pulsed shortwave diathermy, laser, and low-frequency transcutaneous electrical nerve stimulations (TENS). There are alternatives for heating tissues, such as continuous shortwave diathermy, hot packs, and other superficial agents. A series of questions may assist the inexperienced clinician in deciding whether ultrasound is indicated.

BEFORE YOU BEGIN

PARAMETER SELECTION QUESTIONS

1. Have I asked the patient whether or not he or she is allergic to the medication that is planned for use?
2. Have I documented his or her response to the question regarding an allergy to the medication?
3. Is the tissue I am treating superficial (use 3 MHz) or deep (use 1 MHz)?

4. Are the signs and symptoms suggestive of acute inflammation? (Use a 20% duty factor, i.e., a ratio of 1:4, when treating acute inflammation.)

5. What is the transducer BNR? (Consider the potential for "hot spots" in the treatment field.)

6. What is the transducer ERA? (Consider contact between the transducer and tissue surface.)

7. How many areas equivalent to the ERA of the transducer fit into the treatment area? (Use a treatment time of about 5 minutes for each ERA, but remember that the treatment area must not be larger than twice the size of the transducer area for thermal effects.)

8. Is there a clinical diagnosis? Ultrasound is not a global treatment for undiagnosed pain or loss of function. Rather, ultrasound is indicated for treatment of well-defined localized tissue problems. The clinician should have clearly defined treatment goals when ultrasound is being considered.

9. Is stimulation of tissue repair indicated? Acute and subacute inflammation from strains and sprains, bruising, muscle tears, burns, superficial and deep skin wounds, crush injuries, and other similar types of conditions respond positively to low-intensity pulsed ultrasound.

10. Are heat and stretch indicated? Restriction of movement, with or without pain, because of muscle spasm, chronic edema, fibrosis, connective tissue contracture, adhesions, unresolved hematoma, and similar conditions of a chronic inflammatory nature are indications for high-intensity continuous-mode thermal ultrasound.

11. Is ultrasound a time-effective approach to the problem? The clinician has to be with the patient for the duration of treatment. Ultrasound in excess of 15 minutes may not be efficient use of time. Shortwave diathermy is an alternative modality to consider. (Diathermy will be discussed in Chapter 10.)

12. Is the target tissue accessible? Ultrasound is preferentially absorbed by dense tissue; therefore, bone and joint structures should not lie between the target tissue and the path of the ultrasound beam. For example, this would mean selecting an alternative modality if swelling were inside a joint, whereas swelling outside a joint might be an indication for ultrasound. If the patient is unable to maintain a posture that makes the tissue accessible, another modality should be considered. For example, a contracture of the inferior portion of the shoulder joint capsule may be better heated with shortwave diathermy if a patient is unable to abduct the arm sufficiently for an ultrasound approach.

13. Is delivery of ultrasound practical? Either direct contact or a water-immersion technique has to be used. Skin breakdown, risk of infection, tenderness, and presence of dressings, casts, and splints may preclude the use of ultrasound.

14. Is the treatment goal to enhance delivery of topical medication? If difficult tissue contours preclude adequate transducer contact, phonophoresis, iontophoresis may be an alternative solution: for example, over the lateral epicondyle of the humerus or the calcaneal bursa in "bony" individuals.

15. Is ultrasound medically safe for the patient? There are some contraindications that would immediately preclude ultrasound as a choice of treatment. Screening of patients is essential.

Summary

Throughout this chapter there has been a continuing emphasis placed on the importance of understanding the parameters of therapeutic ultrasound and the ability to explain what one is doing in simple terminology to the patient. Ultrasound has been used therapeutically for many years; however, it has been only within the past 20 to 30 years that the technology has significantly changed, permitting more precise delivery and monitoring of acoustical energy. This has enabled researchers to apply and understand more about the effects of specific frequencies of ultrasound, beam characteristics including the BNR, and intensity levels. This research has also made it possible for clinicians and ultimately patients to benefit from what we now know about therapeutic ultrasound and more accurately deliver appropriate parameters to accomplish our treatment goals and prevent potential damage to the underlying tissues. We hope that the research will continue so that the benefits of therapeutic ultrasound will outweigh the confusion that some clinicians still might have regarding the multitude of parameters.

Remember that the selection of parameters can be determined by asking yourself the following questions:

QUESTION	TO DETERMINE THIS PARAMETER
What is the depth of what I am treating?	The frequency
Is what you are treating something superficial	Use 3 MHz.
Is what you are treating something deeper than you can palpate?	Use 1 MHz.
Is what you are treating acute or chronic?	This helps you determine the duty factor (duty cycle).
The more acute the problem, the lower will be the duty factor.	
The more cardinal signs of inflammation that are present, the lower the duty factor.	
This means that if all five cardinal signs are present (Pain, Edema, Heat, Erythema, and Loss of Function), then a duty factor of 10% could be indicated but with the loss of each of the cardinal signs, the duty factor could increase up to a thermal mode of 100% if there was only one remaining sign.	
Treatment time can be based upon the treatment area and the size of the transducer. The treatment area should not exceed twice the size of the transducer; however, the time needs to take into account any duty factor that has been applied. Treatment time can be based upon 2–3 minutes per treatment area that is equal to the ERA of the transducer.	

Review Questions

1. A 30-year-old secretary has been evaluated by the physical therapist following a motor vehicle accident. The PTA used ultrasound to treat the pain and muscle guarding after palpating a small nodule in the upper trapezius. During the treatment, the patient complained of burning sensation under the transducer. What most likely caused the burning sensation?
   a. The BNR of the transducer was too high
   b. Too low of an intensity was used during treatment
   c. Too high of a frequency was used during treatment
   d. a and b

2. Every ultrasound transducer is tested in a lab to determine the quality of the energy as it leaves the head. The surface area of the transducer that is producing acoustical energy 5 mm from the surface of the transducer is referred to as
   a. Beam nonuniformity ratio
   b. Unstable cavitation
   c. Effective radiating area
   d. Acoustical streaming

3. You have been instructed to apply ultrasound for the purpose of deep heating to one of your patients arriving for treatment this afternoon. The department is particularly busy and you observe only one ultrasound unit is not in use for you to familiarize yourself with prior to the treatment session with your patient. Here are the available parameters of this particular unit:

FREQUENCIES	1 MHZ, 2 MHZ, 3 MHZ		
Duty Factors	100%, 50%, 33%, 20%, 15%, 10%, 5%		
BNR	@1 MHz = 6:1	@2 MHz = 10:1	@3 MHz = 4:1
ERA	@1 MHz = 8 cm^2	@2 MHz = 6 cm^2	@3 MHz = 4 cm^2

4. Based upon this information, what would the maximum intensity be that would be considered safe for you to apply if you were using this unit to treat your patient and you did not want to possibly exceed dangerous levels of tissue heating?
   a. There is not enough information to answer the question
   b. 1.5 W/cm^2
   c. 1.0 W/cm^2
   d. 0.8 W/cm^2

5. Based upon this information, which frequency produces the most uniform beam from the crystal?
   a. 1 MHz
   b. 2 MHz
   c. 3 MHz

6. If you were informed that there were three separate transducers for the unit that is described above, would the sizes of the transducers make sense as described above based upon the information provided?
   a. Yes, smaller heads would be for more superficial areas
   b. No, smaller heads would be for deeper tissues
   c. Yes, larger heads would be for smaller areas
   d. No, smaller heads would be for more superficial areas

7. If you were attempting to accomplish the initially stated goal of deep tissue heating, which of the following parameter sets would be most appropriate?
   a. 3 MHz @ 100% with the 4 cm^2 head @ 1 W/cm^2 (depending upon the amount of soft tissue in the Rx area) for at least 5 minutes
   b. 1 MHz @ 100% with the 8 cm^2 head @ 1 W/cm^2 (depending upon the amount of soft tissue in the Rx area) for at least 5 minutes
   c. 3 MHz @ 50% with the 4 cm^2 head @ 1 W/cm^2 (depending upon the amount of soft tissue in the Rx area) for at least 5 minutes
   d. 1 MHz @ 50% with the 8 cm^2 head @ 1 W/cm^2 (depending upon the amount of soft tissue in the Rx area) for at least 5 minutes

8. Ultrasound primarily affects which of the following structures:
   a. The arterioles
   b. The tendons
   c. The cell membrane
   d. The hyaline cartilage in synovial joints

Continued

9. There is a relationship between the power of ultrasound and the intensity of ultrasound. Which of the following statements is most accurate?

a. The intensity of ultrasound is a measure of the electrical energy delivered to each square centimeter of the transducer

b. The power of ultrasound is a measure of the electrical energy delivered to each square centimeter of the transducer

c. The power of ultrasound is a measure of the intensity of the acoustical energy delivered to each square centimeter of the transducer

CASE STUDY

Cindy is a 50-year-old amateur speed trial race-car driver who has been referred to physical therapy for lower back pain and muscle guarding. The pain radiates into the buttocks and down to the left popliteal space. She has a history of lower back strains related to lifting injuries while working as a roofer when she was younger. She is 5 feet tall and weighs 90 pounds. Traction relieves her radiating pain, but heat relieves her muscle guarding.

• Is ultrasound potentially indicated for this patient?
• If yes, answer the following:

Where would you apply it?
What parameters would you use?

What position should the patient be in during treatment?
When in the treatment program would this potentially be indicated?
Why?
What would you expect to occur, and after how many treatments?
How would you be able to determine whether or not it was effective?
How would you document what you did?

DISCUSSION QUESTIONS

1. The patient is a 50-year-old woman with chronic venous swelling of the lower legs. She has an ulcer 20 cm² in area and 2 cm deep on the anteromedial aspect of one leg. The ulcer has not healed in 10 months despite excellent wound cleansing by a visiting nurse and the use of moist dressings.

   a. Select ultrasound parameters that would be suitable to stimulate healing of the ulcer.

   b. Draw on paper a representative 20-cm² ulcer. Calculate the time it would take you to apply ultrasound around the perimeter of the ulcer at the rate of 5 minutes per 5 cm² of treatment area. If you have a 5-cm² transducer face, you can count exactly the number of 5-cm² areas that fit around the ulcer perimeter.

   c. The patient's skin circulation is also compromised in areas close to the ulcer because of severe tissue swelling. How can you use ultrasound to improve the condition of these other areas?

2. A 30-year-old patient suffered a whiplash injury 10 days ago. The present problems are painful muscle guarding of the upper trapezius, limited range of neck movement, and headache that the patient reports starts at the back of the head. As part of the current treatment session you plan to use ultrasound.

   a. Select ultrasound parameters that would be suitable for treating the muscle guarding.

   b. Would you also consider using ultrasound over the spinal joints at the level of the injury? If so, what parameters would you use?

REFERENCES

1. Robertson, VJ, and Ward, AR: Limited interchangeability of methods of applying 1 MHz ultrasound. Arch Phys Med Rehabil 77:379, 1996.
2. Pye, SD, and Milford, C: The performance of ultrasound physiotherapy machines in Lothian region, Scotland. Ultrasound Med Biol 20:347, 1994.
3. Hekkenberg, RT, Oosterbaan, WA, and van Beekum, WT: Evaluation of ultrasound therapy devices. Physiotherapy 72:390, 1986.
4. Williams, AR: Production and transmission of ultrasound. Physiotherapy 73:113, 1987.
5. Hekkenberg, RT, Reibold, R, and Zeqiri, B: Development of standard measurement methods for essential properties of ultrasound therapy equipment. Ultrasound Med Biol 20:83, 1994.
6. Forrest, G, and Rosen, K: Ultrasound: effectiveness of treatments given under water. Arch Phys Med Rehabil 70:28, 1989.
7. Dinno, MA: The significance of membrane changes in the safe and effective use of therapeutic and diagnostic ultrasound. Phys Med Biol 34:1543, 1989.
8. Barnett, SB: Thresholds for nonthermal bioeffects: Theoretical and experimental basis for a threshold index. Ultrasound Med Biol 24:S41, 1998.
9. Nyborg, WL: Ultrasonic microstreaming and related phenomena. Br J Cancer 45(suppl V):156, 1982.
10. ter Haar, GR: Ultrasonically induced cavitation in vivo. Br J Cancer 45(suppl V):151, 1982.
11. Shamburger, RC, et al: The effect of ultrasonic and thermal treatment on wounds. Plast Reconstr Surg 68:860, 1981.
12. Repacholi, MH: Standards and recommendations on ultrasound exposure. In Repacholi, MH, Grandolfo, M, and Rindi, A (eds): Ultrasound: Medical Applications, Biological Effects and Hazard Potential. Plenum Press, New York, 1987.
13. Lehmann, JF: Ultrasound: Considerations for use in the presence of prosthetic joints. Arch Phys Med Rehabil 61:502, 1980.
14. Skouba-Kristensen, E: Ultrasound influence on internal fixation with a rigid plate in dogs. Arch Phys Med Rehabil 63:371, 1982.
15. Krotenberg, R, Ambrose, L, and Mosher, R: Therapeutic ultrasound effect on high density polyethylene and polymethyl methacrylate (abstract). Arch Phys Med Rehabil 67:618, 1986.
16. Sicard-Rosenbaum, L, et al: Effects of continuous therapeutic ultrasound on growth and metastasis of subcutaneous murine tumors. Phys Ther 75:3, 1995.
17. Angles, JM, et al: Effects of pulsed ultrasound and temperature on the development of rat embryos in culture. Teratology 42:285, 1990.
18. CDRH Consumer Information , US Food & Drug Administration Center for Devices and Radiologic Health, March 15, 2005.
19. Dyson, M: Therapeutic applications of ultrasound. In Nyborg, W, and Ziskin, M (eds): Biological Effects of Ultrasound (Clinics in Diagnostic Ultrasound). Churchill Livingstone, New York, 1985.
20. Heckman, JD, et al: Acceleration of tibial fracture-healing by non-invasive, low-intensity pulsed ultrasound. J Bone Joint Surg Am 76-A:26, 1994.
21. Frizzel, LA, Miller, DL, and Nyborg, WL: Ultrasonically induced intravascular streaming and thrombus formation adjacent to a micropipette. Ultrasound Med Biol 12:217, 1986.
22. Williams, AR: Effects of ultrasound on blood and the circulation. In Nyborg, W, and Ziskin, M (eds): Biological Effects of Ultrasound. Churchill Livingstone, New York, 1985.
23. Maxwell, L: Therapeutic ultrasound: Its effect on the cellular and molecular mechanisms of inflammation and repair. Physiotherapy 79:421, 1992.
24. Al-Karmi, A, et al: Calcium and the effects of ultrasound on frog skin. Ultrasound Med Biol 20:73, 1994.
25. Maxwell, L, et al: The augmentation of leucocyte adhesion to endothelium by therapeutic ultrasound. Ultrasound Med Biol 20:383, 1994.
26. De Deyne, PG, and Kirsch-Volders, M: In vitro effects of therapeutic ultrasound on the nucleus of human fibroblasts. Phys Ther 75:429, 1995.
27. Williams, AR, et al: Effects of MHz ultrasound on electrical pain threshold perception in humans. Ultrasound Med Biol 13:249, 1987.
28. Gray, RJM, et al: Temporomandibular pain dysfunction: Can electrotherapy help? Physiotherapy 81:47, 1995.
29. Uygur, F, and Sener, G: Application of ultrasound in neuromas: Experience with seven below-knee stumps. Physiotherapy 81:758, 1995.
30. Lehmann, JF, et al: Effects of therapeutic temperatures on tissue extensibility. Arch Phys Med Rehabil 51:481, 1970.
31. Warren, CG, Lehmann, JF, and Koblanski, JN: Elongation of rat tail tendon: Effect of load and temperature. Arch Phys Med Rehabil 52:465, 1971.
32. Sapega, AA: Biophysical factors in range of motion exercise. Physician Sports Med 9:57, 1981.
33. Knight, CA, et al: Effect of superficial heat, deep heat, and active exercise warm-up on the extensibility of the plantar flexors. Phys Ther 81:1206, 2001.
34. Draper, DO, and Ricard, M: Rate of temperature decay in human muscle following 3 MHz ultrasound: The stretching window revealed. J Athl Train 30:304, 1995.
35. Gammell, PM, LeCroissette, DH, and Heyser, RC: Temperature and frequency dependence of ultrasonic attenuation in selected tissues. Ultrasound Med Biol 5:269, 1979.
36. Draper, DO, et al: Temperature changes in deep muscles of humans during ice and ultrasound therapies: An in vivo study. J Orthop Sports Phys Ther 21:153, 1995.
37. Lentell, G: The use of thermal agents to influence the effectiveness of a low-load prolonged stretch. J Orthop Sports Phys Ther 16:200, 1992.
38. Low, J, and Reed, A: Cold Therapy. Electrotherapy Explained: Principles and Practice. Heinemann Medical, Oxford, 1990, p 203.
39. Waylonis, GW: Physiologic effects of ice massage. Arch Phys Med Rehabil 43:38, 1967.
40. McLachlan, Z, et al: Ultrasound treatment for breast engorgement: A randomised double blind trial. Austral J Physiother 37:23, 1991.
41. Apfel, RE: Acoustic cavitation: A possible consequence of biomedical uses of ultrasound. Br J Cancer 45(suppl V):140, 1989.
42. Fyfe, MC, and Bullock, MI: Acoustic output from therapeutic ultrasound units. Austral J Physiother 32:13, 1986.
43. Lundeberg, T, Abrahamsson, P, and Haker, E: A comparative study of continuous ultrasound, placebo ultrasound and rest in epicondylalgia. Scand J Rehab 20:99, 1988.
44. Balmaseda, MT: Ultrasound therapy: A comparative study of different coupling media. Arch Phys Med Rehabil 67:147, 1986.
45. Docker, MF, Foulkes, DJ, and Patrick, MK: Ultrasound couplants for physiotherapy. Physiotherapy 68:124, 1982.
46. Stevenson, JH, et al: Functional, mechanical, and biochemical assessment of ultrasound therapy on tendon healing in the chicken toe. Plast Reconstr Surg 77:965, 1986.
47. Draper, DO, Castel, JC, and Castel, D: Rate of temperature increase in human muscle during 1 MHz and 3 MHz continuous ultrasound. J Orthop Sports Phys Ther 22:142, 1995.
48. Chan, AK, et al: Temperature changes in human patellar tendon in response to therapeutic ultrasound. J Athl Train 22:130, 1998.
49. Hayes, BT, Merrick, MA, Sandrey, MA and Cordova ML: Three-MHz ultrasound heats deeper into the tissues than originally theorized. J Athl Train 39(3): 230–234, 2004.
50. Ebenbichler, GR, et al: Ultrasound therapy for calcific tendinitis of the shoulder. N Engl J Med 340:1533, 1999.
51. Draper, DO, et al: A comparison of temperature rise in human calf muscle following applications of underwater and topical gel ultrasound. J Orthop Sports Phys Ther 17:247, 1993.
52. Robertson, VJ, and Ward, AR: Subaqueous ultrasound: 45 kHz and 1 MHz machines compared. Arch Phys Med Rehabil 76, 1995.
53. Reed, BJ, et al: Effects of ultrasound and stretch on knee ligament extensibility. J Orthop Sports Phys Ther 30:341, 2000.
54. Draper, DO, et al: Immediate and residual changes in dorsiflexion range of motion using an ultrasound heat and stretch routine. J Athl Train 33:141, 1998.
55. Hasson, S, et al: Effect of pulsed ultrasound versus placebo on muscle soreness perception and muscular performance. Scand J Rehab Med 22:199, 1990.
56. Reed, BJ, and Ashikaga, T: The effects of heating with ultrasound on knee joint displacement. J Orthop Sports Phys Ther 26:131, 1997.
57. Lehmann, JF, et al: Temperatures in human thighs after hot pack treatment followed by ultrasound. Arch Phys Med Rehabil 59:472, 1978.
58. Kimura, IF, et al: Effects of two ultrasound devices and angles of application on the temperature of tissue phantom. J Orthop Sports Phys Ther 27:27, 1998.
59. Wessling, KC, DeVane, DA, and Hylton, CR: Effects of static stretch versus static stretch and ultrasound combined on triceps surae muscle extensibility in healthy women. Phys Ther 67:674, 1987.
60. Robinson, SE, and Buono, MJ: Effect of continuous-wave ultrasound on blood flow in skeletal muscle. Phys Ther 75:145, 1994.
61. Lehmann, JF: Therapeutic temperature distribution produced by ultrasound as modified by dosage and volume of tissue exposed. Arch Phys Med Rehabil Dec:662, 1967.
62. Draper, DO, et al: Temperature change in human muscle during and after pulsed short-wave diathermy. J Orthop Sports Phys Ther 29:13, 1999.
63. Haker, E, and Lundeberg, T: Pulsed ultrasound treatment in lateral epicondylalgia. Scand J Rehab 23:115, 1991.
64. Binder, A, et al: Is therapeutic ultrasound effective in treating soft tissue lesions? BMJ 290:512, 1985.
65. Stratford, P, et al: The evaluation of phonophoresis and friction massage as treatments for extensor carpi radialis tendinitis: A randomized controlled trial. Physiother Can 41:93, 1989.
66. Downing, DS, and Weinstein, A: Ultrasound therapy of subacromial bursitis. A double blind trial. Phys Ther 66:194, 1986.
67. Falconer, J, Hayes, K, and Chang, R: Therapeutic ultrasound in the treatment of musculoskeletal conditions. Arthritis Care Res 3:85, 1990.

68. Holdsworth, LK, and Anderson, DM: Effectiveness of ultrasound used with a hydrocortisone coupling medium or epicondylitis clasp to treat lateral epicondylitis: Pilot study. Physiotherapy 79:19, 1993.

69. Pienimaki, TT, et al: Progressive strengthening and stretching exercises and ultrasound for chronic lateral epicondylitis. Physiotherapy 82:522, 1996.

70. Falconer, J, Hayes, K, and Chang, R: Effect of ultrasound on mobility in osteoarthritis of the knee. Arthritis Care Res 5:29, 1992.

71. Martinez de Alpornoz, P, Khanna, A, Longo UG, Forriol F, and Maffulli, N: The evidence of low-intensity pulsed ultrasound for in vitro, animal and human fracture healing. Br Med Bull;100:39–57. 2011. Epub 2011 Mar 23.

72. Dyson, M, and Smalley, DS: Effects of ultrasound on wound contraction. In Millner, R, Rosenfeld, E, and Cobet, U (eds): Ultrasound Interactions in Biology and Medicine. Plenum Press, New York, 1983.

73. Dyson, M, and Luke, DA: Induction of mast cell degranulation by ultrasound. IEEE Trans Ultrason Ferroelectr Freq Control UFFC-33 2:194, 1986.

74. Young, SR, and Dyson, M: Macrophage responsiveness to therapeutic ultrasound. Ultrasound Med Biol 16:809, 1990.

75. Byl, N, et al: Incisional wound healing: A controlled study of low and high dose ultrasound. J Orthop Sports Phys Ther 18:619, 1993.

76. Young, SR, and Dyson, M: Effect of therapeutic ultrasound on the healing of full-thickness excised skin lesions. Ultrasonics 28:175, 1990.

77. Roberts, M, Rutherford, JH, and Harris, D: The effect of ultrasound on flexor tendon repairs in the rabbit. Hand 14:17, 1982.

78. Enwemeka, CS, Rodriguez, O, and Mendosa, S: The biomechanical effects of low-intensity ultrasound on healing tendons. Ultrasound Med Biol 16:801, 1990.

79. Turner, SM, Powell, ES, and Ng, CSS: The effect of ultrasound on the healing of repaired cockerel tendon: Is collagen cross-linkage a factor? J Hand Surg 14B:428, 1989.

80. Byl, N, et al: The effect of phonophoresis with corticosteroids: A controlled pilot study. J Orthop Sports Phys Ther 18:590, 1993.

81. Kleinkort, JA, and Wood, F: Phonophoresis with 1% vs 10% hydrocortisone. Phys Ther 55:1321, 1975.

82. Wing, M: Phonophoresis with hydrocortisone in the treatment of temporomandibular joint dysfunction. Phys Ther 62:33, 1982.

83. Mourad, PD, et al: Ultrasound accelerates functional recovery after peripheral nerve damage. Neurosurgery 48:1136, 2001.

84. Saad, AH, and Williams, AR: Effects of therapeutic ultrasound on the activity of the mononuclear phagocyte system in vivo. Ultrasound Med Biol 12:1986, 1986.

85. Dyson, M, Franks, C, and Suckling, J: Stimulation of healing of varicose ulcers by ultrasound. Ultrasonics Sep:232, 1976.

86. Eriksson, SV, Lundeberg, T, and Malm, M: A placebo controlled trial of ultrasound therapy in chronic leg ulceration. Scand J Rehab Med 23:211, 1991.

87. Lundeberg, T, et al: Pulsed ultrasound does not improve healing of venous ulcers. Scand J Rehab Med 22:195, 1990.

88. Callam, MJ, et al: A controlled trial of weekly ultrasound therapy in chronic leg ulceration. Lancet 2:204, 1987.

89. Levy, D, Kost, J, Meshulam, Y, et al: Effect of ultrasound on transdermal drug delivery to rats and guinea pigs. J Clin Invest 83:2074–2078, 1989.

90. Byl, NN: The use of ultrasound as an enhancer for transcutaneous drug delivery: phonophoresis. Phys Ther 75:539–553, 1995.

91. Mitragotri, S, Blankschtein, D, and Langer, R: Ultrasound-mediated transdermal protein delivery. Science 269:850–853, 1995.

92. Mitragotri, S, Blankschtein, D, and Langer, R: An explanation for the variation of the sonophoretic transdermal transport enhancement from drug to drug. J Pharm Sci 86:1190–1192, 1997.

93. Cameron, MH, and Monroe, LG: Relative transmission of ultrasound by media customarily used for phonophoresis. Phys Ther 72:142–148, 1992.

94. Benson, HAE, and McElnay, JC: Topical non-steroidal anti-inflammatory products as ultrasound couplants: Their potential in phonophoresis. Physiotherapy 80:74–76, 1994.

95. Benson, HAE, and McElnay, JC: Transmission of ultrasound energy through topical pharmaceutical products. Physiotherapy 74:587–589, 1988.

96. Docker, MF, Foulkes, DJ, and Patrick, MF: Ultrasound couplants for physiotherapy. Physiotherapy 68:124–215, 1982.

97. Simonin, JP: On the mechanisms of in vitro and in vivo phonophoresis. J Control Release 33:125–141, 1995.

98. Mitragotri, S, Edwards, DA, Blankschtein, D, et al: A mechanistic study of ultrasonically-enhanced transdermal drug delivery. J Pharm Sci 84:697–706, 1995.

99. Meidan, VM, Walmsley, AD, Docker, MF, et al: Ultrasound-enhanced diffusion into coupling gel during phonophoresis of 5-fluorouracil. Int J Pharm 185:205–213, 1999.

100. Griffin, JE, and Touchstone, JC: Effects of ultrasonic frequency on phonophoresis of cortisol into swine tissues. Am J Phys Med 51:62–78, 1972.

101. Griffin, JE, and Touchstone, JC: Ultrasonic movement of cortisol into pig tissues. Am J Phys Med 42:77–85, 1963.

102. Griffin, JE, and Touchstone, JC: Low-intensity phonophoresis of cortisol in swine. Phys Ther 48:1336–1344, 1968.

103. Miyazaki, S, Mizuoka, H, Kohata, Y, et al: External control of drug release and penetration. VI. Enhancing effect of ultrasound on the transdermal absorption of indomethacin from an ointment in rats. Chem Pharm Bull Tokyo 40:2826–2830, 1992.

104. Miyazaki, S, Mizuoka, H, Oda, M, et al: External control of drug release and penetration: enhancement of the transdermal absorption of indomethacin by ultrasound irradiation. J Pharm Pharmacol 43:115–116, 1991.

105. Asano, J, Suisha, F, Takada, M, et al: Effect of pulsed output ultrasound on the transdermal absorption of indomethacin from an ointment in rats. Biol Pharm Bull 20:288–291, 1997.

106. Hippius, M, Smolenski, U, Uhlemann, C, et al: In vitro investigations of drug release and penetration-enhancing effect of ultrasound on transmembrane transport of flufenamic acid. Exp Toxicol Pathol 50:450–452, 1998.

107. Hippius, M, Uhlemann, C, Smolenski, U, et al: In vitro investigations of drug release and penetration-enhancing effect of ultrasound on transmembrane transport of flufenamic acid. Int J Clin Pharmacol Ther 36:107–111, 1998.

108. Benson, HAE, McElnay, JC, and Harland, R: Use of ultrasound to enhance percutaneous absorption of benzydamine. Phys Ther 69:113–118, 1989.

109. Oziomek, RS, Perrin, DH, Herold, DA, et al: Effect of phonophoresis on serum salicylate levels. Med Sci Sports Exerc 23:397–401, 1991.

110. Bare, AC, McAnaw, MB, Pritchard, AE, et al: Phonophoretic delivery of 10% hydrocortisone through the epidermis of humans as determined by serum cortisol concentrations. Phys Ther 76:738–745, 1996.

111. Byl, NN, McKenzie, A, Halliday, B, et al: The effects of phonophoresis with corticosteroids: A controlled pilot study. J Orthop Sports Phys Ther 18:590–600, 1993.

112. Conner Kerr, TA, Franklin, ME, Kerr, JE, et al: Phonophoretic delivery of dexamethasone to human transdermal tissues: A controlled pilot study. Eur J Phys Med Rehabil 8:19–23, 1998.

113. Darrow, H, Schulthies, S, Draper, D, et al: Serum dexamethasone levels after Decadron phonophoresis. J Athl Train 34: 338–341, 1999.

114. Ciccone, CD, Leggin, BG, and Callamaro, JJ: Effects of ultrasound and trolamine salicylate phonophoresis on delayed-onset muscle soreness. Phys Ther 71:666–675, 1991; discussion 675–678.

115. Shin, SM, and Choi, JK: Effect of indomethacin phonophoresis on the relief of temporomandibular joint pain. Cranio 15:345–348, 1997.

116. Kleinkort, JA, and Wood, F: Phonophoresis with 1 percent versus 10 percent hydrocortisone. Phys Ther 55:1320–1324, 1975.

117. Klaiman, MD, Shrader, JA, Danoff, JV, et al: Phonophoresis versus ultrasound in the treatment of common musculoskeletal conditions. Med Sci Sports Exerc 30:1349–1355, 1998.

118. Penderghest, CE, Kimura, IF, and Gulick, DT: Double-blind clinical efficacy study of pulsed phonophoresis on perceived pain associated with symptomatic tendinitis. J Sport Rehabil. 7:9–19, 1998.

119. Gogstetter, DS, and Goldsmith, LA: Treatment of cutaneous sarcoidosis using phonophoresis. J Am Acad Dermatol 40:767–769, 1999.

120. Fang, J, Fang, C, Sung, KC, et al: Effect of low frequency ultrasound on the in vitro percutaneous absorption of clobetasol 17-propionate. Int J Pharm 191:33–42, 1999.

121. Harris, DW, and Hunter, JA: The use and abuse of 0.05 per cent clobetasol propionate in dermatology. Dermatol Clin 6: 643–647, 1988.

122. Ueda, H, Ogihara, M, Sugibayashi, K, et al: Change in the electrochemical properties of skin and the lipid packing in stratum corneum by ultrasonic irradiation. Int J Pharm 137:217–224, 1996.

123. Kost, J, Pliquett, U, Mitragotri, S, et al: Synergistic effect of electric field and ultrasound on transdermal transport. Pharm Res 13:633–638, 1996.

124. Ciccone, CD, Leggin, BG, and Callamaro, JJ: Effects of ultrasound and trolamine salicylate phonophoresis on delayed-onset muscle soreness. Phys Ther 71:666, 1991.

LET'S FIND OUT

Lab Activity: Therapuetic Ultrasound

Before testing any piece of equipment, first familiarize yourself with each of the components. Completion of the following chart will assist in providing the information that you need to become oriented with ultrasound equipment prior to utilizing it with patients.

A. Select an ultrasound unit and record the following information:

Manufacturer
Last inspection date or manufacture date
Available frequencies
Available transducer sizes
Effective radiating areas (ERAs)
Available duty cycles
Beam nonuniformity ratios (BNRs):
Locate each of the following components of the ultrasound unit. Describe them in the space provided and inspect them for wear.
Generator
Coaxial cable
Transducer
Timer
Intensity control
Duty cycle control

B. Select a transducer that is waterproof.

- Make a tape ring around the transducer so that you are creating a "well" that is capable of being filled with water.

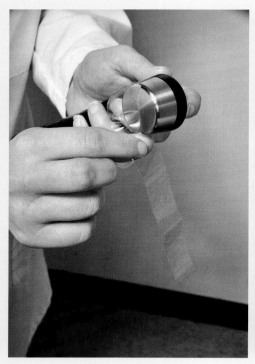 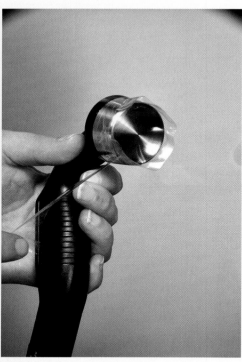

- Pour some tap water into the "well" so that the water depth is about a quarter inch deep.

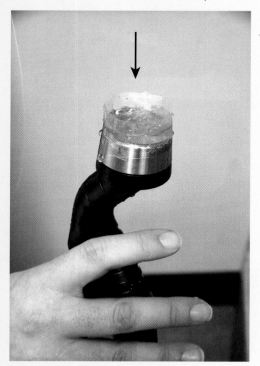

- Set the following parameters: 1 MHz, CW @ 1.5 W/cm².
- Look at the transducer surface; if there is a disturbance in the water, then there is acoustical output from the transducer.

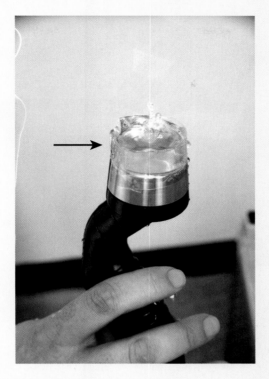

Specifications and their meaning: ERA & BNR

- Look down at the transducer surface from the top, and note how much of the surface of the transducer is producing disturbances in the water.
- This is similar to looking at the ERA of the transducer. Observe the disturbance to see whether it is a high percentage or low percentage of the surface area.
- Look at the surface of the water through the tape from the side. Gently move the water around so that you can see a cross section of the acoustical energy leaving the transducer.

- This is similar to looking at the BNR of the transducer. You are looking for uniformity to the beam. Lower BNRs are represented by fewer peaks and valleys. Higher BNRs are represented by many peaks and valleys, and many irregularities in the beam of energy.

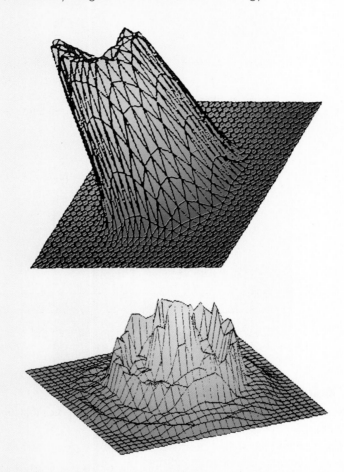

- Since ultrasound is usually administered without the report of any sensation from the patient, it is important to know whether or not there is any acoustical energy leaving the transducer. The water test will physically show you whether or not the transducer is producing and transmitting acoustical energy. *(Some facilities recommend that this exercise be done weekly to ensure that there is US output.)*

LET'S FIND OUT

Lab Activity: Differentiating Parameter Sets for Effective Therapeutic Treatment Interventions With Ultrasound: Thermal, Nonthermal, and Mechanical Effects of Ultrasound

Identify four classmates/patients who have palpable fibrocystic nodules in the upper trapezius that are painful to palpation. You will be comparing various ultrasound treatment parameter sets and reporting your results to your classmates and lab faculty.

Position and drape each patient so that they are comfortably supported and the upper trapezius is at rest. (All patients should be positioned identically for this exercise.)

Patient 1_____

Palpate the upper trapezius and ask the patient to rate the degree of discomfort that he or she experiences during palpation, recording it on a scale of 1 to 10.

Set the following parameters:

- 3 MHz, 50% DF, 1.0 W/cm², for 5 minutes
- Limit the treatment area to the nodule that was palpated.

What should the patient feel during the treatment?

_____

_____

Repalpate the area after treatment and record his or her pain rating and any change that you perceived when you initially palpated the area.

Patient 2_____

Palpate the upper trapezius and ask the patient to rate the degree of discomfort that he or she experiences during palpation, recording it on a scale of 1 to 10.

Set the following parameters:

- 3 MHz, 100% DF, 1.0 W/cm², for 5–8 minutes depending on the transducer size. (5 minutes per treatment area that is equal to the size of the transducer)
- Sonate the entire trapezius.

What should the patient feel during the treatment?

_____

_____

Repalpate the area after treatment and record his or her pain rating and any change that you perceived when you initially palpated the area.

Patient 3_____

Palpate the upper trapezius and ask the patient to rate the degree of discomfort that he or she experiences during palpation, recording it on a scale of 1 to 10.

Set the following parameters:

- 1 MHz, 100% DF, 1.0 W/cm², for 5 minutes for 5–8 minutes depending on the transducer size. (5 minutes per treatment area that is equal to the size of the transducer)
- Sonate the entire trapezius.

What should the patient feel during the treatment?

_____

_____

Repalpate the area after treatment and record his or her pain rating and any change that you perceived when you initially palpated the area.

Patient 4_____

Palpate the upper trapezius and ask the patient to rate the degree of discomfort that he or she experiences during palpation, recording it on a scale of 1 to 10.
Set the following parameters:

- 1 MHz, 50% DF, 1.0 W/cm^2, for 2 minutes
- Sonate only the palpated nodule.

What should the patient feel during the treatment?

_____

_____

Repalpate the area after treatment and record his or her pain rating and any change that you perceived when you initially palpated the area.

Questions

1. What was the rationale behind what you did?
2. Which of these parameter sets produced palpable differences in the upper trapezius?

Patient 1: 3 MHz, 50% DF, 1.0 W/cm^2 for 5 minutes and limit the treatment area to the nodule that was palpated

Palpable difference?

Why or why not?

Patient 2: 3 MHz, 100% DF, 1.0 W/cm^2 for 5–8 minutes depending on the transducer size. (5 minutes per treatment area that is equal to the size of the transducer), sonating the entire trapezius.

Palpable difference?

Why or why not?

Patient 3: 1 MHz, 100% DF, 1.0 W/cm^2 for 5–8 minutes depending on the transducer size. (5 minutes per treatment area that is equal to the size of the transducer), sonating the entire trapezius.

Palpable difference?

Why or why not?

Patient 4: 1 MHz, 100% DF, 1.0 W/cm^2 for 5 minutes, sonating only the palpated nodule.

Palpable difference?

Why or why not?

3. When would 3 MHz potentially be more appropriate than 1 MHz?
4. When would pulsed ultrasound potentially be more appropriate than continuous ultrasound?
5. When would treating the nodule instead of treating the entire muscle potentially be indicated?

Patient Scenarios

Read through each of the following patient scenarios and determine the following:

- Which of the parameter sets for therapeutic ultrasound would potentially be indicated and provide your rationale?
- What application technique you would potentially employ?
- When would ultrasound be contraindicated?
- What precautions would there be for the patient described?
- What additional information, if any, would you need to know prior to applying therapeutic ultrasound to the patient described?
- How would you assess whether or not your selection was appropriate in accomplishing the stated treatment goals?
- How you would position the patient for treatment if ultrasound was deemed appropriate?

A. Betty is a 55-year-old manager of a multimedia theater who has been evaluated by the physical therapist. She seeks relief for pain and muscle guarding in her cervical musculature. She has a prior history that includes osteoarthritis, three cervical strains, and a laminectomy and fusion of C5 and C6. She has no significant other medical history.

B. Cindy is a 50-year-old amateur speed trial race-car driver who has been evaluated by a physical therapist for her lower back pain and muscle guarding. Her pain radiates into the buttocks and down to the left popliteal space. She has a history of lower back strains related to lifting injuries while working as a roofer when she was younger. She is 5 feet tall and weighs 90 pounds. Traction relieves her radiating pain, but heat relieves her muscle guarding. Her x-rays were negative for disc space narrowing, disc herniation, fractures, and stenosis and she has no other significant medical history.

C. Phil is a 40-year-old Federal Express driver who has stopped in to the physical therapy office subsequent to intermittent pain, weakness, and cramping in his dominant left hand thumb. He has a perfect attendance record with FedEx that he would like to maintain but his level of pain and weakness is now a real concern for him. Extension and abduction of the thumb reproduce his pain. There are no fractures, and he describes the onset of the pain as gradual. The hand is edematous with exquisite tenderness over the anatomical "snuff box." Phil is anxious and appears sincere.

D. Jim is a 32-year-old police officer who has been referred to physical therapy by his lawyer for treatment of his right forearm. While on duty he was involved in an automobile accident in which his vehicle collided head-on with another vehicle. He had multiple fractures and contusions that have now healed. His chief complaint centers on his wrist and forearm, which were fractured and pinned with a steel plate between the distal radius and ulna. He has pain with stretching of the supinators into pronation. His incision is well healed and he has normal sensation in the upper extremity. Jim seems unwilling to provide very much information about the circumstances surrounding his accident, but an article in the newspaper has accused him of "playing chicken" while on duty. He appears to have normal range of motion but winces with pain easily and seems to linger in the therapy gym long after his sessions are over.

Documentation

In order for the treatment to be reproduced by another clinician, or for it to be reviewed by another individual who was not there for the treatment, the documentation must include the following:

- The parameters of the treatment
  - Frequency of the ultrasound administered
  - Duty factor
  - Intensity
  - The treatment area
  - Treatment time
- It is not important to recorded the medium, *unless it is something other than ultrasound gel or lotion.*
- If phonophoresis is being used, then it *must* be documented that the patient was asked whether or not he or she was allergic to the medication that was to be administered and the patient's response.
- Position for treatment will be determined by the treatment goals. *The only time it must be recorded is when it is unusual.* If stretching is taking place during the ultrasound administration, then the position and the type of stretch need to be recorded.
- Assessment and reassessment tools must be recorded in the patient record.

Lab Questions

1. How might knowledge of a high BNR alter the application of ultrasound?
2. How might knowledge of a low BNR alter the application of ultrasound?
3. How would the knowledge of the ERA of a unit potentially benefit the clinician?
4. What tissue types absorb the greatest amount of acoustical energy?
5. Where will a patient first report a sensation from ultrasound?
6. Utilizing terminology that a patient would understand, describe how ultrasound works, and why they do not hear it and may not feel it.

7. If you were directed to treat an area with ultrasound that was larger than twice the size of the transducer, and the goal was to produce heat, what would be the most appropriate action to take? Why?

8. What difference would it make if the coupling medium was not acoustically conductive?

9. If a pharmacist "whipped up" a phonophoretic medication for use in the physical therapy department, what would you need to know about the mixture? Why? (Remember that whipping adds air.)

10. Outline the steps necessary for a successful treatment with phonophoresis.

6

Aquatics and Hydrotherapy

Holly C. Beinert, PT, MPT | *Russell Stowers, PTA, MS, EdD*
Robert Babb, PT

Learning Outcomes

Following the successful completion of this chapter, the learner will be able to:

- Describe the physical principles of water.
- Describe the therapeutic benefits of hydrotherapy.
- Describe the components of and care of a whirlpool.
- Describe the benefits of aquatic exercise as a modality.
- Differentiate between the benefits of land and water activities.
- Describe the benefits of hydrotherapy for wound management.
- Describe the techniques for wound care with hydrotherapy.
- Differentiate between the benefits and potential problems of using hydrotherapy for wound care.
- Describe physical principles of water and how it can be therapeutically beneficial for a patient.
  These principles include:
  - Buoyancy
  - Drag
  - Resistance/turbulence
- Compare a buoyant environment with a gravity environment in terms of therapeutic activities for a patient, describing which would be more challenging and which would be more supportive and why.
- Describe the purpose of the components of a therapeutic whirlpool through the identification, adjustment, cleaning, and use of each of these components.
- Problem-solve patient scenario difficulties in using whirlpools for patients with medical diagnoses.
- Explain the advantages and disadvantages of water versus land exercise programs.
- Describe the benefits of buoyancy in therapeutic exercise programs.

Key Terms

Aquatic pools
Aquatic physical therapy
Buoyancy

Débridement
Hydrotherapy

Hydromechanics
Whirlpools

"Is the whirlpool half full or half empty?" —Anonymous

Patient Perspective
"I can move with less pain in the water."

Hydrotherapy, the application of water for therapeutic purposes, has ancient roots and is one of the oldest forms of therapy. Hippocrates, the Greek father of medicine, used contrast baths of hot and cold water to treat various diseases. Europeans have been using warm-water spas for hundreds of years and developed a great deal of the original therapeutic water regimens that are used today. Exercise in water was popular in the polio era, and a resurgence of interest occurred in the 1990s as evidenced by the formation of the Aquatic Section of the American Physical Therapy Association, which defines **aquatic physical therapy** as "treatment time with therapeutic exercises in the water, utilizing supine, prone, vertical, or reclined positions."[1] Today, thousands of clinicians use water for therapeutic purposes every day in their practices. This use has evolved into two different areas: whirlpool treatments and aquatic therapy using aquatic pools. This chapter will define, discuss, and differentiate between the wide variety of therapeutic applications of water.

129

Whirlpools Versus Aquatic Pools

Whirlpools use tanks of water such as a low boy or Hubbard tank (Figs. 6-1 and 6-2). These tanks come in a variety of depths and sizes dependent on the amount of immersion required for the treatment.[2] Whirlpools involve the treatment of one patient at a time in an individual tank. **Aquatic pools** refer to the use of larger pools with more body immersion and potential treatment of more than one patient at a time. Individuals with a true phobia of the water would potentially be able to tolerate whirlpool treatment but not an aquatic pool (Tables 6-1 and 6-2).

Physical Principles and Properties of Water

BUOYANCY

Buoyancy is a force that works in the opposite direction to gravity. Gravity pulls downward; buoyancy pushes upward from the bottom. When an object is placed in water, water displacement occurs because of the upward pressure of buoyancy. The amount of displacement has been described by Archimedes, who stated that an immersed body will experience an upward thrust equal to the weight of the liquid

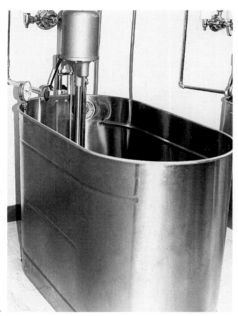
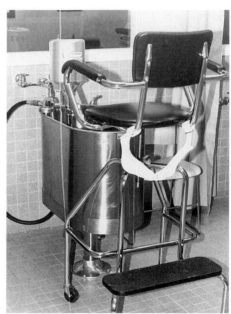
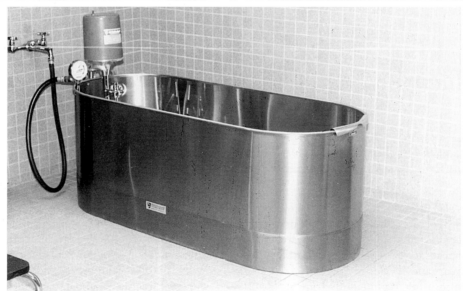

FIGURE 6-1 Various types and styles of whirlpools. (*A*) "High boy" for knees or hips. (*B*) Extremity tank for distal upper or lower extremities. (*C*) "Low boy."
(From Walsh, MT: Hydrotherapy: The use of water as a therapeutic agent. In Michlovitz, SL, ed: Thermal Agents in Rehabilitation, ed 3. FA Davis, Philadelphia, 1996, p 144, with permission.)

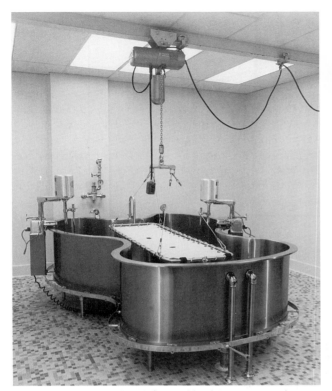

FIGURE 6-2 Hubbard tank for total body immersion. The shape enables full range of motion of both upper and lower extremities in a buoyant environment.
(From Michlovitz, SL ed.: Thermal Agents in Rehabilitation, ed 3. FA Davis, Philadelphia, 1996, p 163, with permission.)

TABLE 6-2 | Contraindications for Use of Whirlpools and Aquatic Pools

CONTRAINDICATIONS	WHIRLPOOLS	AQUATIC POOLS
Edema	X	
Lethargy		X
Unresponsiveness	X	X
Maceration	X	X
Febrile	X	X
Compromised cardiovascular or pulmonary disorder	X	X
Acute phlebitis		X
Renal failure		X
Dry gangrene	X	X
Incontinence		X

TABLE 6-1 | Indications for Use of Whirlpools and Aquatic Pools

INDICATIONS	WHIRLPOOLS	AQUATIC POOLS
Neuromuscular disorders		X
Musculoskeletal disorders	X	X
Cardiovascular disorders		X
Pulmonary disorders		X
Integumentary disorders	X	

displaced.[3] Water is more supportive than air because of buoyancy. There will be greater buoyant forces acting on larger objects, creating more water displacement, than on smaller objects, which will experience less water displacement and less buoyancy. A relative "weightlessness" occurs when a body is immersed in water. The amount of weightlessness depends on the percentage of the body that is below the surface of the water (Fig. 6-3). Buoyant forces support the body, giving the sensation of weightlessness.

This will also be affected by body density, postural alignment, and vital capacity of the lungs. When a patient fully inflates his or her lungs, he or she will be much more likely to float than if the lungs were not inflated. Buoyancy can offer enough support to the extremities, reducing the compressive forces that would be experienced out of the water. Buoyancy can provide opportunities for patients to perform assisted upper or lower extremity exercises or to run with reduced joint compression.

CENTER OF BUOYANCY

The center of buoyancy (COB) and center of gravity (COG) are functionally similar. COB refers to a point when a body is underwater, and the COG refers to a point when a body is out of the water. They represent points or locations on the human body that need to be maintained within a base of support (BOS) to establish and maintain an upright and stable posture. The COG is located just anterior to the sacral vertebrae; the COB is located in the chest region. While a body is submersed in the water, the forces of buoyancy and gravity act in opposite directions to each other. Buoyancy devices or flotation devices can be used to help a patient maintain his or her COB within the BOS to maintain an upright position in the water. Anteriorly placed buoyancy devices will tend to cause extension of the spine to assist in maintaining proper body alignment. For example, a patient who has had a total hip replacement needs to be able to perform buoyancy-supported hip abduction before he or she would be able to perform standing hip abduction.

HYDROSTATIC PRESSURE

Hydrostatic pressure is pressure exerted by water on an object immersed in the water. Pascal's law states that the pressure of a liquid is exerted equally on an object at a given

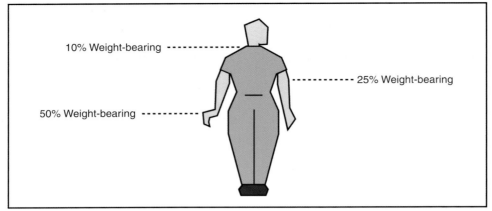

FIGURE 6-3 *Percentage of weight-bearing and immersion at three depths.*

depth, and the object will experience pressure that is proportional to the depth of immersion.[4] Pressure increases 0.433 lb/in.[2] for each foot of depth. This pressure is thought to help control inflammation with water exercise. It will also assist in venous return, heart rate reduction, and a centralization of peripheral blood flow.[5] There is less inflammation when patients who have had anterior cruciate ligament repairs perform their exercises in the water than when they perform their exercises out of the water.[6] Perhaps this is because of reduction of joint compression and shear forces.

Because hydrostatic pressure is proportional to the depth of immersion, exercises will be easier to perform closer to the surface of the water, where the pressure is less.

SPECIFIC GRAVITY

Specific gravity is the weight of a particular substance compared with the weight of an equal volume of water. It is related to the density of an object and therefore is also referred to as relative density. The specific gravity of a person increases when there is increased bone mass and muscle mass and decreases when there are greater amounts of adipose tissue (body fat). An object with a low specific gravity or specific gravity of less than 1.0 will float; an object with a high specific gravity of greater than 1.0 will sink. Water has a specific gravity of 1.0. The human body has a specific gravity of 0.87 to 0.97; therefore, the human body will tend to float just beneath the surface of water. For example, children with chronic debilitating diseases do well in water therapy because they expend little energy to stay afloat and the buoyant forces assist in reducing weight-bearing. Men tend to have lower percentages of body fat than do women[7] and may require more buoyancy-assistive devices than do women to keep them afloat. The lower extremities will have larger bones than the upper extremities and therefore will tend to sink more than the upper extremities.

BEFORE YOU BEGIN

Keep in mind that patients may be able to perform activities in the water that they would not be able to perform on land.

VISCOSITY AND RESISTANCE

Viscosity is a measure of the frictional resistance caused by cohesive or attractive forces between the molecules of a liquid.[5] *Resistance* is created by the viscosity of the liquid and is proportional to the velocity of movement through the liquid. Water has a higher viscosity than air but less than that of oil, so it would be easiest to move through air, then water, then oil. Exercise training in an aquatic environment can result in increased strength, improved cardiovascular responses, and improved VO_2 maximums.[8,9] The amount of resistance in water can be adjusted in several ways to vary the training regimen. Decreasing the length of the lever arm will decrease the resistance in a buoyancy-resisted movement, a movement down toward the bottom of the pool. Adding a "boot" or "paddle" will increase the resistance of an activity, because increasing the surface area of the part to be moved will also increase the resistance. The resistance that water provides inhibits rapid movement and can enable muscle strengthening without the use of weights.

SPECIFIC HEAT

Specific heat is defined as the amount of heat, in calories, required to raise the temperature of 1 gram of a substance by 1°C (one degree). The specific heat of water is 1.0, which is used as the standard for setting specific heat units of other substances. When heat is added to an object, the change in temperature depends on its mass and specific heat. The specific heat or thermal capacity of water is greater than that of air. This will cause more heat loss in the water compared with out of water at the same temperature. Cool or tepid water temperature is best for a long exercise session, whereas warm water is indicated for short-duration exercise and manual techniques. Patients diagnosed with multiple sclerosis will perform better in cooler water, which will assist in keeping their inner core body temperature low, preventing exacerbation of their symptoms that might occur if the exercise were performed out of the water. Patients with arthritis will benefit from warmer water temperatures because of increased circulation and tissue elasticity. Warm-water exercise may increase the core body temperature of obese patients because adipose tissue acts as an insulator, limiting proper heat exchange. Therefore, warmer water temperatures may be inappropriate for obese patients if they will also be exercising in the water, which would also increase the core body temperature.

HYDROMECHANICS OF WATER

Hydromechanics is a term used to refer to movement through water. It is a function of velocity of movement, surface area of the moving object, and direction of the movement of the immersed object. *Turbulence* is a product of several forces acting on an object immersed in water. *Laminar flow*, *drag,* and *resistance* to forward movement all act on the body moving in the water (Fig. 6-4). *Frontal resistance* is encountered initially as a body moves through the water, creating a positive pressure. The resistance is proportional to the velocity: the faster the movement, the greater is the resistance.[3] Progressive resistance in aquatic exercise can be increased by increasing the velocity of movement, by increasing the surface area, or by moving closer to the surface of the water where the turbulence is greater.[10]

Frontal resistance, proportional to the surface area, will offer resistance to initiation of movement as inertial forces

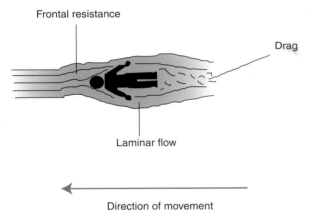

FIGURE 6-4 Various forces that will act on an object as it moves through the water.

are overcome. The greater the surface area, the greater the amount of water is moved; therefore, more drag will be created. *Drag* inhibits movement by resisting forward motion. Quick changes in the direction of movement in water will also encounter greater resistance.

Laminar flow is the horizontal flow of water passing over a body part in motion that creates drag. The more irregular the laminar flow, the greater is the drag of a part. Irregular shapes will alter the laminar flow of the water. Increasing the velocity, surface area, and change in direction will raise the level of effort needed to accomplish a task in the water. Depending on the effort exerted, energy requirements in an aquatic environment have been reported to be 33% to 42% greater at any given workload when compared with land exercises (Table 6-3).

Water Temperature

Temperature regulation is more difficult in water in part because of diminished body surface area that may lose heat. Conversely, cold water could produce a significant amount of heat loss because water conducts heat 25 times faster than air.[12] Therapeutic warmth is considered to be 94°F (34.4°C), which is appropriate for performing therapeutic exercises. Warm water may act as a superficial heating agent and has been reported to elevate pain threshold and decrease muscle spasm.[2] Inappropriate temperature selection could decrease the effectiveness of the therapeutic intervention and possibly cause adverse responses (Fig. 6-5).

BEFORE YOU BEGIN

It is beneficial to consider your thoughts regarding professional attire in the aquatic setting. What would you consider to be professional attire while treating a patient in an aquatic pool? Is it the same as or different from what you would wear to the beach? What should be covered while working with a patient in the pool for both genders? How might your appearance in the pool affect the patient's perception of you?

TABLE 6-3 | Overview of Water Properties and Principles

Buoyancy	Buoyancy helps to support the patient's weight. Joint stress is lessened and the patient may be able to perform water-based exercises with less pain.
Center of Buoyancy (COB)	Center of Buoyancy is functionally similar to Center of Gravity. In order to establish an upright and stable posture, the COB needs to be maintained within the Base of Support. The COB is located in the chest region.
Hydrostatic Pressure	Hydrostatic pressure helps control soft tissue and joint edema.
Specificity of Gravity	The human body tends to float just beneath the surface of the water.
Viscosity and Resistance	Water provides more resistance than air and that resistance can be adjusted in various ways.
Specific Heat	Consider which water temperature will best serve the needs of your patient.
Hydromechanics of Water	Turbulence, laminar flow, drag, and frontal resistance all play a role in a patient's movement through water. The section "Aquatic Therapy Techniques" discusses how these are considered during therapy.

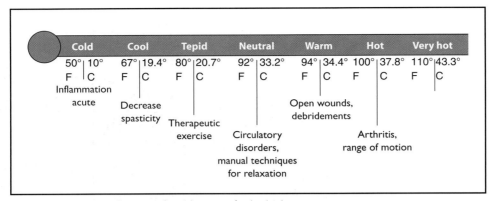

FIGURE 6-5 Water temperatures and potential applications for hydrotherapy.

Aquatic Therapy Equipment

Any Internet search will come up with the vast array of accessories and tools that can be utilized in the pool. When choosing which tool to use, the therapist must consider the goal as well as the patient's ability to safely and appropriately use the tool. Some that can be used are noodles, round and triangular dumbbells, kickboards, collars, ankle weights, resistance cuffs, floats, mats, fins, webbed gloves, belts, water-resistant footwear, and other pool toys and water games.

Foam noodles, dumbbells, and kickboards can be used to provide flotation, improve balance, build strength, and increase resistance. These accessories can be used on the surface of the water as well as under the water. When using triangular dumbbells to increase resistance and strengthening, you can use the points to decrease resistance and the flat surface for added resistance. Kickboards and other tools can be used in a variety of positions including standing, sitting, and kneeling. Collars are used to keep a patient's head above water. Ankle weights and resistance cuffs are used to increase resistance for strengthening purposes. Floats are made of foam and can be specific to the hand, wrist, or any extremity. They can be used either for resistance or to float the intended body part. Mats are available in different sizes and densities. They provide a surface on which patients can move from one position to another. Fins increase resistance and can be used for ankle strengthening. Webbed gloves are typically made of neoprene or silicone and increase the surface area of the patient's hands, thereby increasing the amount of resistance when pushed or pulled under the water. Flotation belts are made of foam and maximize buoyancy. Flotation belts are ideal for deep water exercises. Weighted water belts increase resistance and decrease the effects of buoyancy. Water-resistance footwear is made of foam and increases both buoyancy and drag.

Therapeutic Aquatic Pools

Therapeutic aquatic pools vary in depth and size with water temperature ranges from 86°F to 94°F (30°C to 34.4°C). The therapeutic treatment goals for aquatic pools can be the same goals as those established for therapeutic exercise out of the water. Water immersion eliminates the effects of gravity, so water is an ideal environment for early interventions for many musculoskeletal and neurological conditions. The initial assessment of the patient should be performed on land and then again in the water to ensure that the medium is capable of assisting the patient in meeting negotiated treatment goals. Aquatic rehabilitation should be combined with land techniques to progress the patient functionally because the land environment will ultimately be the goal (Table 6-4 and Fig. 6-6).

TABLE 6-4 | Comparison of Treatment Goals for "Land" Versus Aquatic Exercise

	LAND	AQUATIC
Improving range of motion	Manual stretching	Manual stretching
Improving arthrokinematics	Joint mobilization	Joint mobilization
Improving strength	Open-chain manual resistance	Closed-chain manual resistance
	Resistive equipment	Paddles, boots, boards
Improving balance	Unilateral stance, mini-tramp	Unilateral stance, turbulence challenge
Improving endurance	Bike, treadmill	Deep water walk, run
Improving ambulation status	Parallel bars to crutches to cane	Deep water to shallow water to land

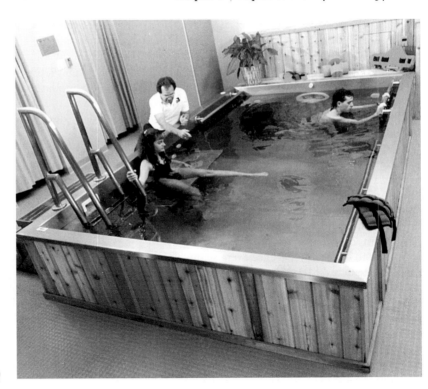

FIGURE 6-6 Patients performing aquatic exercises in a Therafit therapeutic pool. *(Courtesy of Aqua Therapy Systems, Lafayette Hill, PA.)*

Hydrotherapy Techniques

AQUATIC POOLS

Aquatic Pools and Infection Control

Unlike whirlpool treatment, the water is not emptied for aquatic pools following every patient treatment. There are also situations in which there will be more than one patient in the water at the same time. This presents some different considerations for infection control. First, it is recommended that patients shower to remove any excess soil from their skin before entering the aquatic pool. These pools have a filtration system that is either chlorinated or treated in some way to minimize the spread of organisms from one individual to another. It is not safe for a patient who is incontinent or who has an open wound to be immersed in an aquatic pool.

AQUATIC THERAPY TECHNIQUES

Aquatic therapy is a growing area of interest. The growth in commercial popularity is, unfortunately, not matched with effectiveness studies to determine the efficacy of the aquatic environment compared with a land program. Preliminary evidence and intuition lead many clinicians to believe that aquatic therapy is an effective tool for early intervention of acute injuries, for restoring function, for reducing the need for ambulatory assistive devices, for exercise, and for numerous other applications in which gravity-resisted exercise and movement are difficult to perform. Therapeutic pools are sometimes equipped with underwater treadmills, stationary bikes, and various other exercise stations similar to what one would see in a therapeutic gym on land. Any of the strengthening or conditioning treatment goals that are worked on in a land environment can also be done in an aquatic environment. The difference between the two is that the aquatic environment will provide the patient with more support and will decrease compressive forces on weight-bearing joints because of the effects of buoyancy. Despite this advantage, aquatic therapy cannot completely meet all of the goals, because the ultimate goal of restoring function is to return the patient to functionality in the gravity environment of everyday life. Successive progressions from deep water to shallow water within the aquatic environment will enable patients to prepare for gravity as they recover.

BEFORE YOU BEGIN

- Make sure that your patient feels comfortable in an aquatic environment.
- Ask the patient if he or she knows how to swim or has any fear of the water.

DEEP WATER EXERCISE

Deep water exercises are those that take place in an aquatic pool that is deep enough so that the patient's feet do not touch the bottom. The feet are not "fixed" to the bottom; therefore, the exercises that are capable of being performed are termed *open chain*. Depending on the height of the patient, the depth of the water should be at least 5 to 6 feet so that the patient is suspended in the water without touching the bottom. Buoyancy-assistive devices or tethering devices can be worn by the patient to maintain an upright posture in the water so that the lower extremities are free to move without having to try to maintain flotation. Deep ends of

Olympic-size pools or public pools are effective for deep water unloaded exercise. The water temperature should be tepid (80°F to 90°F) (26.7°C to 32.2°C) because active and sometimes aggressive exercise is performed for treatment times that may approach 45 minutes. Deep water exercises can be successful and sometimes compare favorably with land exercise, particularly for patients recovering from stress fractures, because the weight-bearing load is decreased.[14]

"Unloaded" deep water exercises may also be an effective exercise medium during late pregnancy, because the pressure will be relieved from the lower back. Caution needs to be taken, though, regarding the length of immersion and water temperature. Generally, the resting heart rate is lowered when patients are immersed in water. This has an important implication when treating pregnant women with back pain, because exercise on land has been reported to increase fetal heart rates.[15] Results from some studies have indicated that there is an increase in oxygen consumption that occurs in the water compared with doing the same exercises on land.[10,16,17] This is a critical factor for maintaining levels of function and fitness when recovering from a spinal or an extremity injury. Athletes can perform the same amount of cardiovascular work with less strain to their joints because of the increased metabolic demands of exercise in the water, thus maintaining their fitness levels of endurance and VO_2 maximums with "in-water running."[18] Conversely, the cardiac or pulmonary compromised patient may be unduly stressed by in-water exercise.

Full excursion of joints can occur underwater without incurring the forces sometimes contraindicated with land or shallow water exercise. In a limited-space immersion deep water tank, tether cords are used to minimize forward movement in the tank. Full movement and forward progression are encouraged with deep water pool walking or running to facilitate normal movement patterns of the soft tissues. Many sizes and shapes of buoyancy belts or vests exist today to facilitate floating in an upright position. The devices can be adjusted to promote either lumbar extension or flexion, whichever is indicated for the patient.[19]

MIDLEVEL TO SHALLOW-LEVEL EXERCISE

Midlevel (T12 to chin) to shallow-level (knee to T12) water depths permit the body to move over a fixed distal extremity, promoting some weight-bearing. Activities in these depths of water would be considered "closed-chain" activities because there is weight-bearing on the distal extremities. Progression in weight-bearing is accomplished through the use of shallower water depths (Table 6-5). When open-chain exercises are contraindicated, as with an unstable lower extremity or recent joint reconstruction wherein weight-bearing is desired, shallower depths can provide the closed-chain support that is necessary.[20] It has been reported that patients with intra-articular reconstructions had less joint effusion and faster return to perceived functional levels when performing water-based exercise compared with a similar group of patients performing the land exercises alone.[6]

Significant training effects have been reported with closed-chain water exercises. The findings included improved resting heart rates, improved VO_2 maximum measurements, and improved treadmill endurance tests.[16] Additional studies have reported improved VO_2 responses with water calisthenics and closed-chain exercise. Functionally, low-level patients can practice proper movement patterns of step climbing or upper-extremity reaching with the buoyant support of the

TABLE 6-5	The Relationship Between the Depth of Water in an Aquatic Pool and the Types of Activities That Would Be Possible in That Depth		
DEEP WATER 5 FT OR > (UNLOADED, OPEN CHAIN)	**MIDLEVEL WATER, SHOULDER TO NIPPLE (MINIMAL LOAD, CLOSED CHAIN)**	**SHALLOW WATER, ILIAC CREST TO NIPPLE (MODERATE LOAD, CLOSED CHAIN)**
Cardiovascular with joint protection	Wall slides	Land-specific functional movements
Unloaded sport specific	Trunk PNF patterns	Progressive ambulation, balance/proprioceptive challenge
Ambulation without assistive devices	Progressive ambulation to wean from assistive devices	
Unloaded exercises for spine/lower extremity injuries	Plyometrics	Sport-specific challenge
	General flexibility	
	Sport progressive lateral challenge	
	Balance/proprioceptive challenge using turbulence	

PNF = proprioceptive neuromuscular facilitation.

water. To treat patients who have trunk weakness, dynamic stabilization of the trunk can be first addressed in midlevel water using buoyancy and hydrostatic pressure forces for support.[23] Pain with exercise can be minimized in an aquatic environment. For example, for a patient on land, pain can persist throughout a movement if weight is applied, whereas in the water the resistance to movement will stop once movement stops.

BAD RAGAZ TECHNIQUES

Bad Ragaz techniques have been used and refined over the past 60 years. They were introduced at the Bad Ragaz Spa in Switzerland during the late 1950s. Bad Ragaz techniques use a buoyant ring to assist the patient in floating in the water. The ring may be placed around the trunk, under the extremities, or it may support the head and neck.[21] As knowledge of exercise and movement patterns increased, diagonal patterns of movement were developed using Proprioceptive Neuromuscular Facilitation (PNF) patterns of movement and applying them to a water environment.[22] These simple techniques are indicated for many musculoskeletal, neurologic, and arthritic conditions. Manual stretching is performed when there is a restriction in soft tissue movement. The patient's weight can be used to offer the overpressure needed to provide for an effective stretch. The patient is in effect lying supported by the buoyant force of the water, and his or her other body weight can act as resistance because of the drag that it creates to movement (Fig. 6-7). Positioning can be in supine buoyancy assisted, prone buoyancy assisted, or side-lying. Manual skills from massage such as soft tissue mobilization have sometimes been incorporated into buoyancy-supported movements. Aggressive stretching using techniques of Shiatsu massage

have been incorporated into water techniques. Whatever the stretching technique performed, it should be based on a quantifiable dysfunction and have a desired specific outcome. For example, if the glenohumeral joint is hypomobile and the goal is to increase shoulder range of motion, stretching of the joint, long-axis distraction, and joint mobilization can all be applied by the clinician to the patient lying supine supported by the water. Bad Ragaz techniques also use isometric and isotonic exercises for the trunk or extremities. Trunk "pelvic-neutral" exercises have been described and studied developing proximal trunk stability (Fig. 6-8). Progression of exercise involves the addition of distal extremity mobility patterns.[23,24] The Bad Ragaz isometric techniques are often less painful to perform with an unloaded supine position compared with performance on land. For this reason, these exercises are an appropriate starting point for deconditioned patients, such as those with low back pain. The patient will progress appropriately to land activities for functional levels of activity or mobility to return.

HALLIWICK METHOD

The Halliwick Method was developed in the 1950s by James McMillan when he and his wife helped students of the Halliwick School for Crippled Girls in London become independent in the water.[41] The Halliwick Method teaches patients to become independent in the water, while improving both balance and controlled movement. It is taught using a 10-point program consisting of mental adjustment, sagittal rotation control, transversal rotation control, longitudinal rotation control, combined rotation control, upthrust, balance in stillness, turbulent gliding, simple progression, and basic movement.[42]

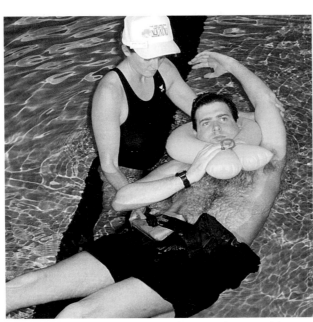

FIGURE 6-7 Patient supported by flotation devices while performing elongation of the left side of the trunk. Buoyancy is supporting the patient.

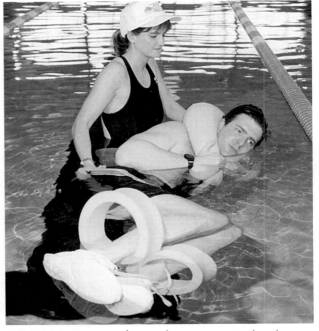

FIGURE 6-8 Patient performing buoyancy-assisted trunk flexion. He is supported by rings, similar to Bad Ragaz rings, as flotation devices.

Mental adjustment requires that the individual learn breath control and adjust to moving around in a body of water. Sagittal rotation control, transversal rotation control, and longitudinal rotation control are three steps during which the learner acquires the ability to control any rotation made about that particular axis of motion. When the swimmer has control of rotation about all three axes, combined rotation control provides the learner with the ability to control any combination of rotations. Upthrust is trusting that the water will support the individual. This step is sometimes referred to as mental inversion, because the swimmer must understand that he or she will float and not sink. Balance in stillness requires both mental and physical control to float while relaxed on the water. During turbulent gliding, the clinician moves the floating swimmer through the water without the use of physical contact. The swimmer must maintain balance. Simple progression and basic movement form the initiation of propulsive movements and swim strokes.[43]

WATSU

In the early 1980s Harold Dull (director of the Harbin School of Shiatsu and Massage in northern California) began to apply the stretches and moves of Zen Shiatsu in warm water. *Watsu* is a form of therapy performed in warm water (around 90°F to 94°F), which combines elements of massage, joint mobilization, Shiatsu, and muscle stretching. The receiver is continuously supported while being floated, cradled, rocked, and stretched. The warm water and nurturing effects of being cradled provide deep relaxation, which can deepen the effects of the applied stretches and massage.[42]

Patient Safety

In an aquatic environment, it is important to remember that patients may not know how to swim. Many people have an innate fear of water and drowning. You will need to reassure the patient regarding safety precautions while in the aquatic environment.

● Check your surroundings and know what is going on at all times.
● Know your equipment.
● Know emergency evacuation procedures for exiting an aquatic environment.

Aside from reassuring the patient, it would benefit the clinician and the patient-therapist relationship to gather a subjective history of the patient specific to water. This might best be done with a patient survey, which can be stored in the patient's chart. Appropriate questions include:

● Which of the following levels would you consider yourself—non-swimmer, beginner, intermediate, advanced?
● Do you feel comfortable submerging your mouth, nose, and eyes underwater?
● Do you feel comfortable getting in and out of the water?
● Are you affected by increased temperatures?
● Do you have any water-related fear? Please rate your fear on a scale from 0 to 10, 0 being no water-related fear and 10 being you refuse to enter the water.

PATIENT EDUCATION

The patient will need to be educated on the need to progress to more functional types of exercises outside of an aquatic pool. There will need to be ongoing education to reassure and reinforce the patient of the aquatic environment and its purpose. Patients must be able to perform functional activities in a land environment to be considered functional.

Patient Perspective

Patients often say they have never felt better than when they are in an aquatic environment.

PATIENTS' FREQUENTLY ASKED QUESTIONS

1. What is the difference between aquatic exercise and aquatic physical therapy?

2. What is the range of pool temperatures for specific kinds of therapy and certain ailments?
3. Can patients with hepatitis B virus infection and other water-borne illnesses participate in aquatic therapy?

CLINICAL DECISIONS FOR AQUATIC THERAPY

The water depth, temperature, and techniques are all important considerations for aquatic therapy. Deep water walking might be appropriate for a patient with a total hip replacement after the sutures have been removed. Midlevel to shallow-level water exercises gradually increase the amount of weight-bearing for a patient; activities might include jumping, running, or walking, using the water to assist or resist the activity. Unilateral balance activities can be accomplished in midlevel water depths, and resistance can be increased by adding turbulence to perturb the balance.

Aquatic Therapy Documentation and Billing

Functional rehabilitation should be carefully documented to record the parameters of care so that its efficacy can be established and the therapeutic program can be adjusted appropriately. A program with progression of exercises from buoyancy-assisted positions to buoyancy-resisted motion is illustrated in Table 6-6. Buoyancy-assisted motions use buoyancy devices to assist agonist muscle groups through the movement; buoyancy-resisted motions are the same motions without the device. These exercises are used

TABLE 6-6 | Documentation and Progression of Hip Abduction in Aquatic Exercise

EXERCISE TYPE	ACTIVITY
Buoyancy-supported passive (supine in water)	Provider provides passive stretch.
Buoyancy-supported active assist (supine in water)	Provider assists movement of the motion while in buoyancy-supported position.
Buoyancy-supported active (supine in water)	Active range of motion.
Buoyancy supra assist	Standing, abduction with buoyancy-assist device on ankle.
Buoyancy-assisted	Standing, abduction.
Buoyancy-resisted	Standing, abduct with increasing speed against resistance.
Buoyancy supra resist	Standing, resistive boot secured, abduct against resistance.
Buoyancy-supported, manual resist (supine in water)	Closed chain, body moves over fixed extremity (fixed by provider).

to improve active motion and function. Buoyancy-resisted motions are performed with the agonistic muscle groups in a direction against the buoyancy of the water, with a supraresistive device added to increase the surface area and increase the resistance. It is imperative that the progression from buoyancy-assisted to buoyancy-resisted activities be documented clearly, as well as the depth and temperature of the water. Items that must be documented include the following:

● Equipment used
● Buoyancy-assisted devices
● Weights used
● Water temperature
● Exercises
● How buoyancy-assisted devices were used
● Where weights were located and their purpose
● Depth of immersion
● Treatment time
● Any significant changes in the vital signs of the patient should also be recorded

Aquatic therapy currently has its own current procedural terminology (CPT) code. Performing physical therapy interventions in water does not automatically constitute aquatic therapy for billing purposes. A therapist who creates a land-based intervention program and then has the patient perform the exercises in water is not necessarily providing aquatic therapy. The patient may still be performing therapeutic exercise and therapeutic activities or participating in neuromuscular re-education, but the use of the aquatic therapy code indicates that skilled therapy is occurring in which thoughtful consideration of water as a medium occurs first, instead of as an afterthought.

Hydrotherapy for Wound Care

EQUIPMENT

Equipment for hydrotherapy involves the use of whirlpools with stainless steel or fiberglass tanks that may be movable or stationary (depending on their size and configuration) and have a turbine, drain, and thermostatically controlled water supply. Whirlpools vary in size, and one is selected for treatment depending on the treatment goal and extremity or area to be treated. The smallest tanks are extremity tanks, which hold approximately 25 gallons of water depending on the manufacturer. They vary in depth from 20 to 25 inches and have one turbine. Full-body tanks are called "low boys," and they resemble a bathtub resting on the floor with enough room for patients to "long-sit" in the tank with their legs outstretched in front of them. Low-boy tanks may hold as much as 200 gallons of water and they also have a turbine for aeration of the water. High-boy tanks are tall and are more appropriate for large body areas. They will hold up to 100 gallons of water. The extremity, low-boy, and high-boy tanks have been used in the treatment of open wounds, peripheral joint stiffness, sprains/strains, and postoperative joint replacements (see Fig. 6-1).

Hubbard tanks are whirlpool tanks that were created to accommodate a patient in a supine position and allow range of movement in both the upper and lower extremities with support from the water (see Fig. 6-2). These tanks may have a deep trough in the center of the tank with parallel bars for in-water ambulation. Patients who cannot be transferred into a low boy or who have too large a surface area for treatment in an extremity tank or low boy are candidates for the Hubbard tank. There are several turbines on Hubbard tanks that can be moved to different positions around the tank so that the turbulence can be directed to more than one area at a time. These tanks have a lifting device to transfer the patient from a gurney into the pool and then out. Often these lifts are hydraulically controlled and may be intimidating to certain patients. It is important to remember this when transferring a patient into any pool.

Consideration should be given for what type of tank should be used to conserve water and optimally perform the treatment. If active wrist exercises are needed, a small extremity tank is well suited for this patient. If the patient is being treated for a decubitus ulcer on the ischial tuberosity, a low-boy or Hubbard tank would be the most appropriate, because an aquatic pool would be contraindicated for this patient.

Turbines

Turbines mix air and water to provide agitation and turbulence to the water in a tank. The mechanical stimulation from the agitation to the skin receptors may promote an analgesic effect. The analgesic effect can be effective for pain reduction in sprains and strains, as well as other conditions. Turbines have several adjustable features, including height, direction of flow, and strength of the aerated flow. The more air that is mixed with the water, the more turbulence will be created in the water. Turbulence may assist in nonspecific débridement of an open wound if indicated. Wound management with hydrotherapy is discussed later in this chapter.

WHIRLPOOLS

The objective of therapeutic intervention for wound care is to provide an optimal wound healing environment. Based on knowledge of the expected progression of wound healing and on thorough assessment of intrinsic and extrinsic factors, treatment should facilitate normal cellular activity. Clinicians need to recognize how treatment will affect cellular function and provide care that will avoid wound trauma.

ADDITIVES TO PREVENT INFECTION

Whirlpools have been used for many years in the treatment of open wounds, fractures, and other orthopedic injuries.[13] To accomplish treatment goals without spreading infection, the tanks and their turbines must be thoroughly disinfected between patients. The most common agents used to prevent or reduce the chance of infection are povidone-iodine, chloramine-T, and sodium hypochlorite (household bleach). The size of the tank and the manufacturer's recommendations will guide the clinician toward the appropriate concentration of an additive. It is important to remember that the tank is not the only potential host for infections; the turbine is also a potential source. It is important to run the turbine with a disinfectant agent in the water so that the air intake valves of the turbine are also disinfected.

Whirlpool Cleaning Procedure

The whirlpool cleaning procedure includes the following:

- Filling and emptying whirlpools
- Know where drain open/closure knob is.
  - Open to drain
  - Close to fill
- Know where your water supply is.
  - Hose
  - Wall mounted
- Disinfecting the tank
- Spray/squirt disinfectant on all inside surfaces of tank (diluted solution).
  - Let set 5 minutes (while turbine is cleaning)
  - Wash with wet cloth
  - Rinse with water
- Spray stainless steel cleaner on outside surface of tank.
  - Do once a day, usually at the end of the day.

- Turbine disinfecting
- Place turbine in bucket.
  - Add one full squirt of full-strength disinfectant to each gallon of water.
  - Turn speed control/aerator to lowest speed or closed, so water filters up through turbine.
  - Fill bucket with water sufficient to cover the air hole on the turbine.
  - Run turbine for a minimum of 5 minutes.
  - Empty cleaning bucket and refill with clean water. Place turbine in bucket and run for an additional 5 minutes to rinse.
- Small tanks into which buckets will not fit
  - Disinfect sides of tank as done previously.
  - Fill tank with water (sufficient to cover air hole on turbine).
  - Close aerator as done previously.
  - Run turbine for 5 minutes.
  - Drain tank and fill with clean water.
  - Run turbine for 5 additional minutes to rinse (Figs. 6-9 and 6-10).
- Disinfecting of other tanks
  - Spray disinfectant on all inside surfaces.
  - Wipe with wet cloth.

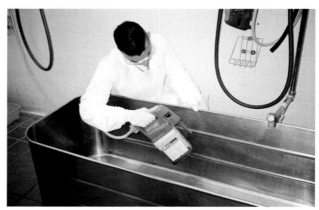

FIGURE 6-9 Gloved clinician has emptied the whirlpool to be cleaned and is spraying cleaner into the tank.

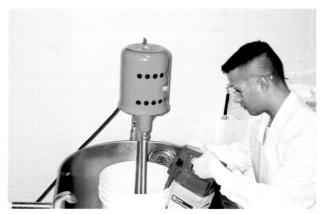

FIGURE 6-10 To clean the turbine, a bucket has been placed under the turbine, filled with enough water to cover the air intake hole. Then cleaner is being added before running the turbine in the bucket for at least 5 minutes.

- Let set 5 to 10 minutes.
- Rinse with clean water.
- Types of cleaners (common)
  - Expose (full strength and diluted)
  - Stainless steel cleaner
  - Cenclean
  - Waxcide
- Exposure to chemicals
- Refer to Material Safety Data Sheet for all cleaners and disinfectants used.

CONSIDERATIONS FOR HYDROTHERAPY TREATMENT

In considering hydrotherapy treatment for wound management, the clinician needs to ask the following questions:

- What are the effects of the treatment?
- When do the effects facilitate healing, and when are they detrimental?
- How should the effects be used?
- Are there other treatment options?

Hydrotherapy can be used for débridement, cleansing, hydration, circulatory stimulation, and analgesia. Care should be given to maintain appropriate patient positioning to guard against increased pressure (Fig. 6-11).

DÉBRIDEMENT

Débridement is the rapid removal of necrotic and devitalized tissue to allow reepithelialization and granulation. Necrotic and devitalized tissue impedes granulation and prevents or slows migration of epithelial cells across the wound.[25,26] Débridement is indicated for wounds with extensive necrotic tissue. This tissue delays healing and provides potential for bacterial growth and infection.[27] Hydrotherapy can be used to débride, soften, and loosen adherent devitalized tissue in preparation for manual or enzymatic débridement (Fig. 6-12).

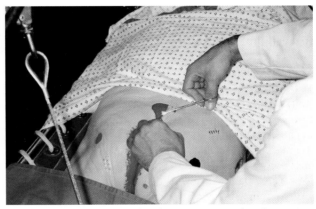

FIGURE 6-12 This patient has been transported to the hydrotherapy area of the department and transferred to a gurney that can be raised and lowered into the Hubbard tank for treatment. As long as the gurney is lowered so that the head is angled above the surface of the water, this position will potentially provide nonspecific débridement to the healing areas without undue pressure.

Hydrotherapy provides nonselective débridement, with removal of viable tissues along with necrotic devitalized tissue and debris. Nonselective débridement may cause injury to new endothelial and epithelial cells, disrupting the formation of new blood vessels (neovascularization) and the formation of new skin (reepithelialization).

MODALITY

The provision of hydrotherapy for wound care may be done with different types of modalities, such as whirlpools, pulsatile lavage, and irrigation. With each, the goals will be the same; however, the modalities will provide different benefits versus disadvantages. For example, if a patient is nonambulatory and has a small wound, pulsatile lavage may be more appropriate than whirlpool treatment.

WHY DO I NEED TO KNOW ABOUT...

HEALING AND HYDROTHERAPY

Hydrotherapy may inhibit the healing process if initiated too soon, as it may inadvertently remove viable tissue along with nonviable tissues.

CLEANSING

Cleansing removes dirt, foreign bodies, exudate, or residue from topical agents and bacteria. Excess exudate, bacterial residue, or foreign substances can prolong the normal inflammatory response and delay the proliferative phase of healing.[28] Dirt and foreign bodies provide a medium for promoting bacterial growth and infection. The critical number for bacteria is considered to be 10^5 organisms/gram of tissue;[30] an excess may result in infection. If there is concern of infection, a culture should be obtained.

Removal of residue from topical agents is done to allow topical antibodies or enzymatic preparations, if used, to

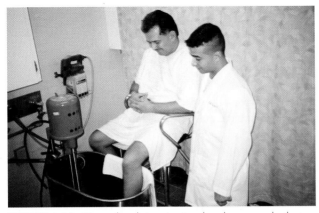

FIGURE 6-11 Once the determination has been made that whirlpool is appropriate to facilitate wound repair, the patient must be positioned so that there is no undue pressure from the side of the tank on the immersed extremity. The towel cushions the calf and the popliteal space has clearance from the edge of the side of the tank.

reach the wound bed. When using cleansing techniques, avoid concentrations of topical agents that might damage new cells.

HYDRATION

Hydration provides a moist wound bed that will proceed more rapidly through the phases of healing.[25,30] Dehydration (desiccation) of the wound may result in an alteration of electrical potentials of skin (e.g., a decreased lateral voltage gradient) and adversely affect epidermal migration.[31]

CIRCULATORY STIMULATION

Increased circulation obtained with hydrotherapy appears to be the result of thermal rather than mechanical effects.[34] Increasing local circulation can facilitate healing by increasing oxygen levels and metabolite removal.

Increasing circulation in an area of venous insufficiency can facilitate circulatory compromise, increase edema, and impede healing. The blood is entering the area and hydrostatic pressure is increased more than the venous system can compensate for.

Mechanical effects of hydrotherapy can be potentially damaging to new endothelial and epithelial cells, slowing healing and decreasing resistance to infection.

ANALGESIA AND SEDATION

Mechanical stimulation of skin receptors, such as occurs with gentle whirlpool agitation, can assist in decreasing pain. Thermal effects can assist with pain relief by increasing circulation in areas of compromised arterial flow.

INTRINSIC AND EXTRINSIC FACTORS

Effective utilization of hydrotherapy for wound healing must consider intrinsic and extrinsic factors. Information obtained and documented should include status of the patient, condition of tissues other than the wound, and description of the wound.

PATIENT STATUS

Important factors in providing treatment include the following:

- Subjective report, especially of pain and sensory changes
- Duration and intensity of symptoms
- Age
- Occupation
- Alcohol and tobacco use
- Systemic conditions
- Medications
  - Previous
  - Current
- Allergy
  - History of the wound
- Mechanism
- Healing progress or lack thereof
- Previous treatment
- Location of wound

CONDITION OF SURROUNDING TISSUES

The area around the wound or even an entire extremity environment is important in optimal wound healing. The area around the wound or extremity tissues should be assessed for the following:

- Color
- Edema
- Temperature
- Areas of pain or sensory changes
- Trophic changes
- Skin integrity
- Pulses

Attention should be given to areas of swelling, redness, increased temperature, and pain. During the early inflammatory phase, these are not unexpected, but prolongation may indicate potential for delayed healing or infection.

DESCRIPTION OF THE WOUND

Wounds may be classified according to type of closure:

- Primary
- Delayed primary
- Secondary intention
- Grafts or flaps
- Delayed
- Chronic stage I–IV

Open wounds can be classified according to the three-color concept of Marion Laboratory.[32] This concept uses a color description of the wound bed tissue in order of severity: red, yellow, or black. Documentation of the color or colors present and percentage of each directs treatment toward the most severe or predominant color.

In addition to the type of closure and description of wound bed, the clinician needs to document and describe the location of the wound; its size, shape, and margins; and the amount, color, consistency, and odor of any exudate.

Facilitation of Healing

INDICATIONS

Indications for hydrotherapy include débridement or preparation for débridement in wounds healing by second intention, stable flaps or grafts, and stage III or IV chronic ulcers with less than 50% necrotic tissue.

Hydrotherapy may also be indicated for cleansing wounds containing excess or malodorous exudate, loose debris or foreign bodies, or localized infection. A venous insufficiency ulcer may benefit from cleansing techniques that avoid dependent positioning and increased tissue temperature. A desiccated wound bed may be moisturized with hydrotherapy techniques. The patient with arterial insufficiency may obtain some pain relief[33] and increased circulation with gentle agitation–warm temperature treatment.

CHECK IT OUT 6-1

Before you begin, we need to first address the precautions and contraindications for using hydrotherapy. It's important to know what they are, but perhaps more important to understand *why* each is either a precaution or a contraindication.

PRECAUTION	WHY?
Healing wounds with granulation tissue	Exposure to forceful water from a turbine in a whirlpool may remove fresh granulation tissue.
Edematous extremities	Placement in a whirlpool would mean placement of the extremity in a dependent position, which may increase edema.
Sensitivity or allergies to additives in water	If there are no patient sensitivities to the additives in the water, water treatment and immersion are safe; if not, the treatment is contraindicated.
Catheter	If the patient has an indwelling catheter, it is usually considered safe for the patient to be in water.
	External catheters are not considered appropriate for water submersion as they may leak or easily become dislodged.
Seizure disorder	If the patient has a seizure disorder that is treated with medication and is stable and water has not been a trigger for an event, then there is little risk. Otherwise, this type of treatment is not appropriate.
Tracheostomy	If a patient is being treated using an extremity tank, there is little risk of water entering the tracheostomy.
	If the patient is going to be placed in a Hubbard tank or aquatic environment, extreme caution should be used to prevent water from entering the tracheostomy.

CONTRAINDICATIONS AND WHY

CONTRAINDICATION	WHY?
Split-thickness skin grafts prior to 3 to 5 days	These grafts hydrate readily and may slough off when immersed in water.
Full-thickness skin grafts prior to 7 to 10 days	This type of graft takes longer before safety with water immersion can be assured. The possibility of the graft sloughing off is of great concern.
Full-body immersion when vital capacity is less than 1,500 mL	If a patient is incapable of inflating the lungs against air pressure, he/she will have more difficulty inflating the lungs against the hydrostatic pressure of water, which will increase his/her difficulty in breathing.
IV line	This type of indwelling device would be difficult to stabilize and maintain at an adequate height to allow the administration of medication. However, a whirlpool treatment might be a viable option.
Colostomy	This type of opening cannot be adequately sealed to prevent leakage into the pool or leakage of water back into the patient. Water immersion in an aquatic environment must not include a colostomy.
Incontinent	Patients who are incontinent should not enter an aquatic environment, where voiding will contaminate the water for others.
Fever	Patients with an active infection who are febrile should not be placed in an aquatic environment in which the water temperature might further increase their core temperature.

Clinical Use of Hydrotherapy Techniques

Whirlpool may be indicated for débridement or preparation for débridement, cleansing, circulatory stimulation, hydration, or analgesia. Clinical hydrotherapy techniques include whirlpool, irrigation or flushing, rinsing, and soaking. The technique used will depend on the desired effect, condition of the patient, and status of the wound and surrounding tissues.

Irrigation or flushing with sterile water or saline in a syringe or Water Pik[34] may be indicated for removing superficial nonadherent cell debris or topical agents. Cleansing of malodorous wounds, removal of exudate, and hydration may also be obtained with alternatives to whirlpool, such as use of a faucet or hose or soaking in a basin. The amount of pressure delivered to tissues with irrigation, rinsing, or flushing is manually controlled and therefore is not consistent, and care must be taken to avoid tissue and wound trauma.

Cleansing or débridement with irrigation, flushing, rinsing, or soaking techniques can be considered as an alternative to whirlpool, more tolerable to a debilitated patient, with avoidance of prolonged dependent positioning, and more efficient in use of time and staff. For example, a cleansing technique other than whirlpool is often appropriate for venous insufficiency ulcers to avoid dependent positioning and increased tissue temperature.

ADDITIVES

Bactericidal additives most frequently used are povidone-iodine, sodium hypochlorite, and chloramine-T (Chlorazine). These agents, unless properly diluted, can be injurious to fibroblasts.[35] Patients may also have sensitivity or allergy to additives, and the open wound provides entrance for systemic absorption.[36]

The clinician needs to consider the effects of an additive and, if necessary for bacterial control of wound infection, use a concentration that is bactericidal without injuring fibroblasts. Often, use of sterile water or saline for irrigation, flushing, or soaking and avoidance of any whirlpool additive will provide the best wound environment.

Recommended dilutions of povidone-iodine are 1:1,000 and of sodium hypochlorite 1:100.[38] Steve and colleagues[37] recommend use of chloramine-T in concentrations of 50 g per 60-gallon tank and 320 g per Hubbard tank. See earlier in chapter under "Additives to Prevent Infection."

TEMPERATURE

Recommended temperature for hydrotherapy application in wound treatment is in the neutral range of 92°F to 96°F (33.5°C to 35.58°C)[33] or no greater than 1°C above skin temperature. Temperature will be based on the indications for hydrotherapy, the condition of the patient, and the area to be treated.

DURATION AND AGITATION

Duration of treatment and amount of whirlpool agitation or force of irrigation or rinsing are determined by the indications for treatment. Considerations are the desired effects, state of the wound and surrounding tissues, and patient tolerance.

There is no absolute standard duration, with soaking, irrigation, or rinsing varying from 1 to 5 minutes, débridement from 10 to 20 minutes, and increasing circulation 20 minutes.[38] A venous ulcer may benefit from 5 minutes or less of rinsing or soaking in tepid water.[36]

When using whirlpool agitation, it is important to remember that increased airflow through the turbine results in increased pressure and that there is increased turbulence toward the water surface.[10] Fragile tissues, such as a split-thickness skin graft at 3 to 5 days or a full-thickness skin graft at 7 to 10 days, should be exposed to only minimal agitation and should not be positioned toward the water surface, due to increased turbulence. Treatment duration initially should be limited to 5 minutes.

POSITIONING

Patient tolerance and comfort and avoidance of circulatory compromise or nerve compression with posturing or restrictive garments must always be considered when positioning a patient for treatment.

AMBIENT TEMPERATURE

A warm environment is important in ensuring patient comfort and avoiding reflex vasoconstriction and compromised wound healing, which can occur with exposure to cool room air.

THEORY BEHIND EFFECTIVENESS

Whirlpool affects the *inflammation phase* of healing.

- Warm water increases vasodilatation of the superficial vessels.
- Increased blood flow brings oxygen and nutrients to the tissues and removes metabolites.
- Increased blood flow brings antibodies, leukocytes, and systemic antibiotics.
- Fluid shifts into the interstitial spaces, leading to edema.
- Softening and loosening of necrotic tissue aid phagocytosis.
- Cleansing and removal of wound exudate control infection.
- Mechanical effects of whirlpool stimulate granulation tissue formation.
- Sedation and analgesia are induced by the warm water.

EXPLANATION TO PATIENT

Clinicians need to remember the importance of the patient as a member of the health care team. Explanation of the problems, goals, precautions, and treatment plan is a vital component of optimal care. Example of education to patient would include discussion of nutrition and how this relates to wound healing, contraindications, and instructions on dressing wound.

Hydrotherapy for Wound Care Documentation and Billing

The purpose of documentation is to provide an accurate record of the treatment that has been rendered. It should contain elements of the treatment technique and specific details of its application if performed in any unusual or uncustomary manner. It should also provide an assessment of the patient's response to the treatment intervention.

For the treatment to be reproduced by another clinician, or for it to be reviewed by another individual who was not there for the treatment, the documentation must include the following:

- Full assessment of the wound pre- and posthydrotherapy
- Type and size of whirlpool tank
- Patient position
- Water temperature
- Treatment time
- Whether agitation was used
- Quantity and type of additive used, if any
- Any significant changes in the vital signs of the patient should also be recorded, along with an assessment and plan based on these changes.
- Patient education and patient's verbal informed consent

Currently, there are separate CPT codes for whirlpool and Hubbard tank. Becoming familiar with the current codes and definitions will assist with accurately billing for the services provided.

Summary

Hydrotherapy use can vary from burn management, active sprains, wound care, and buoyancy-assisted or -resisted exercise. Although specific treatment protocols may vary by facility, the decision to include hydrotherapy for treatment should be based on knowledge of the potential benefits of water as a therapeutic medium and the treatment goals. Wound treatment should be based on knowledge of the biological events in wound healing, effects of techniques used, status of the patient and the wound, and other available options.

Other purposes of hydrotherapy. It can

- Provide phasic stimuli to the skin afferents, continuously reactivating them.
- Increase hydrostatic pressure, which may increase lymphatic circulation.
- Provide a mean for grading exercises (for example, moving a limb with or without turbulence).
- Provide heat or cold to a large part of the body.
- Help to decrease weight-bearing.
- Remove debris and necrotic tissue from wounds and decrease the bacterial load.

Review Questions

1. The relative "weightlessness" that occurs when a body is immersed in water is owing to which of the following?
   a. Buoyancy
   b. Hydrostatic pressure
   c. Specific gravity
   d. Viscosity

2. Which of the following temperature is considered therapeutic warmth?
   a. 92°F
   b. 94°F
   c. 100°F
   d. 110°F

3. Which of the following best describes the type of wound débridement provided by whirlpool hydrotherapy?
   a. Selective débridement
   b. Nonselective débridement
   c. Enzymatic débridement
   d. Sharp débridement

4. Which of the following is a property of water?
   a. Cleansing
   b. Hydration
   c. Specific heat
   d. Circulatory stimulation

5. Your 15-year-old patient sprained her ankle while wearing flip-flops and is coming to you for care in the outpatient clinic where you work. Her ankle is painful and swollen and has a small abrasion on the lateral malleolus from scraping against the concrete. The patient's mother sprained her ankle 20 years ago and remembered receiving whirlpool therapy for her sprained ankle. She is curious to know why whirlpool is not being done for her daughter. Which of the following best explains the reason?
   a. It is not on the doctor's prescription
   b. Her wound is too small for the whirlpool
   c. It takes too long to prepare and clean up the whirlpool
   d. The warmth of the whirlpool and the dependent position of the lower extremity may increase edema and pain

CASE STUDY

Mary is a 72-year-old woman with rheumatoid arthritis affecting mainly her hands, feet, knees, and shoulders. She ambulates with two canes in a flexed posture owing to flexion deformities at her hips and knees. This patient loves heat and finds the pool very soothing. She was admitted 3 weeks earlier with an acute flare-up and is now in the subacute phase.

- What are the goals of hydrotherapy?
- Describe the best method of entry into the pool and the ideal starting position. What treatment approach would you use?
- Because rheumatoid arthritis is a chronic disease for which your treatment is as much preventive as curative, when would you discontinue treatment and with what recommendations?

DISCUSSION QUESTIONS

1. The use of whirlpool agitation provides which method of débridement?

2. Why is nonselective débridement possibly detrimental to wound healing?

3. What alternative method to whirlpool might be more appropriate for the treatment of venous insufficiency ulcer?

4. Is whirlpool treatment indicated for a wound described as having 100% red granulation bed? Why?

5. What precautions should be considered with use of additives in whirlpool treatments?

6. What are some safety issues with aquatic pools?

7. What are some contraindications to aquatic therapy?

8. What is more difficult for a patient with weight-bearing precautions in the aquatic pool—walking in deep water or walking in shallow water? Why?

9. What are some educational issues that would need to be addressed before a patient is discharged from an aquatic environment?

REFERENCES

1. Framroze, A: Aquatic rehabilitation Q & A: Judy A Cirullo PT. Rehab Manag 8:43, 1995.
2. Walsh, M: Hydrotherapy: The use of water as a therapeutic agent. In Michlovitz, SL (ed): Thermal Agents in Rehabilitation, ed 3. FA Davis, Philadelphia, 1996.
3. Skinner, AT, and Thomson, AM: Duffield's Exercise in Water, ed 3. Bailliere Tindall, London, 1983.
4. Bueche, F: Principles of Physics, ed 6. McGraw-Hill, New York, 1994.
5. Johnson, LB, Stromme, SB, Adamczyk, JW, et al: Comparison of oxygen uptake and heart rate during exercises on land and in water. Phys Ther 57:273, 1977.
6. Tovin, BJ, Wolf, SL, Greenfield, BH, et al: Comparison of the effects of exercise in water and on land on the rehabilitation of patients with intra-articular anterior cruciate ligament reconstructions. Phys Ther 74:712, 1994.
7. Wilmore, J, II: Athletic Training and Physical Fitness. Allyn & Bacon, Boston, 1978.
8. Behlsen, GM, Grigsby, SA, and Winant, DM: Effects of an aquatic fitness program on the muscular strength and endurance of patient with multiple sclerosis. Physiotherapy 64:653, 1984.
9. Hanna, RD, Sheldahl, LM, and Tristani, FE: The effect of enhanced preload with head-out water immersion on exercise response in men with healed myocardial infarction. Am J Cardiol 71:1041, 1993.
10. Hellerbrand, T, Holutz, S, and Eubank, I: Measurement of whirlpool temperature, pressure and turbulence. Arch Phys Med Rehabil 32:17, 1950.
11. Costil, D: Energy requirements during exercise in the water. J Sports Med 11:87, 1971.
12. Bullard, RW, and Rapp, GM: Problems of body heat loss in water immersion. Aerospace Med 41:1269, 1970.
13. Toomey, R, Grief-Schwartz, R, and Piper, MC: Clinical evaluation of the effects of whirlpool on patients with Colles' fractures. Physiother Can 38: 280–284, 1986.
14. Clemant, DB, Ammann, W, Taunton, JE, et al: Exercise-induced stress injuries to femur. J Sports Med 14:347, 1993.
15. Katz, VL, McMurray, R, Goodwin, WE, and Cefalo, RC: Nonweightbearing exercise during pregnancy on land and during immersion: A comparative study. Am J Perinatol 7:281, 1990.
16. Routi, RG, Toup, JT, and Berger, RA: The effects of nonswimming water exercises on older adults. J Orthop Sports Phys Ther 19:140, 1994.
17. Cassady, SL, and Nielsen, DH: Cardiorespiratory responses of healthy subjects to calisthenics performed in land versus in water. Phys Ther 72:532, 1992.
18. Fyestone, ED, Fellingham, G, George, J, and Fisher G: Effect of water running and cycling on maximum oxygen consumption and two mile run performance. Am J Sports Med 21:41, 1993.
19. Whann, CM, Chung, JK, Gregory, PC, et al: A new improved flotation device for deep-water exercise. J Burn Care Rehabil 12:62, 1991.
20. Shelbourne, KD, and Wilckens, JH: Current concepts in anterior cruciate ligament rehabilitation. Orthop Rev 11:957, 1990.
21. Boyle, AM: The Bad Ragaz ring method. Physiotherapy 67:265, 1981.
22. Voss, DE, Ionta, MK, and Myers, BJ: Proprioceptive Neuromuscular Facilitation. Harper & Row, Philadelphia, 1985.
23. Cole, A, Eagleston, RE, Moschetti, M, and Sinnett, E: Spine pain: Aquatic rehabilitation strategies. J Back Musculoskel Rehabil 4:273, 1994.
24. Saal, JA: Dynamic muscular stabilization in the non-operative treatment of lumbar pain syndromes. Orthop Rev 19:691, 1990.
25. Hunt, TK, and Van Winkle, W: Wound healing: Normal repair. In Dunphy, JE (ed): Fundamentals of Wound Management in Surgery. Chirugecom, South Plainfield, NJ, 1977, p 40.
26. Albaugh, K, and Loehne, H: Wound bed preparation/debridement. In McCulloch, JM, and Kloth, LC (eds): Wound Healing: Evidence Based Management, ed 4. FA Davis, Philadelphia, 2010.
27. Agency for Health Care Policy and Research: Treatment of Pressure Ulcers: Clinical Practice Guideline No.15. ACHPR Publication No. 95.0625. U.S. Department of Health and Human Services, Rockville, MD, 1994, pp 6–7, 47–53.
28. Kloth, LC, and Miller, KH: The inflammatory response to wounding. In McCulloch, JM, Kloth, LC, and Feedar, JA (eds): Wound Healing: Alternatives in Management. FA Davis, Philadelphia, 1990, p 3.
29. Alvarez, OM, Mertz, PM, and Eaglstein, WH: The effect of occlusive dressings on collagen synthesis and re-epithelialization in superficial wounds. J Surg Res 35:142, 1983.
30. Pollack, SV: The wound healing process. Clin Dermatol 2:8, 1984.
31. Kloth, LC: Electrical stimulation in tissue repair. In McCullough, JM, Kloth, LC, and Feedar, JA (eds): Wound Healing: Alternatives in Management, ed 2. FA Davis, Philadelphia, 1995, p 298.
32. Walsh, MT: Relationship of Hand Edema to Upper Extremity Water Temperature During Whirlpool Treatment on Normals. Master's thesis. College of Allied Health Professions, Philadelphia, 1983.
33. Cazell, JZ: Wound care forum—the new RYB color code. Am J Nursing 1342, 1988.
34. Walsh, MT: Hydrotherapy: The use of water as a therapeutic agent. In Michlovitz, SL (ed): Thermal Agents in Rehabilitation, ed 3. FA Davis, Philadelphia, 1996.
35. Trelstad, A, et al: Water Piks: Wound cleansing alternative. Plast Surg Nursing 9:117, 198.
36. Linneaweaver, W, et al: Cellular and bacterial toxicities of topical antimicrobials. Plast Reconstruct Surg 75:394, 1985.
37. Aronoff, GR, et al: Increased serum iodide concentration from iodine absorption through wounds treated topically with povidone-iodine. Am J Med Sci 279:173, 1980.
38. Steve, L, Goodhard, P, and Alexander, J. Hydrotherapy burn treatment: Use of chloramine-T against resistant micro-organisms. Arch Phys Med Rehabil 60:301, 1970.
39. Borrell, R, et al: Comparison of in vivo temperature produced by hydrotherapy, paraffin wax treatment, and Fluidotherapy. Phys Ther 60:1273, 1986.
40. McCulloch, JM, and Houde, J: Treatment of wounds due to vascular problem. In Kloth, LC, McCulloch, JM, and Feedar, JK (eds): Wound Healing: Alternatives in Management, ed 2. FA Davis, Philadelphia, 1990, p 191.
41. Martin, J: The Halliwick Method. Physiotherapy 67:288–291, 1981.
42. Brody, LT, and Geigle, PR: Aquatic Exercise for Rehabilitation and Training. Human Kinetics, Champaign, IL, 2009.
43. Hastings, P: The Halliwick Concept: Developing the teaching of swimming to disabled people. Interconnections Q J 8, 2010.

LET'S FIND OUT

Lab Activity: Aquatics and Hydrotherapy

This lab activity is designed to familiarize the student/learner with a wide variety of potential application techniques for water to accomplish therapeutic treatment goals. This modality is referred to as hydrotherapy.

Throughout this lab activity, students/learners are instructed to apply or experience various forms of hydrotherapy that are commonly used in the clinic today. Questions accompany each of the exercises. These questions are intended to help the student/learner learn how to incorporate the use of hydrotherapy in clinical practice for the accomplishment of clinical treatment goals.

The lab is divided into two parts: aquatic pools and whirlpools.

Equipment

Whirlpools
Towels
Gowns
Whirlpool tanks (various)
Stethoscope and sphygmomanometer

Aquatic Pools
Access to a therapeutic pool
Paddles (aquatic exercise devices)
Stethoscope and sphygmomanometer
Bathing suits or T-shirts and shorts
Towels
Flotation belts

Lab Activity: Orientation to Therapeutic Aquatic Pools

Experiencing Buoyancy and Resistance in Water

Buoyancy is a force present underwater that is not present on land. It acts in opposition to the force of gravity. For this reason, virtually everything that is limited owing to gravity on land can be performed more easily with the support of buoyancy.

Land
Against gravity
With gravity
Gravity eliminated

Aquatic
Buoyancy assisted
Buoyancy resisted
Buoyancy supported

To facilitate learning about these differences, it will be necessary for you to have access to a therapeutic pool with varied depth from about 2 feet to more than 6 feet. Because you will be exercising in the pool, as would your patients, the pool temperature is an important consideration.

Therapeutic exercise   94°F (±2°F)
Therapeutic heat   104°F (*not appropriate for a pool!*)

1. Have a classmate record your vital signs and a few other pieces of data before and after you enter the water.

	Before Therapy	After Therapy
Heart rate		
Blood pressure		
Respiration		
Pool temperature		
Time		

2. You will be in a therapeutic pool for the following activities. It is suggested that you appoint a classmate to read and record your responses from the activities while you are in the water.

3. Walk in water of various depths and describe the difference each makes in your ease of movement.

Knee Deep: _____

_____

_____

Waist Deep: _____

_____

_____

Shoulder Deep: _____

_____

_____

4. In shoulder-depth water, perform the following activities and describe what happens and why.

Walk Forward: _____

_____

_____

Stop Quickly: _____

_____

_____

Try to Run:

_____

_____

5. Stand in shoulder-depth water and slowly horizontally abduct your right shoulder, stopping at 45 degrees.

• Does your arm have a tendency to move or stop in this position?

_____

_____

• Would this be a gravity-assisted position on land?

_____

_____

• How would you describe the position in the water (buoyancy resisted or buoyancy assisted)?

_____

_____

6. What could you do to increase the amount of resistance to movement that you encounter in the water? Try it. Does it work?

_____

_____

_____

_____

7. If a patient tried your technique to increase the resistance, would there be any additional considerations? If yes, what would they be?

_____

_____

_____

_____

8. What happens when you push your hands down to your sides from the surface of the water with your forearms pronated?

_____

_____

_____

_____

- What happens when you repeat this with your forearms in a neutral position? Why?

  _____

  _____

  _____

  _____

9. Float in the water with your shoulders abducted to 90 degrees. Once you are floating, what happens when you extend your hip?

   _____

   _____

   _____

   _____

   - For what exercise or motion would this position provide buoyancy assistance and resistance?

     _____

     _____

     _____

10. Apply a deep water belt securely around your waist before entering the deep end of the pool. If you have a tendency to sink, you may need to apply more than one belt. Move into the deep end of the pool where the depth of the water exceeds your height. "Walk" in the deep water so that your body remains vertical. Perform the following activities and record your observations below.

	What Happened?	How Much Effort Was Required?	How Much Weight-Bearing Took Place?
Walk forward			
Walk backward			
Ski			
Scissor your legs			
Bring your knees up to your chest			
Lower your knees			

11. Come out of the pool, and record the same data as when you entered the pool in the table in question 1. Also record the following:

    - How long were you in the pool?

      _____

      _____

    - How, if at all, did your vital signs change? Why or why not?

      _____

      _____

      _____

      _____

12. Based on any changes in your vital signs, what impact would similar changes have on patients involved in aquatic pool programs?

    _____

    _____

    _____

    _____

Lab Activity: Whirlpools
Orientation to the Equipment
1. Identify and name each piece of hydrotherapy equipment listed in the table below.

   • Find and label the turbine on each of the whirlpools.

   • Find and label the aeration adjustment on the turbines and locate the breather opening(s).

2. Record your observations of the various kinds of tanks in the table below.

	High Boy	Low Boy	Extremity Tank
How many gallons of water does this tank hold?			
What areas of the body could be treated in this tank?			
Fill and empty the tanks, recording the time to fill and your technique for filling the tank to maintain the water at 104°F.			
While the tank is full, perform the activities listed in Problem-Solving Activities, below.			

Problem-Solving Activity: Transfers and Patient Positioning With Whirlpools
Low Boy
1. Transfer a patient into the low boy from a wheelchair. He or she is non-weight-bearing (NWB) on the left lower extremity (LLE). The patient has no significant past medical history (PMH).

   • What planning is required for you to accomplish this task safely?

   _____

   _____

   _____

   • What else do you need to know about the patient before you transfer him or her into the tank?

   _____

   _____

   _____

   • Of what significance is the water level in the tank prior to transferring the patient into the tank?

   _____

   _____

   _____

   _____

   • What transfer aids, if any, did or would you use?

   _____

   _____

   • Describe the sequence for the transfer and any difficulties that you may have had, outlining how you would approach it the next time.

   _____

   _____

   _____

   _____

2. Adjust the patient's position so that he or she is long-sitting in the low boy. Support the patient's back and arms so that no excess pressure is exerted on him/her. (A towel roll may be used to cushion the extremities from the edges of the tank.)

3. Turn on the turbine and adjust it so that the turbulence is directed at a 45-degree angle to the left side of the tank.

- What sensation does the patient report?

  _____

  _____

- Where does the patient feel the agitation?

  _____

  _____

- Decrease the amount of air that flows into the turbine. How does this change the sensation that the patient has reported?

  _____

  _____

- Increase the amount of airflow to maximum. How does this change the sensation reported by the patient, if at all?

  _____

  _____

4. Adjust the turbine so that it is pointing directly at the patient.
   - What is the patient's response to the adjustment?

  _____

  _____

  _____

   - After 5 minutes of submersion and adjustments to the turbine air flow, recheck the water temperature. Has it changed? If yes, why?

  _____

  _____

5. Prepare your patient to be transferred out of the tank and back into the wheelchair. List the steps that you need to perform.

  _____

  _____

  _____

  _____

6. Repeat the transfer in and out of the low boy until you are comfortable with what you will need to consider to ensure patient and personal safety.

Extremity Tank

1. Position your patient to have his or her right foot treated in the extremity tank. What considerations do you need to make?

  _____

  _____

  _____

2. Adjust the turbine to perform nonspecific débridement to a fragile calcaneal ulcer. What considerations do you need to make, and how would you adjust the turbine?

  _____

  _____

  _____

3. What would change if the patient were being treated for an acute ankle sprain?

_____

_____

_____

4. Describe some of the problems you encountered and how you addressed them.

_____

_____

_____

_____

Patient Transfers in the Hubbard Tank

1. Demonstrate the use of the Hubbard tank and its lift by transferring one of your classmates into the tank. As appropriate for the use of the Hubbard tank itself and for the lift, describe the following:

Patient Instructions:

_____

_____

Indications:

_____

_____

Contraindications:

_____

_____

Precautions:

_____

_____

Cleaning the Whirlpool Tanks

1. Empty and clean each of the tanks that was used and describe the procedure.

_____

_____

_____

_____

2. Where did you find the information for cleaning the tanks?

_____

_____

3. What is the procedure for cleaning the turbines?

_____

_____

_____

_____

4. Why do the turbines need to run while cleaning?

_____

_____

_____

Patient Scenarios

Read through the patient scenarios and determine the following for each:

- Whether hydrotherapy is indicated
- What equipment you would use
- The optimal water temperature
- Whether agitation should be used
- The potential benefits of hydrotherapy

A. Hazel is a slender 80-year-old woman with a left (L) calcaneal pressure ulcer. She has a past medical history (PMH) of diabetes.

B. John is a 25-year-old man status post (s/p) open reduction and internal fixation (ORIF) of the right (R) ankle and spasm of the right calf musculature. His incision is well healed, and he is partial weight-bearing (PWB) on the R leg with crutches. His range of motion (ROM) in dorsiflexion and plantarflexion is limited.

C. Janet is a 60-year-old woman s/p R long-leg cast removal. She lives alone in a first-floor condominium and has been ambulating non-weight-bearing (NWB) on the R leg with a walker. She has good strength throughout her upper extremities (UEs) and lower extremities (LEs). She is anxious to resume her schedule, which included aerobics and bicycling.

D. Mike is a 35-year-old man who experienced a traumatic amputation of his left upper extremity (LUE) above the elbow. The injury occurred 8 weeks ago. He is anxious to resume working. His amputation scar is well healed, and he will be fitted with a prosthesis as soon as the residual limb is toughened up. His UE strength is poor, and he fatigues easily since the injury. He has inquired about a possible home therapy program.

E. Marty is a 55-year-old woman who is 8 weeks s/p transtibial amputation of the RLE secondary to insensate ulcerations as a result of diabetes. She is anxious to be fitted for a prosthesis and to begin ambulation. Her incision is well healed, and she has no other significant PMH.

F. Mary is a 68-year-old obese woman with severe osteoporosis of the hip bilaterally. She was referred to the physical therapy department after a fall that resulted in a compound fracture of the L femur. The fracture has healed. Goals include increasing strength and promoting weight-bearing to prevent further bone loss.

G. Bill is a 45-year-old man s/p 8 weeks lumbar laminectomy who has bilateral muscle guarding of the paraspinal musculature. He is working as an architect and is limited in all spinal movement because of this muscle guarding. He formerly was very active as a triathlete. He needs mobility and aerobic exercises that will allow the paraspinal muscles to relax.

H. Brian is a 22-year-old man with an acute sprain (3 days ago) of the anterior talofibular ligament of the right ankle. His ankle is edematous but pain free. His ankle ROM is limited in all directions by muscle guarding. He is anxious to return to work as a mail carrier.

I. Sharon is a 68-year-old woman s/p R radical mastectomy with decreased shoulder ROM in all directions. Her incisions are well healed, and she is anxious to resume as much activity as possible. She had been an aerobics instructor for a senior citizen center.

J. Jack is a 45-year-old man s/p 4 weeks arthroscopic meniscectomy of the L knee 4 weeks ago. His incision is well healed, and he is now fully weight-bearing (FWB) on the L leg. He complains of weakness and that his knee "gives out" when he descends stairs.

Lab Questions

1. Approximately how long should you allow for the preparation of a whirlpool?
2. What additional considerations are there for positioning and body mechanics with high-boy and low-boy whirlpools?
3. Describe the benefits of nonspecific débridement.
4. Describe the potential adverse effect that a turbine can cause to a healing ulcer and how the harm could be prevented.
5. Your patient has been diagnosed with a spinal cord injury that is now stable at T4. What potential reasons are there to have the patient participate in an aquatic pool program?
6. What additional benefits are derived from deep water activities in an aquatic pool that are not possible through land exercises?
7. Other than ROM in a buoyancy-assisted environment, what are the benefits of aquatic therapy for patients postmastectomy?
8. Describe how flotation devices can be used to increase the level of resistance for an exercise program.

CHAPTER 7

Soft Tissue Treatment Techniques: Traction

Holly C. Beinert, PT, MPT | Burke Gurney, PT, PhD

Learning Outcomes

Following the successful completion of this chapter, the learner will be able to:

- Define the principles of the therapeutic application of traction.
- Describe the theories of cervical and lumbar traction.
- Describe the theories and application of mechanical forms of traction.
- Discuss the clinical uses and safety considerations regarding the use of traction.
- Outline the clinical decision-making in the use of traction as a treatment modality.
- Discuss the importance of appropriate patient positioning techniques for the application of traction by describing the line of pull and the impact of gravity.
- Discuss current theories behind the application of cervical and lumbar traction.
- Demonstrate techniques to decrease the stresses on postural muscles so that a traction force may be successfully applied to the cervical musculature.
- Identify the controls on mechanical traction equipment devices and describe their functions for potential patient application.
- Demonstrate the proper application of supports, belts, and straps to accomplish mechanical traction.
- Demonstrate problem-solving techniques for patient stabilization during the application of manual traction.
- Describe what various forms or traction feel like when applied and relate this experience to a patient.

Key Terms

Angle of pull
Disc herniation
Distraction
Force

Friction
Gravitational traction
Impingement
Intervertebral space

Manual traction
Mechanical traction
Traction

"The human body experiences a powerful gravitational pull in the direction of hope." —Norman Cousins

Patient Perspective
"Will traction affect my height?"

Traction has long been a mainstay for physical therapists when treating a variety of spinal problems. Many causes of spinal pain, as well as weakness, paresthesia, and pain referred from the spine, have traditionally been treated with traction techniques.

There have been mixed reviews from researchers regarding the physiological effects of traction.[1] The findings range from claims of profound changes in spinal occlusion[2,3] to studies showing no statistical differences between traction and bedrest.[4] The negative findings have largely been in studies of specific and/or dated methods such as bed traction.

Like some physical therapy treatments, the use of traction has been a subject of ongoing debate among physical therapists and physicians. Controversy exists regarding optimal techniques, treatment times, positions, frequency, duration, force of pull, angle of pull, and overall efficacy of traction.

The scrutiny of research has helped drive the evolution of traction over the past several decades. Traction no longer means simply mechanical traction performed by traction machines and can include forms such as polyaxial traction, inversion traction, home traction units, and an assortment of manual traction.

A review of the literature in traction is daunting as there exists a seemingly endless variety of treatment techniques and protocols. In attempts to face this problem, several researchers have consolidated the different protocols into useful information,[5-7] such as the general acceptance that supine is preferable to sitting when treating the cervical spine. It also appears that, regarding apparent efficacy, all forms of traction cannot be lumped together. In general, for example, there seems to be a greater body of literature to support the use of cervical traction than the use of lumbar traction.

Some therapists use traction liberally for a number of conditions such as herniated nucleus pulposus and lateral stenosis (a diminution of the intervertebral foramen). Some do not use traction at all. Although controversy remains as to physiological effects, traction has weathered the test of time as a useful treatment for many spinal problems.[1-3,8-12]

Principles of Therapeutic Application

TERMINOLOGY AND DEFINITIONS

Traction

The terms "traction" and "distraction," while related, are not synonymous. The word **traction** is defined as a process of drawing apart or pulling. Traction is a force. The ultimate goal of most traction is distraction, or the separation of bones, usually spinal segments. Two areas of the spine are commonly treated using traction—the lumbar spine (lumbar traction) and the cervical spine (cervical traction). There are many types of traction used in clinics; a partial list is given in Table 7-1.

Distraction

Distraction is defined as the separation of surfaces of a joint by extension without injury or dislocation of the parts.[13] As noted above, distraction is the ultimate goal of traction. When we apply the modality of traction, how do we know for sure that distraction is occurring? While traction can cause distraction, it may not *always* cause distraction.

RELATED PHYSICS

A basic knowledge of the physical principles of traction is necessary to understand the physiology of traction. Principles to be discussed include definitions of force and friction as they pertain to traction.

A **force**, in the simplest sense, is a push or a pull. In the case of traction, it is generated either by the therapist (**manual traction**), by a machine (**mechanical traction**), or by weight (**gravitational traction**). If a therapist places a 100-pound weight on a cable and attaches it by way of a strap onto a patient, the patient will receive traction force of 100 pounds (Fig. 7-1).

Friction is the resistive force that arises to oppose the motion or attempted motion of an object past another with which it is in contact.[14] Friction results from irregularities of the surfaces of the two bodies. The direction of frictional force is always parallel to the surfaces in contact and in the direction opposing motion (Fig. 7-2).

The maximal frictional force on a body resting on another body is proportional to the normal force pushing the

TABLE 7-1	Methods of Traction	
TYPE OF TRACTION	**FEATURES**	**ADVANTAGES/DISADVANTAGES**
Autotraction	This involves the patient using his/her own muscle strength as the traction force, which can be done in different ways. It was first used in Europe and has gained popularity in the U.S. In addition, several home lumbar traction units utilize this method.	**Advantage:** Patient can control parameters such as position and amount of force. Some forms can be done at home. **Disadvantages:** Three-dimensional tables are expensive, have been shown to increase intradiscal pressure.
Cervical traction	Traction applied to the cervical spine by applying a force to move the weight superiorly, or manual technique used to distract the individual cervical vertebra. This can be done manually, with halters, or through Crutchfield tongs, which are inserted directly into the skull.	
Continuous (bed) traction	Traction that is administered for several days to weeks. The traction force is often minimal because of the duration of the treatment. This form of traction has fallen into disuse because of studies indicating that the results are consistent with bedrest alone.	**Advantages:** Can be done at home, inexpensively. **Disadvantages:** Efficacy is questionable.
Elastic traction	Traction by use of elastic devices such as rubber bands.	
Gravity-assisted traction	Uses gravity to facilitate localized traction of target issue. This differs from inversion traction in that the body is not suspended in the air.	**Advantages:** Can be done at home, inexpensively. Does not require healthy cardiopulmonary systems, as does inversion traction. **Disadvantages:** Traction force is limited by body weight.
Head traction	Traction applied to the head in the presence of injury to the cervical vertebra.	

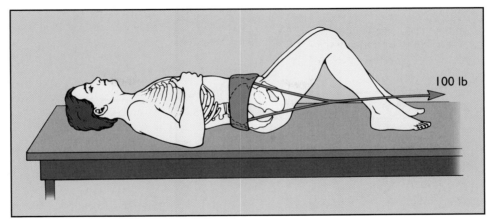

FIGURE 7-1 Patient is positioned supine with 100 pounds of pull.

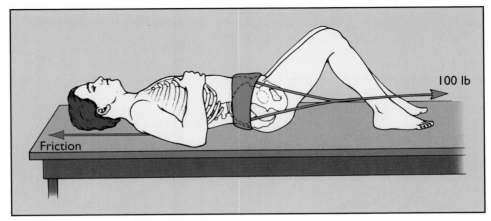

FIGURE 7-2 Patient is positioned with 100 pounds of traction pull, and the force of friction is depicted.

two objects together. For our purposes, the normal force would be the weight of the person on a table. The relationship between the maximal force of friction and the normal force is known as the coefficient of static friction and is designated by m_s.

Expressed mathematically:

$$r_s = \text{maximal force of friction/normal force (weight of person)}$$

The coefficient of static friction has no units and is different for any two objects depending on how irregular the surfaces are between the two objects. It has been shown that the coefficient for static friction between a person and a treatment table is about 0.5.

Therefore, by example, if a person lying on a table weighed 160 pounds (normal force), the force of friction between the person and the table would be 80 pounds (Fig. 7-3).

With lumbar traction, a thoracic harness is often used to keep the upper body from sliding along the table. Therefore, only half (the lower half) of the patient's body weight is involved in the traction. In our example, then, the amount of body weight involved would be 80 pounds, and the frictional force would be 40 pounds. In this case, the force of traction would be 60 pounds (Fig. 7-4).

In most clinics, however, this frictional force is eliminated by use of a split traction table that allows half of the table to glide horizontally on rollers independent of the other half of the table (Fig. 7-5). The use of a split traction table in combination with a thoracic harness ensures that very little force is lost to friction; therefore, the pull of traction can be substantially less.[15] This equipment is necessary only with lumbar traction.

With cervical traction, the coefficient of static friction between the head and the table has been calculated to be 0.62.[16] If the weight of the head were 15 pounds, for example, the traction force would have to be 9.3 pounds to overcome friction.

Theory of Application

BRIEF HISTORICAL PERSPECTIVE

The use of traction may well date back to the time of the Egyptians and is documented at least to the times of Hippocrates (460–376 BC). The original traction table, or *Scamnum Hippocratis* ("the bench of Hippocrates"), was used by Galen (AD 130–200) and others (Fig. 7-6). The Turks have used a traction device for more than 500 years, and the Italians used a traction table in the mid-16th century

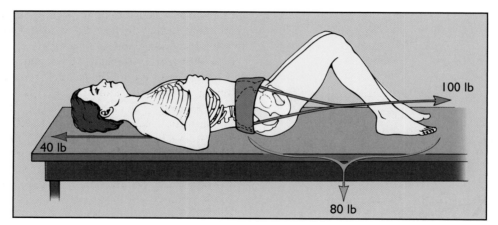

FIGURE 7-3 Patient is positioned supine with 100 pounds of traction pull, and the force of friction is indicated. The resultant pull is equivalent to 60 pounds once the coefficient of friction is calculated into the formula. The weight of the individual was 160 pounds, and 50% of the weight of the individual (80 pounds) was distributed between the legs and pelvis. The coefficient of friction was 50%. Summary: 160-pound patient (80 pounds below the waist), coefficient of friction = 50% or 40 pounds to move the pelvis and legs. Traction force applied = 100 pounds – 40 pounds for the pelvis and legs = 60 pounds of traction force. With the coefficient of static friction of 0.5, the 160-pound patient would have a frictional force of 80 pounds.

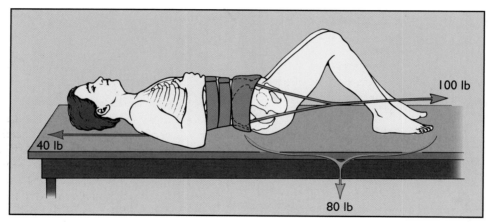

FIGURE 7-4 Patient is positioned supine with 100 pounds of traction pull, and the force of friction is indicated. The resultant pull is equivalent to 60 pounds once the coefficient of friction is calculated into the formula. The weight of the individual was 160 pounds, and 50% of the weight of the individual (80 pounds) was distributed between the legs and pelvis. The coefficient of friction was 50%. Summary: 160-pound patient (80 pounds below the waist), coefficient of friction = 50% or 40 pounds to move the pelvis and legs. Traction force applied = 100 pounds minus 40 pounds for the pelvis and legs = 60 pounds of traction.

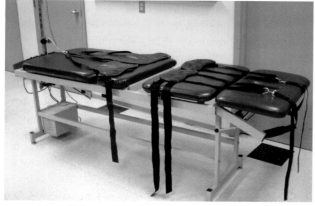

FIGURE 7-5 Split traction table, which lowers the coefficient of friction to close to zero. Traction force to cause movement or separation is greatly reduced through the use of a split table.

that was based on the Hippocratic model.[17] Traction came into disuse for some time based in part on studies challenging its efficacy.

Traction enjoyed a renaissance starting in the 1950s with an orthopedist named James Cyriax and others who developed new and creative approaches to traction treatment. This spurred new research that verified some physiological effects such as vertebral separation and reversal of spinal nerve root impingement.[12] Nerve root **impingement** is compression of a nerve root owing to various causes.

CURRENT TRENDS AND RESEARCH

Modern research involving traction has been under way since at least the 1950s and involves studies of the physical and physiological effects and efficacy of traction and comparisons

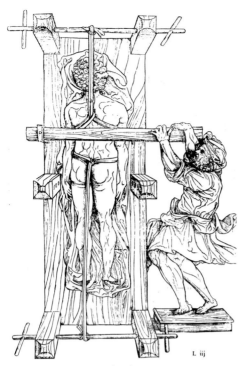

FIGURE 7-6 Hippocratic method.

of different protocols of traction such as optimal patient positioning, intermittent versus continuous pull, angle of pull, and time and frequency of application. Some of the problems that arise when researching traction (and many other modalities) are (1) conclusively defining the population base; (2) objectively measuring variables, that is, pain and dysfunction levels, nerve decompression; and (3) eliminating or accounting for unwanted, for example, confounding, variables.[18] It is probable that the future of traction research will be enhanced by better imaging equipment such as magnetic resonance imaging (MRI) and computerized axial tomography (CAT) scans. This will allow researchers to better categorize their diagnostic groups and better assess physiological changes.

WHY DO I NEED TO KNOW ABOUT...
APPLICATION OF WEIGHT

If distraction of the vertebral bodies is the desired goal, then the amount of weight used must be great enough to overcome friction.

If the weight used is not sufficient to overcome friction, no therapeutic action will occur.

GENERAL TREATMENT GOALS FOR TRACTION

Traction should be used, as are all physical agents, with careful regard to desired physiological effects[1] and should usually be combined with active components of treatment[19] such as strengthening, stretching, postural/proprioceptive training, and patient education. Goals of traction include

reduction of radicular signs and symptoms associated with conditions such as disc protrusion, lateral stenosis, degenerative disc disease, and subluxations (i.e., spondylolisthesis). Other goals of traction include reduction of muscle guarding/spasm via prolonged stretch, reduction of joint pain via neurophysiological pathways (gating mechanism), and increasing range of motion (ROM) via distraction of joint surfaces. Traction has also been used for fracture immobilization. Examples include immobilization of cervical spine fracture via Crutchfield or Burton tongs and immobilization of lower extremity long bones via skeletal or skin traction, that is, Buck's traction or Russell's traction, respectively. Further discussion of traction for fracture immobilization is beyond the scope of this book. The remainder of this chapter addresses the issues of lumbar and cervical traction methods.

✖ BEFORE YOU BEGIN

You need to ask yourself how much the patient weighs so that you can use an appropriate amount of weight for lumbar traction to at least overcome the coefficient of friction.

Cervical Traction

PHYSIOLOGICAL EFFECTS AND CLINICAL USES

Cervical traction is a mainstay in physical therapy treatment for various cervical conditions. As noted earlier, a close review of the literature reveals that clinical efficacy of cervical traction is less controversial than that of lumbar traction. Results of studies have reported cervical traction alone and in conjunction with other modalities to be beneficial in cases of osteoarthritis,[20] cervical radiculopathy,[21-23] disc herniation,[24-26] and tension headaches.[27,28] Cervical radiculopathy is pain originating from the cervical spine, oftentimes referred into the upper extremity. **Disc herniation** is the protrusion of the intervertebral disc from its normal anatomic position. Tension headaches are related to contraction and guarding of the head and neck muscles.

The physiological effects of cervical traction include increasing cervical vertebral separation,[12,25] reducing cervical electromyographic (EMG) activity,[23] reducing nerve conduction disturbances,[29] increasing H reflex amplitude,[22,30] reducing alpha-motor neuron excitability,[31] increasing blood flow to cervical musculature,[32] and restoring cervical lordosis.[33] In contrast, there are studies that show that cervical traction actually increases EMG activity in cervical musculature,[32] has no effect on cervical muscle EMG activity,[34,35] and decreases the H reflex pathway for the soleus muscle.[36]

MECHANICAL TECHNIQUES

Mechanical traction is the use of free weights and traction machines to create a pulling force. Programmable traction units are primarily used because of their versatility. Traditional halters pull from both the occiput and the mandible

(Fig. 7-7). There is evidence that mandibular pull can create and aggravate temporomandibular joint problems.[37] Occipital halters have largely replaced traditional halters (Fig. 7-8). They have no mandibular strap and pull exclusively from the occiput. In addition, some models are capable of pulling the head into side flexion and rotation.

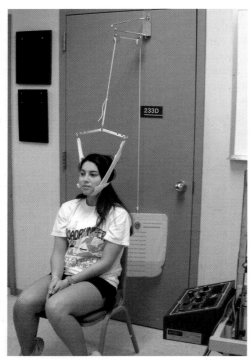

FIGURE 7-7 Traditional halter that pulls from both the occiput and the mandible.

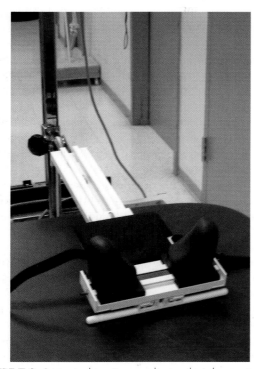

FIGURE 7-8 A cervical traction appliance that does not apply any pressure to the mandible.

Position

Supine position has been shown to be preferable to sitting for most treatments.[38] Research has shown that performing cervical traction in the supine position may be more effective for increasing posterior vertebral separation than cervical traction in the seated position.[100]

Poundage

The head weighs approximately 14 pounds. The poundage used for cervical traction varies according to the source, but it is generally accepted that to produce elongation of the spine, 25 to 30 pounds (11.25 to 13.5 kg) is necessary.[7] Greater amounts produce greater separation only to a point, and excessive traction may produce muscle guarding that can overcome up to 55 pounds of traction force.[12] It appears that the upper cervical spine requires less traction force to cause separation than does the lower cervical spine.[6] Weight approaching 120 pounds was necessary to cause a disc rupture at the C5–C6 level.[40] One study indicates that application of cervical traction can reproduce low back radiculopathy in patients with past episodes,[41] so care should be taken to use the least amount of force that is clinically effective.

> ### BEFORE YOU BEGIN
>
> Make sure that you know what segments that you are trying to separate so that you use appropriate poundage.

Angle of Pull

The **angle of pull** is the angle of the traction force on the target structure, which varies according to target tissue. For maximal perpendicular facet separation, the angle would be 0° at the atlanto-occipital (A/O) joint and increasing amounts of extension to C6–C7 (Fig. 7-9). Prolonged positioning of the neck in extension should be done with discretion, however, as it causes a reduction in the intervertebral separation posteriorly.[42] Beyond that, the relationship between angle of pull and posterior vertebral separation is unclear. Although one study contends that greater amounts of flexion cause greater separation more distally down the cervical spine,[43] another study shows that traction with a neutral spine position actually causes

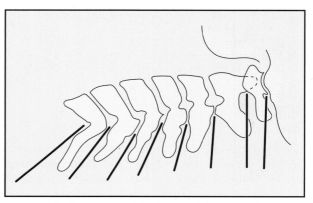

FIGURE 7-9 Orientation of the facets of the cervical spine.

more posterior separation at C6–C7 than the same force of traction performed with 30° of flexion.[42] For increasing the intervertebral space overall, it is generally accepted that about 25° of flexion is optimal.[44]

Intervertebral space is the space between two adjacent vertebrae, which is usually taken up by the intervertebral disc in healthy individuals. A slightly different perspective on the subject was given by the authors of a study that concluded that the maximal force acting on the cervical spine as a whole was obtained with a 35° traction inclination.[16] Too much flexion has been shown to decrease intervertebral space because of encroachment of the ligamentum flavum on the intervertebral foramen.[5,45] For some disc problems, a neutral spine is indicated because it causes the ligaments to be lax and the traction can be transmitted more completely to the disc. Three-dimensional or polyaxial traction is becoming more popular because of its ability to maximally gap vertebral segments unilaterally (Fig. 7-10).

Static Versus Intermittent Traction

While there is little agreement on one over the other, some research provides results that favor intermittent traction over continuous traction for the purpose of pain relief.[99] Intermittent traction seems to be more comfortable for most patients. The shorter the time of pull, the more poundage can generally be tolerated. Muscle relaxation and facet joint capsule stretching applications might respond better to low-load, long-duration stretch (static traction). Facet distraction techniques could best be mimicked by shorter and equal on time and off time (10 seconds/10 seconds), and patients with herniated disc problems to longer on-off times with a ratio of approximately 3:1 (60 seconds/20 seconds) and static pulls.

Facet problems seem to respond better to shorter and equal on time versus off time (10 seconds/10 seconds), and herniated disc problems to longer on-off times with approximately 1:3 ratios (20 seconds/60 seconds), and sustained pulls.

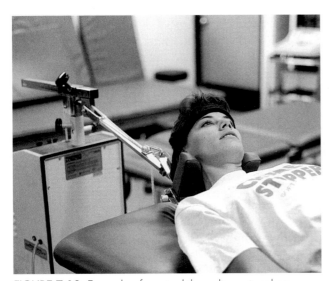

FIGURE 7-10 Example of cervical three-dimensional or polyaxial traction.

Treatment Time

The optimal amount of time that traction is administered ranges from 2 minutes[46] to 24 hours.[47] One study showed that maximal vertebral separation per pull phase occurs after 7 seconds with intermittent traction.[48] One study found that no significant muscular relaxation was found on EMG after 10 minutes of traction and concluded that if muscle relaxation does occur with traction, the effects are not immediate.[35] In general, therefore, the minimum amount of time that traction should be applied to allow full muscular relaxation is 20 to 25 minutes.[7] Treatment time for cervical degenerative joint disease (DJD) should be approximately 25 minutes; for acute disc protrusion, no more than 8 minutes. Traction for longer than 8 minutes with disc protrusions can cause the disc to imbibe excess fluid and increase intradiscal pressure.[6]

Frequency of Treatment

The number of times per week the patient is treated is dependent on type and severity of the problem and duration of relief from traction. The frequency should generally be greater when the problem is more acute, as in the presence of neurological findings.

Other Equipment for Traction of the Cervical Spine

Autotraction

Autotraction of the cervical spine has become more popular recently. The traction force is controlled by the patient through a footboard or other device. This allows constant adjustments to be possible at the patient's discretion and creates an active role of the patient in therapy. The Goodley polyaxial cervical traction unit (E-Z-Em, Westbury, NY) has the advantage of allowing the therapist to administer the line of force through three dimensions. Results using this method have been promising.[8]

Home Units

The use of the "over-the-door" variety of home units has endured despite the necessity to perform the traction sitting (see Fig. 7-7). The maximal weight of these units is 20 pounds. When considering the weight of the head at 14 pounds, this means the maximum force on the cervical spine can be only 6 pounds. It has already been established that 25 pounds is necessary to create a significant distraction of the cervical vertebra. In addition, less cervical muscle activity occurs in supine position than it does in sitting.[35] Despite this, however, there are several studies that show symptomatic relief for patients with spondylosis syndromes[49] and whiplash-type injuries[50] as well as improved pain and ROM in patients with cervical disc herniation.[51]

Other home units are available that allow the patient to be treated in supine and can deliver traction forces sufficient to allow vertebral separation (Figs. 7-11 and 7-12). Traction forces in these units can be generated by gravity assistance, pneumatic pressure, and springs.

Although the supine systems tend to be more expensive, in two separate studies patients seemed to prefer supine pneumatic cervical traction units to the conventional over-the-door counterweight systems[52] and had specific preferences within

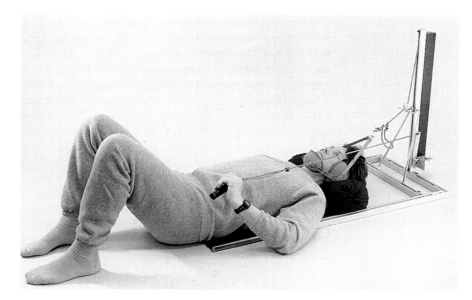

FIGURE 7-11 Home traction unit. *(Courtesy of C-Tract, Granberg International, Richmond, CA.)*

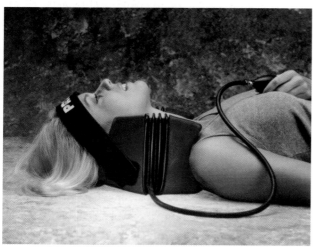

FIGURE 7-12 Pronex system, another type of home traction unit. *(Courtesy of EMPI, St. Paul, MN.)*

the supine models.[53] It seems that if cost is not an issue, supine systems should be a consideration for home use.

MANUAL TRACTION

Cervical manual traction techniques are commonly used by therapists, probably owing to ease in application of a three-dimensional force and the ability to continually assess the patient during treatment. It has been shown that experienced physical therapists are able to apply a reliable force of traction force over repeated trials.[54] Manual traction, like mechanical traction, has been shown to decrease the number of alpha motor neurons firing in upper extremity musculature.[31] Techniques ranging from simple occipital distraction (Fig. 7-13) to various segmental locking techniques in unison with three-dimensional distraction to isolate specific vertebral levels are commonly applied. Specific techniques of manual traction are beyond the scope of this text.

POSITIONAL TRACTION

Positional distraction techniques are inviting because the patient can perform them at home with little to no equipment. The general principle is to place the neck in positions that either enhance limited ROM or maximize intervertebral foraminal space to release impinged tissues. The components of motion to maximally open facets would be forward flexion, contralateral side flexion, and ipsilateral rotation, whereas the components of motion necessary to maximally open up the foramen are forward flexion, contralateral side flexion, and contralateral rotation (Fig. 7-14). The forward flexion position of 15° was found to significantly increase the foraminal volume and isthmus area at C5–C6. Interestingly, this same study showed that adding 25 pounds of traction in this position did little to further increase foraminal opening.[55] Placing one side of the spine in maximal facet or foraminal opening places the other side of the spine in a more closed position, and caution should always be taken to avoid prolonged positions that would place the facet joints or foramen in a closed position.

Procedure for Mechanical Cervical Traction

Before starting a mechanical cervical traction treatment, the following should be done:

1. Review the chart, including diagnosis, indications, contraindications, precautions, and plan of care.
2. Prepare the table, including halter, pillows, draping sheets, call bell, and timer.
3. Preset treatment time, poundage, time on and off, and duration and angle of pull as per plan of care.
4. Explain fully the effects of traction to the patient, answer all questions and concerns of the patient, and obtain verbal informed consent.
5. Use a mouthpiece or soft insert between the teeth if no occipital halter is available to reduce compression forces on the temporomandibular joint (TMJ).
6. Position patient according to desired effect, that is, supine with 25° of cervical flexion in the case of

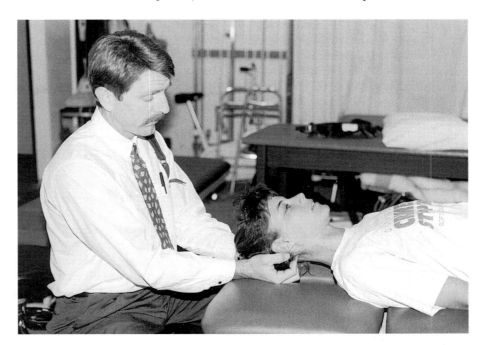

FIGURE 7-13 Proper positioning of both the patient and the clinician for manual cervical traction. Great care must be taken to ensure an appropriate line of pull.

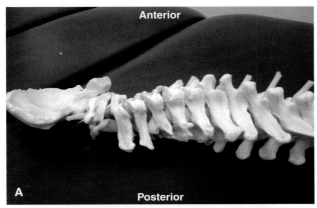

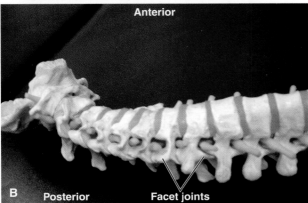

FIGURE 7-14 Positional distraction of the cervical spine. (A) Position of maximal opening of the cervical facets. (B) Position of maximal opening of the intervertebral foramen.

intervertebral foraminal separation. Provide pillows for support and comfort.

7. Adjust the halter according to desired effect. Traditional halters should be positioned so that the patient feels the majority of the pull from the occiput. The posterior (occipital) part of the halter should cradle

the occiput at the level of the inferior nuchal line to both mastoid processes. Place a tissue between the anterior (chin) pad and the chin. If properly applied, the anterior pad should cradle the mandible and be snug to patient's tolerance.

8. Attach halter to spreader bar, and remove all slack from the rope.
9. Double-check all settings.
10. Turn on the machine, and stay with patient at least through one entire cycle to ensure proper setup.
11. Explain the use of the call bell or safety switch before leaving and ensure that it is in the patient's grasp.

Lumbar Traction

PHYSIOLOGICAL EFFECTS AND CLINICAL USES

The evidence regarding the clinical efficacy of lumbar traction is conflicting, owing in part to the wide variety of treatment protocols used and the open range of pathologies for which traction is used.[1] In a recent survey of physical therapists' approach to treatment of low back pain (LBP), use of lumbar traction was infrequent.[56] Studies have found various forms of lumbar traction be to useful alone and in conjunction with other treatments in cases of disc herniation[2,3,10,57–64] and generalized LBP with and without radicular findings.[65–70] Other research has not been supportive of lumbar traction. In several studies, there was no statistically significant difference between patients treated with lumbar traction compared with controls.[4,71–73] A recent systematic review of randomized controlled trials using lumbar traction concluded that the use of traction in LBP remains inconclusive because of the lack of methodological rigor and the limited application of clinical parameters as used in clinical practice.[74]

The physiological effects of lumbar traction include increase in vertebral separation,[75–80] decrease in intradiscal pressure,[81] reduction of disc protrusion,[2,3,59–61] increase in lateral foraminal opening,[82,83] distraction of the apophyseal joints,[61] temporary reduction of scoliosis,[84] temporary increase in lordosis with extension traction,[85] decrease in lumbar paraspinal EMG activity,[86] and temporary increase in stature.[87] In contrast, there are studies that show no decrease in lumbar paraspinal EMG activity with lumbar traction[88] and no reduction of disc protrusion or altered intradiscal pressure.[89]

MECHANICAL TECHNIQUES

Mechanical traction using a traction machine is the most frequently used method. A programmable traction unit is generally used because of its versatility (Fig. 7-15).

Free weights have largely been abandoned owing to the large amount of weight needed.

Position

Lumbar traction has traditionally been performed with the patient in supine position with knees and hips flexed to varying degrees. It has been demonstrated that, during traction, posterior vertebral separation of the lumbar spine increases as hip flexion increases from 0° to 90°.[75] Colachis and Strohm[80] found that with traction in 70° of hip flexion, there is an increase in vertebral separation at all lumbar levels. As with the cervical spine, excessive lumbar flexion can decrease intervertebral foraminal space because of encroachment of the ligamentum flavum on the intervertebral foramen.[5,45]

Current trends include positioning the patient in supine position with hips and knees extended and the prone position, depending on the target tissue and desired effect. Some health care providers prefer prone as a position of choice in cases of LBP involvement.[39] The prone position has the advantage of accessing the back for modalities to be performed concurrently. Studies conclude that prone lumbar traction provided with concurrent heat therapy is more effective in increasing lumbar intervertebral disc spaces than prone lumbar traction alone.[101] It appears that there is no difference in myoelectric activity in back musculature between prone and supine positions.[88]

Poundage

As described under the physics of traction, the poundage necessary to overcome the frictional forces of the lower body (with a thoracic harness, and in the absence of a split traction table) is one-fourth body weight. When using a split traction table, the frictional force is negligible. The protocol for optimal tractional force varies according to source, ranging from 300 pounds[10] to the minimum one-fourth body weight.[5] Maximal tolerance of the T11–T12 discs in cadavers was found to be 440 pounds,[40] although estimates for the lumbar spine in living persons are considerably higher than that. One author contends that based on a review of the literature, there is no relationship between dose (poundage) of traction and response and advocates low dosages.[89] Others suggest that one of the reasons therapists have poor results with lumbar traction is that they use inadequate traction forces.[5] One study showed that patients with LBP showed improvements in pain-free straight leg raise range when 60% and 30% of body weight traction force was used, but no improvement was reported with 10% body weight.[65] Another study showed similar results; most outcome measures of LBP patients improved more with 44% of body weight traction force compared with 19%.[66] As a starting point, then, perhaps Judovich[15] was correct when he proposed that a minimum of one-half body weight be used to have a therapeutic effect.

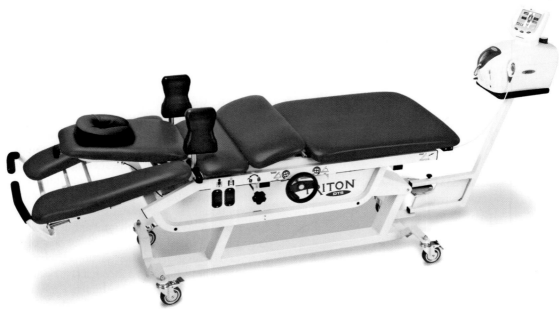

FIGURE 7-15 Commercial mechanical traction unit.
(From Chattanooga Corporation, Chattanooga, TN, with permission.)

Angle of Pull

The angle of the traction force on the pelvis can ultimately determine the low back position during traction and can actually be more important than patient position.[44] To maximize separation, the pull of the traction should occur perpendicular to the surfaces acted upon. In the case of the upper lumbar discs, then, the angle of the pull of the rope should be relatively horizontal. In the case of the L5–S1 level, however, there is a normal 30° lumbosacral angle (Fig. 7-16) posterior to the transverse plane. To ensure a pull as close to perpendicular as possible, the patient should either be placed in supine with maximal hip flexion to minimize the shearing angle or, better still, placed in prone with a 30° angle of pull (Fig. 7-17). Perhaps this is why in several studies traditional angles of pull had minimal effects of joint separation at the L5–S1 level. Colachis and Strohm[80] found that, with supine traction, the least amount of increase in vertebral separation occurred at the L5–S1 interspace. Similarly, Kane et al[82] found that with gravity traction mean intervertebral foraminal separation was significant at all levels except L5–S1.

With the use of modern harnesses, a pull can be generated in the lumbar spine to promote either lordosis or kyphosis depending on the relative placement of the two halves of the harness. Therefore, supine with knees and hips straight with a lordosis pull might be indicated in cases of a disc protrusion, whereas supine with knees and hips bent to 90° with a kyphosis pull might be indicated in the case of lateral stenosis secondary to spondylosis.

Unilateral traction has the advantage of allowing side flexion and rotational forces to occur. This can be of use in cases of lateral disc protrusion or unilateral foraminal stenosis, to name two. Unilateral traction can be performed by either positioning the patient askew to the line of force or applying the traction pull on one side without the use of a spreader bar (Fig. 7-18).

Static Versus Intermittent Traction Force

As with cervical traction, the physiological differences of static versus intermittent traction force are poorly understood, although intermittent traction allows the therapist to use greater traction forces. One study concludes that

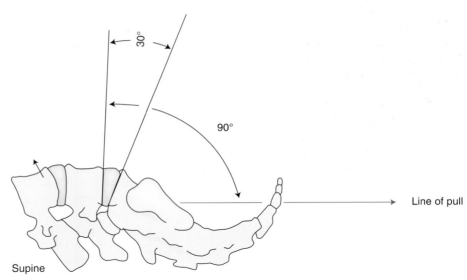

FIGURE 7-16 The 30° lumbosacral angle.

Supine

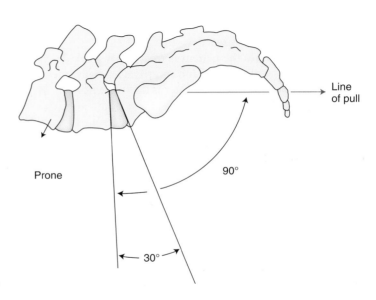

FIGURE 7-17 Lumbopelvic area in prone, with a 30° angle of pull and its perpendicular orientation to L5–S1.

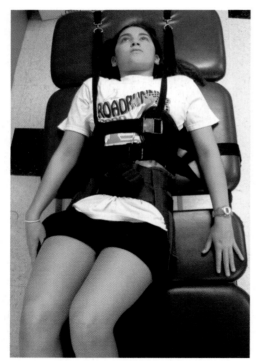

FIGURE 7-18 Unilateral pull of lumbar traction force.

there is no significant difference in magnitude of myoelectrical activity between static and intermittent lumbar traction.[88] Muscle relaxation and facet joint capsule stretching applications might respond better to low-load, long-duration stretch (static traction). Facet distraction techniques could best be mimicked by shorter and equal on time and off time (10 seconds/10 seconds), and herniated disc problems to longer on-off times with approximately 1:3 ratios (20 seconds/60 seconds), and static pulls.

Treatment Time

The length of time for treatment depends on the desired effect and tends to be shorter for disc herniations (8 minutes or less) and longer for spondylosis (about 25 minutes). Traction for longer than 8 minutes with disc protrusions can cause the disc to imbibe excess fluid and increase intradiscal pressure.[6]

Frequency of Treatment

The number of times the patient is treated per week depends on the type of problem and severity. Generally, the more severe the problem, the greater is the frequency.

Other Equipment for Traction of the Lumbar Spine

Autotraction

The term "autotraction" can be used in the broad definition to mean any form of traction where the patient uses his or her own muscle force to generate the traction force, but autotraction is also used to mean a specific type of traction that uses a table that is capable of pivoting on three dimensions. The patient uses his or her own muscle power to create the traction force, so the patient, with the therapist's guidance, can create a varied three-dimensional traction treatment. This latter type of autotraction has gained

support in parts of Europe and the United States. There are several studies addressing the clinical efficacy of autotraction. Autotraction was shown to reduce the incidence of surgery in a population of LBP patients compared with controls at 6 months postintervention.[62] In one study, the use of autotraction compared with sustained mechanical traction showed significantly better results,[57] although the methods of this study have been questioned.[90] Another study comparing autotraction with manual traction showed them to be equally successful.[58] These studies sound favorable; however, the use of autotraction has been shown to increase intradiscal pressure, probably due to the patient creating a contraction of his or her abdominal musculature.[91]

Gravity-Assisted Traction Including Inversion Traction

Gravity-assisted traction is the use of body weight as a distractive force, and it is used both in the clinic and as a home treatment. Various devices have evolved, including inversion traction, where the weight of the suspended body, either fully or from the waist down, is used as a tractive force. Both inversion techniques create a lumbar traction force of about 40% of body weight. This method of traction is acceptable only in patients without cardiopulmonary or cardiovascular compromise or hypertension, as it has been shown to raise both systolic and diastolic blood pressure significantly and to increase oxygen uptake.[76,92,93]

Inversion traction has been shown to have effects similar to mechanical traction, including vertebral separation[76,80] and intervertebral foraminal separation.[82] Patients can also be suspended without being inverted in various ways by use of harnesses that allow the lower body to exert a traction pull on the lumbar spine. This type of gravitational traction reduces the possible cardiovascular concerns and has been shown to increase intervertebral space by greater than 3 mm at all levels between L2 to S1.[78] In one study, noninversion gravitational traction was shown to be efficacious for use with LBP patients without true disc herniation but ineffective with those patients with a diagnosis of extruded disc.[67] A more recent study shows this type of traction to be superior to bed rest in pain reduction and objective gains in subjects with radicular pain.[68]

In other studies using noninversion gravitational traction, lumbar lengthening has been measured as well as lordosis reduction.[77]

Home Units

Many of the home units for lumbar traction use the patient's own muscle strength as a traction force and therefore would be considered autotraction. In addition, various other home units use traction force from gravity, hydraulics, spring loaded, and various other mechanical systems (Fig. 7-19).

Manual Traction

Manual traction techniques can be as simple as providing a simple longitudinal traction force to locking techniques used in unison with three-dimensional pulls to create joint-specific traction in any desired direction.

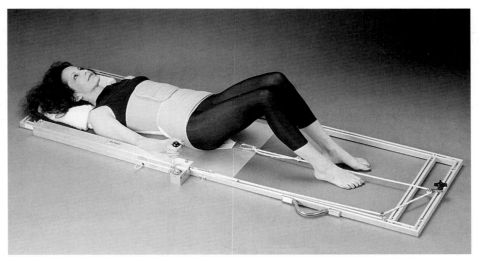

FIGURE 7-19 An "E-Z track" traction unit.
(Courtesy of Granberg International, Richmond, CA.)

Positional Traction

Positional traction is used frequently in the lumbar area by therapists because it can be done at home and requires little or no equipment. The forces can be three-dimensional and can be significant, because the weight of the legs can be used as the traction force. The components of motion to maximally open facets would be forward flexion, contralateral side flexion, and ipsilateral rotation, whereas the components of motion necessary to maximally open up the foramen are forward flexion, contralateral side flexion, and contralateral rotation. One study confirmed radiographically that the lumbar neuroforamen is increased by an average of 4 mm with positional distraction.[83] As with the cervical spine, the position that either enhances limited ROM or maximizes foraminal size should be encouraged and positions that create a closed-packed position over a prolonged period of time should be avoided.

Procedure for Lumbar Traction

Before initiating lumbar traction, the following should be done:

1. Review the chart, including diagnosis, indications, contraindications, precautions, and plan of care.
2. Prepare the table, including harnesses, pillows, draping sheets, call bell, and timer. Always use a split traction table if available.
3. Preset treatment time, poundage, time on and off, and duration and angle of pull as per plan of care.
4. Explain fully the effects of traction to the patient, answer and discuss all patient's questions and concerns, and obtain verbal informed consent.
5. Remove clothing from around belt sites, and drape patient appropriately. Position patient according to desired effect, that is, supine with knees and hips flexed to 45°. Provide pillows for support and comfort.
6. Adjust harnesses according to desired effect. Place a folded towel between patient's abdomen and traction harness. Attach traction (pelvic) harness first; the superior part should be in line with the umbilicus. The

countertraction (thoracic) harness should then be positioned so that the superior part fits snugly around ribs 8, 9, and 10. If properly applied, the two belts should overlap slightly and be snug to patient's tolerance.
7. Attach harness to spreader bar, and remove all slack from the rope.
8. Double-check all settings.
9. Turn on machine and wait for one complete cycle so that all of the slack is taken up; release catch of split table (during off cycle if using intermittent traction).
10. Explain the use of the call bell or safety switch before leaving and ensure that it is within the patient's reach.

✖ BEFORE YOU BEGIN

Make sure that you ask patients if they need to use a restroom to relieve themselves before securing the traction harnesses.

Clinical Uses and Safety Considerations for Traction

INDICATIONS AND EFFECTS
Herniation of Disc Material

Traction has been a treatment for impingement or irritation of nerves secondary to a variety of causes, including disc material contacting the spinal nerve roots. There is a measurable increase in intervertebral space with traction to both the cervical[11,12,18,25,48] and lumbar[2,10,59,75–80] spine. The debate to date revolves around how much separation occurs with specific distractive forces. There are studies that seem to indicate that the application of traction can reverse spinal obstruction secondary to disc protrusion.[2,3,25,60] It has been proposed that in the presence of increased volume of the disc, intradiscal pressure would be lessened. In other words, the negative pressure that should accompany the increased volume should "suck" the disc material back into the disc.[9,25,60,61,81] This is generally accepted, although one study found that intradiscal pressure either remains the same or actually increases during the application of different forms of traction.[91] In summary, although the precise mechanisms of action are unclear, traction has been found to be effective in treatment of herniated discs.[2,10,11,18,24–26,48,59–64]

Degenerative Joint Disease

With DJD of the spine, there are at least two clinically significant occurrences: (1) a decrease of intervertebral space with an associated decrease of the intervertebral foraminal space and (2) osteophyte production into the intervertebral space coming from the facet joint and the vertebral body. Collectively, this progression leads to lateral stenosis, which is a reduction of the intervertebral foraminal size. As mentioned, traction has been shown to increase intervertebral space and, with it, the size of the intervertebral foramen. Although the increase in foraminal size seen with traction should return to pretreatment size after the treatment is over, the decrease in pain can last for a prolonged time. Once the nerve is decompressed, perhaps the swelling in the nerve subsides and the existing foraminal size is sufficient to accommodate the smaller-diameter nerve. Traction has been shown to be an effective treatment for impingement of the spinal nerve secondary to spinal stenosis.[5–7,9,10,17,20,82,85]

Muscle Guarding

In the presence of spinal pain, be it cervical, thoracic, or lumbar secondary to muscle spasm or guarding, traction can be of use to cause a slow, prolonged stretch of the muscles. Although some sources state that prolonged stretch via traction can cause a reflex inhibition of the muscle,[31,47,86] others disagree.[32,34,35,88] Possible explanations include Golgi tendon organ involvement, a "resetting" of the muscle spindle to a longer length, a stretching of joint receptors or even skin receptors,[94] and relaxation of nociceptive reflexes.

Joint Hypomobility

In studies discussed earlier, it has been shown that traction is capable of vertebral separation in both the cervical and lumbar spines. This separation would have to occur at both the intervertebral bodies and the facet joints. In the presence of generalized decreased spinal ROM, therefore, spinal traction will mobilize the joints by moving the articular surfaces on each other and distract the surfaces and decrease articular pressure.[61] In addition, intermittent traction should have the effect of increasing synovial fluid production and thus nutrifying the cartilage as well as firing mechanoreceptors to "gate" the pain transmission. Treating patients with specific areas of hypomobility would be difficult with generalized traction; however, manual traction or three-dimensional traction might be indicated in this case.

Facet Impingement

The facet joints have a capsule that can theoretically become impinged within the joint space.[95] Traction techniques, especially in combination with positions that maximize specific joint separation, will cause a decompression of the facet joints and thus could be of some use in treating impingements.[61] Although standard mechanical traction could be used for this condition, polyaxial autotraction, positional traction, and manual traction would be the preferred methods because of their ability to isolate specific joints.

PRECAUTIONS AND CONTRAINDICATIONS FOR THE USE OF TRACTION

Before you begin, we need to first address the precautions and contraindications for traction. It's important to know what they are, but perhaps it is more important to understand *why* each is either a precaution or a contraindication. See Box 7-1 for a list of questions to elicit information on possible contraindications.

PRECAUTION	WHY?
Joint hypermobility (spinal)	The pull that is applied with traction may exacerbate joint instability unless it is carefully monitored.
Pregnancy	The lumbar belts that must be applied to administer mechanical lumbar traction may be inappropriate depending on the delivery date.
Acute inflammation (spinal)	After an acute injury, there may be muscle guarding, which would impair the patient's ability to relax during the application of traction. This may lead to minor muscle tearing, which could increase the patient's symptoms.
Claustrophobia	Patients who have difficulty with confinement or closed spaces may experience increased muscle guarding during the application of mechanical traction.
Temporomandibular joint dysfunction	The cervical halter used for these patients must be one that does not apply any pressure on the mandible or mechanical cervical traction may exacerbate their TMJ dysfunction.
Cardiac or respiratory insufficiency	Inversion traction and mechanical lumbar traction can have adverse effects on cardiac and respiratory function.[96]
Patients whose symptoms increase with traction	Traction should be terminated and the patient reevaluated.
Patients with blood pressure issues	Decreases in both systolic and diastolic blood pressure were seen in patients undergoing cervical traction.[98]

CONTRAINDICATION	WHY?
Spinal infection	The possibility exists that infection could be spread through the use of spinal traction.
Rheumatoid arthritis	The integrity of the joint is compromised by the disease process. The addition of a traction force may further increase joint instability without providing any relief for the patient.
Osteoporosis	The application of mechanical traction may cause fragile bone to fracture either through the pull of the traction or the tightness of the straps.
Spinal cancer	Increasing circulation to the spinal structures through the use of spinal traction may encourage the spread of the malignancy via seeding.
Cardiac or respiratory insufficiency or recent ophthalmic surgery	Inversion traction is the only form of traction contraindicated in these patients because it increases internal pressure.
Spinal cord pressure secondary to central disc herniation	Patients with major involvement of the intervertebral disc, including central disc herniation, will receive no sustained benefit from externally applied traction.

Hernia all around (handwritten annotation)

SPECIAL CONSIDERATIONS FOR THE APPLICATION OF TRACTION

Patients must be given a shut-off button (if available) or call button to use in case of emergency.

PATIENT EDUCATION

As with all treatments, the patient should be as completely informed as possible regarding the effects and goals of traction treatment. Patient compliance markedly increases when patients understand the treatment they are to receive. A spinal model with spinal nerves and drawings of the physical effects are useful tools for traction education. For example, the therapist, upon explaining the effects of cervical traction to treat lateral stenosis, might use a finger to represent a nerve and form an "O" with the finger and thumb of the other hand to represent the foramen, then pass the "nerve" through the "foramen," demonstrating the normal relationship.

BOX 7-1 | Contraindications and Clinical Decision-Making

During the patient's treatments, certain questions can help prevent problems from arising. The following are examples of some of the questions to ask patients that could yield valuable information. Questions to rule out contraindications and precautions include the following:

1. Is your pain in both legs (arms)? *Contraindication—* spinal tumor or central spinal cord impingement
2. Are you having problems going to the bathroom? *Contraindication—* spinal cord tumor or central spinal cord impingement
3. Have you had any swelling or pain in other joints for no reason (without a traumatic event)? *Contraindication—* rheumatoid or other systemic inflammatory disorders
4. Tell me about any bones that you have broken. *Contraindication—* osteoporosis
5. Have you had a fever or sweating and unusual tiredness as of late? *Contraindication—* spinal infection
6. Is your pain worse at night, do you have any changes in your appetite, sleep patterns, etc.? *Contraindication—* spinal tumor
7. When did you last injure your back or neck? *Precaution—* acute inflammation, avoid excessive forces in traction
8. Does all movement hurt your back or neck or specific movements and do you experience any excessive popping, clicking, or other noises with movement? *Precaution—* hypermobility, avoid excessive forces in traction
9. Do you get short of breath easily? *Precaution—* respiratory insufficiency, avoid inversion traction
10. Do you have high blood pressure? *Precaution—* cardiac insufficiency, avoid inversion traction
11. Do you have popping or clicking in your jaw, jaw pain, or frequent headaches? *Precaution—* TMJ dysfunction
12. Have you ever received traction before, and if so, did it aggravate your condition? *Contraindication/ precaution—* all of the above

---

Inflammation of the nerve might be represented by using two fingers side by side. Radiculopathy can be represented by making the "O" too small for the nerve. Next, the therapist might show on a spinal model how distraction can increase the size of the foramen to allow the nerve unimpeded passage. If the therapist prescribes positional distraction for a patient, the effect of positional distraction on the diameter of the foramen can be represented by making the "O" larger to depict the position used for positional distraction.

Patient Perspective

Remember that your patient may not understand what you are going to do with him or her. He or she might even have images of "the rack" in his or her mind when you mention the word "traction." Be calm and provide patient education in terms that are easily understood. Some patients may not realize how claustrophobic they are until after they have been set up with mechanical traction. For this reason it is critical to check on the patient within the first 5 minutes and also to provide access to a call system should it be necessary.

PATIENTS' FREQUENTLY ASKED QUESTIONS

1. **Will I be taller after traction?**
2. **Why are the straps so tight?**
3. **Can I read while I have traction for my neck?**
4. **What do I do if I need to use the restroom while I am receiving traction?**
5. **Why did the pain that went down in my leg go up into my back after traction? My back didn't hurt before.**

If the patient is to be given a home traction device or technique to perform, the therapist should demonstrate the use of it and have the patient demonstrate the use to the therapist. Have the patient bring the device to the next treatment (or use a similar model available in the clinic) and demonstrate the proper use again. These "pop quizzes" will give the therapist valuable information regarding compliance and will alert one to improper use of the modality. Improper use of traction units and improper traction positioning can aggravate many conditions.

BILLING

Billing for mechanical traction can be done by using the mechanical traction Current Procedure Terminology (CPT) code. Billing for manual traction can be done using the manual therapy code. Items that must be documented when using traction as an intervention are as follows:

- Area to be treated (cervical vs. lumbar)
- Goal of traction
- Patient position
- Angle of pull
- Poundage
- Static vs. intermittent (on: off times)
- Duration
- Patient response
- Patient education and informed consent

PATIENT POSITIONING AND DRAPING CONSIDERATIONS

Patient positioning is especially important when dealing with problems for which traction is indicated.

Although there remains controversy about extension versus flexion when treating the spine, patient comfort is paramount. As mentioned earlier, if the patient is in an uncomfortable position and is muscle guarding, the strength of the spinal muscles will overcome any desired physiological effects of traction. Because patient position greatly affects intradiscal pressure,[38] it is of particular importance for patients with disc herniations.

Lumbar Spine

Prone positions tend to increase lumbar extension (lordosis) of the spine with a relative anterior wedging of the disc, decrease intervertebral foraminal space, and increase weight-bearing forces on the facets (closed-packed position). Prone positioning might be indicated with disc bulges without total dissociation of the nuclear material. It would be contraindicated with severe osteoarthritis with lateral stenosis.

The supine position without leg support can also create lumbar extension (lordosis), which has the same effects as above. Supine with knees and hips flexed creates flexion of the lumbar spine and produces a relative posterior wedging of the disc, increased intervertebral foraminal space, and decreased weight-bearing forces on the facets. Excessive lumbar flexion has actually been shown to decrease intervertebral space, probably because of the movement of the ligamentum flavum into the foraminal space.

Cervical Traction

When performing cervical traction, positioning is usually performed either sitting or supine. As mentioned earlier, there is less muscle activity in the paraspinals when supine compared with sitting, and therefore this appears to be the position of choice if the patient can tolerate it. Prone positioning creates an extension bias and should be avoided unless the therapist can create a neutral spine with supports. The supine position maintains an approximately neutral cervical spine in patients with normal thoracic kyphosis. Patients with excessive kyphosis or a dowager's hump are apt to experience a position of excessive cervical lordosis when supine without at least one pillow for support. A position of slight hip and knee flexion during cervical traction prevents lumbar lordosis in persons with tight hip flexors and can relax the patient to ensure greater efficacy.

Patient draping should be consistent with room temperature and patient modesty and expose only the skin necessary to perform techniques effectively.

Documentation

As with other modalities, it is important to document the parameters administered to a patient. When using traction, this is particularly important. The following parameters must be documented:

- Patient position (e.g., supine, knees flexed or extended, prone, sitting)

- Type of traction
  - mechanical
  - intermittent
  - sustained
  - manual
- Amount of force in pounds
- Duration
  - hold time
  - rest time
- Attachments
  - Saunders cervical traction (Empi)
  - cervical halter
  - over-the-door home unit
  - total treatment time

It is also important to document the patient's initial complaint before traction and his or her response to the traction. Traction is commonly applied to relieve radicular symptoms. Record whether the goal was accomplished subsequent to the application of traction. Sometimes a patient will report a decrease in symptoms during traction but a return of the symptoms once the traction force is released. This must also be documented.

Summary

Traction has endured as a treatment technique for hundreds of years because of its ease of application and versatility. Although traction is not a panacea, it can be an effective treatment technique for a variety of spinal disorders and can be used with a modicum of equipment both in the clinic and in the home setting. Although there is a plethora of research that substantiates the efficacy of certain traction methods, there is also a body of literature to refute the physiological effects and clinical efficacy of traction, most notably lumbar traction. Either way, more research needs to be done to validate (or invalidate) specific methods of traction treatment in all of its applications.

Review Questions

1. Which of the following best defines the term "traction"?
   a. The separation of joint surfaces
   b. A force that draws apart or pulls apart joint surfaces
   c. A piece of physical therapy equipment
   d. It is the same as friction
2. Which of the following is *not* a general treatment goal of traction?
   a. Reduction of radicular signs and symptoms
   b. Reduction of muscle guarding
   c. Reduction of pain
   d. Reduction of range of motion
3. Which of the following positions is the preferred position for cervical traction?
   a. Supine
   b. Prone
   c. Sitting
   d. Hook-lying
4. Which of the following percentages of body weight is necessary to overcome the frictional forces of the lower body (with a thoracic harness and in the absence of a split traction table)?
   a. One-eighth body weight
   b. One-fourth body weight
   c. One-half body weight
   d. Three-quarters body weight
5. Which of the following is *not* a potential contraindication for the use of traction?
   a. Osteoporosis
   b. Spinal cancers
   c. Low back pain
   d. Rheumatoid arthritis

CASE STUDY 1

Ellen is a 68-year-old left-handed woman who complains of neck pain, predominantly on the left side. She has no specific underlying cause but seems to remember falling about 8 years ago and experiencing some pain in her neck for a week or so afterward. She has pain with extension and side flexion to the left. She reports that her left arm often feels heavy and clumsy but denies sensory changes. She says, "It's not as bad in the morning and gets worse as the day goes on," and she reports problems looking overhead and doing her sewing. Your examination reveals she has limitations with extension, side flexion left, and rotation to the right. She has somewhat diminished reflexes on the left triceps compared with the right and has a 4/5 wrist extension on left when compared to right. She has decreased right side glide to the right in slight extension of C6 on C7 and has tenderness over her left C6–C7 facet with deep pressure. Her radiograph shows some degenerative changes at this level with some spurring of the facet joint encroaching on her lateral foramen. She also exhibits some tightness in her upper trapezius, anterior scalenes, and levator scapula on both sides. The category she falls under using the *Guide to Physical Therapist Practice*

is impaired joint mobility, motor function, muscle performance ROM, and reflex integrity associated with spinal disorders with the interventions to include intermittent mechanical traction. You elect to start with supine traction with 25° of flexion 15 seconds on, 5 seconds off with 20 pounds of traction for 15 minutes on the first treatment to assess efficacy.

Patient education includes using a step stool to ensure the work space is at eye level or below; self-ranging of the neck with emphasis on flexion and side flexion right; stretching of the upper trapezius, scalenus, and levator scapula; and instruction in use of a home cervical traction unit. She has been instructed to use an over-the-door unit in sitting, while facing the door with 15 pounds of force for 20 minutes in the morning. In addition, she has been given information on the anatomy of the cervical spine including the lateral foramen, and she has been shown how the nerve in her lower neck is being pinched owing to the bony changes in her spine and how to maximally open up the lateral foramen using the position of forward flexion, side bending right, and rotation right (see Fig. 7-14). She was instructed in the use of pillows and positioning to facilitate this position.

CASE STUDY 2

Henry is a 27-year-old carpenter with a history of LBP that started with an episode about 3 months earlier, when he was reaching across a sawhorse to lift some wood off a shelf. He felt immediate pain in the right side of his low back. He went to the emergency department, where they took a radiograph, which was negative, and gave him some NSAIDs and muscle relaxants. He stated the pain kept getting worse and he started developing pain shooting into the posterior leg to the back of the knee. He went to see his primary care physician, who ordered an MRI, which was also negative for disc herniation. The physician sent him to the therapist, who found that the patient had a negative straight leg raise test on the right, pain and limitations with forward bending, pain-free extension, painful rotation and side bend left. The patient also complained of some discomfort with posterior-anterior glides at L4–L5, which did reproduce his pain in the low back and leg. Joint plays revealed a hypomobility in facet opening at L4–L5 and L5–S1 on the right. Segmental passive ROM revealed a failure of the L4–L5 facet to open on the right. There was no evidence of changes in sensation, reflexes, or strength in the lower extremity.

The category the patient falls under using the *Guide to Physical Therapist Practice* is "Impaired joint mobility, motor function, muscle performance, range of motion and reflex integrity associated with spinal disorders" with the interventions to include static mechanical traction. The therapist elects to perform mechanical traction in supine starting with one-half body weight to cause a therapeutic effect of joint separation. He sets the patient in 90° of flexion of the hips and knees to ensure posterior pelvic tilt and reduction of lumbar lordosis and the angle of pull at 20° above horizontal to maximize facet separation. The therapist elects to do static traction to promote a reduction in muscle guarding and to induce a possible elongation of scar tissue that may have formed at the facet joint capsule.

Patient education for this patient would include an understanding that positional traction in left side-lying with a pillow under his left hip, knees to chest, and left rotation can maximize the separation of his facet joints on the right. He is told to maintain this position for at least 30 minutes at least once a day.

DISCUSSION QUESTIONS

1. Why would position make a difference in the treatment outcome when using either cervical or lumbar traction?

2. Of what significance is the presence of a lordosis in the lumbar spine if lumbar traction is used?

3. How does knowledge of the coefficient of friction influence your decision regarding the amount of traction required to cause distraction of the joint surfaces?

4. How would you explain the purpose of cervical traction to a patient who was referred for treatment with a diagnosis of a cervical strain with radiating pain and paresthesia in the right upper extremity following an automobile accident?

5. Describe the differences between the use of an occipital pull harness and a typical head halter for cervical traction.

REFERENCES

1. Pellecchia, GL: Lumbar traction: a review of the literature. J Orthop Sports Phys Ther 20:262–267, 1994.
2. Mathews, J: Dynamic discography: a study of lumbar traction. Ann Phys Med 9:275, 1968.
3. Gupta, R, and Ramarao, S: Epidurography in reduction of lumbar disc prolapse by traction. Arch Phys Med Rehabil 59:322, 1978.
4. Pal, B, et al: A controlled trial of continuous lumbar traction in the treatment of back pain and sciatica. Br J Rheumatol 25:181, 1986.
5. Saunders, H: Lumbar traction. J Orthop Sports Phys Ther 1:36, 1979.
6. Saunders, H: The use of spinal traction in the treatment of neck and back conditions. Clin Orthop Rel Res 179:31, 1983.
7. Harris, P: Cervical traction: review of literature and treatment guidelines. Physical Therapy 57:910, 1977.
8. Walker, G: Goodley polyaxial cervical traction: a new approach to a traditional treatment. Physical Therapy 66:1255, 1986.
9. Larsson, U, et al: Auto-traction for treatment of lumbagosciatica. Acta Orthop Scand 51:791, 1980.
10. Cyriax, J: The treatment of lumbar disc lesions. Br Med J 2:1434, 1950.
11. Judovich, B: Herniated cervical disc. Am J Surg 84:649, 1952.
12. Bard, G, and Jones, M: Cineradiographic recording of traction of the cervical spine. Arch Phys Med Rehabil August:403, 1964.
13. Taber's Cyclopedic Medical Dictionary, ed 21. FA Davis, Philadelphia, 2009.
14. Hewitt, P: Conceptual Physics, ed 11. HarperCollins, New York, 2009.
15. Judovich, BD: Lumbar traction therapy—elimination of physical factors that prevent lumbar stretch. JAMA 159:549, 1955.
16. Pio, A, et al: The statics of cervical traction. J Spinal Disord 7:337–342, 1994.
17. Natchev, E: A Manual of Auto-traction Treatment for Low Back Pain. Folksam, Stockholm, Sweden, 1984.
18. Goldie, I, and Reichmann, S: The biomechanical influence of traction on the cervical spine. Scand J Rehabil Med 9:31, 1977.
19. Tan, JC, and Nordin, M: Role of physical therapy in the treatment of cervical disc disease. Orthop Clin North Am 23:425–449, 1992.
20. Gilworth, G: Cervical traction with active rotation. Physiotherapy 77:782–784, 1991.
21. Moetti, P, and Marchette, G: Clinical outcomes from mechanical intermittent cervical traction for the treatment of cervical radiculopathy: a case series. J Orthop Sports Phys Ther 31:207–213, 2001.
22. Abdulwahab, SS: The effect of reading and traction on patients with cervical radiculopathy based on electrodiagnostic testing. J Neuromusculoskeletal System 7:91–96, 1999.
23. Lee, MY, Wong, MK, Tang, FT, Chang, WH, and Shiou, WK: Design and assessment of an adaptive intermittent cervical traction modality with EMG biofeedback. J Biomech Eng Trans ASME 118:597–600, 1996.
24. Constantoyannis, C, et al: Intermittent cervical traction for cervical radiculopathy caused by large-volume herniated discs. J Manipulative Physiol Ther 25:188–192, 2002.
25. Chung, TS, et al: Reducibility of cervical disc herniation: evaluation at MR imaging during cervical traction with a nonmagnetic traction device. Radiology 225:895–900, 2002.
26. Saal, JS, et al: Nonoperative management of herniated cervical intervertebral disc with radiculopathy. Spine 21:1877–1883, 1996.
27. Fitz-Ritson, D: Therapeutic traction: a review of neurological principles and clinical applications. J Manipulative Physiol Ther 71:39–49, 1984.
28. Stone, RG, and Wharton, RB: Simultaneous multiple-modality therapy for tension headaches and neck pain. Biomed Instrum Technol 31:259–262, 1997.
29. Hattori, M, Shirai, Y, and Aoki, T: Research on the effectiveness of intermittent cervical traction therapy, using short-latency somatosensory evoked potentials. J Orthop Sci 7:208–216, 2002.
30. Haraoka, K, and Nagata, A: Modulation of the flexor carpi radialis H reflex induced by cervical traction. J Phys Ther Sci 10:41–45, 1998.
31. Brandman, L, Rochester, L, and Vujnovich, A: Manual cervical traction reduces alph-motoneuron excitability in normal subjects. Electromyogr Clin Neurophysiol 40:259–266, 2000.
32. Nanno, M: Effects of intermittent cervical traction on muscle pain. Flowmetric and electromyographic studies of the cervical paraspinal muscles. Nihon Ika Daigaku Zasshe 6(12): 137–147, 1994.
33. Harrison, DE, et al: A new 3-point bending traction method of restoring cervical lordosis and cervical manipulation: a nonrandomized clinical controlled trial. Arch Phys Med Rehabil 83:447–453, 2002.
34. Jette, DU: Effect of cervical traction on EMG activity of upper trapezius. Phys Ther 65:730, 1985.
35. Murphy, MJ: Effects of cervical traction on muscle activity. J Orthop Sports Phys Ther 13:220–225, 1991.
36. Hiraoka, K, and Nagata, A: The effects of cervical traction on the soleus H reflex amplitude in man. Jpn J Phys Fitness Sports Med 47:287–294, 1998.
37. Shore, A, et al: Cervical traction and temporomandibular joint dysfunction: report of case. J Am Dent Assoc 68:4, 1964.
38. Deets, D, et al: Cervical traction: a comparison of sitting and supine positions. Physical Therapy 57:255, 1977.
39. Sood, N: Prone cervical traction. Clin Manag 7:37, 1987.
40. DeSeze, S, and Levernieux, J: Les traction vertebrales. Semin Hip Paris 27:2075, 1951.
41. LaBan, M, et al: Intermittent cervical traction: a progenitor of lumbar radicular pain. Arch Phys Med Rehabil 73:295, 1992.
42. Wong, AM, et al: The traction angle and cervical intervertebral separation. Spine 17:136–138, 1992.
43. Hseuh, TC, et al: Evaluation of the effects of pulling angle and force on intermittent cervical traction with the Saunder's Halter. J Formos Med Assoc 90:1234–1239, 1991.
44. Saunders, H: Evaluation, Treatment, and Prevention of Musculoskeletal Disorders, ed 4. WB Saunders, Philadelphia, 2004.
45. Maslow, G, and Rothman, R: The facet joints, another look. Bull NY Acad Med 51:1294, 1975.
46. Frazer, H: The use of traction in backache. Med J Aust 2:694, 1954.
47. Crue, BL, and Todd, EM: The importance of flexion in cervical halter traction. Bull Los Angeles Neurol Soc 30:95, 1965.
48. Colachis, SC, and Strom, BR: Cervical traction: relationship of traction time to varied tractive force with constant angle of pull. Arch Phys Med Rehabil 46:815, 1965.
49. Swezey, RL, et al: Efficacy of home cervical traction therapy. Am J Phys Med Rehabil 78:30–32, 1999.
50. Olson, VL: Whiplash-associated chronic headache treated with home cervical traction. Phys Ther 77:417–424, 1997.
51. Baker, P, and Marcoux, BC: The effectiveness of home cervical traction on relief of neck pain and impaired cervical range of motion. Phys Ther Case Rep 2:145–151, 1999.
52. Waylonis, GW, et al: Home cervical traction: evaluation of alternative equipment. Arch Phys Med Rehabil 63:388–391, 1982.
53. Venditti, PP, et al: Cervical traction device study: a basic evaluation of home-use supine cervical traction devices. J Neuromusculoskeletal Syst 3: 82–91, 1995.

54. Sailors, ME, et al: Force reproduction in submaximal manual cervical traction applied by experienced physical therapists. J Manual Manipulative Ther 5: 27–32, 1997.

55. Humphreys, SC, et al: Flexion and traction effect on C5-C6 foraminal space. Arch Phys Med Rehabil 79:1105–1109, 1998.

56. Li, LC, and Bombardier, C: Physical therapy management of low back pain: an exploratory survey of therapist approaches. Physical Therapy 81:1018–1028, 2001.

57. Tesio, L, and Merlo, A: Autotraction versus passive traction: an open controlled study in lumbar disc herniation. Arch Phys Med Rehabil 74:871, 1992.

58. Ljunggren, A, et al: Autotraction versus manual traction in patients with prolapsed lumbar intervertebral discs. Scand J Rehabil Med 16:117, 1984.

59. Mathews, W, et al: Manipulation and traction for lumbago sciatica: physiotherapeutic techniques used in two controlled trials. Physiother Pract 4:201, 1988.

60. Onel, D, et al: Computed tomographic investigation of the effect of traction on lumbar disc herniations. Spine 14:82, 1989.

61. Goldish, G: Lumbar traction. In Tollison, CD, and Kriegel, M (eds): Interdisciplinary Rehabilitation of Low Back Pain. Williams & Wilkins, Baltimore, 1989.

62. Tesio, L, et al: Natchev's auto-traction for lumbago-sciatica: effectiveness in lumbar disc herniation. Arch Phys Med Rehabil 70:831–834, 1989.

63. Weinert, AM, and Rizzo, TD: Nonoperative management of multilevel lumbar disc herniations in an adolescent athlete. Mayo Clin Proc 67:137–141, 1992.

64. Guvenol, K, et al: A comparison of inverted spinal traction and conventional traction in the treatment of lumbar disc herniations. Physiother Theory Pract 16:151–160, 2000.

65. Meszaros, TF, et al: Effect of 10%, 30% and 60% body weight traction on the straight leg raise test of symptomatic patients with low back pain. JOSPT 30:595–601, 2000.

66. van der Heijden, GJM, et al: Efficacy of lumbar traction: a randomized clinical trial. Physiotherapy 81:29–35, 1995.

67. Oudenhoven, RC: Gravitational lumbar traction. Arch Phys Med Rehabil 59:510–512, 1978.

68. Moret, NC, et al: Design and feasibility of a randomized clinical trial to evaluate the effect of vertical traction in patients with a lumbar radicular syndrome. Manual Ther 3:203–211, 1998.

69. Werners, R, et al: Randomized trial comparing interferential therapy with motorized lumbar traction and massage in the management of low back pain in a primary care setting. Spine 24:1579–1584, 1999.

70. Corkery, M: The use of lumbar harness traction to treat a patient with lumbar radicular pain: a case report. J Manual Manipulative Ther 9:191–197, 2001.

71. Beurskens, AJ, et al: Efficacy of traction for nonspecific low-back pain. 12-week and 6-month results from a randomized clinical trial. Spine 22:2756–2762, 1997.

72. Beurskens, AJ, et al: Efficacy of traction for nonspecific low-back pain: a randomized clinical trial. Lancet 346:1596–1600, 1995.

73. Borman, P, et al: The efficacy of lumbar traction in the management of patients with low back pain. Rheumotol Int 23:82–86, 2003.

74. Harte, AA, et al: The efficacy of traction for back pain: a systematic review of randomized trials. Arch Phys Med Rehabil 84:1542–1553, 2003.

75. Reilly, JP, et al: Effect of pelvic-femoral position on vertebral separation produced by lumbar traction. Physical Therapy 59:282–286, 1979.

76. Gianakopoulos, G, et al: Inversion devices: their role in producing lumbar distraction. Arch Phys Med Rehabil 66:100–102, 1985.

77. Janke, AW, et al: The biomechanics of gravity-dependent traction on the lumbar spine. Spine 22:253–260, 1997.

78. Tekeoglu, I, et al: Distraction of lumbar vertebrae in gravitational traction. Spine 23:1061–1063, 1998.

79. Twomey, LT: Sustained lumbar traction, an experimental study of long spine segments. Spine 10:146–149, 1985.

80. Colachis, SC, and Strohm, BR: Effects of intermittent traction on separation of lumbar vertebrae. Arch Phys Med Rehabil 50:251–258, 1969.

81. Ramos, G, and Martin, W: Effects of vertebral axial decompression on intradiscal pressure. J Neurosurg 81:350–353, 1994.

82. Kane, MD, et al: Effect of gravity-facilitated traction on intervertebral dimensions of the lumbar spine. JOSPT 6:281–288, 1985.

83. Creighton, DS: Positional distraction, a radiological confirmation. J Manual Manipulative Ther 1:83–86, 1993.

84. Hales, J, et al: Treatment of adult lumbar scoliosis with axial spinal unloading using the LTX3000 Lumbar Rehabilitation System. Spine 27:E71–E79, 2002.

85. Harrison, DE, et al. Changes in sagittal lumbar configuration with a new method of extension traction: nonrandomized clinical controlled trial. Arch Phys Med Rehabil 83:1585–1591, 2002.

86. Falkenberg, J, et al: Surface EMG activity of the back musculature during axial spinal unloading using an LTX 3000 Lumbar Rehabilitation System. Electromyogr Clin Neurophysiol 41:419–427, 2001.

87. Bridger, RS, et al: Effect of lumbar traction on stature. Spine 15:522–524, 1990.

88. Letchuman, R, and Deusinger, RH: Comparison of sacrospinalis myoelectric activity and pain levels in patients undergoing static and intermittent lumbar traction. Spine 18:L1361–L1365, 1993.

89. Krause, M, et al: Lumbar spine traction: evaluation of effects and recommended application for treatment. Manipulative Ther 5:72–81, 2000.

90. Trudel, G: Autotraction. Arch Phys Med Rehabil 75:234–235, 1994.

91. Andersson, G, et al: Intervertebral disc pressures during traction. Scand J Rehabil Med 9:88, 1983.

92. Ballantyne, B, et al: The effects of inversion traction on spinal column configuration, heart rate, blood pressure, and perceived discomfort. J Orthop Sports Phys Ther 7:254, 1986.

93. LeMarr, J, et al: Cardiorespiratory responses to inversion. Phys Sport Med 11: 51, 1983.

94. Katavich, L: Neural mechanisms underlying manual cervical traction. J Manual Manipulative Ther 7:20–25, 1999.

95. Paris, S: The spine: etiology and treatment of dysfunction including joint manipulation. Course notes, 1979.

96. Quain, BM, and Tecklin, JS: Lumbar traction: Its effect on respiration. Phys Ther 65:1343–1346, 1985.

97. Simmers, TA, et al: Internal jugular vein thrombosis after cervical traction. J Internal Med 241:333–335, 1997.

98. Balogun, JA, et al: Cardiovascular responses of healthy subjects during cervical traction. Physiother Canada 42:16–22, 1990.

99. Graham, N, Gross, A, and Goldsmith, C: Mechanical traction for mechanical neck disorders: a systematic review. J Rehabilitation Med 38:145–152, 2006.

100. Fater, D, and Kernozek, T: Comparison of cervical vertebral separation in the supine and seated positions using home traction units. Physiotherapy Theory Pract 24:430–436, 2008.

101. Cevik, R, Bilici, A, Bukte, Y, et al: Effect of new traction technique of prone position on distraction of lumbar vertebrae and its relation with different application of heating therapy in low back pain. *J Back Musculoskeletal Rehab* 20:71–77, 2007.

LET'S FIND OUT

Lab Activity: Traction

This lab activity is designed to demonstrate the principles of therapeutic traction that are currently practiced in clinical environments. Learners will become familiar with the treatment goals, positioning, apparatus, and techniques that are commonly employed. Learners will administer and receive various forms of traction and learn the importance of proper positioning for both the patient and the device or individual applying the traction. This lab activity also covers what to document and how important appropriate patient instruction is to treatment success.

Equipment

mechanical traction unit (with instruction manual)	Saunders cervical traction appliance
	goniometer
belts and straps for traction unit	foot stool
cervical traction head halter	pillows
treatment table	towels

Mock Cervical Traction Model Setup (Optional)

empty plastic gallon milk container	string plum bob
level (small plastic bubble level)	protractor
cloth straps (about 3 yd)	adhesive tape

Lab Activity: Orientation to Patient Positioning for Traction

Traction can be defined as a process of pulling or drawing apart. This process involves pulling or separating joint surfaces. Traction can be applied manually or mechanically. Regardless of the technique, patient positioning to accomplish the goal is an integral part of the process. Without proper positioning, the line of pull may not be capable of accomplishing the separation desired.

Supine

1. Have one of your classmates lie supine on a plinth without any pillows. Position them so that there is a straight line along midline bisecting their right and left sides.

   - What was/were your point(s) of reference to determine that they were "straight"?

     _____

     _____

     _____

   - Is the patient comfortable in this position?

     _____

   - What is the position of the lumbar spine? (Is there a lordosis?)

     _____

     _____

   - What is the position of the cervical spine?

     _____

2. Position your classmate so that they have a flat lumbar lordosis and a neutral cervical lordosis (Figs. 7-20 and 7-21).

  • Describe what you had to do to accomplish this.

  _____
  _____
  _____
  _____

  • Is the patient comfortable in this position?

  _____

  • Is the patient still "straight" with a bisecting midline?

  _____

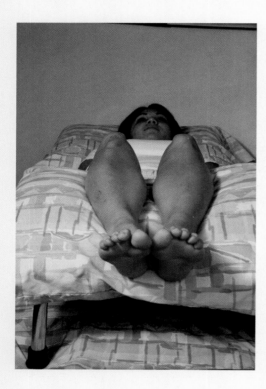

FIGURE 7-20 Patient positioned supine with midline in proper alignment with all bony landmarks.

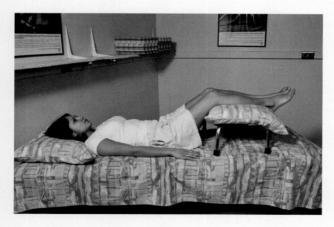

FIGURE 7-21 Patient positioned in supine with a flat lumbar lordosis as viewed from the side.

- How long does it take to position the patient so that he or she has both a flat lordosis and a neutral cervical spine?

_____

3. Grasp the humerus of your classmate (the patient), superior to the distal epiphysis, so that you can apply gross distraction/traction to the right upper extremity.

- What happens to the alignment of the patient?

_____

_____

- How much traction force did it take for the alignment to shift (a lot, some, hardly any)?

_____

4. Have another classmate (patient) stabilize the acromion process of the scapula and trunk while you distract the humerus.

- What happens to the alignment of the patient?

_____

_____

_____

- How much traction force did it take for the alignment to shift (a lot, some, hardly any)?

_____

- What purpose would stabilization serve when applying traction?

_____

_____

_____

Sitting

1. Have one of your classmates sit in a chair that has a straight back (armrests optional). He or she should be positioned so that the feet are flat and firmly touching the floor in an erect posture with a straight line running from the external auditory meatus of the ear through the acromion process, the spine, and the greater trochanter.

- Describe what you had to do to accomplish this.

_____

_____

_____

- What tools did you use to assess the patient's position?

_____

_____

- Is the patient comfortable in this position?

_____

- How long did it take to accomplish this position?

_____

- While you were recording your answers, did the patient shift position? If yes, how?

_____

_____

- If your goal was to relieve the pressure of the head on the cervical spine created by gravity, where would the "pull" need to come from?

  _____

  _____

  _____

- How would you stabilize the rest of the body?

  _____

  _____

  _____

2. Select one of the cervical head halters and inspect it. Determine which is the mandibular strap and which is the occipital strap. With the classmate (patient) seated, place the halter on him or her. There should be some kind of adjustment that can be made between the mandibular and occipital straps. Adjust the straps with a hand on each side of the head. Gently pull upward to take up the slack in the straps; do not try to relieve the weight of the head.

   - If your goal was to relieve the weight of the head, what direction or angle should the traction pull toward?

     _____

     _____

   - Why is it important not to have the pull come from the mandible?

     _____

     _____

   - How difficult is it to adjust the line of pull to accomplish an occipital pull? What do you need to do?

     _____

     _____

     _____

3. What would the rationale be for an occipital pull? What would be accomplished?

   _____

   _____

   _____

   _____

4. What is/are the treatment goal(s) of cervical traction?

   _____

   _____

   _____

   _____

5. How would you know if a patient was responding favorably to the application of cervical traction? How would his or her symptoms change?

   _____

   _____

   _____

   _____

Mock Cervical Traction Setup (Optional)

1. Fill an empty gallon milk container with water and recap it, securing the cap with a ring of adhesive tape. The bottle will represent the head for this exercise. The handle of the milk bottle represents the posterior upper cervical spine as it comes from the base of the occiput. The cap of the bottle is inferior to the chin.

2. Place a ring of adhesive tape around the base of the occiput, and around the entire head (bottle) so that it bisects the head just below the nose. The line of tape should be perpendicular to the seam on the container (Fig. 7-22).

3. Place another line of tape on the anterior seam on the container. This will be an additional reference point for positioning.

4. Attach the level to one side of the container so that it is parallel to the seam and perpendicular to the occipital tape ring.

5. You will note that handling the container full of water is not easy. The weight of the gallon container is approximately 8 lb, which actually is less than the weight of the human head.

6. You will also note that resting the container on the table so that the seam is facing up and is aligned is not easy either. The human head is much the same. The patient will have a tendency to turn the head to one side to rest as it does not easily balance in neutral (Fig. 7-23).

7. Take the cloth tape and make a cervical halter similar to the prefabricated one that you previously inspected and worked with. Start by making a loop that is about 24 inches long when folded. Make two tape rings for this loop; they will represent the metal D-rings that you held on the prefabricated cervical halter (Fig. 7-24).

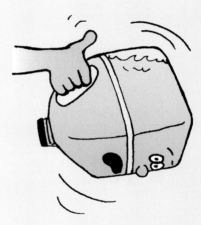

FIGURE 7-22 Gallon water container filled, capped off, and marked with tape to indicate the position of horizontal midline and the occiput.

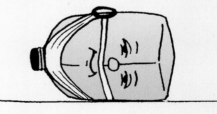

FIGURE 7-23 Gallon water container lying on its side and wearing a cervical head halter.

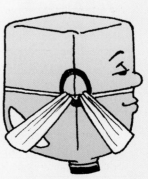

FIGURE 7-24 Gallon water container in erect posture and wearing a cervical head halter.

8. Build an occipital strap and a mandibular strap with tape so that the bony prominences of the head ("container") will have a place to catch on to.

9. Apply your cervical halter to the container. Determine what angle the line of pull should be to relieve the weight of the head while maintaining the level in a fixed position (Fig. 7-25).

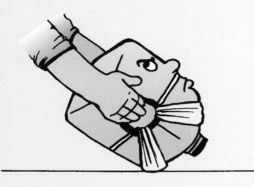

FIGURE 7-25 Manual adjustment of the line of pull on the halter to attempt to pull from the occiput.

Manual Cervical Traction Demonstration

1. Ask one of your lab instructors to demonstrate manual cervical traction with the patient in a seated and a supine position.

   • Which position appeared "easier" for the clinician? Why?

   _____
   _____
   _____

   • Which position appeared more comfortable for the patient? Why?

   _____
   _____
   _____

2. Cervical traction is usually applied in the supine position. Why do you think this is?

   _____
   _____
   _____
   _____

3. Ask one of the lab instructors to set up the Saunders cervical traction appliance by attaching it to a mechanical traction unit (Refer to Fig. 7-8).

   • Before a patient is positioned on the plinth, what can you predict about the position in which the appliance will place the cervical spine?

   _____
   _____
   _____

   • Inspect the appliance. What is the purpose of the small sled on which the occiput rests?

   _____
   _____
   _____

   • Inspect the straps and supports for the appliance. What is the purpose of the temporal/frontal strap?

   _____
   _____
   _____

• How is the mandible treated with this appliance? Is there any support for it or pull on it?

_____
_____
_____

4. If you were to give your seated cervical traction patient a magazine to pass the time while he or she were in traction, what would happen to his or her positioning?

_____
_____

5. If you were to instruct a supine patient to "just get up" after a traction force had been applied and released, what would happen to the intradisc pressure?

_____
_____
_____

6. Why would the position of the patient prior to the application of a traction force make a difference?

_____
_____
_____
_____

7. How much force would it take to overcome the weight of the head?

Sitting _____

_____
_____

Supine _____

_____
_____

8. When your patient was supine and you were using the cervical appliance, what happened when you tried to adjust the angle of pull to the occiput? Did you have any difficulty maintaining alignment of the cervical spine? Why and why not?

_____
_____
_____
_____
_____

9. The cervical spine has two individual curves. Of what significance are they when applying cervical traction?

_____
_____
_____
_____

10. What muscles maintain the normal cervical curves?

_____
_____
_____
_____

11. Which muscles tend to guard following a cervical strain? What impact, if any, would guarding in these muscles have on the curves of the cervical spine?

_____

_____

_____

_____

Lumbar Traction Demonstration

1. Observe while one of your lab instructors demonstrates manual lumbar traction with the patient in a supine position with hips and knees flexed.

   • What problems do you see for the clinician in maintaining this level of traction?

   _____

   _____

   _____

   • Which form of traction appeared to be more comfortable for the patient? Why?

   _____

   _____

   _____

   • How much traction force was the clinician able to apply manually, and how reproducible would this be from clinician to clinician? Why?

   _____

   _____

   _____

   _____

2. Lumbar traction is usually applied with mechanical devices. Why do you think this is?

   _____

   _____

   _____

3. Observe while one of the lab instructors sets up the thoracic and lumbar traction belts and straps and attaches them to the mechanical traction unit.

   • Before a patient is positioned on the plinth, what can you predict about the position in which the appliance will place the lumbar spine?

   _____

   _____

   _____

   _____

   • Inspect the setup. Why were straps applied to the thoracic and lumbar areas?

   _____

   _____

   _____

   • Why was padding added to the straps?

   _____

   _____

• Why were the hips flexed? What did this do to the lumbar spine?

_____

_____

_____

_____

4. If you were to instruct a supine patient to "just get up" after a traction force had been applied and released, what would happen to the intra-disc pressure?

_____

_____

5. Why would the position of the patient prior to the application of a traction force make a difference?

_____

_____

_____

_____

6. How much force would it take to overcome the weight of the lower half of the body in the supine position?

_____

_____

• If you are using a traction table that splits, does this make a difference? If so how?

_____

_____

_____

_____

7. What happens to the pressure on the lumbar spine when the angle of pull is adjusted?

_____

_____

_____

_____

8. Which muscles tend to guard following a lumbar strain? What impact, if any, would guarding in these muscles have on the curves of the lumbar spine?

_____

_____

_____

_____

9. Apply lumbar traction to a classmate, and have a classmate apply lumbar traction to you. Use the poundage suggested by your lab instructor. Record your observations regarding how the traction felt.

Your Observations

_____

_____

Classmate's Observations

_____

_____

10. What instructions did your lab instructor provide to the sample patient that you would use in the future? Why?

_____

_____

_____

_____

11. It is important to ask a patient whether or not he or she needs to use the restroom before the application of lumbar traction. Why do you believe that this would be an important consideration?

_____

_____

_____

Patient Scenarios

A. If you were instructed to apply cervical traction for the reduction of cervical muscle pain and guarding in a patient who had unilateral guarding of the upper trapezius on the right, what, if anything, about the treatment setup would change? Why?

B. Matt is a 45-year-old construction worker who injured his back while installing a steel grate to cover a drainage basin. He has no other significant past medical history. His back and leg pain occurred after he let go of the grate when he attempted to straighten up. He now has radicular symptoms in the left leg from the buttocks down to the lateral malleolus. His strength and sensation are normal. His primary complaint is that of pain down the back of his leg. He is anxious to return to work. Would traction of some form be indicated? If yes, how? If not, why? What additional considerations might there be for this patient?

C. Sue was referred to therapy for evaluation and treatment of her cervical pain symptoms. Her physician recommended that traction be considered along with other palliative modalities to relieve her discomfort and improve her mobility. This physician is eager to discuss treatment options for this patient with the evaluating therapist . Sue was injured in an automobile accident in which her car was struck from behind. She has bilateral guarding in all cervical muscles. She recently underwent a mandibular reduction to correct horizontal alignment of her incisors. What additional considerations are there for this patient? Would traction be contraindicated? Why or why not?

D. Will has been referred to therapy by his family physician for lumbar traction to relieve questionable lumbar radiculopathies that appear to be transient. Will injured his back while working, and he has not yet returned to work. He works as an architect. His complaints of pain and numbness vary. Some days the paresthesia is located in the right foot and other days it is in the left foot. Traction was suggested to determine if centralization of the pain would be possible. There were no signs of fracture. After examination and discussion, traction was initiated to determine whether or not it would provide any sustained benefit.

One day after receiving his first treatment with traction, Will returns to the clinic for another treatment. He states that his symptoms subsided following the traction. Today, his paresthesia is behind his left knee, but he also complains of pain in the right buttocks. When setting up the lumbar belts, you ask him whether he needs to use the restroom before receiving traction. Will declines and states that he has not been able to urinate for about the past 12 hours. What course of action should you take? Why?

Lab Questions

1. Describe how your body mechanics might change if you performed manual cervical traction while a patient was seated in a chair and while lying supine.

2. If cervical and lumbar traction are performed to relieve radiculopathies, what is the goal of appendicular manual traction?

3. Of what significance is hand placement of the individual who is stabilizing the patient during a manual traction treatment?

CHAPTER 8

Soft Tissue Management Techniques: Compression and Edema Management

Holly C. Beinert, PT, MPT | Joy C. Cohn, PT CLT-LANA

Learning Outcomes

Following the successful completion of this chapter, the learner will be able to:

- Discuss the pathophysiology of edema and identify different types of edema.
- Discuss the specific interventions to address edema.
- Discuss the factors that determine the appropriate intervention for edema reduction.
- Discuss the clinical decision-making process for determining the effectiveness of the chosen intervention for edema reduction.
- Demonstrate edema assessment techniques for the upper and lower extremity, including use of a volumeter and tape measure.
- Demonstrate patient positioning for, clinical application of, and removal of an intermittent compression device for edema reduction in the upper and lower extremity.
- Demonstrate the monitoring of pedal, popliteal, and radial pulses on classmates and indicate the clinical relevance of these for patient populations with edematous extremities.

Key Terms

Lymphatic system
Interstitial space

Primary lymphedema
RICE

Secondary lymphedema

"Such bees! Bilbo had never seen anything like them. 'If one were to sting me,' He thought 'I should swell up as big as I am!'" —J.R.R. Tolkien, The Hobbit

Patient Perspective

"I thought I could put my cancer behind me, but now this swelling is a daily reminder."

Edema is an abnormal accumulation of fluid in the **interstitial space**, which is the fluid-filled areas that surround cells. This is a seemingly simple definition, but it in fact reflects a very complex interaction between physiological and anatomical facts. Edema can present as an acute event in a localized area of the body as is commonly seen, for example, after a sports injury. Or an individual may experience a more sustained effect and less-localized swelling of a limb, for example, as a consequence of treatment for cancer. The intervention required can be very different in these two instances. As is true in all areas of practicing physical therapy, a precise understanding of the mechanisms giving rise to the edema is critical to determining the appropriate intervention.

Pathophysiology of Edema

Fluid travels through the body in three major pathways—the circulatory system, the lymphatic system, and in the interstitial spaces between the cells. The circulatory system has a "pump"—the heart—that pushes the fluid through an extensive network of vessels divided into an arterial side and a venous side. These sides are divided by the capillary bed in the interstitial spaces where fluid and nutrients leave the capillary bed on the arterial side and fluid and byproducts of metabolism are reabsorbed on the venous side. In the normal state, 90% of the fluid that filters out of the capillary bed on the arterial side is reabsorbed on the venous side.[1] The 10% of the remaining fluid and all proteins and other debris are removed by the lymphatic vessels that lie in intimate contact with the capillaries in the interstitial space. The removal of proteins along with the excess fluid cannot be emphasized too strongly because [italics added] *"this removal of proteins from the interstitial spaces is an essential function without which we would die within about 24 hours."*[2] Fluid and proteins in the interstitial space are held primarily in a "gel matrix" that serves several purposes: it acts as a spacer between the cells, it prevents excessive movement of the fluid into the lower body when we stand, and it prevents the rapid spread of bacteria through the tissues.[2]

The **lymphatic system** (Fig. 8-1) is analogous to a sewer system and is not often thought of unless the "water backs up into the street" and edema becomes clinically symptomatic. It serves three important functions in the body: (1) regulation of fluid balance through transport of fluid

187

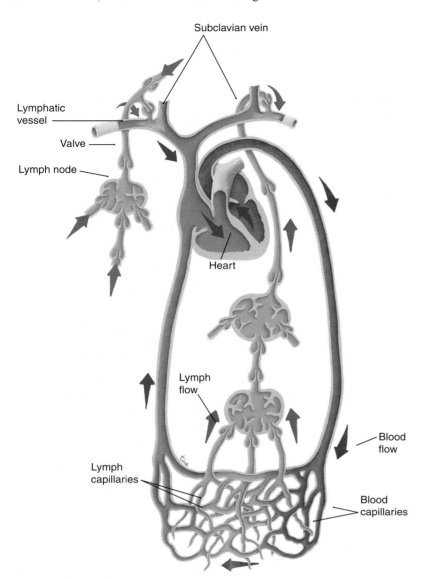

FIGURE 8-1 Lymphatic system.
(From Scanlon, V, and Sanders, T: Essentials of Anatomy and Physiology, 5th edition. Philadelphia: F. A. Davis, 2007.)

and proteins, (2) defense against infection/cancer as a part of the immune system, and (3) transport of digested fat from the gut. It is a system with a one-way flow from the periphery to its termination at the jugular angles just above the heart where the lymph fluid is returned to the circulatory system. The vessels of the lymphatic system gradually progress from fragile, very superficial capillaries to deeper "collectors" that lie in parallel to the deep veins in returning fluid to the circulatory system. The absorbing lymphatic capillaries are vessels with walls of endothelial cells in a single layer. They are anchored into the tissues by fine filaments. Fluid enters these vessels through gaps between the cells that are opened by the anchoring filaments in response to changes in local tissue pressure from movement or an increase in the hydrostatic pressure in the tissue space. These gaps are larger than those in the blood capillaries and also allow proteins and debris to be absorbed. The deeper lymphatic vessels have valves like the veins that prevent backflow. They also have intrinsic muscle in their

walls and pulsate in response to being stretched or from stimulation from the autonomic nervous system to help propel fluid toward the heart. Lymph transport relies on several extrinsic mechanisms because there is no intrinsic pump (the heart) as in the circulatory system. These include the musculoskeletal pump, respiratory pressure changes, the intrinsic pulsation of the deep lymphatic vessels, close proximity to the pulsating arteries, and gravity. All of these mechanisms should be kept in mind when treating an individual with edema.

The lymphatic system normally transports approximately 2 to 2.5 liters of fluid per day and 80 to 200 g of protein back to the circulatory system.[3] The fluid is filtered through nodes that are responsible for the removal of foreign substances and are the site of lymphocyte activity to fight infection. It has the capacity to increase its flow up to 10 times the normal volume of fluid carried as the hydrostatic pressure increases,[1] but not for the long term.

Types of Edema

Edema becomes apparent when the interstitial fluid has reached a level at least 30% above normal.[2] Owing to the capacity of the lymphatic system to increase its flow rate by 10-fold and because the gel matrix is able to absorb 30% to 50% more fluid than in the normal state before free fluid accumulates, if edema is apparent, it represents, at least in the short term, a failure of the normal compensatory mechanisms in the tissues.

Localized acute edema usually occurs because of tissue injury in response to trauma of a mechanical, infectious, or toxic nature. This causes inflammation that is characterized by localized redness, warmth, swelling, and pain. The patient may be unable to move comfortably or bear weight on the affected limb. The edema in this case is caused by a substantial increase in the capillary permeability, allowing large quantities of fluid and protein to escape the capillaries and flood the interstitial space. Actual bleeding with hematoma formation is also possible. The capillary permeability is changed by actual trauma to the vessels, the inflammatory response to an injury, and the secondary release of chemicals that not only stimulate the healing response but also increase capillary permeability.[4] The edema fluid has a relatively low protein content in this situation. An acute edema usually occurs in conjunction with a normal venous and lymphatic system. This type of edema usually resolves in a limited time frame (weeks to months), although more extensive injuries may progress to a more chronic form. The therapist's intervention focuses on enhancing the normal physiological mechanisms to resolve the edema via venous and lymphatic return. Examples of this type of edema would include a sports injury to soft tissue or a joint, a wound in the skin, a localized infection, or a reaction to an insect or snake bite (Table 8-1).

Acute edema of a widely affected area of the body is usually the result of metabolic disease states such as malnutrition or liver, kidney, or heart disease. Congestive heart failure (CHF) is a good example. In this instance, there is increased capillary pressure because of a venous obstruction from pooling of blood in the veins as the heart fails to adequately pump.[2] CHF causes a soft, symmetrical swelling in the legs. The causes of cardiac failure are complicated, and the treatment of this type of edema requires the skilled care of a physician and is beyond the scope of this chapter.

Chronic or progressive (slow or rapidly accumulating) edemas can be more accurately described as lymphedemas. This type is the result of venous and/or lymphatic obstruction. The edema fluid in this instance has high protein content because of the slow accumulation of proteins in the absence of adequate clearance by the lymphatics. The lymphatic return is limited because of obstruction or failure because of overload in compensating for a lack of adequate venous return. It must be remembered that the lymphatics are the only mechanism to remove protein from the tissues. This type of edema can often be painless and only mildly warm in relation to the contralateral limb. Other symptoms common to this type of swelling include heaviness,

TABLE 8-1	Types of Edema	
TYPE	**SIGNS AND SYMPTOMS**
Acute	Rapid onset after known injury Redness Warmth Painful to palpation or movement Localized
Venous	Slowly progressive Moderate warmth Dusky color or brownish staining of skin Achy pain as day progresses Normal contours of leg are lost
Lymphatic	Slowly progressive Mild warmth Color changes rare Usually painless Sensation of fullness or heaviness in limb Soft and pitting or hard Asymmetrical in comparison of limbs
Systemic edema (heart, kidney, and generally pitting	Abdominal swelling (ascites) Generalized, varying edema (liver disease) Bilateral, symmetrical edema
Toxic	Acute
	Localized
	Itchy or painful
	Redness
	Nonpitting

warmth, aching, stiffness, tight/shiny skin, loss of skin folds, and inability to wear clothing or jewelry on the affected limb. Lymphedema can be divided into two varieties. **Primary lymphedema** is a congenital lack of adequate lymphatic drainage. The lymphatic vessels are usually either malformed or reduced in number. There are several presentations (Box 8-1). **Secondary lymphedema** is the result of an acquired injury to the venous or lymphatic system. There are many known causes. Lymphedema is frequently associated with fibrotic skin changes. The fibrosis is the result of increased fibroblast activity in response to the high level of proteins in the tissues. The therapist's intervention in this case is aimed at enhancing the remaining venous and lymphatic return to reduce the lymphedema volume, modifying chronic changes in the soft tissue, and teaching strategies to reduce the reaccumulation of fluid.

EXAMINATION OF PATIENT

In the American Physical Therapy Association's *Guide to Physical Therapist Practice*,[23] the practice pattern "6H–Impaired Circulation and Anthropomorphic Dimensions Associated with Lymphatic System Disorders" addresses all of the pertinent data that should be included

BOX 8-1 | Types of Lymphedema[5]

Primary Lymphedema
- Milroy's disease (presents at birth)
- Lymphedema praecox (presents at adolescence)
- Lymphedema tarda (presents after age 30)

Secondary Lymphedema
Lymphatics damaged by:

- Trauma
- Surgery
- Infection
- Obstruction by tumor
- Radiation therapy
- Obstruction by parasite
- Paralysis of a limb
- Chronic venous insufficiency

in a thorough examination. Certain aspects of the initial examination warrant particular attention once general demographics and social, employment, and living environments and habits have been considered.

1. *Timing of symptoms of edema*: When did the swelling begin? Is there an event that precipitated the edema? Has the swelling improved, worsened, or remained unchanged? Is the edema worse as the day goes on? Is the edema gone first thing in the morning?
2. *Medical/surgical history*: Includes history of cancer treatment, other medical conditions, all surgical procedures, and history of previous injury
3. *Pain*: Intensity, quality, and what causes an increase or a decrease
4. *Self-treatment*: Has the patient self-treated or received any treatment up until now and with what response?
5. *Medications/tests*: Has the patient taken any over-the-counter or prescribed medications? Has the patient had any medical tests; if so, what were the results?
6. *Functional limitations*: What functional limitations does the patient report?

The results of this part of the examination can help to classify a generalized limb edema as lymphedema and allow determination of whether it is a primary or secondary lymphedema. Lymphedema is characterized by stages, each of which describe the amount of progression (Box 8-2).

BOX 8-2 | Stages of Lymphedema[14]

Stage I   Reversible: edema reverses with elevation, pitting edema with pressure
Stage II Irreversible: edema remains with elevation. Increased fibroblast activity owing to proteins causes fibrosis in the tissues. Minimal pitting to pressure
Stage III Elephantiasis: extensive tissue hardening, papillomas (wart-like growths), and huge limb size

Tests and measures to document the particular impairments of the patient are chosen based on the initial interview of the patient, but in the presence of edema, they should always include the following:

- Musculoskeletal survey including range of motion (ROM), strength, stability of joints, and posture
- Neurological status including sensation and signs of neural tension
- Skin integrity including color, breaks or irritations in the skin, presence of scars, tattoos demarcating an area of previous radiation therapy, and temperature
- Edema including circumferential measurements or volumetric measurements, pitting or nonpitting, and extent of edema
- Cardiovascular/circulatory status including blood pressure, pulses, heart rate, rubor with dependency, and venous filling time
- Wounds, if any, described by size, depth, presence of drainage, odor, appearance of the depth of the wound, and appearance of the immediate skin area
- Functional status and activity level including whether the patient has difficulty with clothing or shoes, reaching overhead, ambulation, or transfers

Anthropomorphic characteristics of the limb or area of the edema can be documented by circumferential measurements or volumetric measurements. A simple body diagram is also very useful. Measurements should ideally always be taken at the same time of day and by the same person. Circumferential measurements are taken with a nonstretch tape measure of a material that can be easily cleaned with alcohol between uses. The tape must have a lead at the beginning meaning that the zero mark must be easily discerned and not hidden or missing. All measurements must be taken at reproducible landmarks that should be documented or at regular intervals. Casley-Smith and Casley-Smith[5] describe taking measurements at 4- or 10-cm intervals with no loss in accuracy or reproducibility. This has become a commonly used method in lymphedema management because it is inexpensive, it can be accomplished in any location, and it is convenient. This method is sensitive to varying degrees of change in a limb. These measurements can used to obtain a calculated volume by a truncated cones method.[5] The measurements can be used to calculate a rough estimate of the difference in volume between two limbs by summing all of the measurements of each limb and comparing the sum for the affected to the unaffected side. A percentage difference can also be calculated. This very simple method allows the therapist to learn how the limb changes over time in comparison with the opposite limb with little error compared with more rigorous mathematical determinations of volume.[5] The comparisons can be expressed as a percentage difference.

A volume measurement can also be obtained by use of a volumeter that follows the principle of water displacement (Fig. 8-2). This method is excellent when assessing the edema in a hand or foot/ankle injury because of the irregular surfaces. This method requires a volumeter

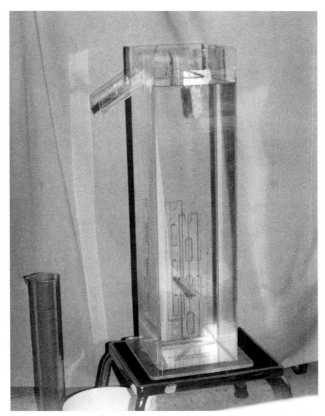

FIGURE 8-2 A volumeter is generally constructed of Plexiglas with a spout. It is filled with water until a small amount runs out of the spout and stops.

designed for the hand or foot filled preferably with tepid or lukewarm water. The patient immerses the body part to a standard depth, and the water displaced is collected as it runs out of a spout (Fig. 8-3A). The volume of fluid displaced is measured[22] (Fig. 8-3B). This method is less convenient, not easily transportable, and more expensive as the clinic must own a volumeter. In addition, it provides only one measure of change in the body part and is not sensitive to varying amounts of change in different parts of the limb. However, this "total volume" can be used to make direct comparisons over time to assess overall response to treatment. Either method (water displacement or calculated volume) is acceptable as they have been shown (for the upper extremity at least) to have concurrent validity though they are not interchangeable.[24,25] Measurement of and comparison to the contralateral limb gives information as to a "normal" value for the individual being treated.

The quality of the edema is important to note. An acute edema with a large sudden increase in fluid in the tissue space will "pit" when the skin is pressed with a finger. This occurs because, with pressure, the fluid flows through the gel matrix away from the area of pressure and then returns to the original location within 5 to 30 seconds. A scale used commonly by physicians rates pitting edema on a 1-to-4 scale (Box 8-3). With longstanding edema or inflammation, the gel matrix becomes fibrotic due to macrophage activity and will be firm and no longer "pit" with pressure.

Palpation of the skin also serves to provide information concerning thickening in the skin and soft tissue. Attempting

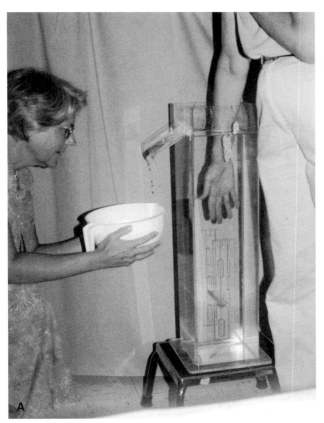
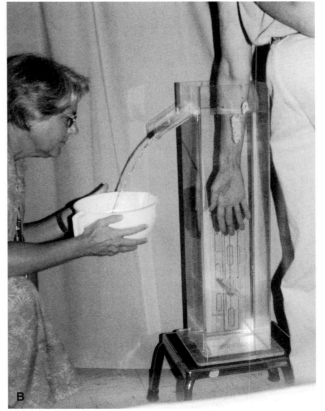

FIGURE 8-3 The patient inserts the limb slowly (A), and the water displaced by the limb is collected and measured (B).

> **BOX 8-3 | Pitting Edema[26,27]**
>
> 1+ = Edema is barely detectable.
> 2+ = A slight indentation is visible when the skin is depressed.
> 3+ = A deeper fingerprint resolves in 5 to 30 seconds.
> 4+ = The limb is swollen to 1.5 to 2 times its normal size.

to lift a skin fold in comparison to the corresponding contralateral area of the body can give a sense of the skin turgor. This is particularly helpful if assessing areas such as the trunk for edema. Stemmer's sign[28] is a diagnostic tool used in the physical examination. If a skin fold cannot be lifted off the dorsum of the hand or foot, it is considered to be a positive Stemmer's sign for lymphedema. However, if negative, it does not eliminate lymphedema as a diagnosis.

GOALS AND EXPECTED OUTCOMES

The American Physical Therapy Association's *Guide to Physical Therapist Practice* "Pattern 6H" covers the wide range of possible goals to be set in addressing the impairments, functional limitations, and disabilities identified during the initial examination. Goals and outcomes specific to reduction of edema could include the following:

- Increased ROM
- Decreased pain
- Decreased edema, lymphedema, or effusion
- Improved skin integrity
- Normal tissue temperature
- Independent management of symptoms achieved by patient/caregiver
- Risk of recurrence reduced through patient education
- Adequate edema control achieved with appropriate device if indicated
- Patient/caregiver able to correctly don/doff and care for devices

In the treatment of a stage II lymphedema, the literature demonstrates that complete resolution of the swelling is rarely achieved owing to the chronic tissue changes that accompany a lymphedema in this stage. An outcome with an edema volume reduction of 50% or better is expected. This reduction, if maintained by consistent self-management, can be expected to continue to improve, but more slowly, over time.[5]

Management of Edema

INTERVENTIONS FOR EDEMA

Interventions for edema include RICE therapy, exercise, aquatic physical therapy, electrical stimulation, massage, and complete decongestive therapy (CDT) for the treatment of lymphedema. Acute localized edema resulting from a traumatic injury is best treated immediately after injury to minimize the extent of bleeding and edema fluid accumulation. This is important to minimize the proteins that accumulate in the tissues. The protein-rich fluid, or exudate, can determine the extent of the inflammatory reaction that occurs, and the greater the inflammatory reaction, the greater is the risk of a chronic, fibrotic change in the tissues.

RICE THERAPY

RICE therapy has been the intervention of choice since the 1950s in the first 24 to 72 hours after injury.[4] RICE stands for Rest, Ice, Compression, and Elevation of the affected body part.

Rest

Rest, for the most part, is important to limit the blood flow to the area during the time period that there is excessive capillary permeability and increased pain with movement. The time period for rest, however, is very brief.

Ice

The application of ice or cold to the tissues causes a number of important physiological effects: decreases in the local tissue temperature, inflammation, metabolic rate, circulation through vasoconstriction, and pain with treatments lasting more than 2 to 3 minutes in duration.[35] Continuous application of ice is generally limited to time periods of 10 to 20 minutes because extended applications of cold can cause a reflex vasodilation or tissue damage.[4] The application of cold can take many forms: ice massage, a chemical or gel ice pack, an iced towel, an ice bath, or whirlpool. An ice bath or whirlpool is not the treatment of choice in many situations because it does not allow elevation of the body part and is less practical in many settings. Contraindications to the use of cold include intolerance to cold (ask patient about previous experiences), history of Raynaud's phenomenon, ischemic tissue (frostbite injury likely without adequate blood flow), and decreased sensation. Use cold with caution in a patient with a recent open wound/incision or active bleeding. While compression technique will be discussed below, it has been found that the combination of ice and compression may have better results than the use of ice alone. Knobloch et al measured microcirculation in the Achilles tendon and found that recovery of blood flow was increased in the group receiving both ice and compression, as compared with the group receiving ice alone.[36]

Compression

Compression increases the hydrostatic pressure in the tissues, decreasing ultrafiltration out of the damaged capillaries and increasing the absorption of fluid by the veins and fluid and proteins by the lymphatic vessels.[9] Compression can be accomplished by intermittent compression devices, compression bandaging, compression garments, or a combination compression/cold device. Intermittent compression devices are most commonly air-inflated sleeves that fit over the limb. The sleeves can have only one chamber or various numbers of multiple chambers that fill sequentially.[8] The parameters that can commonly be controlled by the therapist include inflation pressure, on-time/off-time cycle, and total treatment time. Inflation pressures are usually set between 30 and 100 mm Hg. There is a potentially significant problem associated with setting the pressure above the patient's diastolic pressure, as this could occlude the arterial blood supply. Therefore, most manufacturers recommend staying below this level. Recommended pressures are in the range of 30 to 60 mm Hg for the upper extremity and 40 to 80 mm Hg in the lower extremity. Many authors recommend staying at or below 30 to 40 mm Hg pressure in all instances because of inaccurate control of the actual pressures created by the devices[8] or because of the potential damage to the delicate, superficial lymphatics.[9] One author reports complete closure of lymphatic vessels at pressures of 75 mm Hg.[10]

There is no published research regarding the on-time/off-time cycle. In many devices this is not even adjustable. The range of settings could be from 30 seconds on/30 seconds off up to 4 to 5 minutes on/1 to 5 minutes off. Some of these ratios seem to relate more to the time necessary to fill all chambers sequentially than to any actual physiological reason. Patient comfort could probably be used as a deciding factor. The total treatment time recommended also varies widely.[7] Times can range from 30 minutes up to 6 to 8 hours repeated over 2 to 3 days.[11] In practical terms, treatment times range from 30 minutes up to 1 hour. Circumferential measurements should be taken before and after a session of intermittent compression to evaluate the response. The choice of a single-chamber pump as opposed to pumps with multiple chambers is also not clear. There is a theoretical advantage in a pump with multiple chambers that fill sequentially as they ascend the limb. This would then be pushing edema fluid along through the limb. This advantage has not been proved.[12,13] It has been recommended that a trial of different pumps be completed before long-term use at home.[7] The contraindications for use of an intermittent pump include CHF, active infection, unstable fractures, recent thrombophlebitis, and pulmonary emboli.

Compression can also be applied with bandaging or garments. The intent of static external compression is to decrease ultrafiltration by increasing hydrostatic pressure, to decrease the present edema by improving the musculoskeletal pump, and to soften fibrotic tissue.

Compression bandaging is available in three varieties: short stretch, medium stretch, and long stretch (Table 8-2). Short stretch bandages provide a low pressure at rest and a high pressure when the limb is working (Fig. 8-4). Long stretch bandages provide a high pressure at rest because of the increased elasticity but a lower pressure when the limb is working because of the "give" inherent to the bandage. Short stretch bandages are preferable to reduce edema because they provide a better pumping effect in combination with the muscles when the patient moves (Fig. 8-5). Long

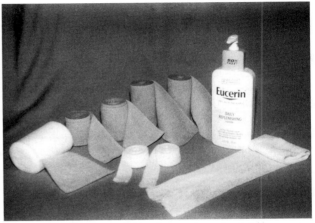

FIGURE 8-4 Short stretch bandages of varying widths are used to conform to a limb and apply a low resting pressure and high working pressure. Padding materials and soft elastic gauze are included to protect bony prominences and to add pressure to fingers or toes.

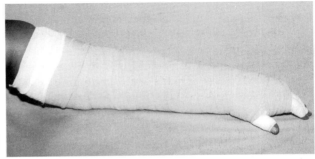

FIGURE 8-5 A completed compression bandage for an upper extremity from the fingers to the axilla.

stretch bandages are inexpensive and frequently adequate for acute, localized swellings. A long stretch bandage should always be removed at night and replaced by elevation of the limb to avoid arterial occlusion. Arterial occlusion is possible at night because of decreased limb perfusion with elevation, decreased perfusion without assistance from the musculoskeletal pump, and the danger of rolling or shifting of the bandage, which can produce a tourniquet effect. An Unna boot is a type of very short stretch bandage that can be applied to the leg. It is a zinc oxide–impregnated gauze bandage that keeps the skin moist while creating a "soft cast" on the limb, thereby improving the musculoskeletal pump and preventing additional fluid accumulation. It is frequently used in managing the edema associated with a venous wound and can be left in place for up to 1 week. Another bandaging scheme to manage edema with wounds is to combine short and medium stretch bandages in layers used in the same way as Unna boots. All bandaging should include adequate padding of bony areas by felt, foam, or soft cotton to prevent excessive pressure and skin breakdown. Contraindications to the use of bandaging include active infection, recent thrombophlebitis or pulmonary embolus without adequate anticoagulation, and CHF. Precautions for bandaging include arterial disease, diabetes mellitus, decreased sensation, and metastatic disease.

TABLE 8-2	Compression Bandages	
Short stretch	<70% stretch
Medium stretch	70% to 140% stretch
Long stretch	<140% stretch

Types: short, Comprilan (BSN Medical, Charlotte, NC), Rosidal (BSN Medical, Charlotte, NC); medium, Coban; long, Ace bandages.

Elevation

Elevation of the body part alone can decrease the edema in an ankle.[6] Elevation allows gravity to assist both the veins and the lymphatic vessels to carry excess fluid and proteins away from the area of injury. Elevation also decreases the hydrostatic pressure in the tissues.[7] Elevation of the body part above the level of the heart is commonly recommended if practical. Elevation has not been shown to help except in the early stages of swelling.[7] The contraindication to elevation is an ischemic limb, because this increase in hydrostatic pressure in the limb will further reduce arterial flow to the limb.

Compressive garments are similar in action to bandaging and are used to maintain a limb size and to prevent reaccumulation of fluid during the day when a limb is dependent. They are a compromise compared with short stretch or inelastic supports, which allow greater freedom of movement and comfort. Compression garments cannot be expected to reduce a chronic edema.[7,15] They are more appropriately fitted to a limb once the edema volume has reduced and reached a plateau. A randomized, controlled study of compression bandaging followed by compression garments versus compression garments alone demonstrated that the combination therapy led to double the reduction achieved by compression garments alone.[16] A compression garment is manufactured to place the most pressure at the wrist or ankle and then progressively less through the remainder of the limb[17] (see Fig. 8-5). This is described as a gradient pressure on the limb. Compression garments are available as off-the-shelf sizes and as custom made. The off-the-shelf garments *must* fit correctly at the wrist or ankle as this is the location at which the maximum compression is applied. A custom-made garment is much more expensive but essential if a limb is disproportionate, such as a small ankle with a very large calf, or irregular in size. There are many other factors that should be considered when choosing a garment for a patient (Box 8-4). The compression class chosen varies by the limb and degree of edema. For treatment of a lymphedema, generally an arm sleeve/glove is prescribed in a compression class I or II and a leg garment in compression class II or III (Table 8-3). After an acute injury such as an ankle fracture, many patients can benefit from a compression class I knee-high garment to control the swelling in the rehabilitation phase

TABLE 8-3 | Compression Classes for Medical-Grade Garments[1,17]

Class I	20 to 30 mm Hg	Minor varicose veins, minor varicosities of pregnancy, mild lymphedema of the arm
Class II	30 to 40 mm Hg	Significant varicose veins with edema, post-traumatic swelling, postphlebitis swelling, significant varicosities of pregnancy, lymphedema of the arm
Class III	40 to 50 mm Hg	Chronic venous insufficiency, status postvenous ulcers, lymphedema of the arm or leg
Class IV	50 to 60 mm Hg	Lymphedema

after immobilization. The contraindications for compression garments are acute thrombophlebitis/infection, cardiac edema, malignant lymphedema (relative), arterial disease (relative), and acute vascular blockages.[17,18] Garments should be used with caution in patients with active cancer, decreased sensation, or arterial compromise.

EXERCISE

Exercise enhances venous and lymphatic flow.[4,5,19] Exercise in combination with compression of any kind further enhances the musculoskeletal pump.[20] This can include isometric exercises during intermittent compression pumping, walking with a compressive bandage on the lower leg, simple arm exercises while wearing a compression bandage or compressive sleeve, or specific exercise programs designed for patients with lymphedema.[5] Exercise programs for lymphedema management usually are performed in a specific sequence in which more central regions are exercised before the more distal portions of the limb. This allows more central reservoirs to be emptied before edematous areas are exercised.[5] Elevating the limb while performing exercise enhances edema reduction. Aerobic exercises are often prescribed for patients with edema. An athlete with an acute injury may wish to maintain his or her level of fitness while recovering. An individual with a chronic lymphedema may be deconditioned because of a decreased level of activity. Aerobic exercise is accompanied by an increased heart rate and respiratory rate. Lymph flow is enhanced by both the pressure differential in the thorax that occurs with breathing and increased pulsation of the arteries.[21] Exercise such as active ROM can provide more powerful edema reduction when used in combination with other edema-reducing modalities, such as ice. Yanagisawa et al measured the cross-sectional area of a baseball pitcher's rotator cuff 24 hours after pitching and found that the cross-sectional area was significantly less in the group receiving both ice and exercise, as compared with the group receiving only ice and the group receiving only exercise.[37]

BOX 8-4 | Factors to Consider in Choosing a Compression Garment[18]

- Coverage
- Compression class
- Appearance
- Custom-made versus off the shelf
- Material or fabric
- Construction
- Suspension
- Skin condition/sensitivity/wounds
- Ability of patient to don/doff
- Cost and source of payment

AQUATIC PHYSICAL THERAPY

Aquatic therapy is particularly beneficial for individuals with leg swelling of nonmetabolic origin and with a stable cardiovascular system. Water exerts a gradient compression on a body when immersed, with the most distal portions of the limb under greatest pressure. For example, an individual with a 32-inch inseam standing in groin-deep water has a pressure of 60 mm Hg exerted on the foot/ankle.[5] Combined with the musculoskeletal pump activity with exercise, an individual with acute edema could experience a notable difference in swelling after an aquatic therapy session. The edema reduction is often considered a side benefit to the ease of movement achieved because of the reduction in weight-bearing and active assistance for joint motion from buoyancy. Excessive warmth, however, can have a deleterious effect because of an increase in local blood flow. Increased blood flow adds to the hydrostatic pressure in the tissues and can cause increased ultrafiltration into the interstitial space, leading to more edema volume.

ELECTRICAL STIMULATION

Electrical stimulation can be used to achieve rhythmic contraction of muscles in an area of localized edema, thereby enhancing the musculoskeletal pump. Electrical stimulation below the threshold to elicit muscle contraction can also be used to repel proteins. Proteins and plasma in the interstitial space have a negative polarity, and when treated with negative polarity, they are repelled, causing a movement from the local area of edema. As the water is attracted to the proteins, it is also shifted from the area (see Chapter 13). This treatment is most easily used for hand edema.[22]

MASSAGE

Massage is effective in reducing swelling.[32,33] Retrograde massage, sports massage, and specialized massage as a component of complete decongestive therapy to treat lymphedema may be incorporated into a treatment session to decrease edema. Massage as a treatment intervention is discussed in more detail in Chapter 9.

COMPLETE DECONGESTIVE THERAPY

Complete decongestive therapy (CDT) is the current interventional program used to treat patients with lymphedema. Treating this patient population requires specific knowledge and experience in addition to entry-level professional education. Both physical therapists and physical therapist assistants may become certified lymphedema specialists. CDT is a two-phase program. Phase I includes skin care, manual lymphatic drainage, bandaging, and exercise.[34] These patients will eventually be fitted with compression garments. Phase II also includes skin care and exercise. The therapist will provide manual lymphatic drainage as needed. Compression garments are likely to be worn during the day and bandaging at night.[34]

DOCUMENTATION

When documenting edema management interventions, measurements of the edema should be taken before and after the intervention. The method of edema measurements, whether circumferential or done with a volumeter, should be consistent from measurement to measurement. Documentation of the interventions provided should include enough details and parameters, making the intervention easily reproducible by another clinician. For instance, whether the patient uses a device outside of the department setting or receives treatment in the clinic, it is important to document the settings of the device. In addition, edema is a cyclic event, which means that it is important to reexamine the patient at the same time of day for every session. It is helpful to record comparisons with the unaffected extremity to note differences. Patient response to the application of the device should also be recorded. Some patients may experience an increased urgency to urinate after intermittent compression. This should be documented. If fluid intake and output are monitored by nursing staff, then plans should include the measurement of urine produced following intermittent compression. The goal of edema reduction should be tied to the functional skills that the clinician is hoping to improve. Finally, all patient education regarding edema reduction and self-management should be documented.

PATIENT EDUCATION

In any instance in which edema is treated, it is essential to educate the patient about self-care measures to achieve timely reduction in the edema. Providing the patient with an "owner's manual" description of how swelling occurs and what can be done to reduce it gives the patient a sense of control and usually results in better adherence to the suggested treatments. Take-home instructions written in layperson's terms and in the patient's language greatly enhance understanding and follow-through. Family members or caregivers are always encouraged to attend a treatment session to learn how to assist the patient with his or her edema management.

Lymphedema is not a well-understood condition among physicians. Lymphedema as a consequence of treatment for cancer is well understood by most surgeons and oncologists, who usually refer their patients promptly for treatment; however, not all patients receive or comprehend timely information in risk-reduction measures after treatment for cancer. Individuals with congenital forms of lymphedema often see many physicians before receiving an accurate diagnosis. Information accessible to the general public regarding lymphedema was even harder to obtain, until recently. The advent of the widespread use of the World Wide Web has made it easier to obtain information. Many patients come for their first visit with a large file of printouts from their Internet searches. It is extremely important to help patients understand that they must be careful to consider the source of any information obtained from the Internet. Two excellent sources of information about lymphedema are the Lymphoedema Association of Australia and the National Lymphedema Network (Box 8-5). In recent years, there have been several excellent texts published on lymphedema and treatment as well.

Of special concern to people at risk for lymphedema is how to prevent it from developing. There is no research to date that demonstrates that lymphedema can be prevented. There are several known factors that do increase the risk of lymphedema in women who have been treated for breast cancer[29]: radiation therapy of the axilla, an axillary node dissection, and obesity. Despite a lack of research in this area, a number of lists of "dos and don'ts" have been developed as guidelines based on an understanding of normal physiology and the pathophysiology of lymphedema.[30] The most well known of these lists is the "18 Steps to Prevention" published by the National Lymphedema Network for people at risk for upper extremity or lower extremity lymphedema. In practice, these lists are frequently very upsetting to patients, because they seem overwhelming. In our practice, we have developed a somewhat condensed version for patients with breast cancer that we believe puts more emphasis on understanding the "why" of risk reduction.[31]

Summary

The presence of edema can have a negative impact on a person's ROM, strength, pain level, skin integrity, function, and body image. While edema in and of itself is not a diagnosis, it is a sign that something is wrong. It is important to understand that there are many different types and causes of edema, along with a variety of interventions. Knowing which interventions are appropriate for each individual's edema reduction is vital. Clinicians will measure the amount and location of edema so that the effectiveness of the chosen intervention can be determined and adjusted if necessary. Because the presence of edema can have a negative impact on so many factors, patients tend to be very appreciative of their therapists when edema reduction interventions are successful.

Review Questions

1. Which of the following usually occurs with acute edema that occurs in conjunction with a normal venous and lymphatic system?
   a. Low-protein edema
   b. High-protein edema
   c. Protein-rich edema
   d. Lymphedema

2. Which of the following is the only mechanism that removes protein from the interstitial space?
   a. Circulatory system
   b. Lymphatic system
   c. RICE
   d. Surgery

3. Which of the following best describes the type of massage that can reduce edema?
   a. Scar massage
   b. Transverse friction massage
   c. Effleurage
   d. Retrograde massage

4. Which of the following diagnoses would be most likely to benefit from complete decongestive therapy for edema management?
   a. Acute ankle sprain
   b. Postmastectomy with lymphedema
   c. Total knee replacement with infection
   d. Congestive heart failure

5. You are setting the parameters for your patient's intermittent compression device. You took her blood pressure when she arrived in the clinic and it was 120/80 mm Hg. When deciding which compression pressure to set the device at, you determine which of the following?
   a. It shouldn't be over 120 mm Hg, so you set the device to 100 mm Hg
   b. It shouldn't be under 120 mm Hg, so you set the device to 140 mm Hg
   c. It shouldn't be over 80 mm Hg, so you set the device to 60 mm Hg
   d. It shouldn't be under 80 mm Hg, so you set the device to 100 mm Hg

Patient Perspective

PATIENTS' FREQUENTLY ASKED QUESTIONS

1. **What is the cause of the swelling?**
2. **How do I reduce the swelling effectively?**
3. **How do I keep the swelling from returning?**

CASE STUDY 1

Acute Ankle Sprain

Patient Description

The patient is a 40-year-old accountant who sustained an acute inversion injury of the right ankle playing basketball with friends 2 days ago. He was been sent to your clinic after a fracture has been ruled out by an x-ray examination in the emergency department. He was treated immediately with ice and elevation, which he continued at home. He presents with significant nonpitting edema and ecchymoses in the region of the lateral malleolus and lateral foot. The ankle is painful to palpation over the anterior talofibular ligament. A figure-of-eight girth measurement is 2.8 cm larger than on the opposite ankle. His active ankle dorsiflexion and plantarflexion are limited and painful, and he is unable to bear weight on that extremity without crutches.

Diagnosis

Acute ankle sprain (inversion)

Plan of Care

Intermittent compression

Compressive bandaging/compressive ankle support
Active range-of-motion exercises
Progressive weight-bearing as tolerated
Balance/proprioceptive training
Return to work and leisure-specific activities

Intervention

After completion of the initial examination, the patient was positioned with the right lower leg elevated. A length of stockinette was applied from the toes to the knee, and a three-chamber sequential compression boot was slipped on over the extremity. The limb was treated for 30 minutes at a pressure setting of 30 to 40 mm Hg adjusted to the patient's pain tolerance. The patient was encouraged to gently pump the foot inside the boot and to use the calf muscle during the off time of the pump cycle. Post-treatment figure-of-eight measurements were taken. The patient was compressively bandaged with a low stretch bandage with a posterior kidney-shaped malleolar pad behind the lateral malleolus. An alternative method for compression is a thermoplastic ankle stirrup brace with a built-in air bladder for compression. The stirrup brace is preferable if the patient can tolerate weight-bearing because it combines compression with protective medial lateral stability. The patient is given written take-home instructions, including the following:

- Ambulate as tolerated (with appropriate assistive device if needed).
- Elevate and continue to ice for 20 minutes at a time.
- Perform gentle ankle pumps four or five times per day.
- Wear bandage/ankle support full time when not in bed.

The patient attended six additional sessions during the next 2 weeks, with gradual resolution of the edema/inflammation and decreased pain with AROM/weight-bearing. Intermittent compression was discontinued after two additional sessions, and strengthening exercises were gradually added and progressed. Functional skills to improve balance and proprioception were added as tolerated, and the patient was to be weaned from his ankle support as tolerated when AROM and strength returned to normal.

CASE STUDY 2

Postmastectomy Lymphedema

Patient Description

The patient is a 56-year-old woman who was treated for breast cancer 4 years earlier with a right lumpectomy/axillary node dissection, followed by chemotherapy for six cycles and radiation therapy to the right breast/chest wall and axilla. The patient saw her oncologist last week with a complaint of 2 weeks of swelling in her right hand and difficulty buttoning the cuff of her blouse. The patient states that the swelling is better but not gone when she arises and that it is worse as the day goes on, with an achy discomfort in the forearm by the end of the working day as a secretary. The patient is right-handed. Highlights of her examination were as follows: After disrobing to the waist, the patient was examined. It was observed that the patient had a dropped right shoulder with moderate protraction of the right scapula. Her active ROM was limited to 0 to 150 degrees of right shoulder flexion, 0 to 160 degrees of shoulder abduction, and 0 to 70 degrees of shoulder external rotation. All other ROM measurements were within normal limits. The patient reported "pulling" in the right breast and axilla with all extremes of ROM. Strength was graded as either 4 or 4/5 in all muscle groups of both upper quadrants. Inspection of the skin revealed a healed but puckered and relatively immobile lumpectomy incision in the upper lateral quadrant of the right breast and swelling of the posterior axillary region compared with the left. Tattoos delineating the radiation field were sought and noted.

Continued

CASE STUDY 2—cont'd

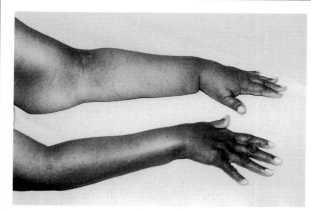

Clinical presentation of a woman with a postmastectomy lymphedema of the left upper extremity. This represents a stage II secondary lymphedema caused by damage to the lymphatic drainage of the left arm because of removal of lymph nodes in the left axilla and subsequent radiation therapy.

Circumferential measurements of both arms were taken using the most distal wrist crease as the 0 mark and measuring every 4 cm distal (to the metacarpal joints) and proximal (to the axilla). Each finger was individually measured just distal to the metacarpophalangeal joint. The patient had a 10% difference (right larger than left).

Diagnosis
Early stage II lymphedema of the right upper extremity and trunk secondary to breast cancer/lumpectomy

Plan of Care
- Education re: diagnosis and pathophysiology
- Education re: reduction of risk and skin care
- Postural and flexibility exercises
- Diaphragmatic breathing exercises
- Lymph drainage massage
- Compressive bandaging of the right upper extremity
- Instruction in a home exercise program for increased lymphatic flow
- Scar modification
- Fitting of compression garment at end of treatment

Intervention
After completing the initial examination, the patient was provided with written educational material on lymphedema and its treatment, and the plan of care was discussed. The patient was instructed in gentle postural and flexibility exercises to address the limited ROM and postural faults seen. The patient

was scheduled to be seen two or three times a week during the next 3 weeks.

At the next session later that week, the patient was instructed in how to moisturize the skin with a low pH lotion and then apply a lightweight compression bandage (see Fig. 8-5) to be worn full time and removed for showering. The patient was also instructed in a simple exercise program of diaphragmatic breathing and gentle massage of adjacent regional lymph nodes combined with movement of the limb. The goal of exercise was to enhance the musculoskeletal pump through movement combined with compressive support from bandaging. The patient was encouraged to supplement her exercise with a 15- to 20-minute walk at a moderate pace to enhance the effect of the respiratory pressure change on lymphatic flow.

At the next session, the patient's arm was remeasured and a reduction to 6% larger than the left arm was seen. Manual lymphatic massage and gentle mobilization of the lumpectomy scar were initiated, the arm was bandaged again, and the exercise program was reviewed. The ROM of the right shoulder had improved by 10 degrees in flexion, abduction, and external rotation. A small, high-density foam pad was cut, and after it was covered with stockinette, it was tucked into the patient's bra on the lateral chest wall to provide a gentle compression to the posterior axilla. The patient was encouraged to very gently mobilize the lumpectomy scar after showering every day.

At subsequent visits, her exercise program was advanced to include strengthening exercises with 2- to 3-pound free weights. After five sessions, measurement demonstrated a reduction of the lymphedema to the right arm being only 2% larger than the left with minimal swelling over the dorsum of the hand. As the patient is right-handed, a small differential in size was expected because of the increased muscular development of a dominant limb. The patient was fitted with a compression sleeve of 20 to 30 mm Hg from the wrist to the axilla and a gauntlet of the same compression to place pressure on the dorsum of the hand. She was instructed in donning/doffing of the sleeve and care of the garments. She was instructed to wear the garment daily. She was to remove it at night and replace with compression bandaging. All of these instructions were given in written form. The patient was scheduled for a follow-up visit in 1 week and instructed to call immediately if any unusual swelling was experienced.

In 1 week's time, the patient returned with full active ROM of the right arm, improved posture, and a stable limb size and demonstrated she was independent in all aspects of self-management. She was instructed to replace her compression garments every 4 to 6 months.

CASE STUDY 3

Edema Following Patellar Surgery
Patient Description

The patient is a 72-year-old retired male schoolteacher who fell 6 weeks ago and had a comminuted fracture of the left patella. He was treated by surgical repair and an immobilizer for 4 weeks. He began physical therapy 2 weeks ago to regain ROM and strength and was progressing well. When he started therapy, he had minimal nonpitting edema at the ankle. As he used the immobilizer less and was on his feet more, he began to notice increased swelling at the end of the day. This afternoon, he demonstrates +2 pitting edema to the mid-calf without pain. The other leg is not swollen. He states that there was no swelling when he got up this morning. Despite a low level of suspicion for a deep vein thrombosis, the patient was referred back to his surgeon because of the change in his status.

Diagnosis
Mild venous insufficiency

Plan of Care

Fitting of knee-high compression garment
Instruction in donning, care, wearing, and replacement
  schedule

Intervention

After the patient had a negative Doppler ultrasound study, he was referred back to continue his physical therapy. He was scheduled for an early morning appointment when his edema was minimal and measured and fit with a 20 to 30 mm Hg knee-high garment. Owing to limited knee ROM, he was unable to reach his foot to don his garment independently, so his wife was instructed in don/doff skills. He was instructed to remove the garment at night. He was encouraged to wear his garment daily for at least 1 to 2 months and then to have his need for continued compression therapy reassessed. He continued the rehabilitation of his patellar fracture without further edema.

DISCUSSION QUESTIONS

1. Your patient has come to physical therapy today and is in the waiting area. You observe that the patient is sitting with his legs outstretched and crossed, supported by his ankles on the chair in front of him. He was scheduled to see you for treatment of an acute ankle sprain/strain with pronounced edema. He had also previously reported knee and back pain. During this patient's last visit, you had instructed him in the proper use of axillary crutches with weight-bearing as tolerated (WBAT), and you had also instructed him to keep his leg elevated.
   a. What patient education needs to be revisited and why?

   b. What do you expect to find when you reassess edema for this patient and why?
   c. How could you prevent this in the future?

2. You observe a patient who has been scheduled for physical therapy for lymphedema following a mastectomy; she is wearing spandex clothing. Is this something that is of concern to you as a clinician? Why or why not?

BIBLIOGRAPHY
Recommended Books on Lymphedema

Modern Treatment for Lymphedema, ed 5, by Judith R. Casley-Smith and J. R. Casley-Smith, Lymphoedema Association of Australia, Adelaide, Australia, 1997.

Textbook of Lymphology for Physicians and Lymphedema Therapists, by M. Foldi, E. Foldi, and S. Kubik, Urban and Fischer, Munich, Germany, 2003.

A Primer on Lymphedema, by Deborah G. Kelly, Prentice Hall, Upper Saddle River, NJ, 2002.

Lymphedema: Diagnosis and Therapy, ed 3, by H. Weissleder and C. Schuchhardt, Viavital Verlag GmbH, Koln, Germany, 2001.

Lymphedema: A Breast Cancer Patient's Guide to Prevention and Healing, by Jeannie Burt and Gwen White, Hunter House, Alameda, CA, 1999.

Researching the Literature

An essential reference for understanding and treating lymphedema is Textbook of Lymphology for Physicians and Lymphedema Therapists, by M. Foldi, et al.

This book can be ordered through the National Lymphedema Network at www.lymphnet.org.

REFERENCES

1. Foldi, M, and Foldi, E: Foldi's Textbook of Lymphology for Physicians and Lymphedema Therapists, ed 2. Urban & Fischer, Munich, Germany, 2007.
2. Guyton, AC, and Hall, JE: Textbook of Medical Physiology, ed 12. WB Saunders, Philadelphia, 2010, p. 306.
3. Weissleder, H, and Schuchhardt, C: Lymphedema: Diagnosis and Therapy, ed 3. Viavital Verlag, Koln, Germany, 2002, p 26.
4. Leadbetter, WB, Buckwalter, JA, and Gordon, SL: Sports-Induced Inflammation. American Academy of Orthopaedic Surgeons, Park Ridge, IL, 1990, p 12.
5. Casley-Smith, JR, and Casley-Smith, JR: Modern Treatment for Lymphoedema, ed 5. The Lymphoedema Association of Australia, Adelaide, Australia, 1997, p 55.
6. Sims, D: Effects of positioning on ankle edema. J Orthop Sports Ther 8:30–33, 1986.

7. Brennan, MJ, DePompolo, RW, and Garden, FH: Focused review: postmastectomy lymphedema. Arch Phys Med Rehabil 77:S74–S80, 1996.

8. Segers, P, Belgrado, JP, LeDuc, A, LeDuc, O, and Verdonck, P: Excessive pressure in multichambered cuffs used for sequential compression therapy. Phys Ther 82:1000–1008, 2002.

9. Foldi, E: Editorial: Massage and damage to lymphatics. Lymphology 28:1–3, 1995.

10. Miller, GE, and Seale, J: Lymphatic clearance during compressive loading. Lymphology 14:161–166, 1981.

11. Pappas, CJ, and O'Donnell, TF: Long term results of compression treatment for lymphedema. J Vasc Surg 16:555–564, 1992.

12. Klein, MJ, Alexander, MA, Wright, JM, Ward, LC, and Jones, LC: Treatment of adult lower extremity lymphedema with the Wright Linear Pump: statistical analysis of a clinical trial. Arch Phys Med Rehabil 69:202–206, 1988.

13. Zanolla, R, Monzeglio, C, Balzarini, A, and Martino, G. Evaluation of the results of three different methods of post mastectomy lymphedema treatment. J Surg Oncol 26:210–213, 1984.

14. Foldi M, and Foldi, E: Lymphoedema (translation from German: Das Lymphodem, ed 5.) Lymphoedema Association of Victoria Inc, Victoria, Australia, 1993, pp 48–49.

15. McCulloch, JM, and Kloth, LC (eds): Wound Healing: Evidence Based Management, ed 4. FA Davis, Philadelphia, 2010, p 599.

16. Badger, CMA, Peacock, JL, and Mortimer, PS: A randomized, controlled, parallel-group clinical trial comparing multilayer bandaging followed by hosiery versus hosiery alone in the treatment of patients with lymphedema of the limb. Cancer 88:2832–2837, 2000.

17. Hohlbaum, GG: The Medical Compression Stocking. Schattauer, Stuttgart, 1989, pp 34, 56.

18. Cohn, JC, and Lowry, AL: It's all in the stocking. Rehab Management June/July:36–40, 2002.

19. Mortimer, PS. Managing lymphedema. Clin Exp Derm 20:98–106, 1995.

20. LeDuc, O, Peters, A, and Bourgeois, P: Bandages: Scintigraphic demonstration of its efficacy on colloidal protein resorption during muscle activity. Progr Lymphol 12:421–423, 1990.

21. Wittlinger, H, and Wittlinger, G: Textbook of Dr. Vodder's Manual Lymph Drainage, ed 7. Karl F. Haug Verlag, Heidelberg, Germany, 2003.

22. Villeco, J, Mackin, EJ, and Hunter, JM: Edema: Therapist's Management in Rehabilitation of the Hand and Upper Extremity, ed 5. Mosby, St Louis, 2002, p 192.

23. Guide to Physical Therapist Practice, rev ed 2.,APTA, 2003.

24. Karges, JR, Mark, BE, Stikeleather, SJ, and Worrell, TW: Con_current validity of upper extremity volume estimates: Comparison of calculated volume derived from girth measurements and water displacement volume. Phys Ther 83: 134–145, 2003.

25. Megens, AM, Harris, SR, Kim-Sing, C, and McKenzie, DC: Measurement of upper extremity volume in women after axillary dissection for breast cancer. Arch Phys Med Rehabil 82:1639–1644, 2001.

26. Guyton, AC, and Hall, JE: Textbook of Medical Physiology, ed 12. WB Saunders, Philadelphia, 2010.

27. Kelly, DG: A Primer on Lymphedema. Prentice Hall, Upper Saddle River, NJ, 2002, p 37.

28. Weissleder, H, and Schuchhardt, C: Lymphedema: Diagnosis and Therapy, ed 3. Viavital Verlag, Koln, Germany, 2002, p 34.

29. Rockson, SG: Precipitating factors in lymphedema: Myths and realities. Cancer 83:S2814–S2816, 1998.

30. Ridner, SH: Breast cancer lymphedema: pathophysiology and risk reduction guidelines. Oncol Nursing Forum 29:1285–1293, 2002.

31. Cohn, JC: Lymphedema: Understanding and decreasing your risks. Living Beyond Breast Cancer Newsletter Fall 2000. Available at: www.lbbc.org/docs/nlfall00.pdf.

32. Zainuddin, Z, Newton, M, Sacco, P, and Nosaka, K: Effects of massage on delayed-onset muscle soreness, swelling, and recovery of muscle function. J Athletic Training 40:174–180, 2005.

33. Coban, A, and Sirin, A: Effect of foot massage to decrease physiological lower leg oedema in late pregnancy: a randomized controlled trial in Turkey. Int J Nurs Pract 16:454–460, 2010.

34. O'Sullivan, SB, and Schmitz, TJ: Physical Rehabilitation, ed 5. FA Davis, Philadelphia, 2006.

35. Hocut, J, Jaffe, R, Rylander, C, et al: Cryotherapy in ankle sprains. Am J Sports Med 192:316–310, 1982.

36. Knobloch, K, Grasemann, R, Spies, M, et al: Midportion Achilles tendon microcirculation after intermittent combined cryotherapy and compression compared with cryotherapy alone: a randomized trial. Am J Sports Med 36: 2128–2138, 2008.

37. Yanagisawa, O, Miyanaga, Y, Shiraki, H, et al: The effects of various therapeutic measures on shoulder range of motion and cross-sectional areas of rotator cuff muscles after baseball pitching. J Sports Med Phys Fitness 43:356–366, 2003.

LET'S FIND OUT

Lab Activity: Edema Management

This lab activity focuses on therapeutic techniques for the management of edema. Clearly, there are multiple causes of edema, and it is a complex problem for both the patient and the clinician. Students/learners will practice assessment techniques for edema, because without accurate measurement of the edema it is impossible to determine whether or not the technique used proved effective. Part of the lab activity also focuses on treatment techniques with the use of intermittent compression devices.

Equipment

vinyl tape measure	thermometer
goniometer	marking pen
upper extremity volumeter	sphygmomanometer
foot volumeter	intermittent compression device
catch basin for water	upper and lower extremity appliances
large graduated cylinder	for compression device
stethoscope	disposable stockinette

Precautions and Why

Precaution	Why?
Diuretics	Patients taking diuretics may need more frequent breaks for voiding.
Decreased cognitive ability	If the patient is capable of communicating discomfort, cold, and tingling sensations, then this application is considered safe.

Contraindications and Why

Contraindication	Why?
Acute pulmonary edema	Intermittent compression causes the movement of fluids through the circulatory system. If the system is already compromised, this application is not considered safe.
Acute localized infection	A localized infection can be spread through the circulatory system if intermittent compression is applied to the treatment area.
Congestive heart failure	Intermittent compression causes the movement of fluids through the circulatory system. If the system is already compromised, this application is not considered safe.
Acute deep vein thrombosis without medical management and follow-up	Compression is intended to cause the movement of fluids. A thrombus may become dislodged and move to the heart, lungs, or brain, causing additional complications.

Lab Activity: Edema Assessment Using a Tape Measure

1. Select two classmates/patients of different body sizes. You will take circumferential measurements of their right and left upper extremities. Position the patients so that they are supine, with the extremity to be measured first elevated and supported. For you to measure the extremity, you will need to support both the distal and proximal aspects.

2. Clean the tape measure with alcohol. Using a pen, place a mark on the bicipital crease of the elbow.

3. Using the tape measure, place a mark on the skin every 1.5 inches moving proximally to the axilla from the elbow and distally every 1.5 inches to the wrist (Fig. 8-6). A small mark is preferred as some inks may cause allergic reactions or injure fragile skin.

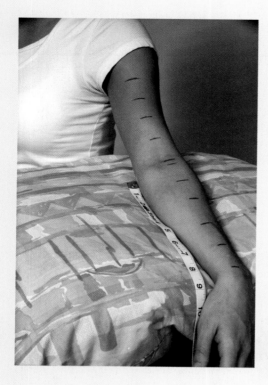

FIGURE 8-6 Upper extremity with markings made every 1.5 inches starting from the bicipital crease and moving proximally and then distally.

4. Record your and your partner's measurements in the table below. Start with the distal measurements and work proximally.

Right UE	Your measurements										
	Partner's measurements										

Left UE	Your measurements										
	Partner's measurements										

5. Compare the measurements of the patient's right and left arm. Compare your measurements to those of your lab partner's.

6. Switch places with the patients and repeat the process of measurement. Compare your findings.

Edema Assessment With a Volumeter

1. Select two classmates/patients who will have the volume of their feet and ankles assessed with a volumeter.

2. Fill the volumeter with water to the "start line." The water should be warm (above 99°F [37°C]). Record the temperature of the water (Fig. 8-7).

Water Temperature:

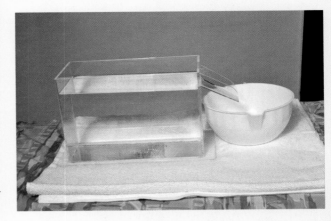

FIGURE 8-7 Water-filled volumeter with a water catch basin placed underneath the spout.

3. Inspect the foot to be immersed. Make sure that it is clean and there are no open lesions.

4. Position the catch basin so that it is below the spout of the volumeter (Fig. 8-8).

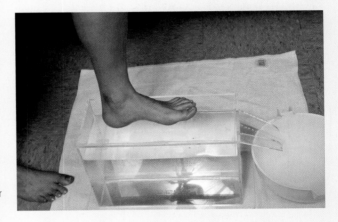

FIGURE 8-8 The standing patient is about to lower her foot and ankle into the water-filled volumeter.

5. Have the patient stand so that his or her foot is flat on the bottom of the volumeter. Water will flow out the spout into the basin (Figs. 8-9 through 8-11).

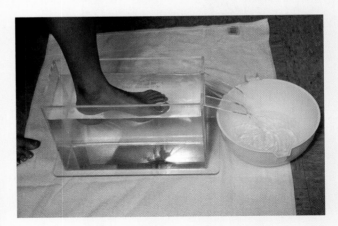

FIGURE 8-9 The patient is lowering her foot and ankle into the water-filled volumeter. The catch basin is collecting the displaced water.

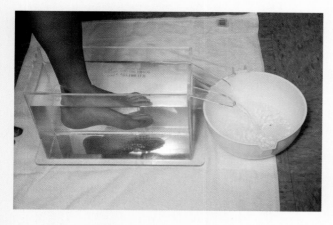

FIGURE 8-10 The patient is lowering her foot and ankle into the water-filled volumeter. The catch basin continues to collect the displaced water.

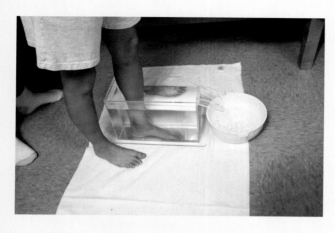

FIGURE 8-11 The plantar surface of the patient's foot is in contact with the bottom of the volumeter.

6. Have the patient remove his or her foot and resume sitting on a treatment table.
7. Measure and record the volume of displaced water using a graduated cylinder (Figs. 8-12 and 8-13).

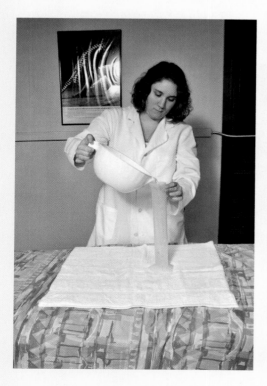

FIGURE 8-12 The clinician takes the water catch basin to measure the volume of water displaced.

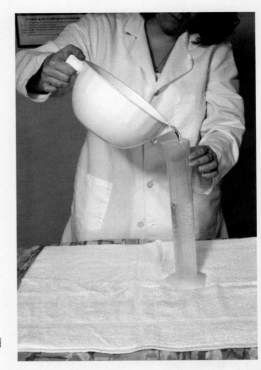

FIGURE 8-13 The displaced water is measured in a graduated cylinder to determine the volume.

Volume:

8. Empty the water, clean the volumeter, and refill it. Repeat these steps, but this time use cold water, approximately 40°F.

9. Record your measurements and observations.

Water Temperature:

_____

Volume:

_____

Observations:

_____

_____

Orientation to Intermittent Compression Devices

1. Read the instruction manual for the device. Locate the controls on the device that will adjust the inflation pressure, the deflation pressure, on time, off time, and treatment time. Select a classmate/patient to receive intermittent compression to the lower extremity.

2. Position and drape the patient so that he/she will be comfortable during the procedure. Inspect the extremity for open lesions, hematomas, etc.

3. Measure the extremity from the knee to about 9 inches proximal to the knee using the same technique as for the upper extremity (Figs. 8-14 and 8-15).

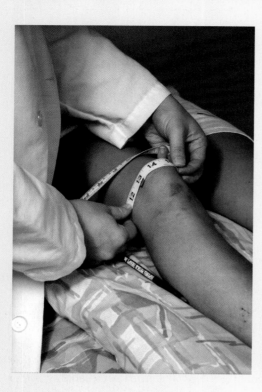

FIGURE 8-14 Circumferential measurement of the superior aspect of the knee is made using a tape measure.

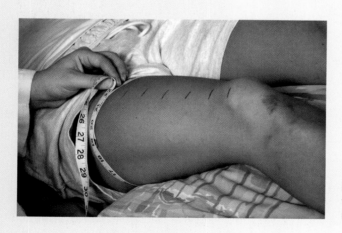

FIGURE 8-15 Sequential markings are placed on the thigh every 1.5 inches starting at the superior border of the patella and moving proximally.

4. Record your and your partner's measurements in the tables below. Start with the distal measurements and work proximally.

Right LE	Your measurements									
	Partner's measurements									

Left LE	Your measurements									
	Partner's measurements									

5. Monitor and check the pedal and popliteal pulses. Record your observations.

_____

_____

6. Take and record the resting heart rate and blood pressure.
   Resting Heart Rate:

_____

   Resting Blood Pressure:

_____

7. Apply a stockinette to the extremity. Make sure that there are no folds or creases.
8. Apply the lower extremity appliance. Re-check the patient's position and ensure that the leg is elevated and supported (Figs. 8-16 and 8-17).
9. Check the inflation and deflation pressures on the device. Set the inflation pressure to 50 mm Hg and the deflation pressure to 20 mm Hg.

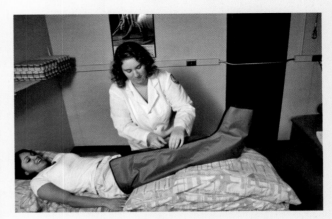

FIGURE 8-16 The clinician ensures that there are no wrinkles within the appliance and that the patient is properly positioned for application of intermittent compression to the lower extremity.

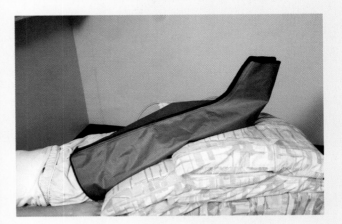

FIGURE 8-17 The patient's lower extremity is positioned for intermittent compression with pillows to assist in elevating the distal extent of the limb.

Special Considerations When Administering Intermittent Compression

- Inflation pressure must be kept below the patient's diastolic pressure so that vessels are not occluded during the compression phase.
- Patients must be encouraged to move fingers and toes during the off times to encourage circulation in the distal extremities.

10. Set the on time to 20 seconds and off time to 6 seconds. (If you cannot individually set these parameters or the device has preset parameters, select the preset parameter that is closest to this ratio, and record your settings.)

11. Start the device. Stay until the inflation is complete and the device has gone through two complete cycles. Let the device run for 15 minutes. Check the patient to make sure that he/she is comfortable.

12. Once the time is up, deflate the appliance, remove the appliance, remove the stockinette, and quickly re-measure the extremity. Record your post-treatment findings and observations in the chart in question 4 and calculate the differences, if any.

13. Repeat so that other classmates have the opportunity to feel the compression appliance as it inflates and deflates.

Patient Scenarios

Read through the patient scenarios and determine the following for each:

- Whether or not intermittent compression would be indicated
- If you decided that it was not indicated owing to a lack of information, what additional information you would need to know
- If indicated, what a realistic expectation of the treatment would be
- If indicated, how treatment would be applied
  - patient position
  - patient instruction
  - additional considerations
- How you will assess whether or not your parameter selections were appropriate
- When intermittent compression would be contraindicated
- When edema assessment techniques should be employed
- Which edema assessment technique would be the most appropriate

A. Todd has been referred to therapy for an injury to his left ankle as a result of his falling from a ladder. He works as a roofer. His ankle is now edematous, particularly anterior to the lateral malleolus. Todd fell 3 weeks ago but didn't seek medical attention until now because he didn't want to miss work. No fractures were noted by the physician. Todd has a long history of ankle sprains and strains, approximately one per year for the past 10 years. Other than being diabetic, he has no other significant medical history. His chief complaint is that he is unable to wear his work boots owing to the swelling. He has no complaints of pain.

B. Karen is a legal secretary who was referred to therapy for lymphedema secondary to a radical mastectomy on the left. Karen was diagnosed with breast cancer approximately 6 months ago. Since the surgery, she has had bouts of depression and has been unable to work. She is now undergoing chemotherapy, and her physician has assured her that there were no signs of active cancer in the surrounding tissues. Her left arm is so edematous that she has difficulty lifting it, which makes work impossible.

C. Inga is a hairdresser who has been having a great deal of difficulty with fluid retention in both legs. She is on her feet all day and rarely has a chance to sit down. She is 5 months pregnant with her first child. Inga has been referred to therapy for edema reduction. She has no significant medical history.

D. Keith is a college student who is returning to school after retiring from another career. He has three grown children who live with him and his wife. One of his daughters is pregnant, and she has been having a difficult time with the pregnancy. Keith is obese and has a classic type A personality. Thus far, his GPA is a 4.0. Keith saw a physician because of the sudden accumulation of fluids in all his extremities.

Lab Questions

1. What is the rationale for marking off the bicipital crease as a starting point for measurement of the upper extremity?

2. What potential reasons are there for using a vinyl tape measure?

3. Of what potential significance is hand dominance in the assessment of edema? Were there differences between your dominant and nondominant hand?

4. What is the potential reason for differences in the measurements that you took and that another classmate recorded?

5. If you noted differences, how will you address this in the future and what does it mean to your practice?

6. Why does the time of day make a difference in edema measurements?

7. What information does the tape measure provide that the volumeter does not?

8. What information does the volumeter provide that the tape measure does not?

9. Was there any difference in the volumeter readings for the warm water versus the cold water? Why or why not?

10. What sensations did the patient report while the intermittent compression device was operating?

11. Were there any differences between pretreatment and post-treatment measurements? What explains this?

12. What is the rationale for a deflation pressure on this type of device?

13. Why were relatively low pressures used? Why not use a pressure that more closely resembles the blood pressure of the patient?

14. What explains the connection between urination and edema?

CHAPTER 9

Soft Tissue Management Techniques: Massage

Holly C. Beinert, PT, MPT

Learning Outcomes

Following the successful completion of this chapter, the learner will be able to:

- Define soft tissue massage.
- Differentiate between the services of a massage therapist and a physical therapist or physical therapist assistant.
- Identify the indications, contraindications, and precautions for the various types of soft tissue management.
- Explain the treatment techniques for scar massage, trigger point release, myofascial release, transverse friction massage, and classic massage.
- Demonstrate the ability to prepare for a massage intervention by gathering all necessary supplies, setting up the environment, and preparing for the patient.
- Demonstrate effective communication skills while gathering subjective information from the patient.
- Discuss the types of questions needed to ask a patient prior to initiating soft tissue management techniques.
- Demonstrate a thorough visual inspection of the treatment area for contraindication, precautions, and documentation purposes.
- Demonstrate competence in the performance of classic massage, scar massage, and transverse friction massage.
- Discuss the elements required of trigger point deactivation techniques.
- Demonstrate completion of the treatment intervention and assessment of treatment efficacy.
- Demonstrate the ability to document the treatment provided.

Key Terms

Active trigger point
Contraindication
Craniosacral therapy
Effleurage
Impairment

Latent trigger point
Manual lymph drainage
Myofascial release
Palpation
Petrissage

Precaution
Scar
Tapotement
Transverse friction massage
Trigger point

> *"When one is out of touch with oneself,*
> *one cannot touch others."* —Anne Morrow Lindbergh

Patient Perspective
"When do I get my massage?"

The clinician's hands are vital tools that play an important role in the rehabilitation process. Studies indicate that patient satisfaction rates are higher when clinicians use hands-on techniques as part of the physical therapy plan of care.[1,2] Soft tissue management using massage techniques requires the clinician to have a sound understanding of anatomy and physiology, as well as confident and competence use of his or her hands as a modality. Like all other physical therapy skills, massage techniques require practice and continual assessment of outcomes to determine effectiveness.

Defining Soft Tissue Massage

When used as a physical therapy intervention, massage is the use of the clinician's hands to purposefully manipulate the patient's soft tissue(s) to promote healing and restore function.[3]

Historical Perspectives

The origin of massage began prior to recorded history and it can be found in every culture in the world[3] (Figs. 9-1 and 9-2). It is the most natural and instinctive means of relieving pain and discomfort.[4] Shiatsu originated from the ancient civilizations of Japan and Ayurveda from the ancient civilizations of India. The forefathers of Western massage were Pehr Henrik Ling (1776–1839) and Johann Georg Mezger (1838–1909), from Sweden and Amsterdam respectively. Mezger coined the French terms "effleurage," "petrissage," "friction," and "tapotement" to describe the four main techniques of soft tissue massage. Since then, the practice of massage has grown considerably. As communication among cultures has increased, so has the sharing of massage practice techniques. Today, massage techniques from all cultures can be found in the United States.

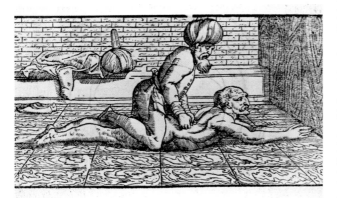

FIGURE 9-1 Ancient woodcut showing one man massaging another's back.
(From U.S. National Library of Medicine, Images from the History of Medicine, originally from Avicenna arabum Medicorum Principis. Venetiis: Juntas, 1595.)

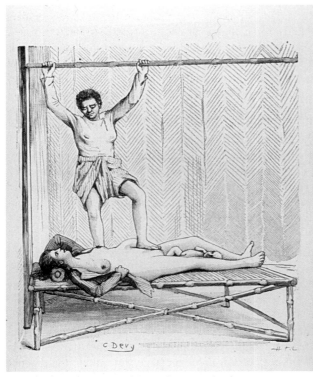

FIGURE 9-2 Massage of the belly using the feet.
(From U.S. National Library of Medicine, Images from the History of Medicine, originally from Witkowski, GJ: Histoire des accouchements chez tous les peuples. Paris, Steinheil, 1887, Figure 425, p. 602, Georges Devy, artist.)

Common Approaches Used in Physical Therapy

ALEXANDER TECHNIQUE

Frederick Matthias Alexander was a Shakespearean actor who developed a technique to restore his loss of voice. With the use of mirrors, he was able to find a relationship between his head and neck posture and his ability to project his voice. The Alexander Technique emphasizes proper posture and dynamic balance by improving kinaesthetic awareness.[3]

CONNECTIVE TISSUE MASSAGE

In the 1940s, German physical therapist Elizabeth Dicke (1884–1952) developed connective tissue massage. Elizabeth herself began experiencing leg pain and was put on bedrest by physicians who were considering a lower extremity amputation. While in bed, she started to experience low back pain and instinctively started to superficially stroke her low back. She noted that sensation in the leg began to return. She eventually recovered and avoided the amputation. She then developed an entire system of connective tissue massage techniques, which are thought to affect vascular and visceral reflexes related to a variety of pathologies and disabilities.[4]

CRANIOSACRAL THERAPY

Craniosacral therapy was developed by John Upledger, Doctor of Osteopathy, along with William Sutherland, a fellow osteopath. In 1970, during surgery Upledger observed a rhythmic movement of the spinal cord that was independent of the patient's heartbeat and respiration.[4] **Craniosacral therapy** is a gentle use of light touch to feel the rhythmic motion theoretically created by the movement of cerebrospinal fluid.[4] Craniosacral therapy is based on the theory of movement occurring at the sutures of the cranium, rhythmic motion of cerebrospinal fluid, and its impact on health. This noninvasive approach finds and corrects cerebral and spinal imbalances or blockages that may cause sensory, motor, or intellectual dysfunction by realigning the bones of the skull and stretching related tissues, such as the dura mater. Upledger has added the concept of SomatoEmotional Release (SER), which is the storing of negative emotions in traumatized tissue.[3]

CYRIAX

Dr. James H. Cyriax (1905–1985) was an English orthopedic surgeon who developed transverse-friction massage, sometimes called cross-friction massage or deep-friction massage.[4] This method uses friction techniques applied in a specific manner to create a stretching and broadening effect in fibrous tissue of muscles and tendons. Transverse friction is applied to reduce unwanted fibrous adhesions in an effort to restore mobility and reduce pain.

FELDENKRAIS

The Feldenkrais method is relatively new to the massage scene, becoming popular during the 1970s and 1980s. It was developed by Moshe Feldenkrais (1904–1984), an engineer, mathematician, physicist, and judo master. After injuring his knee, Moshe developed a system of passive movement reeducation patterns performed by a practitioner on a recipient. He also developed Awareness Through Movement, which is active movement reeducation patterns performed on the floor.[3]

MANUAL LYMPH DRAINAGE

While techniques related to enhancing lymphatic function were developed in the 1800s, it was Emil and Astid Vodder who developed the Vodder method of manual lymph drainage (MLD) in the 1930s. Manual lymph drainage is now one of many components of complete decongestive therapy (CDT), a holistic approach to treating lymphedema. **Manual lymph drainage** consists of gentle techniques applied superficially to enhance movement of lymph fluid into superficial vessels and through the lymphatic system, which in turn reduces edema and improves immune function and healing.[3]

NEUROMUSCULAR THERAPY (TRIGGER POINT)

Neuromuscular therapy is a form of massage in which trigger points are located and deactivated using trigger point pressure release. A **trigger point** is an irritable band of contracted muscle tissue that causes pain at the trigger point and in its referral zone. Pressure is applied to the trigger point, followed by stretching of the muscle. Janet Travell, MD (1901–1997) made trigger point therapy well known during her treatment of presidents Kennedy and Johnson in the 1960s.[3]

ROLFING

Ida Rolf (1896–1979), a biochemist, developed Rolfing, an approach to myofascial manipulation with the goal of creating better alignment and posture.[3] In a healthy body, the spine and body segments are correctly aligned, allowing the organs to function properly. Once poor postural habits are formed, the body loses its normal, healthy alignment. This can cause structural problems, muscle tension, and decreased organ function. Rolfing is usually done in a series of 10 one-hour treatment sessions in which the rolfer will use heavy pressure on various portions of the body.[4]

SWEDISH MASSAGE

Swedish massage is a form of traditional Western massage. Standard massage techniques learned in physical therapy programs including effleurage, petrissage, tapotement, friction, and vibration have their origins in Swedish massage.[3] It uses a system of long strokes and techniques on the more superficial layers of muscles, combined with active and passive movements of the joints. It is primarily used for full-body sessions and promotes general relaxation, improves blood circulation and range of motion (ROM), and relieves muscle tension. It can also be used as a preparatory massage in physical therapy to relax the patient and tissues prior to performing other, more specific, techniques.

TRAGER

Developed by Milton Trager, MD (1908–1997), the Trager approach provides oscillatory tissue mobilization to improve the mobility of fascia and other mechanical structures, as well as neurological inhibition to decrease resting muscle tone. This is combined with relaxation and movement exercises called mentastics.[3]

Clinical Considerations

PERSONAL APPEARANCE

Personal appearance plays a large role in the patient/client's impression and perception of a health care provider, but it can also affect the intervention and outcome. Because the hands are the primary tools for providing soft tissue massage techniques, special attention should be given to them. When performing massage or manual therapy, it is very important to maintain short fingernails that do not extend past the tips of the fingers. Fingernails should be smooth to avoid scratching the patient/client's skin. Oftentimes, soft tissue techniques require the clinician to apply deep pressure with the fingers, which can result in patient discomfort or skin breakage if the fingernails are too long.

Hands should be odor free, clean, and warm prior to implementing hands-on techniques. Health care providers who smoke should pay special attention to the removal of hand odor prior to touching the patient/client. All clinicians should perform a proper hand wash prior to and after every session. Depending on the goal of the manual therapy technique, the clinician may choose to warm up his or her hands prior to touching the patient. Finally, rings, watches, and bracelets should be removed to ensure that they do not scratch or break the client's skin.

If the clinician has long hair, it should be secured to ensure that the hair does not touch the patient. Owing to the close proximity of clinicians to patients, perfume should either not be worn or used in moderation, giving consideration to patients' possible allergies and intolerances.

ENVIRONMENT

Preparation of the environment and the patient is an essential first step to massage. Although physical therapists and physical therapist assistants are typically not providing massage to the entire body for an extended period of time, mechanisms to promote proper body mechanics and comfort should be taken. Treatment tables with firm surfaces are preferred and are commonly found in physical therapy clinics. If an adjustable height table is available, it should be used when providing soft tissue techniques.

Anticipating the need for pillows, bolsters, linens, and lubricant will maximize efficiency during the workday. A barrier such as a sheet placed between the patient and the treatment table will increase patient comfort as well as cleanliness of the environment. Pillows and bolsters should be available to support the patient as needed. Towels should be close by to remove any excess lubricant at the conclusion of the treatment (Fig. 9-3).

Some manual therapy techniques are most effective without lubricant, while others require it to decrease friction between the therapist's hands and the patient's skin, which may cause irritation. Many types of lubricants are available, such as lotions, creams, gels, oils, or powders. While many massage therapists employ oils, the majority of physical therapy clinics use lotions and creams for the soft tissue work they do in a limited area of the body.

PATIENT POSITIONING AND DRAPING

When selecting the patient position for soft tissue techniques, the therapist will need to consider the goal of the intervention, the treatment area, and patient comfort. Pillows, bolsters, and rolled towels are then used to support the body as needed. Common placements in the supine position include support under the knees to reduce stress on the lumbar spine and under the head if needed (Fig. 9-4). Common support in the prone position is placed under the ankles and abdomen to reduce lumbar strain. When the

patient is prone, face cradles or removable openings in a treatment plinth can ensure that the patient is able to breathe without restriction (Fig. 9-5). In the side-lying position, patients may prefer to have a pillow placed between the legs (Fig. 9-6).

Once the clinician has determined which area of the body will benefit from soft tissue management techniques, he/she needs to discuss the plan of care with the patient. The patient should be informed of exactly which articles of clothing will need to be removed and why or which types of clothing should be worn (i.e., shorts instead of long pants) and why. The clinician should always leave the patient in a private area while he/she gets dressed and undressed, providing a sheet, towel, or gown for the patient to use in place of clothing. It is the clinician's responsibility to maintain the patient's dignity, modesty, and comfort level at all times by providing draping that exposes only the area that is being treated.

BODY MECHANICS

When providing many physical therapy interventions, the position and use of the clinician's body has the potential to create strain and injury in the health care provider. Paying close attention to your own health and body mechanics is a habit that should be made a priority and practiced

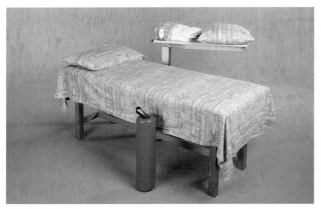

FIGURE 9-3 A prepared treatment plinth with supplies next to it.

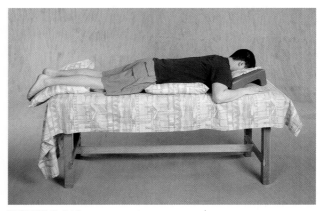

FIGURE 9-5 Proper patient position with support in a prone position.

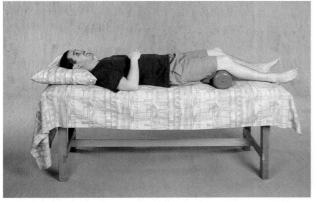

FIGURE 9-4 Proper patient position with support in a supine position.

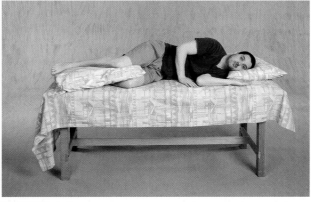

FIGURE 9-6 Proper patient position with support in a side-lying position.

continually. Proper body mechanics during the application of soft tissue massage will help to reduce fatigue and pain. Posture should be upright with both feet remaining in contact with the floor. Bending should occur at the knees instead of the back and care should be taken to avoid unnecessary twisting of the lumbar spine. To get closer to the target tissues, weight should be shifted forward on the legs instead of bending at the back or reaching with the arms. The clinician's joints should be held in neutral and the soft tissue intervention should be stopped if unable to avoid hyperextension of the wrist and fingers. Finally, the clinician should first attempt to shift his or her body weight with the goal of increasing manual pressure before increasing upper extremity muscle contractions. As Scrooge McDuck says, "Work smarter, not harder."

Starting to Palpate

Palpation is "perception by the sense of touch."[5] It is the ability to sense, using one's hands, the conditions, and changes in the body. The hands act as the tool, allowing the clinician to identify bony structures, muscles, skin, and fascia. Experienced clinicians use their hands to inform them of conditions such as tightness, tenderness, adhesions, spasms, muscle guarding, and trigger points.[4] It is a skill that requires patience, practice, and concentration. In physical therapy, the ultimate goal of palpation is to identify local areas of dysfunction. Once the area of dysfunction has been identified through the art of palpation, the clinician employs soft tissue management techniques in an effort to improve tissue mobility to restore function.

Competence in palpation skills requires strong foundational knowledge of functional human anatomy. Most people can tell the difference between confident, experienced hands and the novice. When developing this skill, relax your hands and use a soft touch. It may help to close your eyes so that you can concentrate on the information being sensed by your hands.[6] An essential component to competence is the opportunity to conduct palpation and soft tissue techniques under the direct guidance of experienced clinicians.

Effects of Massage

While the physical and mental benefits of massage are numerous, the effects of massage can differ from one person to another, depending on the type of massage techniques provided and the needs of the recipient.[3] Some massage techniques have a known stimulating effect, while others have a relaxing effect. Choosing the appropriate technique to meet the client's needs is part of the clinical decision-making process. Physical effects of massage include increases in metabolism, increased healing, muscle relaxation, and improved lymphatic function. Massage has a beneficial effect on one's immunity.[7,8] It also helps to prevent and relieve muscle cramps and spasms, and improves blood and lymph circulation.[9] At the tissue level, massage will enhance tissue repair and scar formation and can break up adhesions. The skeletal system benefits from massage via the promotion of joint function, optimal ROM, and proper skeletal alignment.[10] Massage often plays a role in pain management by improving superficial and deep blood circulation and activating the neural-gate mechanism. Massage has been shown to reduce blood pressure and heart rate, producing psychological effects such as increased mental clarity, reduced anxiety and stress, and a promotion of feelings of general well-being.[11,12,13] Studies show that massage used on infants can improve growth and development.[3, 4]

Indications, Contraindications, and Precautions

Soft tissue techniques can address many impairments that patients may present with in a physical therapy setting. According to the Nagi model of disablement, an **impairment** includes any loss or abnormality of physiological, anatomical, or psychological structure or function.[14] Impairments include decreased ROM, decreased strength, poor posture, edema, and pain. Limited ROM can be caused by many soft tissue dysfunctions, which in turn can be improved by soft tissue massage interventions.[15,16,17] Soft tissue dysfunctions that may limit ROM include adhesions; scarring;, restrictions in fascia, skin, ligaments, joint capsule, muscles and tendons; trigger points, guarding, and spasm. Limited strength can be caused by muscle strains, tears, trigger points, and tendinopathies. Poor posture and edema can be addressed with soft tissue management techniques. Pain is an impairment itself, but it can also be caused by any and all of the other impairments listed above. Therefore, addressing the primary impairments through soft tissue management and other appropriate physical therapy interventions can indirectly alleviate pain.

A **contraindication** is a medical reason not to provide massage techniques to an individual.[3] A **precaution** is any condition that *may* render a particular line of treatment inadvisable. Tables 9.1 and 9.2 list common contraindications and precautions to soft tissue techniques in general. Endangerment sites are areas of the body at which the potential for causing harm is greater. When performing soft tissue techniques in these areas, caution is required. Endangerment sites include the anterior neck, eyes, trachea, xiphoid process, axilla, kidneys, umbilicus, vertebral column, elbow, inguinal area, popliteal fossa, and major veins in the extremities.[3,18,19]

Soft Tissue Massage Techniques

CLASSIC MASSAGE

Classic massage techniques use a variety of superficial strokes including effleurage, petrissage, and tapotement.

Effleurage

Effleurage includes strokes applied by sliding and gliding the hands over the body. Effleurage can be performed superficially or deeply. Superficial effleurage is the most commonly used stroke in classic massage. It is used to begin and end a session and to transition between other types of

TABLE 9-1 | Contraindications to General Massage

CONTRAINDICATIONS	WHY?
Acute conditions requiring emergency medical care	Acute complexity requires emergency medical care
Fever	Fever may be a sign of acute inflammation or systemic distress
Acute inflammation	Massage may spread inflammation
Skin conditions	Avoid skin conditions that are contagious or that may be worsened by applying pressure
Blood poisoning and infections	Massage increases circulation in both the lymphatic and circulatory systems
Malignancy	Massage increases circulation in both the lymphatic and circulatory systems
Bleeding and bruising	Possible disruption of tissues already damaged

TABLE 9-2 | Precautions for General Massage

PRECAUTIONS	WHY?
Recent surgery	The doctor needs to be contacted regarding recent surgery
Burns	Extremely fragile skin
Recent fractures	The stability of the fracture site will need to be discussed with the doctor
Decreased sensation	Patients may not be able to provide accurate feedback
Increased sensitivity to touch	Be aware of the patient's reaction to massage and adjust accordingly
Cardiovascular disorders	These patients may be on medications and increased circulation may or may not be desired
Edema	Some causes of edema (such as lymphedema) may be an indication for massage. Other causes may be a precaution or contraindication
Osteoporosis	Bones are brittle and fracture more easily

strokes. Superficial effleurage is used to spread the lubricant over the treatment area, allows the patient to become comfortable with the clinician's touch, and provides information regarding the patient to the clinician. Information provided by this initial stroke includes skin temperature and texture, muscle tone, and sensitivity. Effleurage can be provided using the palm of the hand, fingers, thumbs, knuckles, or forearm. Slow, superficial, repetitive strokes can promote relaxation, both of the body and mind. Deep effleurage requires more pressure than superficial effleurage. Because it has the mechanical effect of stretching muscle and facia, strokes are applied in the same direction as the muscle fibers. Because it has the ability to increase venous and lymphatic circulation, the deep effleurage strokes usually occur in the same direction as the venous or lymphatic flow.[4] While there are numerous effleurage strokes available, Table 9-3 presents three for practice with corresponding Figures 9-7 through 9-9.

TABLE 9-3 | Examples of Effleurage Strokes in Classic Massage

Shingles effleurage	Shingles effleurage is an alternating stroke that uses two hands. One hand is always in contact with the body. Both hands move in the same direction. One hand begins as the other is about to end the stroke, which gives the perception of unbroken contact.[3] (Fig. 9-7)
Bilateral tree stroking	Bilateral tree stroking requires the use of two hands working simultaneously on both sides of the back. The hands start either at the neck and move distally or at the low back and move proximally. The hands are placed at midline and move simultaneously in a lateral direction before being brought back to midline.[3] (Fig. 9-8)
Horizontal stroking	Horizontal stroking is a technique often employed over large areas. While both hands are moving in reverse of each other, they are moving in the same overall direction.[3] (Fig. 9-9)

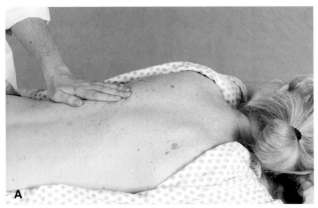

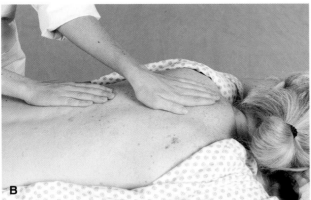

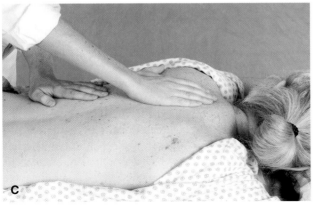

FIGURE 9-7 Shingles effleurage technique being performed. A, One hand begins to travel along the determined soft tissue path. B, The second hand begins to travel along the same soft tissue path, following the first hand. C, While the second hand continues along the soft tissue path, the first hand comes around and begins the path again, providing a feeling of continuous motion.

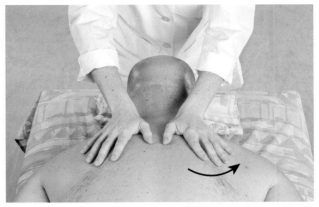

FIGURE 9-8 Bilateral tree stroking effleurage technique being performed.

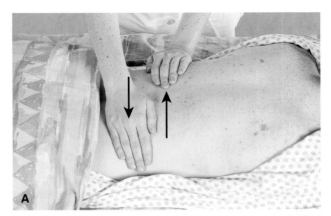

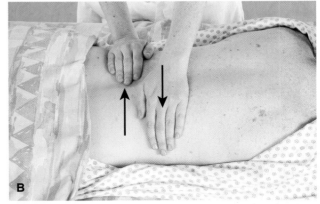

FIGURE 9-9 Horizontal stroking effleurage technique being performed. A, The right hand moves away from the clinician while the left hand moves toward the clinician. Both hands move parallel to one another in opposite directions. B, The hands then reverse roles, creating alternative back-and-forth motion.

Petrissage

Petrissage is a kneading motion that, like deep effleurage, has both mechanical and circulatory effects. Petrissage can break up adhesions located in superficial and deep muscle and fascia, while providing an elongation effect to the same tissues. Petrissage is performed by lifting the skin and underlying soft tissue from its normal resting state, and then pressing, rolling, squeezing, and kneading it prior to releasing it. When working on a large area, two hands work together in an alternating, rhythmic pattern.

When working on a smaller area, one hand may be able to lift and knead the tissue between the fingers and thumb. Petrissage may be the classic massage stroke of choice at the point at which the following effects are desired: improved mobility in the superficial and deep muscle and fascia, improved circulation, and cellular nutrition.[4] Table 9-4 and Figures 9-10 through 9-12 outline three specific petrissage techniques.

TABLE 9-4 | Examples of Petrissage Strokes in Classic Massage

Basic two-handed kneading	With basic two-handed kneading, each hand looks like Pac Man trying to eat the yellow dots! Using the entire hand, each hand alternates lifting, squeezing, and releasing the soft tissue.[3] (Fig. 9-10)
Circular two-handed petrissage	Circular two-handed petrissage is best performed on large, flat areas, such as the back. The hands should be flat on the body. Each hand moves in a clockwise circle (one starting at 12:00 and the other at 6:00) so that at 3:00 and 9:00 the skin is pressed between the two hands.[3] (Fig. 9-11)
Skin rolling	Skin rolling requires a minimal amount of lubricant, as too much will make this quite difficult. The skin is lifted up between the thumb and first two fingers, and then pushed forward by the thumbs. It is like creating a wave on the ocean, which is then rolling forward. This technique is also considered a myofascial release technique. It stretches skin and fascia while increasing superficial circulation.[3] (Fig. 9-12)

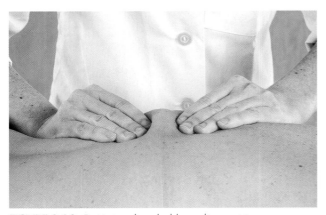

FIGURE 9-10 Basic two-handed kneading petrissage technique being performed.

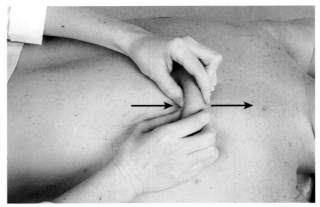

FIGURE 9-12 Skin rolling petrissage technique being performed.

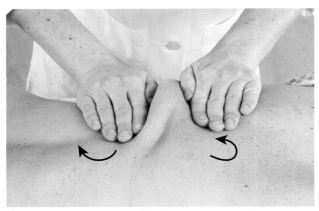

FIGURE 9-11 Circular two-handed petrissage technique being performed.

Tapotement

Tapotement consists of percussion movements performed in a rapid, alternating manner. Minimal force is required and the practitioner's wrists should remain relaxed while performing these strokes. The hands can be held in various positions, such as a loosely held fist, a cupped hand, or an open hand. Tapotement has a stimulating effect on the area. It can increase local blood flow and increase muscle tone. Tapotement should feel pleasant to the patient and not painful.[3,4] Three tapotement

movements have been described in detail in Table 9-5 and illustrated in Figures 9-13 through 9-15.

Cherkin et al found that classic massage techniques improved function and decreased pain in patients with chronic low back pain after 10 weeks.[20] Numerous other studies have evaluated the efficacy of classic massage techniques and found positive results.[21–27] Classic massage techniques have also been proved to play a large role in the reduction of swelling and delayed onset muscle soreness (DOMS) after exercise-induced DOMS.[28]

SCAR MASSAGE

Scars have the ability to limit ROM and function. A **scar** is an adhesion of the skin, which may or may not adhere to the underlying tissues. While there is no one specific scar massage technique, the mechanical action of various massage techniques separates tissues and breaks up adhesions.[3] Lifting, broadening, and applying shear forces can break up adhesions created by skin scarring, which may lead to increased skin, muscle, and joint flexibility.[3] Soft tissue techniques that provide a mechanical effect should be chosen, such as kneading, petrissage, skin rolling, deep transverse friction, and myofascial techniques (Fig. 9-16). These are considered effective in loosening scar tissue by breaking up adhesions between the scar tissue and underlying tissue.[29–31] Because the overall goal of scar massage is to achieve normal ROM, performing scar massage in conjunction with

TABLE 9-5 | Examples of Tapotement Strokes in Classic Massage

Hacking	During hacking, the hands should face one another with the forearms in neutral. The clinician should hold the wrists, hands, and fingers loosely while striking the body with the ulnar side of the wrist and hand in an alternating manner between right and left. Be careful when using this technique over the kidneys.[3] (Fig. 9-13)
Rapping	Rapping uses a lightly closed and loosely held fist. The forearms are held in pronation and the loose wrists and hands are alternately rapped on the body with light force.[3] (Fig. 9-14)
Cupping	Cupping strokes are performed with the hands "cupped" and the thumb held against the first metacarpal. The palmar sides of the cupped hands are alternately struck, creating a hollow sound.[3] (Fig. 9-15)

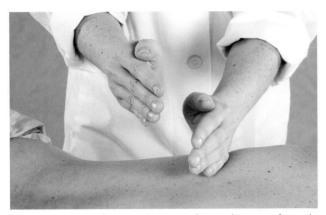

FIGURE 9-13 Hacking tapotement technique being performed.

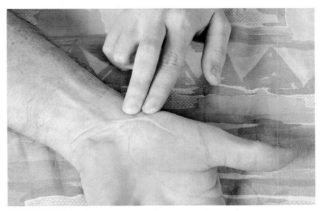

FIGURE 9-16 Scar massage being performed.

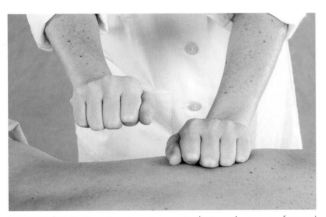

FIGURE 9-14 Rapping tapotement technique being performed

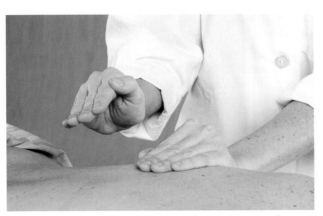

FIGURE 9-15 Cupping tapotement technique being performed.

ROM exercises is effective in stretching the scar tissue and achieving the goals.

TRIGGER POINT DEACTIVATION

Travell and Simons define a **trigger point** (TrP) as "a focus of hyperirritability in a tissue that, when compressed, is locally tender and, if sufficiently hypersensitive, gives rise to referred pain and tenderness."[32] Trigger points are palpated as a palpable nodule in muscle tissue, skin, scars, ligament, joint capsule, and fascia. Trigger points are classified as active or latent. **Active trigger points** are always tender, even when there is no pressure being applied to them. Active trigger points prevent full lengthening of the muscle, weaken the muscle, and refer pain when compressed directly.[3] When pain radiates from the trigger point to another area of the body, it is usually not associated with a nerve or dermatome.[4] "The pattern of referred pain is generally characteristic of a specific TrP and the referral areas are very predictable."[4] Travell and Simons have mapped the referred pain areas for common trigger points in *Myofascial Pain and Dysfunction*.[32] **Latent trigger points** are painful only when pressure is applied to them.[32] Even though latent trigger points are not associated with pain, they often cause stiffness and limited ROM. These are the most common.

According to Beck, nearly 70% of common trigger points are located at the site of known acupuncture points.[4] Locating a trigger point requires palpating the taut band of tissue while asking for verbal feedback from the patient. The patient will be able to provide you with information regarding the location of the trigger point (for example,

"You are almost on it"), the amount of pain they are feeling, and the presence of pain referral.[3]

Once you have identified the exact location of the trigger point, deactivation techniques can be chosen. While we will only discuss the manual techniques for deactivating trigger points, they are not the only intervention options. Nonmanual techniques include injections, dry needling, acupuncture, and spray-and-stretch.[4] The manual technique used to deactivate trigger points is trigger point pressure release, which can be used in conjunction with transverse friction massage. These manual techniques are followed up by stretching and elongation of the tissue that contains the trigger point.

Trigger point pressure release was originally referred to as ischemic compression. However, it has been found that to deactivate a trigger point, there is no need to exert enough pressure to cause ischemia to tissues that are already deprived of adequate oxygen. Trigger point pressure release uses the hands, olecranon process, or other handheld tools to compress the tissue at the site of the trigger point. When heldheld tools are employed to provide the pressure, the fingers must palpate first to accurately identify the trigger point. Pressure is held at the site of the trigger point for 20 to 60 seconds, causing the sarcomeres to lengthen.[33] Pressure should be gradually increased to the point at which the patient reports pain (Fig. 9-17).

Trigger point release can oftentimes be performed by the patient, depending on the location of the trigger point and the tools available. Clinical tools such as the Thera Cane (Fig. 9-18) can assist patients in performing the release independently. Studies have shown that when trigger point deactivation techniques are added to a self-stretching protocol for the treatment of plantar heel pain, the results are superior short-term outcomes.[34] Other studies have shown that trigger point deactivation can immediately increase ROM associated with the treated muscle.[35–37]

WHY DO I NEED TO KNOW ABOUT...

Knowing the referred pain areas of common trigger points can assist the clinician in differentiating between trigger points, neuropathies, and other referred pain sources.

MYOFASCIAL RELEASE

Myofascial release (MFR) is a term used to describe a set of soft tissue techniques aimed at relieving soft tissue from the abnormal grip of tight fascia.[38] Myofascial release stretches the fascial system of the body. This can break up fascial adhesions, thereby relieving mobility restrictions and pain, which can lead to postural deviations and functional limitations. Fascia is connective tissue found throughout the body and is the mechanism by which everything in the body is connected. Subcutaneous fascia

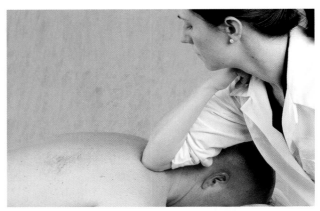

FIGURE 9-17 Trigger point release being performed with olecranon process to prone patient in the upper trapezius muscle.

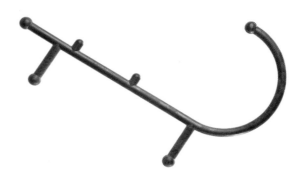

FIGURE 9-18 Thera Cane.
(Courtesy of Thera Cane, www.theracane.com.)

is the layer of connective tissue located between the skin and the deep fascia, whereas the deep fascia holds muscles and organs in place. Because all fascia is connected, a restriction in one area can affect other areas, both adjacent and removed from the area of restriction.

All myofascial release techniques aim to stretch fascia, either locally or more generally. The most common types of myofascial releases performed in physical therapy clinics are myofascial spreads and myofascial mobilizations. Myofascial spreading affects subcutaneous fascia and release local restrictions by placing the hands side by side over the area of restriction and then pulling apart (Fig. 9-19). The tissues are spread until resistance is felt and the clinician maintains this tension until the resistance yields, at which point the hands can be spread even further apart. Myofascial mobilizations include techniques in which tissues are rolled against the subcutaneous fascia, such as skin rolling. Skin rolling is also considered a form of petrissage and can be found in Table 9.4 and Figure 9-12. Skin rolling stretches superficial fascia in the treatment areas and increases local circulation.

One research study aimed to compare outcomes for patients with lateral epicondylitis. The control group received

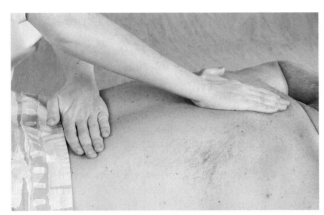

FIGURE 9-19 Myofascial spreading technique being used on a prone patient.

sham ultrasound while the other received myofascial release. They concluded that MFR is more effective for the treatment of lateral epicondylitis.[39] Use of myofascial therapy once weekly has been shown to reduce anxiety and improve quality of sleep and life.[40]

TRANSVERSE FRICTION MASSAGE

Transverse friction massage (TFM), popularized by James Cyriax, produces a myriad of benefits. Studies have compared Cyriax's approach with the treatment of lateral epicondylalgia with phonophoresis and concluded that TFM is a superior treatment approach.[44]

Transverse friction massage is a repetitive, specific, nongliding technique that produces movement between the fibers of connective tissue.[43] It is indicated for any condition in which mobility has been compromised by irregular tissue remodeling, sprains, strains, and chronic repetitive strain injuries such as tendonitis, tenosynovitis, and plantar fasciitis.[43] In TFM superficial friction creates vasodilation of the capillaries, while deep friction can increase blood and lymph circulation. Transverse friction massage breaks up fascial adhesions, softens scar tissue, and causes a mild therapeutic inflammation. This mild inflammatory response can initiate a protective cellular response that promotes repair. When an adhesion is located within a muscle or tendon, stresses are not equally distributed through the tissues as they tend to build up around the adhesion, leading to pain. Breaking up an adhesion can allow the muscle and tendon to share contractile stresses and forces, leading to a decrease in pain perception.[41,42]

Because of the nature of TFM, it is particularly important that the clinician's fingernails be kept short. Because there is no gliding of the clinician's hands over the patient's skin, no lubrication is indicated for this technique. The clinician's fingers and patient's skin must move simultaneously to avoid skin injury and the friction must be provided perpendicular (or transverse) to the striations of the muscle or tendon fibers. According to Cyriax, when applying TFM to a tendon or ligament, the tissue should be on stretch, while a muscle belly should be placed on slack.[42] The point of contact is very specific and palpation should occur to single out the exact area within the tissue that is at fault, typically the most tender area. The pad of the second digit (pointer finger) should be used for small areas, with the third digit (long finger) reinforcing the second digit. The depth of pressure should remain with the patient's pain tolerance and be only deep enough to engage the tissue of interest. The clinician then moves back and forth over the tissue, attempting to sweep over as much of the involved tissue as possible without slipping off and onto healthy tissue (Fig. 9-20). This technique is performed at a relatively quick speed of two to three cycles per second for anywhere between 5 and 20 minutes, depending on the acuity of the injury.[45]

Thorough and clear communication with patients is extremely important when providing friction as a soft tissue technique owing to its risk of producing local tissue damage and its tendency to cause discomfort. Once the tissue needing friction has been identified, the clinician can gently palpate the tissue to determine where it is most tender, by eliciting patient feedback. Because this technique can be painful, that needs to be clearly communicated to the patient before initiating so that the patient can give informed consent to proceed. Discussing the purpose and goal of the treatment technique will help the patient to understand why the clinician has chosen this intervention. It is also beneficial to discuss with the patient how many minutes the clinician plans on doing TFM and that the pressure can and will be adjusted if the patient desires. To make the treatment more tolerable, experienced clinicians naturally engage these patients in stimulating conversations during this one-on-one treatment session.

Patient Perspective

Patients need to know ahead of time if any discomfort is to be expected during the soft tissue technique planned. They also need to be informed of the rationale for choosing the specific soft tissue technique being performed. While the effectiveness of *all* patient outcomes is enhanced with cultural awareness, the use of hands-on techniques requires an acute awareness of cultural differences on the part of the clinician.

Patients' Frequently Asked Questions

1. **Why does the pain shoot up toward my head when you press on that spot on my back?**
2. **Why is my arm so red after you do that transverse friction massage technique?**
3. **It feels so good when you are massaging it, but the pain returns shortly after you stop. Why is that?**

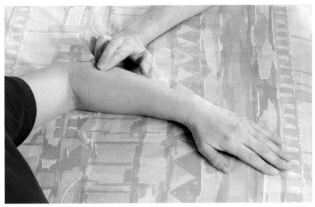

FIGURE 9-20 Close-up of proper finger position for TFM on patient's forearm.

Documentation and Billing

Separate current procedural terminology (CPT) codes exist for massage and manual therapy techniques. Massage includes effleurage, petrissage, and tapotement strokes. Manual therapy techniques include skilled manual therapy such as mobilization, manual lymphatic drainage, and manual traction. Items that should be included when documenting soft tissue techniques include the following:

- The specific area that is being treated
- The specific soft tissue technique that is employed
- The length of time that the service was provided (to quantify the intervention)
- Relate the purpose of the chosen soft tissue technique to the goal
- The patient response to the intervention, including the integrity of the skin

Clinical Decision-Making

Once the initial examination of a patient is complete, the physical therapist completes the evaluation, which includes determining functional goals. Once the functional goals have been identified, the treating clinician determines which impairments need to be addressed to succeed in meeting the goals set forth. When the impairments have been identified, the clinician can determine which are likely to respond favorably to soft tissue techniques. By reviewing any possible contraindications and precautions, the clinician can identify which soft tissue techniques will be most effective for the patient. To maximize the patient's adherence to the physical therapy plan of care, it should be reviewed with the patient and explained that the soft tissue techniques will be used for specific goals and that other interventions have been identified as well (i.e., therapeutic exercise, neuromuscular reeducation, and other modalities).[43]

Summary

Providing effective soft tissue techniques can be a very rewarding experience for all parties involved. Effective use of the hands as tools can elevate the quality of care provided as well as patient outcomes. Growth and expertise occur only when the clinician seeks the input of other, more knowledgeable clinicians and continually assesses his or her effectiveness, adjusting manual techniques accordingly. Physical therapists and physical therapist assistants tend to be very nurturing people who spend a lot of time and energy working with their patients. Maintaining your own physical health is paramount to being able to help others, so becoming the client yourself to receive a massage may be the prescription needed to keep up the good work.

Review Questions

1. Which of the following best defines the term "soft tissue massage"?
   a. Using your hands to move soft tissue
   b. Sending a message to the softer parts of the body
   c. Providing a relaxing experience for a patient
   d. An additional service that your patient can purchase out of pocket at the end of the session

2. Which of the following does not need to be considered prior to giving a patient a massage?
   a. The length of your fingernails
   b. The length of your hair
   c. The presence of rings and watches
   d. The presence of earrings

3. In which of the following situations would massage be safe to perform?
   a. Open wounds
   b. Acute flare-up of rheumatoid arthritis
   c. Acute pneumonia
   d. Pregnancy

4. The majority of trigger points are located at which site?
   a. The musculotendinous junction
   b. Acupuncture sites
   c. The dominant upper extremity
   d. The external auditory meatus

5. All patients will enjoy the soft tissue management techniques you provide.
   a. True
   b. False

CASE STUDY 1

Betsy is a right-hand-dominant nurse who works at an asthma and allergy doctor's office. Lately, she has been giving up to 100 allergy injections each day. She is in physical therapy with complaints of right elbow pain near the lateral epicondyle. The physical therapist has determined that the repetitive wrist extension required to give shots to her patients has resulted in lateral epicondylitis.

- Which soft tissue treatment technique would be best suited for Betsy?

- How many minutes would you plan on providing your chosen soft tissue intervention?
- Are there any other modalities that you might consider using in conjunction with a hands-on approach?

CASE STUDY 2

Betsy turns out to be a repeat customer. She was so happy with your treatment of her lateral epicondylitis last year, that she has returned again, this time with complaints of right-sided neck pain. Her employer decided to switch over to electronic medical records, so Betsy has been spending a tremendous amount of time hunched over her computer at work, entering data for existing patient charts. She has decreased ROM in left cervical side-bending and a dull ache and palpable nodule in her right upper trapezius.

- Which soft tissue treatment technique would be best suited for Betsy?

- How many minutes would you plan on providing your chosen soft tissue intervention?
- Are there any other modalities that you might consider using in conjunction with a hands-on approach?

DISCUSSION QUESTIONS

1. What types of palpation skills are required of a clinician who employs soft tissue techniques?

2. What are some contraindications to classic massage?

3. If a patient asked you what the difference is between massage therapy and physical therapy, how would you explain it?

4. What is the ultimate goal of scar massage as it relates to impairments and functional limitations?

5. What are considered to be normal effects of transverse friction massage?

REFERENCES

1. Lewis, M: Patient satisfaction . . . "In good hands." Physiotherapy Frontline 15(3):20, 2009.
2. Saunders, C: Manual therapy for low back pain. Patient Care 35(10):12–23, 2001.
3. Benjamin, PJ, and Tappan, FM: Handbook of Health Massage Techniques, ed 4. Pearson Prentice Hall, Upper Saddle River, NJ, 2005.
4. Beck, MF: Theory & Practice of Therapeutic Massage, ed 5. Cengage Learning, Clifton Park, NY, 2010.
5. Stedman's Concise Medical Dictionary for the Health Professions, ed 4. Lippincott Williams & Wilkins, New York, 2001.
6. Biel, A: Trail Guide to the Body, ed 4. Books of Discovery, Boulder, CO, 2010.
7. Arroyo-Morales, M, Olea, N, Ruiz, C, Luna del Castillo, JD, et al: Massage after exercise. Response of immunologic and endocrine markers: a randomized single-blind placebo-controlled study. J Strength Cond Res 23(2): 638-644, 2009.
8. Rapaport, MH, Schettler, P, and Bresee, C: A preliminary study of the effects of a single session of Swedish massage on hypothalamic-pituitary-adrenal and immune function in normal individuals. J Alternative Complementary Med 16(10):1079–1088, 2010.
9. Sefton, JM, Yarar, C, Berry, JW, and Pascoe, DD: Therapeutic massage of the neck and shoulders produces changes in peripheral blood flow when assessed with dynamic infrared thermography. J Alternative Complementary Med 16(7):723–732, 2010.
10. Dommerholt, J, and Huijbregts, P: Myofascial Trigger Points: Pathophysiology and Evidence-Informed Diagnosis and Management. Jones & Bartlett, Boston, 2011.
11. Sturgeon, M, Wetta-Hall, R, Hart, T, et al. Effects of therapeutic massage on the quality of life among patients with breast cancer during treatment. J Alternative Complementary Med 15(4):373–380, 2009.
12. Hemmings, B, Smith, M, Graydon, J, and Dyson, R: Effects of massage on physiological restoration, perceived recovery, and repeated sports performance. Br J Sports Med 34:109–114, 2000.
13. Arroyo-Morales, M, Olea, N, Martinez, M, Moreno-Lorenzo, C, et al: Effects of myofascial release after high intensity exercise. A randomized clinical trial. J Manip Phys Ther 21:217–223, 2008.

14. American Physical Therapy Association: Guide to Physical Therapist Practice, ed 2. Phys Ther 81:1, 2001.

15. Arroyo-Morales, M, Olea, N, et al: Psychophysiological effects of massage—myofascial release after exercise: a randomized sham-control study. J Alternative Complementary Med 14(10):1223–1229, 2008.

16. Wiktorsson-Moller, M, Oberg, B, Ekstrand, J, and Gillquist, J: Effects of warming up, massage, and stretching on range of motion and muscle strength in the lower extremity. Am J Sports Med 11:249–252, 1983.

17. van den Dolder, PA, and Roberts, DL: A trial into the effectiveness of soft tissue massage in the treatment of shoulder pain. Aust J Physiotherapy 49:183–188, 2003.

18. Fritz, S: Fundamentals of Therapeutic Massage. Mosby-Lifeline, St. Louis, MO, 1995.

19. Salvo, SG: Massage Therapy. WB Saunders, Philadelphia, 1999.

20. Cherkin, DC, Sherman, KJ, Kahn, J, et al. A comparison of the effects of 2 types of massage and usual care on chronic low back pain a randomized, controlled trial. Ann Intern Med 155:1–9, 2011.

21. Furlan, AD, Imamura, M, Dryden, T, and Irvin, E: Massage for low back pain: an updated systematic review within the framework of the Cochrane Back Review Group. Spine 34:1669–1684, 1976.

22. Cherkin, DC, Eisenberg, D, Sherman, KJ, Barlow, W, Kaptchuk, TJ, Street, J, et al: Randomized trial comparing traditional Chinese medical acupuncture, therapeutic massage, and self-care education for chronic low back pain. Arch Intern Med 161:1081–1088, 2001.

23. Hernandez-Reif, M, Field, T, Krasnegor, J, and Theakston, H: Lower back pain is reduced and range of motion increased after massage therapy. Int J Neurosci 106:131–145, 2001.

24. Preyde, M: Effectiveness of massage therapy for subacute low-back pain: a randomized controlled trial. CMAJ 162:1815–1820, 2000.

25. Field, T, Hernandez-Reif, M, Diego, M, and Fraser, M: Lower back pain and sleep disturbance are reduced following massage therapy. J Bodywork and Movement Ther 11:141–145, 2007.

26. Kumnerdee, W: Effectiveness comparison between Thai traditional massage and Chinese acupuncture for myofascial back pain in Thai military personnel: a preliminary report. J Med Assoc Thai 92:117–123, 2009.

27. Little, P, Lewith, G, Webley, F, Evans, M, Beattie, A, Middleton, K, et al: Randomised controlled trial of Alexander technique lessons, exercise, and massage for chronic and recurrent back pain. BMJ 337:884, 2008.

28. Zainuddin, Z, Newton, M, Sacco, P, and Nosaka, K. Effects of massage on delayed-onset muscle soreness, swelling, and recovery of muscle function. J Athletic Training 40(3):174–180, 2005.

29. Ward, RS: Physical Rehabilitation. In Carrougher, GJ (ed): Burn Care and Therapy. CV Mosby, St. Louis, MO, 1998.

30. Miles, WK, and Grigsby, L: Remodeling of scar tissue in the burned hand. In Hunter, JN, et al (eds): Rehabilitation of the Hand. CV Mosby, St. Louis, MO, 1984.

31. O'Sullivan, SB, and Schmitz, TJ: Physical Rehabilitation, ed 5. FA Davis, Philadelphia, 2007.

32. Simons, DG, Travell, JG, and Simons, LS: Travell and Simons' Myofascial Pain and Dysfunction: The Trigger Point Manual. Volume 1: Upper Half of Body, ed 2. Lippincott Williams & Wilkins, Baltimore, 1999.

33. Simons, D: Review of enigmatic MTrPs as a common cause of enigmatic musculoskeletal pain and dysfunction. J Electromyogr Kinesiology 14:95–107, 2004.

34. Renan-Ordine, R, Alburquerque, F, et al. Effectiveness of myofascial trigger point manual therapy combined with a self-stretching protocol for the management of plantar heel pain: a randomized controlled trial. J Orthop Sports Phys Ther 41(2):43–50, 2011.

35. Grieve, R, Clark, J, Pearson, E, et al: The immediate effect of soleus trigger point pressure release on restricted ankle joint dorsiflexion: A pilot randomised controlled trial. J Bodywork Movement Ther 15:42–49, 2011.

36. Wu, S, Hong, C, You, J, Chen, C, Wang, L, and Su, F: Therapeutic effect on the change of gait performance in chronic calf myofascial pain syndrome: a time series case study. J Musculoskeletal Pain 13(3):33–43, 2006.

37. Grieve, R: Proximal hamstring rupture, restoration of function without surgical intervention: a case study on myofascial trigger point release. J Bodywork Movement Ther 10:99–104, 2006.

38. Juett, T: Myofascial release—an introduction for the patient, Phys Ther Forum 7(41):7–8, 1988.

39. Ajimsha, MS, Chithra, S, and Thulasyammal, RP: Effectiveness of myofascial release in the management of lateral epicondylitis in computer professionals. Arch Phys Med Rehabil 93(4):604–609, 2012.

40. Castro-Sanchez, AM, Mataran-Penarrocha, GA, Granero-Molina J, et al: Benefits of massage myofascial release therapy on pain, anxiety, quality of sleep, depression, and quality of life in patients with fibromyalgia. Evidence Based Complementary Alternative Med, 2011, doi:10.1155/2011/561753.

41. Cyriax, J, and Coldham, M: Textbook of Orthopedic Medicine. Vol 2: Treatment by Manipulation, Massage and Injection, ed 11. Bailliere-Tindall, London, 1984.

42. Cyriax, J: Deep massage. Physiotherapy 63:60–61, 1977.

43. Andrade, CK, and Clifford, P: Outcome-Based Massage. Lippincott Williams & Wilkins, Baltimore, 2001.

44. Nagrale, AV, Herd, CR, et al: Cyriax physiotherapy versus phonophoresis with supervised exercise in subjects with lateral epicondylalgia: a randomized clinical trial. J Manual Manipulative Ther 17(3):171–178, 2009.

45. Kessler, RM, and Hertling, D: Friction massage. In Hertling, D, Kessler, RM (eds): Management of Common Musculoskeletal Conditions, ed 3. Lippincott-Raven, Philadelphia, 1996.

LET'S FIND OUT

Lab Activity: Soft Tissue Management Techniques: Massage

This lab activity is designed to demonstrate the soft tissue management techniques that are currently practiced in clinical environments. Student/learners will practice preparing and positioning the patient, applying soft tissue management techniques, providing the rationale for the use of each, and describing the components used to assess treatment efficacy. Students/learners will administer and receive various forms of soft tissue massage and learn the importance of proper positioning for both the patient and the individual applying the technique. This lab activity also covers what to document and how important appropriate patient instruction is to treatment success.

Equipment

plinth   sheets and towels
lubricant

Lab Activities

Classic Massage

1. Gather all necessary equipment.
2. Prepare yourself for a hands-on treatment intervention by tying up long hair; assessing fingernail length; removing watches, rings and bracelets; and performing proper hand hygiene technique.
3. Discuss the rationale for preparing your hair and hands:

_____
_____

4. What types of questions would you need to ask a patient prior to performing soft tissue massage?

_____
_____
_____
_____

   What types of information would *you* need to provide to the patient prior to touching them?

_____
_____
_____

5. Position the patient prone.
   A. How should you position your patient's head and neck? What is your rationale?

_____

   B. What could you do to position the patient to protect his or her lower back?

_____
_____

6. Drape the patient from shoulders to feet and then expose the area to be treated by undraping the back to the level of the posterior superior iliac spine (PSIS).
   A. What is the rationale behind draping the patient in this manner?

_____
_____

7. Assess the treatment area.
   A. What can be observed about the treatment area after you expose it?

_____
_____

B. You are about to touch the patient. Describe techniques that you can use to test the patient's perception of light touch and circulation?

_____

_____

_____

8. Apply therapeutic massage.
   A. Outline which type of stroke you will start and end with and your rationale for your selections.

   _____

   _____

   B. If you provide pressure with your strokes, will you coincide the pressure with the patient's inspiration or expiration?

   _____

   C. Choose at least two effleurage strokes, two petrissage strokes, and two forms of tapotement. Perform at least 10 strokes of each to your patient.
9. When the treatment is complete, what additional steps need to be taken to complete the treatment?

   _____

   _____

10. How would you assess treatment efficacy?

   _____

   _____

   _____

11. Document this treatment session.

   _____

   _____

   _____

   _____

Scar Massage
1. Which types of massage techniques have you practiced that have the mechanical effects necessary to break up scar tissue?

   _____

2. In which direction should your chosen scar massage technique be provided?

   _____

3. Either locate a real scar on your lab partner that is more than 1 year old and is fully healed or identify a tissue in which you can imagine a scar being located. Perform the scar massage for 5 minutes while maintaining proper body mechanics.
4. If your lab partner really had a scar in the tissue you chose, which joint and motion would be limited in range? How would you stretch it?

   _____

   _____

Transverse Friction Massage

1. Allow your lab partner to choose one of the following tissues to receive 2 minutes of TFM:

    a. proximal wrist extensor tendons

    b. proximal peroneus longus

    c. supraspinatus

2. Practice explaining to your lab partner what TFM is and why you have chosen that particular soft tissue intervention. Make sure that you include what you expect for them to feel.

3. Before you begin, make sure that you are in a position to maximize proper body mechanics, including proper use and protection of your hands and fingers.

4. Which position should you ask your lab partner to assume to maximize exposure of the tissue you are treating? Should you place the tissue on stretch or on slack? Why?

_____

_____

_____

5. In which direction will you be providing the force of friction?

_____

6. Even though your lab partner may not have dysfunction in the tissue you are about to treat, you will still be able to identify the specific and localized area that needs to be treated. How will you do this?

_____

_____

7. Were you able to concentrate on your treatment intervention while holding a pleasant conversation with your lab partner? Yes/No

8. On a scale from 0 to 10, 0 being no fatigue and 10 being maximal fatigue, how tired are your fingers after 2 minutes of performing TFM? Why?

_____

_____

Trigger Point Release

1. List nonmanual and manual techniques for the treatment of trigger points:

_____

_____

_____

2. Which manual technique would you apply?

_____

3. Describe how you would perform this technique.

_____

_____

_____

4. What would you have the patient do immediately after the manual technique you identified above?

_____

Patient Scenarios

A. Ruth is a 67-year-old woman who received a total knee replacement on the right side 2 weeks ago. She presents to physical therapy with limited ROM of the right knee and decreased strength in the right quadriceps, hamstrings, and gastrocnemius. She complains of pain rated as a 4 on a scale of 1 to 10 and minimal swelling in the right foot. She has a 5-inch-long scar along the anterior aspect of her right knee and she is concerned with her inability to climb stairs and drive her car. Which of the above are impairments and which are functional limitations? Which of her impairments may benefit from a soft tissue technique?

B. Billy is a 32-year-old man who has recently taken up jogging. He runs outside in his neighborhood and he is complaining of right thigh pain. The physical therapist examines and evaluates Billy to discover that he has iliotibial band (ITB) syndrome. Which soft tissue management technique(s) would be most appropriate for Billy? Why?

C. Amy is the new mother of an 8-week-old baby girl. Amy has been experiencing left neck and shoulder pain for 4 weeks. Amy reports that she has been folding and unfolding a heavy stroller and lifting it into and out of her SUV multiple times a day. She has been losing sleep because she has been spending half the night in the glider in her daughter's room. The other day she put the baby into her crib and just as she was lowering her down, she felt a sharp pain in her left upper trapezius, which shot up toward her head. This is what brought her to physical therapy. Which soft tissue management technique(s) would be most appropriate for Amy? Why?

Lab Questions

1. When would a patient with low back pain benefit from a pillow placed under the abdomen (in a prone position)?

2. When would a patient with low back pain benefit from the absence of a pillow under the abdomen (in a prone position)?

3. Although they are different interventions, which treatment goals are common to scar massage, transverse friction massage, and trigger point release?

CHAPTER 10

Electromagnetic Radiation: Diathermy, Ultraviolet, and Laser

Barbara J. Behrens, PTA, MS

Learning Outcomes

Following the successful completion of this chapter, the learner will be able to:

- Define the uses of light, ultraviolet (UV), and diathermy in clinical practice.
- Outline the physical properties of electromagnetic (EM) energy of various wavelengths.
- Outline the EM spectrum in terms of therapeutic light and energy sources that can be used as potential treatment interventions in physical therapy.
- Describe the application of diathermy as a potential treatment intervention in physical therapy.
- Discuss the production of laser light and how it differs from other forms of light.
- Discuss the potential uses for laser and UV as potential treatment interventions in physical therapy.
- Discuss the role of the U.S. Food and Drug Administration (FDA) as a regulatory agency and the influence of their guidelines involving investigational devices that are introduced into the physical therapy clinical environment.

Key Terms

Absorption
Actinotherapy
Beam divergence
Biostimulation
Coherence
Diathermy
Dipole

EM radiation
Institutional review board (IRB)
Investigational device exemption
  (IDE)
Laser
Monochromatic
Nanometers

Nonionizing
Photosensitive
Reflection
Refraction
UV
Wavelength

"Science does not know its debt to imagination." —Ralph Waldo Emerson

Patient Perspective

"That's not the same type of laser that I've seen them use in movies is it, where they vaporize people?"

The patient perspective as captured in the question above is important to keep in mind as one thinks about employing therapeutic interventions. We never really know what a patient might be thinking when we first approach him or her with the concept of what we want to use. Although as clinicians we might think that something our patients have said is funny, our patients might have a completely different reaction to what we say. For example, lasers may bring images of ray guns or light sabers to your patients and they might think of them only in terms of destructive tools, not therapeutic modalities. The image of Darth Vader or some other action hero may be what they perceive as the most common use for lasers or laser tag, but they certainly do not see them as a treatment intervention. Patient education becomes crucial to help your patients understand what to expect from these types of therapeutic interventions that are so different from the other, more commonly applied physical agents discussed in previous chapters.

Sunlight is perhaps one of the most primitive examples of a physical agent. It provides illumination in the dark and warmth from the cold. Continuous study of its differentiating characteristics has led to the development and refinement of several forms of treatment modalities that utilize different forms of EM radiation (EMR) including diathermy various forms of light, namely ultraviolet (UV), and laser. The term EMREM can be a frightening one for those who do not understand its meaning; however, all it means is radiation such as x-rays, microwaves, gamma rays, UV light, visible light, infrared (IR) radiation, and radio waves.

EM Radiation

EM radiation has magnetic and electric fields that are perpendicular to each other and also to the direction in which they are traveling. Unlike electrical energy, EMREM travels without a specific conductor or a supporting medium. It can travel through the air, which is why it can be so puzzling and also spark so much imagination in the minds of moviemakers. Figure 10-1 illustrates the EM spectrum.

Figure 10-2 illustrates the path in which EM energy may travel, which is different from the path that other forms of energy—those that travel strictly through a conductor—travel.

This chapter discusses and outlines the uses of these types of physical agents including diathermy, UV, and cold laser in terms of their indications, application techniques, and safety considerations. It is not intended to be an in-depth study of the theoretical basis for any of these modalities, but is merely an overview for clinicians should they have the opportunity to use the techniques.

Diathermy and laser represent modalities that may not be as commonly in use as other physical agents in clinical facilities in the United States today, for very different reasons. Lasers have been considered investigational devices by the U.S. Food and Drug Administration (FDA), and are therefore restricted in their use with humans to specific applications and diagnoses. Investigational status of a modality is a classification assigned to any new modality application for human use. There is a process that any new modality introduced within the United States must go through to ensure both the safety and the efficacy for human use. Laser will be discussed in terms of the process involved with an investigational modality as well as its applications as reported in the literature. Diathermy has not been as commonly used owing to the number of

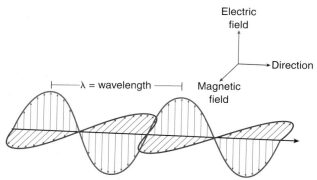

FIGURE 10-2 The path of EM energy generates an EM field that is perpendicular to the direction of the energy source and the source itself.

precautions and contraindications that are primarily a result of the mode of delivery of the modality. The results that were accomplished when diathermy was applied were favorable but clinicians tended not to use it and opted for other physical agents that did not use EM fields to accomplish the results that they sought.

ELECTROMAGNETIC FIELDS AND DIATHERMY

The EM fields that are used therapeutically are those that are applied externally to the body from the *nonionizing* radiofrequency part of the EM spectrum. This is important to note. Our DNA is the backbone of our genetic makeup. Disruption of the sequence of the amino acid chains that make up our DNA could significantly alter how our body functions. This is the basis for radiation treatment for such conditions as cancer, in which the goal is to do just that. X-rays are a form of ionizing energy, which is why such caution must be taken when we are exposed to them.

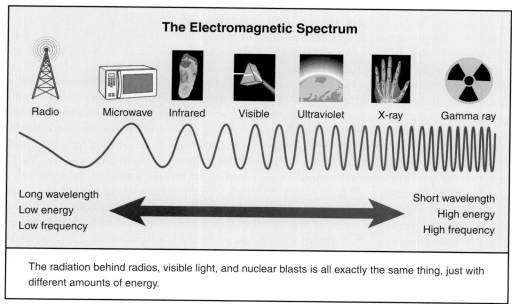

FIGURE 10-1 The EM spectrum. Each of the colors of light is represented by a specific wavelength, which is measured in nanometers (nm). The visible range is indicated.

Nonionizing means that this form of energy does not have the ability to change the chemical structure of the tissue with which it interacts; however, it affects the tissue, and the forms that we use therapeutically have been shown to promote tissue healing.[1-3] There is insufficient energy to depolarize a motor nerve to cause a muscle to contract or to cause sensory perception. The amplitude used with this form of energy is also insufficient to interfere with the patterns of orbiting electrons of the individual molecules. In other words, there is no mutation taking place of one's DNA when this form of treatment is being applied. However, there is sufficient energy, depending upon the mode of application, to produce a heating effect.

Diathermy is a term that literally means "to heat through" and involves the use of EM energy passing through and being absorbed by the body and then converted into heat. The term is used to encompass application techniques using EM fields, which include both contiuous and pulsed short-wave diathermy and nonthermal applications of pulsed EM fields and pulsed radio frequency energy. All of these forms of EM energy are externally applied to effect a change in the healing of soft tissues. They are modalities that had been in use within the past 20 to 30 years, grew unpopular because of technical issues related to leakage,[4,5] and have started to enjoy a resurgence of interest because of the promising results seen with

technologically advanced systems that have addressed some of the problems of the past.[6] Depending upon the type of setting in which someone practices, these forms of EM fields may be the modality of choice for the patient population if it includes wound repair. See Table 10-1 for a list of the EM devices, the acronyms associated with them, and potential uses.

The primary difference between the various devices in this category is based upon the wavelength of the device in the EM spectrum. Since the demand for the use of our airwaves has increased exponentially within the past several decades, and the Federal Communications Commission (FCC) regulates what frequencies can be used for various purposes including the transmission of radio, television, radar, cell phone use, and medical applications, there are tight controls on what frequencies are available. It is interesting to note that this is not a simple regulatory issue for just one nation. The regulation of EMR frequencies relies upon the cooperation of all nations of the world since air, space, communication, and navigation rely so heavily upon the airwaves. If there were no treaties among the various nations, there would be a tremendous amount of interference that would make radio frequency communication virtually useless.[7] The frequencies and wavelengths that the FCC has approved for medical applications are listed in Table 10-2.

TABLE 10-1 | EM Device Acronyms and Their Potential Applications

DEVICE	ACRONYM	THERMAL?	POTENTIAL APPLICATION
Pulsed EM Field	PEMF	No	Tissue healing
Pulsed Radio Frequency	PRF	No	Tissue healing
Pulsed Short-Wave Diathermy	PSWD	No	Tissue healing
Continuous Short-Wave Diathermy	CSWD	Yes	Tissue **heating**, not healing
Microwave Diathermy	MWD	Yes	Tissue **heating**

TABLE 10-2 | Types of EM Radiation and Their Approved Federal Trade Commission Characteristics

TYPE OF EM RADIATION	WAVELENGTH	FREQUENCY (MHz)	POTENTIAL APPLICATIONS
SWD/PRFR	22 meters	13.56	Decrease: pain, muscle guarding, promote deep tissue heating
SWD/PRFR	11 meters	27.12*	
SWD/PRFR	7.5 meters	40.68	
MWD	33 meters	915.00	
MWD	12 centimeters	2450.00	

*Most commonly use frequency for SWD and PRFR
Key: Short-Wave Diathermy = SWD
     Pulsed Radio Frequency Radiation = PRFR
     MicroWave Diathermy = MWD

PHYSIOLOGICAL EFFECTS OF DIATHERMY

Diathermy can be applied in either a pulsed or continuous mode. Whenever the energy is pulsed, this is referring to a temporary but consistent interruption in the "on" time. A continuous stream of energy has a different effect on the tissue than that of a pulsed form of energy. Pulsed short-wave diathermy (SWD) may produce heat and continuous SWD (CSWD) may also produce heat in the treatment field. The determining factor is the power output of the device and the ability of the energy to pass through the body.

Unlike superficial forms of heat that were conductive heat sources, diathermy is a form of heat that works by conversion. Since it has the ability to pass through human tissues and influence those that it encounters, that influence is what we need to understand.

Human tissues contain significant amounts of water, which is a **dipole** molecule. This means that the water molecule is more positive on one end and negative on the other end (Fig. 10-3).

Once exposed to specific frequencies of CSWD, these dipole molecules are literally ionically pushed around, which leads to internal friction as they attempt to rotate back to return to their original state.

This oscillation and friction may cause what are referred to as eddy currents within the underlying tissues. Eddy currents are closed loops of induced current circulating in planes perpendicular to the source of the EM energy (Fig. 10-4).

This dipole rotation also affects other tissues that are adjacent to the water-containing molecules and creates more heat within the tissues. The heating that occurs with diathermy is one that happens from within the tissues. There is no sensation of heat on the superficial structures and no mass on the surface as was perceived with hot packs.

TYPES OF DIATHERMY APPLICATIONS

Diathermy can be applied via either an electric field method or a magnetic field method. Selection of one method over another is based upon the composition of the

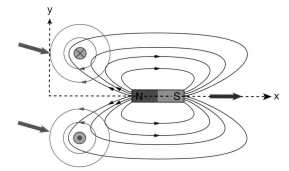

FIGURE 10-4 Eddy currents as a result of an applied induction EM field.

underlying tissue, availability of devices, and treatment goals. The difference between the two is the way in which the energy is delivered to the treatment area. This determination may be made based upon the device that is available in the clinic.

Diathermy With an Electric Field

The introduction of EM energy into human tissues through the creation of an electric field is what has been previously described with dipole rotation. The heating that is created from this form of diathermy is nonuniform, in great part owing to the lack of uniformity of the tissues. Human tissues are composed of skin, connective tissue, muscle, fat, and bone. Each of these tissues has a different water content or concentration of dipoles. Since the dipoles rotate in response to EM energy introduction, which in turn creates heat, the amount of heat produced is highly dependent upon the concentration of tissues that are conductive within the field. For example, muscle and skin are good conductors but fat and bone are poor conductors. The differences in tissue types that the EM energy encounters in effect dissipate the energy or spread it out.

Those tissue types that have the greatest number of dipole molecules also have the greatest ability to store charge. In the case of EM energy this is in the form of heat from the movement of ions. *Those tissues with the greatest water content or ability to carry charge are the most likely to heat up quickly.* This is vitally important to realize when applying diathermy to a patient. The presence of any metal in the treatment field is contraindicated as the metal is highly conductive and would heat up first, long before superficial tissues would perceive discomfort. See Table 10-3 for a summary of different tissue types and their relative conductivity of EM energy.

The applicators for this form of diathermy are referred to as capacitive applicators. They may be placed parallel to the structure that is being treated or medial and lateral to the structure so that the current passes through the joint and soft tissues. Regardless of the placement of the applicators, a towel needs to be placed on the surface of the skin to absorb moisture. Remember that moisture is highly conductive and any collection of moisture could lead to an uncomfortable burning sensation.

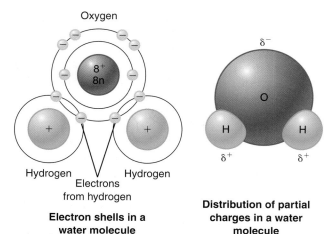

Electron shells in a water molecule

Distribution of partial charges in a water molecule

FIGURE 10-3 Water: An example of a polar molecule in which one end is more positively charged and the other end is more negatively charged.

TABLE 10-3	Tissues and Relative Conductivity to EM Radiation
MOST CONDUCTIVE	**IMPLANTED METALS**
	Oil
	Distilled water
	Adipose tissue
	Bone
	Muscle
	Skin
	Blood
Least Conductive	

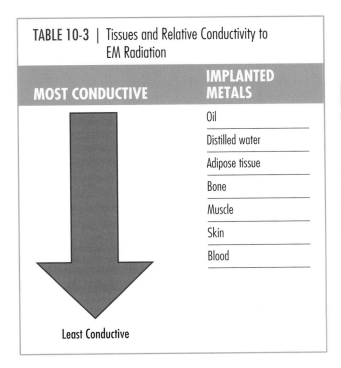
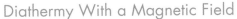

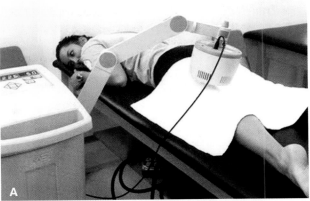

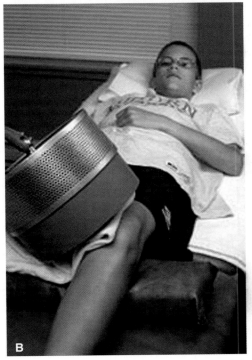

FIGURE 10-5 Magnetic field diathermy application.

Diathermy With a Magnetic Field

When diathermy is applied using a single drum applicator, a magnetic field passes through the tissues and causes the creation of eddy currents close to the surface of the drum. There is subsequently less heating deeper within the tissues, but it is most intense within the superficial muscles, which tend to have higher blood content and consequently greater electrical conductivity.[8] Figure 10-5 illustrates an induction electrode, which is a single drum applicator that is used to induce eddy currents within the underlying tissues.

Regardless of the type of applicator used, diathermy has specific precautions because of the mode of delivery, which must be observed. Metal in the treatment area is dangerous for the patient as it is easily heated by SWD at sufficient levels to cause a burn to the patient. This is true for metal implants deep within the tissue and jewelry that the patient might have worn into the clinic that day. Metal implants are considered a contraindication and jewelry must be removed prior to the application of diathermy. See Tables 10-4 and 10-5 for the precautions and special considerations to the use of diathermy.

CLINICAL APPLICATION CONSIDERATIONS FOR DIATHERMY

It is important to understand when employing diathermy as a treatment modality that the patient becomes part of the circuit that must be "tuned" for treatment. The patient's varying tissue types all contribute to the circuit that is created once the diathermy is turned on. Once the circuit of the patient is adjusted to the circuit created by the diathermy unit itself, the amount of heat is determined by the power delivered to the diathermy device.

Modern devices are most commonly self-tuning, but older devices required manual tuning by the clinician. This, along with other previously mentioned variables, makes the measurement of the amount of EM energy delivered to the patient virtually impossible. This is why clinicians must rely on the patient's subjective responses to heat as the dosage response. See Table 10-6 for diathermy dose levels.

Diathermy can be applied either as a thermal or a nonthermal modality, which means that it can be indicated for both acute and chronic conditions. The common indications for heat are also indications for diathermy. However, unlike hot packs, diathermy heats from the inside out without the need for a heavy mass on the surface of the skin. Diathermy is also different than ultrasound, which is a spot treatment technique. Diathermy is capable of treating larger treatment areas more efficiently than ultrasound and

TABLE 10-4 | Precautions to Diathermy and Why

PRECAUTIONS	WHY
Remove contact lenses when applying SWD around the head, face, or eyes.	The EMR causes eyes to dry out easily, making contact lenses uncomfortable.
The skin exposed to the treatment should be covered by at least 0.5 inch of toweling.	Moisture will collect on the surface of the skin, which will need to be absorbed to prevent burning.
Do not allow perspiration to collect in the treatment field.	Perspiration is conductive, which is prone to heat production.
Thick adipose tissue in the treatment area	Adipose is prone to overheating.
It is difficult to heat only localized areas.	Water pathways within the tissues dissipate heat formed in the treated area.
Never allow the skin to come into direct contact with the heating unit or cables.	Moisture will collect on the skin, which will be prone to heat production.
If the cable method is used, do not allow the cables to touch each other.	Cables that touch each other would not have to pass current through the patient.
If electrode pads are used, space them at least the distance of their diameter apart.	Deeper fields are created by spacing electrodes farther apart, causing deeper penetration of the current.
A deep, aching sensation may be a symptom of overheating the tissues.	Diathermy works from the inside out so symptoms of overheating are from within.
Overheating of the patient's tissues may cause tissue damage without any immediate signs.	Diathermy works from the inside out, so symptoms of overheating are from within.
The SWD energy scatters 2 to 3 feet from the source energy should be maintained to ensure the operator's safety.	EMR travels through the air so care must be taken with other devices and clinicians who might be affected in the area.

TABLE 10-5 | Special Considerations for Diathermy and Why

CONTRAINDICATIONS TO DIATHERMY	WHY
Remove all jewelry, clothing, coins, and other metallic items from the patient.	ERM from diathermy will cause heat production in any metal within the treatment field that is sufficient to cause a burn.
For personal safety, the clinician should remove any rings, watches, bracelets, and clothing with metal zippers or grommets.	ERM from diathermy will cause heat production in any metal within the treatment field that is sufficient to cause a burn. Zippers on jeans should not be metal and if they are, the patient should wear a gown.
There must be no metal within the immediate treatment area.	ERM from diathermy will cause heat production in any metal within the treatment field that is sufficient to cause a burn. This includes metal implants such as intra-uterine devices (IUDs), body-piercings, surgical clips, and staples.
Keep the patient out of reach of any metal objects (e.g., outlets, pipes).	Metal objects can serve as a ground and potentially be harmful.

TABLE 10-6 | Dose Levels for Diathermy

DOSE	LEVEL	SENSATION/RESPONSE	POTENTIAL APPLICATIONS
I	Lowest	Just below the point of any sensation of heat	Acute inflammation
II	Low	Mild heating sensation	Subacute inflammation
III	Medium	Moderate heating	Resolving inflammatory process
IV	Heavy	Vigorous heating but comfortable	Chronic conditions

is an unattended treatment technique. See Table 10-7 for the Indications for Diathermy and Check it Out 10-1, at the end of the chapter, a short laboratory exercise dealing with the application of diathermy.

PULSED EM FIELDS FOR BONE TISSUE REPAIR

Pulsed electromagnetic field (PEMF) signal devices were designed for bone growth stimulation and pulsed radio frequency (PRF) signals for the treatment of soft tissue wounds. Both of these application techniques rely on an inductive coupling of the signal to the target tissue without having to physically touch the area eliminating direct contact with the wound itself. These forms of therapy represent new and emerging forms of therapy within the United States.[9]

Light as a Therapeutic Modality

Both laser (an acronym for "light amplification by the stimulated emission of radiation") and UV can be administered to a patient to accomplish specific therapeutic treatment goals. However, they represent very different forms of light and are handled quite differently. The characteristics of light must be explained before the application of light can be fully understood. This section discusses the characteristics of light that differntiate it from the other modalities that have been explained thus far in this text.

CHARACTERISTICS OF LIGHT

Light has unique qualities in terms of a form of energy and it is described, in part, by its wavelength and frequency. When an electrical stimulation waveform is described, it is described by what it looks like during each individual event

of its own time, in other words, how long it takes for the cycle of the wave to repeat itself (wavelength), how many times it occurs in a second (frequency), and by its shape. Light also has a wavelength but that wavelength is used to describe where it falls on the EM spectrum or the color that it produces within the visible spectrum. Techniques employing light take into consideration the physical properties of reflection, refraction, and absorption.

Wavelength

The spectrum of visible light is made up of light of many different wavelengths, each represented by its own specific color. **Wavelength** is the distance between the beginning and the end of a single wave cycle. The wave cycle referred to is the oscillation of EM energy, which occurs in an orderly and predictable pattern of a sine wave.

Wavelengths are measured in **nanometers** (nm), or billionths of a meter. The visible spectrum of wavelengths occurs between 400 and 800 nm. All visible colors from violet to red have wavelengths within this range. Wavelengths from 180 to 400 nm represent UV nonvisible light and wavelengths from about 800 to 1,500 nm are considered IR. **UV** occurs on the EM spectrum just adjacent to visible violet light. IR occurs just beyond the visible red wavelengths. The spectrum of wavelengths is presented in Figure 10-6.

LET'S THINK ABOUT IT...

Here's another example of why everything you learned in kindergarten was important. Think back to the first time you saw a rainbow. What is the sequence of the colors in a rainbow? Each color represents a different wavelength of light.

Frequency

The frequency of a color of light is inversely proportional to its wavelength. The higher the frequency, the shorter the wavelength. The frequency and resultant wavelength influence the absorption of the light source. Higher-frequency, shorter-wavelength light has a tendency to be absorbed at a more superficial level than light of longer wavelengths.[10,11] See Table 10-8 for a comparison of the two.

Two bands of UV are commonly used. They are referred to as UV-A and UV-B. The two forms of UV differ in their frequency and wavelength. UV-B has a higher frequency and therefore a shorter wavelength (250 to 320 nm) than UV-A (320 to 400 nm). Both UV-A and UV-B are used clinically with different responses.[4] UV-B from unfiltered sunlight or simulated sunlight can be potentially harmful to human skin. UV-B may cause degenerative and neoplastic changes in the skin and modification of the immunologic system of the skin, so prolonged unmonitored exposure is not recommended.[16] UV-C is a third band of UV that has been discussed in the literature. UV-C, which has a wavelength of 250 nm, has been used to promote wound débridement bactericidal effects and tissue regeneration.[16]

TABLE 10-7	Indications for Diathermy	
INDICATION	**HOW**
Pain	• Reduction in larger areas of the body • Joints
Muscle guarding	• Reduction in areas too large for US or that cannot tolerate the weight of a hot pack
Inflammation	• Nonacute stages use higher dose levels • Acute stages use lower dose levels
Soft tissue tightness	• Joint stiffness & joint contractures prior to ROM activities and stretching
Reflex heating	• To increase blood flow to extremities by heating the low back
Pelvic inflammatory disease (PID)	• Improve delivery of medication to pelvic cavity
Herpes zoster	• To promote healing of herpes zoster vesicles

Wavelength (metres)

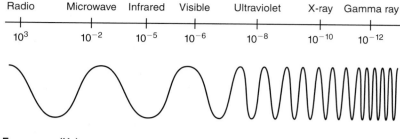

Frequency (Hz)

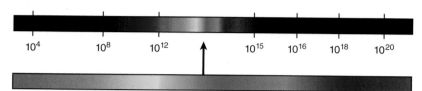

FIGURE 10-6 The EM spectrum of visible light.

TABLE 10-8	The Relationship Between Wavelength Depth of Penetration, Frequency, and Absorption		
FREQUENCY	**WAVELENGTH**	**DEPTH/ ABSORPTION**
High	Shorter	Superficial
Low	Longer	Deeper

The frequency of a color of light is inversely proportional to its wavelength. The higher the frequency of the light, the shorter its wavelength will be. The frequency and resultant wavelength influence the absorption of the light source. Higher-frequency, shorter-wavelength light has a tendency to be absorbed at a more superficial level than has light of longer wavelength.

PHYSICAL PROPERTIES OF LIGHT

Light, like sound, travels in a sine wave pattern and has specific properties such as reflection, refraction, and absorption.

Reflection

Reflection refers to the phenomenon of throwing back a ray of radiant energy from a surface. Light has the ability to bounce off different surfaces. The degree of reflection is reduced as the treatment angle approaches 90 degrees.

Refraction

Refraction refers to a bending of energy that is related to the source of the energy, referred to as the incident angle of the energy delivered. The light source may be redirected off a surface at an angle. For example, when a flashlight is pointed at a mirror it will reflect the light back to the flashlight if the flashlight is perpendicular to the surface of the mirror. If the angle is not perpendicular, the light will be refracted or *bent* in another direction. The incident angle determines the direction of the redirected light; it also influences the delivery of energy to the treatment tissue.

Absorption

Absorption is a substance's ability to take in light or radiant energy. The intensity of the light source will decrease as it passes through a substance. Window blinds typically absorb a great deal of light and allow only a small amount of light through, which is at a much lower intensity once it passes through into a room. Absorption is inversely related to penetration. If an energy source is absorbed by whatever it is passing through, then it will not penetrate deeply. If the energy source is not absorbed, reflected, or refracted, it may penetrate to a much greater depth. In order for a light source to have a physiological effect, it must be absorbed by the tissue.

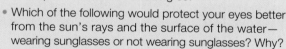

LET'S THINK ABOUT IT...

You are about to take a day off and have decided to go to the beach or to a local pool, and it's perfect weather for doing so!

- Which of the following would protect your eyes better from the sun's rays and the surface of the water — wearing sunglasses or not wearing sunglasses? Why?
- What color would you wear if you wanted to feel cooler in the sun — black or white? Why?

INCIDENT ANGLE AND DOSAGE

Light may be either reflected, refracted, or absorbed, depending on its wavelength, the incident angle of the source, and the type of material receiving the light source. If the given wavelength can be absorbed by a substance or tissue, the absorption intensity will also depend upon the distance from the source. Doubling the distance with radiant light sources typically increases the spread of the light source so that it covers a larger area. By increasing the size of the area but not changing the intensity of the source, it is the same as decreasing the intensity per unit area. If, for example, the treatment area was 1 cm², and the source was 10 cm away from the surface, moving the source a distance of 20 cm from the surface will increase the coverage to 4 cm² and provide 25% of the intensity per given area. This is known as the inverse square law: Doubling the distance will decrease the intensity to 25% of the original amount. If the intensity of a radiant heat source is too great, increasing the distance from the patient will significantly decrease the intensity (Fig. 10–7).

LET'S THINK ABOUT IT...

- Point a flashlight at something and focus the light so that there are crisp edges from the beam.
- Measure how far away from the object it was and record that distance.
- Now move the flashlight back so that it is twice the distance away from whatever it was pointing to.
- What happens to the crispness of the edges and brightness of the light when you now turn it on?
- How large an area is it now covering? Is it larger, smaller, or the same size? Why?

The incident angle becomes an important consideration in the use of light as a therapeutic modality. To maintain a constant dosage from treatment to treatment, the distance from the source must be constant. If a patient is being treated with a radiant source of energy such as a heat lamp and feels uncomfortable, then increasing the distance from the source of the energy will make the patient more comfortable. It is important to note that the increase in distance will significantly alter the delivered dosage.

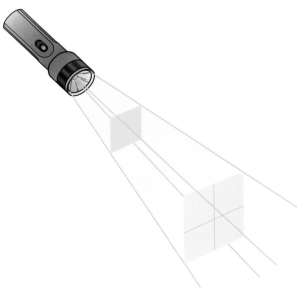

FIGURE 10-7 The inverse square law: Increasing the distance will decrease the intensity by the square of the distance. If the distance from the flashlight is doubled, then the light will cover four times the area but be one-fourth of the brightness or intensity of the original.

Ultraviolet

UV light has been used as a treatment modality for dermatological conditions, such as psoriasis and in the prepartion of wound beds for healing, or to kill harmful bacterial pathogens including methicillin-resistant *Staphylococcus aureus* (MRSA). UV falls just beyond the visible portion of the EM spectrum and is therefore not visible to the naked eye. UV follows the principles that have been described for light. The absorption of UV is also dependent upon the wavelength, with absorption being greater for shorter wavelengths. Shorter wavelengths tend to penetrate less deeply than longer wavelengths, but this is also dependent upon the thickness of the epidermis and the amount of melanin in the skin.[10] Melanin is a significant factor in the protection of human skin from the effects of UV.[15]

PHYSIOLOGICAL EFFECTS OF UV

UV is used predominantly to promote an erythemal response, which occurs within 12 hours of exposure to the UV. Photon energy is absorbed by pigmenting molecules of the skin, for example, melanin. The absorbed energy may induce photochemical reactions and release energy into the surrounding molecules of the skin, promoting various biochemical reactions and potentially having an impacton the immune system.[10,16–18]

AN OVERVIEW OF THE APPLICATION TECHNIQUE FOR UV

The following information is intended to serve as a brief guide to the application of the modality, potential reasons for its application, and safety considerations for its application. It is not intended to be an in-depth study of UV.

Treatment Goals With UV

The treatment goals of UV include:

- Erythemal response within 12 hours of initial exposure
- Pigmentation-thickening of the stratum corneum of the skin
- Destruction of bacteria in wounds and ulcers

See Table 10-9 for a short summary of UV-C application times required to kill MRSA and *Pseudomonas*.

Safety Considerations

Following are safety considerations for the use and application of UV:

- Patients who are photosensitive should not be treated with UV. UV is a photon energy source that may not be tolerated well by individuals who are specifically **photosensitive**. These individuals typically burn easily when exposed to sunlight.
- Patients with pellagra, a niacin-deficiency dermatitis, should not receive UV. UV exposure may reduce the effectiveness of Langerhans cells of the epidermis. The Langerhans cells are capable of activating T lymphocytes and may be involved in the promotion of contact dermatitis.[16]

TABLE 10-9	UV–C Exposure Times Required to Produce 99.9% Kill	
	PSEUDOMONAS	MRSA (METHICILLIN-RESISTANT STAPHYLOCOCCUS AUREUS)
In vitro		
3 seconds	x	
5 seconds		x
In vivo		
30 seconds		x

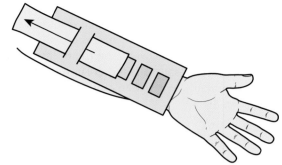

FIGURE 10-8 A method that can be used to determine a minimal erythemal dosage (MED). The patient should be draped so that no skin is exposed except for the forearm. This piece of cardboard is made so that there are several openings, as well as a slide cover that can be pulled up to reveal one opening at a time. The most distal opening will receive the longest exposure time, and the most proximal opening will receive the least amount of exposure time.

- Patients who have dermatitis secondary to systemic lupus erythmatosus (SLE) should not receive UV. Sunlight is said to induce skin lesions in patients with SLE and to exacerbate the systemic manifestations of the disease.[17,18]
- Patients with active tuberculosis should not receive UV, as it may exacerbate the disease process.[12]
- Patients with a fever or acute diabetes should not receive UV, as it may exacerbate the disease process.[12]
- Skin rarely exposed to light may respond more dramatically to UV. Areas such as the genitals may respond adversely to UV and therefore should receive one-third to one-half the dosage of the rest of the body.[14]
- Some medications are photosensitizing and cause reactions to UV. Topical antihistamines, phenothiazine, sulfonamides, hexachlorophene, and topical bleaches are considered photocontact allergens that will respond adversely to UV.[18] Some antibiotics and some diuretics photosensitize the patient. Patients who are taking these medications should not receive UV if the medication has been identified as a photosensitizing drug.[14]
- Both the patient and the clinician should wear protective eye gear with UV (unprotected exposure to UV may promote the formation of cataracts and conjunctivitis).

Dosage

In order to establish a minimal erythemal dosage (MED)—the exposure time necessary to produce a mild erythema that lasts up to 48 hours—the UV lamp should be placed approximately 60 to 90 cm from the patient at a 90-degree angle to the surface being treated. The steps involved in determining the dosage level are illustrated in Figure 10-8 and outlined in Box 10-1.

Because of the application techniques of UV and the importance of accurate dosimetry, patient education is important. A patient must understand that the purpose of the MED test is to determine just how much exposure time is necessary based on his or her skin sensitivity. The UV

BOX 10-1 | Minimal Erythemal Dosage (MED) Procedure

1. Drape patients so that only a small area of the forearm is exposed.
2. Give patients protective polarized goggles to wear and instruct them not to look at the UV lamp when it is ON.
3. Cover the exposed forearm with a prepared piece of UV-opaque cardboard that has a total of four to six openings in it. Each of the openings should be about 1 cm² and 1 cm apart, preferably of different shapes. Cover the openings with an additional piece of UV-opaque cardboard of equal size.
4. Allow the lamp to warm up according to the manufacturer's instructions.
5. Place the lamp perpendicular to the area being tested and a distance of 60–80 cm from the test site.
6. Do not look at the light without protective eye goggles.
7. Open the shutters of the lamp and expose the first opening for 30 seconds, then expose the second opening for an additional 30 seconds, etc.
8. Close the shutters of the lamp.
9. Turn the lamp off.
10. Instruct the patient to monitor the forearm every 2 hours and note which opening or shape appeared pink/red first and when it faded.

Dosimetry

MED = time necessary to produce erythema

1st degree dose = 2.5 MED to produce erythema for up to 48 hours

2nd degree dose = 5 MED to produce erythema for up to 72 hours

3rd degree dose = 10 MED to produce erythema and blistering (limit to small surface area of exposure)[12,14]

used in the clinic is not for tanning purposes, and exposure should be carefully monitored. Proper patient education is outlined in Box 10-2.

Improper dosage may cause either no therapeutic effect or potential skin damage. Appropriate documentation is also an important part of the treatment. Details that should be included in the documentation are outlined in Box 10-3.

LONG-TERM EFFECTS OF EXPOSURE TO UV

Lifetime exposure to UV-B radiation has been well accepted as a causative factor related to various forms of skin cancers.[15] Therapeutic dosage levels that are administered do not fall within the same prolonged exposure levels. However, over the course of a lifetime it is important to be aware that UV-B is known to cause the cancers listed in Box 10-4

Laser

> ### BOX 10-2 | Patient Education for Testing and Treatment With UV
>
> 1. Wear goggles during entire exposure time (cataracts may develop if UV is viewed without proper protection).
> 2. Observe and monitor skin condition following exposure to UV.
> 3. Keep skin moisturized following exposure to UV.
> 4. Pigmentation changes are to be expected and are considered a normal response following exposure to UV. The time of the appearance of the pigmentation change should be recorded and reported to the therapist at the next visit.
> 5. Prolonged and repeated exposure to UV may promote premature aging of the skin and is not recommended.

> ### BOX 10-3 | Documentation for Treatment With UV
>
> 1. Record the patient's response to previous exposures to UV (time and appearance of erythema, any adverse sensitivities to the UV or applied agents).
> 2. Document the UV lamp that was used by recording the brand name, model, and serial number if there is more than one UV lamp in the department. This is important because the age of the lamp and manufacturer specification differences may produce variations in the predictability of results.
> 3. Record the distance from the lamp to the patient (consistently using the same units, which may be either cm or in.).
> 4. Record the incident angle of the lamp to the patient (this should be 90 degrees to promote uniformity and the most predictable results for the response).
> 5. Draping procedures should be noted indicating the exact area of exposure and any irregularities of the surface of the skin, (e.g., bony prominences or other irregular contours of the treatment area.)

> ### BOX 10-3 | Documentation for Treatment With UV—cont'd
>
> 6. Document the exposure time in seconds.
> 7. Document the appearance of the skin following the exposure to the UV.
> 8. Document that you asked the patient if he or she had any allergies to any topically applied moisturizers or medications prior to their application and that the patient denied any allergies.
> 9. Document the use of any topically applied moisturizers or medications following exposure to UV.

> ### BOX 10-4 | Effects of Exposure to UVB
>
> • Increased incidence of skin cancer in experimental animal models with hours of exposure
> • Increased incidence of skin cancer in those individuals who have lighter skin and live at or near the equator
> • Increased incidence of skin cancer in those individuals who both work outdoors and have lighter skin
> • Increased incidence of skin cancer in those tissue areas that have been continually exposed to UVB

Laser is an acronym for "light amplification by the stimulated emission of radiation." It consists of photons of light moving in the same direction at the same frequency and same wavelength.[12] The use of light for therapeutic purposes is not new to clinical practice, but the technology that enables the light source to have such specific characteristics as laser is relatively new to physical medicine. Laser is the first modality to be introduced in the United States since the passage of the law in 1976 requiring the FDA's Bureau of Radiologic Health to regulate this kind of device for human use. The FDA is an agency within the Department of Health and Human Services and is responsible for overseeing medical products and tobacco, foods, global regulatory operations, and policy for the protection of the public. Prior to 1976 there was no specific regulatory agency or testing required for medical devices prior to their being marketed for human use to the general public. Before that time, those devices received what is commonly referred to as "grandfathered" status, indicating that they did not go through the FDA approval process that is now in place, which requires that devices be safe and effective, appropriately tested, and labeled prior to being used and marketed to the general public. Ultrasound and many of the forms of electrical stimulation devices that are commonly used today have been in use for many years and are considered grandfathered devices.

LASER LIGHT PRODUCTION

Laser light production is quite different from what we normally think of as the production of light emanating from something such as a lightbulb. A laser involves a contained chamber or environment that houses an active medium of excitable atoms of either a gas, liquid, or solid. When electrical energy is introduced into the active medium, a molecular excitation occurs. Electrons in the outermost energy level of the active medium are elevated to the next level, resulting in unstable molecules in the active medium. These unstable molecules need to shed energy to accommodate the degradation of the electrons to their original and stable position. The energy that they release in this process is in the form of photons of energy, which pass through the active medium, further exciting it and creating a situation known as population inversion or an active photon emission process.[13,14]

The chamber that houses the active medium is sometimes referred to as the resonant cavity. This resonant cavity has mirrors at each end that are virtually parallel to each other. One of the mirrors is completely reflective and the other is partially reflective, allowing a small percentage of the photon energy (light) to be emitted from the cavity or chamber. The light that exits is what is we refer to as the laser light, which has the unique characteristics that are described next.

CHARACTERISTICS OF LASER LIGHT

Laser light is further differentiated from white light by the fact that laser light is monochromatic and coherent, and exhibits low beam divergence. Laser light is of one specific wavelength and is therefore one color, that is, **monochromatic**. Because the photon emission is the result of the excitation of an isolated active medium, the emitted light has one specific wavelength. White light is made up of many different wavelengths, or many different colors, as evidenced by refracting white light through a prism; it exits the prism as a rainbow of colors of the visual spectrum. Laser light entering a prism would be identical on exit because it is monochromatic.

Coherence

Coherence refers to the precise nature of the laser wavelength in the way it travels. Each individual photon emitted from a laser is emitted precisely in phase with every other photon. Laser light is a phase-related form of energy. All emitted photons travel in the same direction, creating a parallel beam profile (Fig. 10-9). The significance is that all the peaks and valleys of the sine wave pattern are occurring at precisely the same time.

Beam Divergence

Beam divergence refers to the relative parallelism of the beam. The more parallel (collimated) the beam, the greater is the concentration of energy in a localized area. There is a minimal divergence or spreading apart of the photons from a laser. They are easily focused into well-contained areas.[14] This property of laser light enabled the first accurate measuring system for recording the distance to the moon. Part of the mission for NASA's Apollo 11 was the Laser Ranging Retroreflector experiment. A series of corner-cube reflectors were deployed to the moon's surface. This is a special type of mirror having the property of always reflecting an incoming light beam back in the direction it came from. Laser beams are used because they remain tightly focused for large distances. Pulsed laser from Earth was focused on them and they reflected the light back to the incident source. Because the speed of light is known, the distance could be

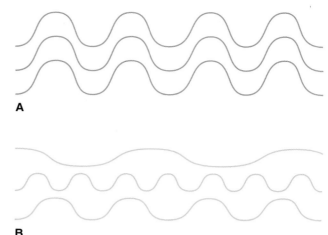

FIGURE 10-9 The property of beam coherence. (A) Laser light is a coherent light source of one specific wavelength. Therefore, the sine waves occur completely parallel to each other. (B) White light is made up of many different colors of light, so it is physically impossible for the sine waves to be perfectly parallel.

calculated based on the time required for the laser beam to return. After having traveled approximately 239,000 miles in space, the laser beam had spread out to a diameter of a little less than 12.5 miles because of its low beam divergence.[4,12,13] Considering the distance, the precision that is required for aiming the beam is comparable to using a rifle to hit a moving dime that is 3 kilometers (approximately 2 miles) away (Fig. 10-10).

These characteristics enable lasers to be focused into microscopic points, yielding enormous energy densities in the area of the focus for many medical and nonmedical applications. The combination of fiber optic and laser technologies has enabled clinicians to easily handle and direct the incident beam regardless of the dimensions of the resonant cavity of the active medium. Gaseous lasers such as carbon dioxide (CO_2) and carbon dioxide yttrium-aluminum-garnet (YAG) lasers use fiber optics to transmit the laser beams for arthroscopic surgical procedures.[15]

LOW-POWER LASERS IN CLINICAL PRACTICE

Clinicians in the United States have reported beneficial effects from two specific lasers, helium neon (HeNe) and gallium arsenide (GaAs). Both of these lasers are considered

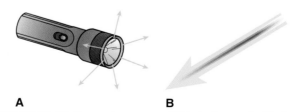

FIGURE 10-10 Beam divergence. (A) Light from a flashlight, which is made up of many different wavelengths, will spread out in all directions. (B) Laser light has very low divergence properties; it does not tend to spread out.

low-power (cold) lasers, because their maximum power levels are not capable of producing a thermal response. HeNe lasers produce a wavelength of 632.8 nm and fall within the visible spectrum of light, emitting a brilliant red light. GaAs semiconductor diode chip lasers produce a wavelength of 910 nm, which does not fall within the visible spectrum of light. For this reason GaAs lasers are referred to as IR lasers (910 nm is considered IR in the EM spectrum).[11,16–18,20]

HeNe and GaAs lasers are considered low-power lasers, since typically the total peak power is less than 1 milliwatt (mW) and they produce no significant heat in the treated tissues. Surgical lasers are considered high-power lasers, and their effects are associated with damaging changes to cells and tissues through thermal effects.[20,42] The power of a laser device is preset within the device along with the wavelength, based on the active medium or type of laser and power source.

Lasers have been used in a wide variety of applications since their development in the early 1960s.[45] Their uses range from industrial applications, such as very accurate drills, scanning devices in supermarkets, and compact disc (CD) players, to medical applications in many fields including but not limited to dermatology, ophthalmology, gynecology, urology, dentistry, and physical medicine.[24–33] Lasers are the first devices in the United States to be introduced after the 1976 Title 21 Foods and Drugs, Chapter 1 FDA Dept. of Health and Human Services Subchapter H, Medical Devices Part 890 Physical Medicine Devices, Subpart A, General Provisions Section 890.3, effective dates of requirement for premarket approval requirements. The manufacturer of any new device to be introduced into the marketplace must apply for approval through the FDA and demonstrate the device's safety and efficacy before commercial distribution can commence.[45] Prior to any device receiving FDA premarket approval, the manufacturer must also go through the processes identified by the FDA and certain protocols for permission to use the devices must be followed. Until a device receives either approval or clearance from the FDA, it is considered investigational and can be used only as a part of a study and not for general population until the safety and efficacy of the device have been established.

The investigational status also restricts claims that can be made regarding the application of the device until such time as full premarket approval from the FDA is obtained. This approval process will be referred to throughout this section.

Proposed Indications

Low-power lasers have been reported in the literature to have specific therapeutic effects for tissue healing and pain management for both acute and chronic pain.[25–27] A 2010 publication that marked the 50th anniversary of the discovery of laser discussed the broad-reaching effects that have been noted in the literature, including applications in neurorehabilitation that range from its benefit for patients with strokes, traumatic brain injuries, degenerative central nervous system disease, spinal cord injury, to peripheral nerve injury.[44]

Safety Considerations

Lasers used for physical rehabilitation have few contraindications because they are low-power lasers with low emitted energy. The FDA has classified these devices as insignificant risk devices that are generally safe. Despite this, there are some precautions to the use of the devices because of the potential for the enhancement of the growth of tissues on a cellular level, sometimes referred to as **biostimulation**. The following list outlines the additional precautions:

- Pregnant women should not be treated with biostimulative lasers.
- Unclosed fontanels of children should not be treated with biostimulative lasers.
- Areas with cancerous lesions should not be treated with biostimulative lasers.
- Direct laser application over the cornea is to be avoided.

Regulatory Processes and Safety of Low-Power Lasers.

The FDA classifies low-power lasers as Class III medical devices, which are devices represented to be life sustaining or life supporting, those implanted in the body, those presenting potential or unreasonable risk of illness or injury, or those new or modified devices not substantially equivalent to any devices marketed before May 28, 1976 (date of enactment of the Medical Device Amendments).[19,46]

Lasers were introduced to American clinicians in the early 1980s for the treatment of pain and the enhancement of tissue healing.[20] Lasers are among the first medical devices proposed for use by therapists to go through the premarket approval (PMA) process for safety and efficacy, as outlined by the Center for Devices and Radiological Health of the FDA. Lasers were introduced after May 28, 1976. Many clinical trials to date have been poorly designed.

This chapter addresses the laser modality and the regulatory issues surrounding its use to inform clinicians of the process required for the use of the devices. It is ultimately the responsibility of the clinician to make sure that any newly introduced modality has met the regulatory guidelines set forth by the FDA, despite what a manufacturer of the device may claim.

As Class III medical devices, low-power or cold lasers require PMA prior to mass distribution and human use. Claims have been made regarding the benefits of laser biostimulation for the acceleration of tissue healing and the reduction of pain by numerous European researchers for the last 15 to 20 years. These claims are in the process of being tested today throughout the United States, Canada, and China.

Proposed Effects

Preliminary studies suggest that laser biostimulation has an effect on type I and type III procollagen mRNA levels, which seem to enhance wound healing by optimizing scar formation.[20-22] Researchers have also reported favorable results for pain relief, improvement in grip strength and tip pinch strength in the treatment of patients with rheumatoid arthritis, enhancement of experimental pain thresholds,[25,26] and tissue repair.[16–18] Despite the reports of favorable findings by numerous investigators, analysis of the research designs has indicated that some of the studies were poorly controlled or monitored.[31]

Institutional Review Board

Clinicians who wish to conduct research with low-power lasers are required to submit a protocol to an **institutional review board (IRB)**, or human subject committee, which will review the use of the technique with humans. The IRB is a committee or group assembled to approve the initiation of new research protocols and conduct periodic review of biomedical research involving human subjects. Their primary purpose is to assure the protection of the rights and welfare of human subjects. Studies may be sponsored or funded by a facility or a manufacturer. The sponsor of the investigation bears the responsibility for the conduct of the investigation, but does not actually perform the investigation. Manufacturers of the devices have served in this capacity over the past 15 to 20 years. If the devices are being used under the supervision of an IRB, with a well-defined protocol, then the device is considered investigational and can be used with human subject participants within the scope of the study as an **investigational device exemption (IDE)**.[45]

Low-power lasers have been considered nonsignificant-risk devices since their output is not capable of causing a burn. They are, however, investigational devices that require the approval of an IRB for use within a well-defined protocol with informed consent of the patient before they can be used.

Documentation for IRBs

Each institution has its own procedure designed to protect the human subjects in the study. General guidelines for information submitted to an IRB include:

- A well-defined protocol outlining the diagnoses and patient population
- Members of the research team and any financial relationship to the manufacturer
- Plan for periodic review of the results of the investigation
- Informed consent forms for patients describing the purpose of the study and potential risks

The future of low-power laser as a therapeutic modality is uncertain but promising as a result of conflicting reports in the literature regarding dosage requirements and the wide variety of wavelengths available. Until uniformity of dosage documentation exists and more well-controlled clinical trials have been performed, clinicians are encouraged to keep an open but critical eye and mind on the use of the modality.

TREATMENT TECHNIQUE WITH LASER

Protocols are based on the amount of energy delivered to the patient measured in joules per square centimeter, which is calculated by a formula encompassing the time of exposure, the power of the laser, and the size of the treatment area. Low-power (biostimulative) lasers provide no sensation to the patient and have no intensity setting, so treatment dosage is determined by the aforementioned factors. Since the variety of devices in use is so vast, and lasers are available in single and multiple beam applicators, specific treatment parameters are still being determined at the time of this writing.

LASER DOSAGE

The dosage of lasers is commonly reported in the literature in joules/cm². Therapeutic ranges are dependent upon the treatment goal. A joule is equivalent to 1 watt per second. Since lasers deliver milliwatts of output or thousandths of a watt, the dosage is determined by the time of exposure. If there is more than one beam or laser diode, then that would double the output or decrease the time of exposure by half. See Box 10-5 for an example.

DOCUMENTABLE PARAMETERS

In order for clinical results to be duplicated with any modality or treatment plan, the parameters of the treatment need to be documented. Each of the individual modalities or techniques will have their own specific sets of variables that must be recorded. Laser is no different from other modalities in terms of the need for accurate documentation for reproducibility of results. The specific parameters that must be recorded for a laser treatment are listed in Table 10-10.

Therapeutic Uses of Light

This chapter has outlined two very different sources of therapeutic light. Their use in clinics will vary greatly depending on many factors, including the patient population, the types of conditions treated most often within the facility, and whether or not the facility is participating in an investigational study.

For lasers to become more clinically available and acceptable, well-designed, controlled studies must demonstrate parameters, application techniques, and their effectiveness. These studies, whether negative or positive, need to be published and reviewed. Proven efficacy of the techniques will facilitate greater availability of the devices for clinical use.

BOX 10-5 | Calculation of Joules

Laser dosage is measured in joules/cm² and a joule = 1 watt/sec.

- If we had a 10 watt laser, it would take 1 second to deliver 10 joules of energy.

  This would be a very short and unrealistic treatment time.

- Most therapeutic lasers deliver mW of intensity.
- It would take a 10 mW laser 100 seconds to deliver the same energy as a 50 mW laser would in 20 seconds.
- However, in physical therapy we use low-level laser therapy (LLLT), which is nonthermal.
- Higher power lasers produce heat, which is not what we are attempting to do.

TABLE 10-10 | Parameters Recorded for the Documentation of Laser Treatment Interventions

Type of laser used	HeNe, YAG, GaAs, etc.
Wavelength of laser	632.8nm, 1032 nm, etc.
Power of the laser	Milliwatts or watts
Size of the treatment area	Number of square centimeters
Time of exposure	Seconds, minutes
Number of diodes	Single or multi-diode delivery
Joules of energy	Delivered to the patient per Rx

Actinotherapy, which is the therapeutic use of UV, has been used for many years, but has seen limited use in the recent past perhaps because of the cumbersome nature of determining the appropriate dosage for a patient and the emergence of new medications. Pharmacological interventions are rarely without side effects, and not all patients can ingest medications without difficulty. UV represents a potential safe treatment option for many patients with skin disorders. It should not be overlooked or discredited as a treatment option.

Summary

Throughout this chapter, light as a therapeutic modality has been presented and has included a variety of sources including UV, diathermy, and laser. Each of these forms of EM energy has specific characteristics that differentiate it from the others, but they all share a common application advantage over other treatment interventions. EM energy travels through the air and works by conversion not conduction. Virtually all of the other therapeutic heating agents that are commonly used have a primary mechanism of action in common, which is that they must touch what they are treating. EM energy is perhaps most exciting as a treatment intervention for the future because of its ability to be used without touching the skin. This significantly decreases any potential for cross-contamination of patients and also allows these forms of treatment to be used with patients who do not have a protective outer layer of skin or who could not tolerate the weight of other heating modalities. The future is particularly bright regarding the potential for what research with these devices might yield.

Review Questions

1. Which of the following statements best reflects how laser light differs from other forms of light?
   a. Laser is an acronym and white light is not an acronym
   b. Laser light is monochromatic and white light is multichromatic
   c. Laser light is noncollimating and white light is collimating
   d. Laser light is ionizing and white light is nonionizing

2. The application of diathermy as a potential treatment intervention in physical therapy is based upon which of the following?
   a. As a conductive heat source
   b. As a convective heat source
   c. As a heat source that works by conversion
   d. Diathermy is not a heat source

3. Which of the following represents a potential use for UV as a treatment intervention in physical therapy?
   a. Preparing of wound beds for healing
   b. Psoriasis
   c. Killing MRSA
   d. UV is not a potential treatment intervention in physical therapy

4. Which of the following statements most accurately represents the role of the U.S. Food and Drug Administration (FDA) as a regulatory agency and its influence involving devices that are introduced into the physical therapy clinical environment?
   a. The FDA is a regulatory commission that has no impact on what is done in the clinical environment
   b. The FDA controls what devices can be sold in the United States
   c. The FDA assures public safety by requiring that prior to being approved, devices must be proved safe and effective
   d. The FDA is a regulatory agency that delays progress requiring paperwork before products can be marketed in the United States

5. What does a rainbow have to do with the EM spectrum?
   a. A rainbow has nothing to do with the EM spectrum
   b. A rainbow is an example of the visible wavelengths of light in the EM spectrum
   c. A rainbow is a myth
   d. A rainbow represents each of the colors of the EM spectrum and is identical to the light that a laser is capable of producing

DISCUSSION QUESTIONS

1. Describe the differences between laser light and UV.

2. Outline the process necessary for the approval of any new modality for human use.

3. What are the differences between radiant energy sources and nonradiant energy sources?

4. Describe the production of laser light, and explain why some are visible and some are not visible light sources.

5. Discuss the potential benefits of UV in clinical practice.

6. What are the precautions for the application of a luminous light source?

7. You are treating a patient with UV. The distance from the lamp to the patient is 36 inches, and his or her exposure time for an MED is 90 seconds. What would potentially be the exposure time necessary to provide an MED if the distance from the lamp were doubled? If the lamp were moved to 18 inches from the patient?

8. Explain the relationship between the incident angle of a light source and the target tissue.

REFERENCES

1. Kloth, LC, Berman, JE, Nett, M, Papanek, PE, and Dumit-Minkel, S: A randomized controlled clinical trial to evaluate the effects of noncontact normothermic wound therapy on chronic full-thickness pressure ulcers. Adv Skin Wound Care 15(6):270–276, 2002.

2. McCulloch, J, and Knight, CA: Noncontact normothermic wound therapy and offloading in the treatment of neuropathic foot ulcers in patients with diabetes. Ostomy Wound Manage 48(3):38–44, 2002.

3. Alvarez, OM, Rogers, RS, Booker, JG, and Patel, M: Effect of noncontact normothermic wound therapy on the healing of neuropathic (diabetic) foot ulcers: an interim analysis of 20 patients. J Foot Ankle Surg 42(1):30–35, 2003.

4. Lerman, Y, Jacubovich, R, and Green, MS: Pregnancy outcome following exposure to shortwaves among female physiotherapists in Israel. Am J Ind Med 39(5):499–504, 2001.

5. Sheilds, N, O'Hare, N, and Gormley, J: An evaluation of safety guidelines to restrict exposure to stray radiofrequency radiation from short-wave diathermy units. Phys in Med Bio 49(13):2999–3015.

6. Leitgeb, N, Omerspahic, A, and Neidermayr F: Exposure of non-target tissues in medical diathermy. BioEMs 31:12-19, 2010. doi:10.1002/bem.20521

7. Electronic Code of Federal Regulations Title 47: Telecommunication Part 2— Frequency Allocations And Radio Treaty Matters; General Rules And Regulations. Web site: http://ecfr.gpoaccess.gov/cgi/t/text/text-idx?c=ecfr&sid=5a4fe2fc8f23563f06fc775318439fbc&rgn=div5&view=text&node=47:1.0.1.1.3&idno=47#47:1.0.1.1.3.2.214.5

8. Tiktinsky, R, Chen, L, and Narayan, P: Electrotherapy: yesterday, today and tomorrow. Haemophilia 16:126–131, 2010.

9. Assiotis, A, et al: Pulsed EM fields for the treatment of tibial delayed unions and nonunions: a prospective clinical study and review of the literature. J Orthop Res 7:24, 2012.

10. Kitchen, SS, and Partridge, CJ: Review of UV radiation therapy. Physiotherapy 77:423, 1991.

11. Scott, BO: Clinical uses of UV radiation. In Stillwell, GK (ed): Therapeutic Electricity and UV Radiation, ed 3. Williams & Wilkins, Baltimore, 1983, pp 228–262.

12. Kahn, J: Physical agents—electrical, sonic and radiant modalities. In Skully, RM, and Barnes, MR (eds): Physical Therapy. JB Lippincott, Philadelphia, 1989, pp 894–897.

13. Patil, UA, and Dhami, LD: Overview of lasers, Indian J Plast Surg 41(Suppl): S101–S113, 2008.

14. Kollias, N, et al: New trends in photobiology (invited review). Photoprotection by melanin. Photochem Photobiol 9:135, 1991.

15. Kubo, Y, Murao, K, Matsumoto, K, and Arase, S. Molecular carcinogenesis of squamous cell carcinomas of the skin. J Med Invest 49(3–4):111–117, 2002.

16. Baadsgaard, O: In vivo UV irradiation of human skin results in profound perturbation of the immune system. Arch Derm, 127:99, 1991.

17. Nussbaum, EL, Biemann, I, and Mustard, B: Comparison of ultrasound/UV-C and laser for treatment of pressure ulcers in patients with spinal cord injuries. Phys Ther 74(9):812–823, 1994.

18. Nived, O, Johansson, I, and Sturfelt, G: Effects of UV irradiation on natural killer cell function in systemic lupus erythematosis. Ann Rheum Dis 51:726, 1992.

19. Golan, TD, et al: Enhanced membrane binding of autoantibodies to cultured keratinocytes of systemic lupus erythmatosus. Clin Invest 90:1067, 1992.

20. Taber's Cyclopedic Medical Dictionary, ed 17. FA Davis, Philadelphia, 1993, p 1501.

21. Kleinkort, JA, and Foley, RA: Laser: A preliminary report on its use in physical therapy. Am J Acupunct 12:51, 1984.

22. Asimov, I: Understanding Physics. Dorset Press, New York, 1988, pp 99–101.

23. Nave, CR, and Nave, BC: Physics for the Health Sciences, ed 3. WB Saunders, Philadelphia, 1985, pp 348–352.

24. Miller, F: College Physics, ed 4. Harcourt Brace Jovanovich, New York, 1977, pp 680–684.

25. Corson, SL: Uses of the YAG laser in laporoscopic gynecologic procedures. Obstet Gynecol Clin North Am 18:619, 1991.

26. Goldman, JA, et al: Laser therapy of rheumatoid arthritis. Lasers Surg Med 1:93, 1980.

27. Gogia, PP, Hurt, BS, and Zirn, TT: Wound management with whirlpool and IR cold laser treatment—a clinical report. Phys Ther 68:1239, 1988.

28. King, CE, et al: Effect of helium-neon laser auriculotherapy on experimental pain threshold. Phys Ther 70:24, 1990.

29. FDA: Fact sheet—laser biostimulation. Clin Manag 7:40, 1987.

30. Lam, TS, et al: Laser stimulation of collagen synthesis in human skin fibroblast cultures. Lasers Life Sci 1:61, 1986.

31. Lyons, RF, et al: Biostimulation of wound healing in vivo by helium-neon laser. Ann Plast Surg 18:1987.

32. Sapiera, D, et al: Demonstration of elevated type I and type II procollagen mRNA levels in cutaneous wounds treated with helium-neon laser—proposed mechanisms for enhanced wound healing. Biochem Biophys Res Commun 138:1123, 1986.

33. US Department of Health and Human Services Public Health Service, Food and Drug Administration: Investigational Device Exemptions, Division of Small Manufacturers Assistance, Office of Training and Assistance, Rockville, MD, February 1986.

34. Enwemeka, CS: Laser photostimulation. Clin Manag 10:24, 1990.

35. Snyder-Mackler, L, et al: Effects of helium-neon laser irradiation on skin resistance and pain in patients with trigger points in the neck or back. Phys Ther 69:336, 1989.

36. King, CE, et al: Effect of helium-neon laster auriculotherapy on experimental pain threshold: Phys Ther 70:24, 1990.

37. Snyder-Mackler, L ,and Bork, CE: Effects of helium-neon laser irradiation on peripheral sensory nerve latency. Phys Ther 68:223, 1988.

38. Kramer, JF, and Sandrin, M: Effect of low-power laser and white light on sensory conduction rate of the superficial radial nerve. Physiother Can 45:165, 1993.

39. Basford, JR, et al: Low-energy helium neon laser treatment of thumb osteoarthritis. Arch Phys Med Rehab 68:794, 1987.

40. Waylonis, GW, et al: Chronic myofascial pain: Management by low-output helium-neon laser therapy. Arch Phys Med Rehab, 69:1017–1020, 1988.

41. Beckerman, H, et al: The efficacy of laser therapy for musculoskeletal and skin disorders: A criteria-based meta-analysis of randomized clinical trials. Phys Ther 72:483, 1992.

42. Fonseca, PA, et al: Effects of light emitting diode (LED) therapy at 940 nm on inflammatory root resorption in rats. Lasers Med Sci, 2012. doi:10.1007/s1013-012-1061-z

43. Bjordal, JM, et al: Low-level laser therapy in acute pain: a systematic review of possible mechanisms of action and clinical effects in randomized placebo controlled trials. Photomed Laser Surg 24(2):158–168, 2006.

44. Hashmi, JT, et al: Role of low-level laser therapy in neurorehabilitation. PM R 2(12 Suppl 2): S292–S2305, 2010.

45. U.S. Food and Drug Administration Medical Devices, Device Advice: Comprehensive Regulatory Assistance, How to Market Your Device. Retrieved from http://www.accessdata.fda.gov/scripts/cdrh/cfdocs/cfcfr/CFRSearch.cfm?fr=890.3

LET'S FIND OUT

Application Techniques for Shortwave Diathermy

Shortwave diathermy is a treatment modality that has been used for many years. Diathermy has the ability to elevate internal tissue temperatures in relatively large treatment areas. It is capable of accomplishing this goal without placing anything but a towel on the surface of the skin. Owing to the increased number of precautions associated with its use, clinicians have not always used the modality in situations in which it may be appropriate. Recent research has yielded further support for the use of diathermy as both a thermal and nonthermal treatment modality. This exercise focuses on the thermal application techniques for diathermy and the sensations that are common with this application. Nonthermal application techniques would use the same principles for setup, but there would be no reported sensation from the patient.

A. Select one of your classmates to be a patient who will have continuous thermal shortwave diathermy applied to the medial aspect of the knee.

- Review the contraindications for diathermy prior to setting up your patient.
- Inspect the area, check the skin for irregularities and sensation, and document your observations.

_____

_____

_____

_____

- Position your patient so that he or she will be supported and comfortable for the 15-minute treatment time.
- Drape the knee with a towel so that the towel is in contact with the skin.
- Familiarize yourself with all of the unit's controls.
- Position the treatment applicator(s) (drum, plates, or cables). Turn the unit ON.

	Initially	After 3 Minutes	After 6 Minutes	After 9 Minutes	After 12 Minutes
Ask your patient to describe how the knee feels.					
Did your patient perspire at all during the treatment time? If yes, what did you do?					
Does he or she report any difference in sensation between the medial and lateral aspect of the knee?					

- Turn the unit OFF. Remove the treatment applicator(s). Unplug the unit from the wall outlet.

Reassess your patient and document your observations.

_____

_____

_____

B. Select one of your classmates to be a patient who will have pulsed nonthermal shortwave diathermy applied to the anterior aspect of the shoulder.
   - Review the contraindications for diathermy prior to setting up your patient.
   - Inspect the area, check the skin for irregularities and sensation, and document your observations.

_____

_____

_____

_____

   - Position your patient so that he or she will be supported and comfortable for the 15-minute treatment time.
   - Drape the shoulder with a towel so that the towel is in contact with the skin.
   - Familiarize yourself with all of the unit's controls.
   - Position the treatment applicator(s) (drum, plates, or cables). Turn the unit ON.
   - Select a pulsed nonthermal mode of treatment.

	Initially	After 3 Minutes	After 6 Minutes	After 9 Minutes	After 12 Minutes
Ask your patient to describe how the shoulder feels.					
Did your patient perspire at all during the treatment time? If yes, what did you do?					
Does he or she report any difference in sensation between the anterior or posterior aspect of the shoulder?					

   - Turn the unit OFF. Remove the treatment applicator(s). Unplug the unit from the wall outlet.

Reassess your patient and document your observations. _____

_____

_____

Diathermy Application Questions

1. What potential advantages are there for thermal treatment interventions with diathermy?

_____

_____

2. What potential advantages are there for nonthermal treatment interventions with diathermy?

_____

_____

3. What types of patients do you think would benefit from thermal treatment interventions with diathermy? What is your rationale for your choices?

_____

_____

4. What types of patients do you think would benefit from nonthermal treatment interventions with diathermy? What is your rationale for your choices?

_____

_____

5. What type of sensation did the continuous diathermy produce? What type of sensation did the pulsed diathermy produce?

_____

_____

6. How would you explain this form of treatment to a patient in the future?

_____

_____

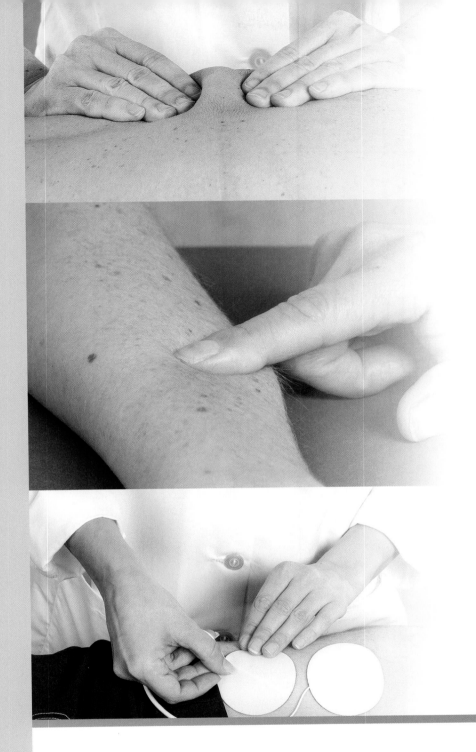

Electrical Stimulation for Therapeutic Treatment Goals

CHAPTER 11

Foundations of Electrical Stimulation and Iontophoresis

Cheryl A. Gillespie, PT, DPT, MA | *Peter C. Panus, PT, PhD*
Barbara J. Behrens, PTA, MS

Learning Outcomes

Following the successful completion of this chapter, the learner will be able to:

- Understand the basic concepts, terminology, and physiology of electrical stimulation and be able to differentiate among them.
- Guide the selection of optimal current parameters for effective and safe delivery of electrical stimulation to accomplish therapeutic treatment goals.
- Describe the use of electrical stimulation for medication delivery including the ionic properties of direct current.
- Outline the procedures for phoretic delivery of medications differentiating between iontophoretic drug delivery and an injection.
- Understand adjustment of treatment parameters to meet the needs and responses of individual patients to the application of electrical stimulation to accomplish therapeutic treatment goals.
- Demonstrate clinical decision-making skills regarding whether or not to apply electrical stimulation to accomplish therapeutic treatment goals.
- Differentiate between the available parameters of electrical stimulation devices and describe the differences among them to a peer.
- Describe the relationships between technical terminology and sensory responses to electrical stimulation and accurately match each term with the sensation that it produces.
- Describe the principles behind the application of electrodes for electrical stimulation to elicit a comfortable level of stimulation and discuss what can be done to improve patient comfort.
- Demonstrate the adjustment of various parameters on electrical stimulation devices to intentionally elicit sensory, motor, and fast pain responses and accurately document the parameters so that the response can be duplicated by a peer.

"Every beat of the heart, every twitch of a muscle, every stage of secretion of a gland is associated in some way with electrical changes."[1] —A. Watkins

Patient Perspective

"That's not going to electrocute me is it? I remember watching horror movies on TV where they used things like that!"

The use of electrical stimulation for the accomplishment of a therapeutic goal is not a new concept to clinicians; however, it is something that is quite a new concept to the patients being treated. Clinicians need to keep that in the forefront of their thoughts both when discussing the use of electrical stimulation with their patients and when applying it to them. This will potentially help decrease some patient anxiety with the concept, which has been around for literally thousands of years. One of the first applications is attributed to Luigi Galvani (AD 46), who used torpedo fish (electric ray) for the treatment of gout and chronic headaches. Fortunately, we have come a long way since then in our understanding of effective use of electrotherapeutic modalities in current practice.

This chapter will use the standardized electrotherapeutic terminology defined by the American Physical Therapy Association's Section on Clinical Electrophysiology and Wound Care.[2] Use of standardized terminology is essential for consistent communication of the parameters of treatment in research and practice. Unfortunately, some of the manufacturers of electrical stimulation devices do not follow the standard that is described. For this reason it is imperative that all clinicians fully understand the equipment that they are working with prior to ever attempting to apply it to a patient. Activities to foster that understanding are supplemented throughout this and other chapters in this text.

Application of Electrical Stimulation

The history of electricity and electrotherapeutics is well documented by numerous authors.[3–7] Two fields have emerged from this early research and use of electricity. Electrotherapy uses electricity to treat disease and dysfunction. Electromyography (EMG) is used to diagnose disease by interpreting the response of nerves and muscles to applied forms of electrical stimulation. EMG combined with the diagnostic procedures of nerve conduction studies (NCV) have enabled biomedical technology to flourish. Manufacturers have been developing more highly technical and versatile electrical stimulation units with microprocessors that enable highly sophisticated levels of function. Small portable stimulators have augmented electrical stimulation for home use, initially for pain management and now for many conditions requiring neuromuscular stimulation. The demand for the development and improvement of neural prostheses for implantation for multiple patient populations significantly increased subsequent to the increased numbers of war veterans returning home without one or more limbs, advances in robotics, acceptance of the technology, and the desire to return to the workforce.

Therapeutic Treatment Goals

Electrical stimulation is most commonly described by the goal for its application. Those goals are most often communicated in the form of acronyms, which are identified in APTA's *Guide to Physical Therapist Practice.*[8] Table 11-1,

TABLE 11-1 | Acronyms and Treatment Goals Explained

ACRONYM	EXPLANATION	TREATMENT GOAL
EMS	Electrical muscle stimulation	Stimulation of denervated muscle to maintain muscle viability
ESTR	Electrical stimulation for tissue repair	Uses electrical stimulation for edema reduction, enhancement of circulation, and wound management.
NMES	Neuromuscular electrical stimulation	Is stimulation of innervated muscle to restore muscle function and includes muscle strengthening, reduction of muscle guarding and spasticity, atrophy prevention, enhancement of range of motion, and muscle reeducation.
FES	Functional electrical stimulation	Activates muscles with electrical stimulation to perform functional activities
TENS	Transcutaneous electrical nerve stimulation	Stimulation for pain management

containing the most commonly used acronyms, is included for easy reference.

Electrical muscle stimulation (EMS) involves the stimulation of denervated muscle to maintain muscle viability. Electrical stimulation for tissue repair (ESTR) uses electrical stimulation for edema reduction, enhancement of circulation, and wound management. Neuromuscular electrical stimulation (NMES) is stimulation of innervated muscle to restore muscle function and includes muscle strengthening, reduction of muscle guarding and spasticity reduction, atrophy prevention, enhancement of range of motion (ROM), and muscle reeducation. Functional electrical stimulation (FES) activates muscles with electrical stimulation to perform functional activities. NMES and FES are often used interchangeably but really represent two different applications of electrical stimulation. NMES can be used to evaluate the patient for long-term management with electrical stimulation, which usually incorporates the use of a neural implant.[9] FES uses neural implants to improve function and includes such devices as cardiac pacemakers,[10] electrophrenic respirators,[11] dorsal column stimulators,[11-13] and visual and auditory implants.[11] Neural implants are also used to manage urinary and anal incontinence[11,14,15] and substitute for orthotics.[11] Transcutaneous electrical nerve stimulation (TENS) has become synonymous with stimulation for pain management. This application of electrical stimulation is usually associated with a group of small, battery-powered electrical stimulators called TENS units that were developed specifically to achieve this goal. Because TENS is the application of electrical stimulation across the skin, all stimulators are really TENS units and can be used for pain management, providing they have appropriate current parameters. The commercial TENS units have the advantage of portability.

Characteristics of Electricity

Electricity is most often described by its *strength* (**charge**), *rate of flow* (**current**), *driving force* (**voltage**), and *opposition* (**resistance/impedance**). Table 11-2 presents a review of these terms.

The relationship between current, voltage, and resistance is defined by **Ohm's law** and is illustrated in Figure 11-1. Current flow is directly proportional to voltage. An increase in voltage when resistance remains constant will increase current. Current flow is inversely proportional to resistance. An increase in resistance when voltage is constant will decrease current. The magnitude of current therefore increases when voltage increases or resistance decreases. High resistance requires high voltages to produce necessary current flow in the tissues below.[16]

TABLE 11-2 | Terminology of Electricity

ELECTRICITY	WATER
Electron	Water drop
Coulomb	Gallon of water
Current	Water flow
Voltage	Water pressure
	Low voltage: in old house
	High voltage: Waterpik (water flosser)
Resistance (impedance)	Water pipe: Narrow pipe
	Hair clog

$$Current = \frac{Voltage}{Resistance}$$

$$Voltage = \frac{Current}{Resistance}$$

$$\frac{Voltage}{Resistance} = Current$$

FIGURE 11-1 The relationships in Ohm's law.

Excitable tissues and nonexcitable biological tissues possess an inherent resistance. Excitable tissues include nerve, skeletal muscle, smooth muscle, and cardiac muscle in which there is the ability of neurons and neurotransmitters to conduct signals. The opposition to current flow in the body is more accurately described by the term "impedance" rather than "resistance." The body's opposition essentially results from the combination of resistive and capacitive reactance properties of tissue. **Capacitance** is the ability to store charge in an electric field and oppose change in current flow. Nerve and muscle membranes are examples of capacitors. The body tissues also function as resistors and model a parallel or series arrangement. When resistors are in series, there is only one pathway for electricity to flow and that is through each resistor in turn. When resistors are in parallel, the current has a choice of pathways and will always flow through the path of least resistance. Skin and adipose tissue function as resistors in series, whereas muscle, blood, tendon, and bone act like resistors in parallel.[17] Electric current therefore takes the path of least resistance once skin and subcutaneous tissues have been penetrated.

Tissue impedance varies throughout the body and conductivity depends on the water content of tissue. High water content decreases impedance and improves conductance. Healthy skin contains a thin layer of water containing salt, yet it offers one of the highest impedances (1,000+ V)[18] to current flow because the outer layer of the skin, the **epidermis**, contains little fluid. The amount of moisture in the deeper layers is determined by age and the number of sweat glands. Skin resistance is also inversely proportional to its temperature.[19] Heat increases moisture and surface salt content, which promotes conductivity. Bone, fat, tendons, and fascia are also poor conductors with low water contents of 20% to 30%.[20] The intracellular components of nerve and muscle have high water contents of 70% to 75%,[20] but their membranes have a high capacitive reactance that opposes charge movement.

Impedance can dramatically influence the ability to electrically generate an adequate response in underlying muscle. A greater intensity of current would be necessary to obtain a motor response in an area covered by adipose tissue (such as the gluteus maximus muscle) compared with an area with little fat (such as the anterior tibialis muscle). Increasing the current intensity to a level sufficient to drive current through the adipose to the nerve may make the sensation of the stimulation unbearable for the patient. This may rule out stimulation as a treatment option, or limit its effectiveness. Minimizing impedance is important for all applications of electrical stimulation because this allows current intensity to be reduced and so increase patient comfort. Cleaning the skin surface with alcohol prior to electrode application will remove dirt and body oils and will decrease impedance; removing excess body hair beneath electrodes will also reduce impedance, as will warming the region to be stimulated or warming the electrode gel.

Impedance changes in the presence of injury and disease. It increases with edema, ischemia, atherosclerosis, scarring, and denervation and decreases in open wounds and abrasions.[19]

Characteristics of Current Flow

Current will flow under two conditions: (1) when there is a source of energy creating a difference in electrical potential and (2) when there is a conducting pathway between the two potentials. In therapeutic electrical stimulation, a charge transfer occurs between the electrical generator and the biological tissue at the electrode interface.[21] Electron flow converts to ionic flow in the body.[22] Sodium chloride (NaCl) ions are examples of charge carriers in the body.

Ionic flow occurs because of the elementary law underlying electrophysics. This is a law that you learned early on in life but probably did not know why. This law states that *like charges repel, unlike charges attract.*[1] Positive ions (cations) are repelled from the positive electrode and migrate toward the negative electrode (cathode), whereas the negative ions (anions) migrate toward the positive electrode (anode). At rest the nerve is positively charged on the outside and negatively charged on the inside; nerves will become hyperpolarized (less excitable) under the anode and more excitable under the cathode (Fig. 11-2). Although both the anode and cathode are necessary to form a complete circuit, the cathode is often referred to as the active electrode because nerve activation (excitation) takes place more easily under this electrode.

Chemical reactions occur at the interface between the electrode and tissue during the transfer of charge.[23] Sodium ions (Na^+), which are positively charged, migrate toward the negative pole and combine with water, forming the base sodium hydroxide (NaOH). This chemical reaction increases the alkalinity of the area and promotes liquefaction of proteins and the softening of tissues.[17] Chloride ions (Cl^-), which are negatively charged, migrate to the positive pole and combine with water, forming hydrochloric acid (HCl). This chemical reaction increases the acidity of the area, thus promoting coagulation of proteins and the hardening of tissues.[17] Circulation is enhanced as the body attempts to neutralize the

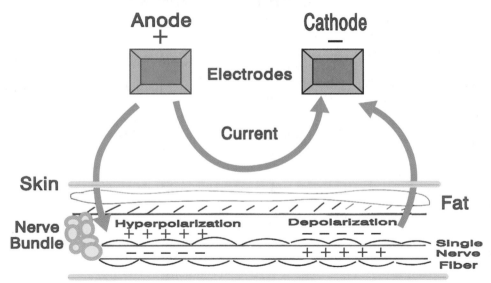

FIGURE 11-2 The flow of current from surface electrodes to an underlying motor nerve is shown. Hyperpolarization takes place under the anode because positive ions are driven away from this electrode into surrounding tissues. Depolarization, which can lead to an action potential, takes place under the cathode.

changes in the pH.[16] The magnitude of the chemical reaction depends on how long the current flows and how much current flows per square centimeter of surface area. Large charge accumulations occur when the current is too strong. This could potentially cause tissue damage such as burns. Small charge accumulations are advantageous to certain electrical stimulation treatments such as wound and fracture healing. Figure 11-3 illustrates current flow and the chemical reactions occurring with electrical stimulation.

Stimulator Outputs

The output of any commercial electrical stimulation machine can be classified as constant-current or constant-voltage. Stimulation units have a safety feature that sets an

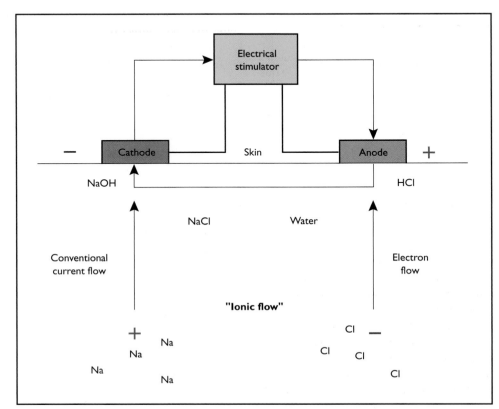

FIGURE 11-3 Concepts of current and ionic flow with application of electrical stimulation.

upper and lower range limit to resistance. This prevents excessive current or voltage output increases when there are large changes in resistance (clinical manifestation of Ohm's law). The selection of a *constant-current* or a *constant-voltage* output for treatment depends on the type of commercial units available in the clinic, and sometimes this is not a choice. If both types of outputs are available, the choice then depends on clinician preference or the therapeutic goal. There are advantages and disadvantages to both types of output.

CONSTANT-CURRENT STIMULATORS

A *constant-current* stimulator produces a current that does not vary and is independent of resistance. This generator maintains the same current output regardless of changes in resistance. The voltage output increases or decreases to maintain a constant current flow. The mechanism is similar to cruise control in a car. The car speed (current) is preset and the accelerator (voltage) maintains this constant speed even when the car is going up and down hills (resistance).

The advantage of stimulation with constant current output is consistency of the physiological response. The quality of the muscle contraction, for example, remains the same throughout the treatment when current level is constant as long as treatment parameters are such that muscle fatigue is avoided or at least minimized.

The disadvantage of this output is the effect on the tissue when resistance changes. Impedance increases as electrode size decreases. Electrode size is decreased with loss of electrode contact or electrode drying. This changes conductivity and increases impedance. The voltage increases to maintain the same level of current flow, which is now focused in a smaller area. The result can be pain with potential for tissue damage.

Clinicians can easily determine on themselves whether a machine has a constant-current or constant-voltage output by slowly peeling the electrode away from the skin surface. The machine is a constant-current stimulator if the current sharpens and starts to bite. The machine's output is constant voltage if the current lessens when the electrode is peeled away from the skin.

CONSTANT-VOLTAGE STIMULATORS

A *constant-voltage* machine produces voltage that does not vary. The current output increases or decreases depending on changes in resistance. This mechanism is similar to conditions of normal driving. The car will decrease speed (current) as it negotiates a steep hill (resistance) or increase speed going down the hill if the same amount of pressure is maintained on the accelerator (voltage).

A constant-voltage stimulator has the advantage of decreased current levels with increased resistance preventing discomfort or damage.

The disadvantage of this output is that the quality of the response, such as muscle contraction, will change with resistance. Current will also increase when initial skin impedance is overcome and resistance decreases. Constant voltage can be a problem if there are large decreases in

resistance. The current could increase to levels causing injury to tissue. See Figure 11-4 for an example using Ohm's law to depict how constant-current and constant-voltage stimulators compare.

Current Classification

Although electrical stimulation treatments are often referred to and documented by the type of commercially named current used, the clinician must be aware of the actual classification of current being produced by the unit. This knowledge is much more important for determining the most appropriate current effective for the treatment intervention. All therapeutic electrical stimulation units use one of three generic forms of current: (1) direct current (DC), (2) alternating current (AC), or (3) pulsatile (pulsed) current (Fig. 11-5).

Commercial generators are often named by the manufacturer and include high-volt pulsed current (HVPC), interferential (IFC), Russian stimulation, variable muscle stimulator (VMS), TENS, and microelectrical nerve stimulator (MENS) units.

DIRECT CURRENT

Direct current (DC) is a continuous unidirectional flow of charged particles with a duration of at least 1 second. One electrode is always the **anode** (positive) and one electrode is always the **cathode** (negative) for the period of stimulation. One electrode always receives current from the machine and current is returned to the machine by the other electrode. The polarity of a given electrode is determined by a polarity switch selection on the electrical stimulation

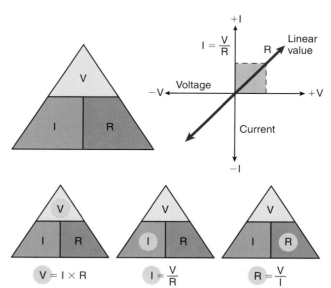

FIGURE 11-4 Ohm's law showing a comparison of constant current and constant voltage stimulators.
$I = V/R$, where I represents the Current and V represents Voltage and R represents Resistance
The formula needs to be presented with V as a constant and then with R as a constant to show the change in I (using numbers!).

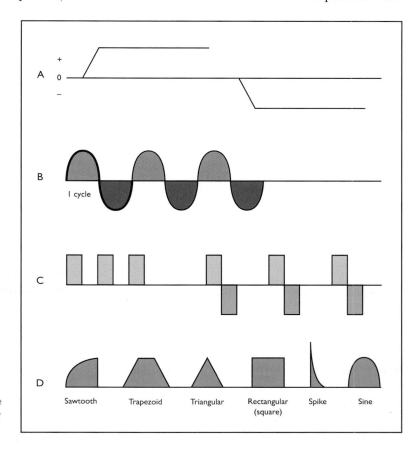

FIGURE 11-5 Types of current. **(A)** Direct current. **(B)** Alternating current. **(C)** Pulsatile current. **(D)** Common waveform shapes for pulsed current.

unit. Because one electrode is always positive and one is always negative, there is an accumulation of charge, as previously discussed. This accumulation of charge is called a chemical or polarity effect. DC has a strong chemical effect on the tissues and can be delivered continuously to promote absorption of medication through the skin, which is referred to as **iontophoresis**, or it can be interrupted to stimulate denervated muscle (EMS). DC is the only current form capable of these two treatment protocols. Iontophoresis is covered later in this chapter.

ALTERNATING CURRENT

Alternating current (AC) is an uninterrupted bidirectional flow of charged particles changing direction at least once a second. AC can also be delivered in an interrupted form, sometimes referred to as bursts. Each electrode becomes positive for one phase of the cycle and then negative as the current reverses. Since the electrodes are continuously changing their polarity, charges do not build up in the tissues.

AC is no longer directly used to stimulate tissue. Several commercial stimulators, including interferential and Russian, use AC as their base or carrier current, which is then modified and delivered to the patient in the form of beats or bursts, respectively.

PULSATILE CURRENT

Pulsed or **pulsatile current** can take on the directionality characteristics of AC or DC current. It is defined as the unidirectional (like DC) or bidirectional (like AC) flow of charged particles periodically ceasing for less than 1 second (milliseconds or microseconds) before the next electrical event. This small interruption in current, or charge movement, between successive pulses differentiates pulsatile current from AC and DC current forms. Pulsatile current is composed of individual pulses of short duration delivered in a continuous series called a **pulse train**. This pulse train can be delivered continuously or interrupted as in the AC and DC current forms. Each individual pulse is composed of one or more phases.

Pulsatile current has a negligible chemical effect in the tissues and the amount of effect depends on whether the pulse is unidirectional, like DC, or bidirectional, like AC. A cathodal or anodal effect will occur under each electrode when the pulse is unidirectional. When the pulse is bidirectional, one phase of the pulse has anodal characteristics and one phase of the pulse has cathodal characteristics, so the polarity effect is neutralized.

CURRENT CHARACTERISTICS

Pulsatile current is the most commonly generated and clinically used current form, and therefore is the emphasis of discussion for the rest of this chapter.

Manipulating the characteristics of both the single pulse and the pulse train are important for customizing treatment protocols. Table 11-3 lists the characteristics of the single pulse and the pulse train.

TABLE 11-3 | Characteristics of Pulsatile Current

SINGLE PULSE	PULSE TRAIN
Waveform	Interpulse interval
Amplitude	Frequency
Rise time/decay time	Duty cycle
Intrapulse interval	On-off time
Duration	Ramp time
Charge	Total current

DESCRIBING A SINGLE PULSE

The single pulse for electrical stimulation is actually an event and it can be described in terms of the characteristics of how it occurs. For example, the characteristics relate to how long it takes for it to occur or "by time," how strong the event is when it is measured or "by amplitude," and a relationship between the two or a "time/amplitude-dependent characteristic."[2]

WAVEFORM

Waveform is a visual representation of the pulse or event. It is a spatial drawing depicting the shape of the pulse, reflecting **amplitude** (*strength*) and **duration** (*length of time*) that the pulse or event takes place within.

Pulses are classified by the number of phases they have; for example, there are monophasic, biphasic, and polyphasic waveforms. A **monophasic** waveform means that the entire event takes place either above or below isoelectric zero, which means that the pulse is either positive or negative. **Isoelectric zero** is the demarcation between positive and negative where there is no net charge. It can also sometimes be referred to as baseline. **Biphasic** waveforms have two phases with one above and one below the isoelectric zero demarcation. Biphasic waveforms can either be balanced, where there would be no net charge, or unbalanced, where there would be either a positive or negative charge remaining. **Polyphasic** waveforms have multiple phases occurring above and below isoelectric zero. Figure 11-6 summarizes the three waveforms.

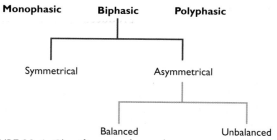

FIGURE 11-6 Classification of waveforms.

An additional description is often added to the waveform (Fig. 11-7), such as square wave or spiked pulse. The body does not distinguish between a square or trapezoid shape, but it does respond to the amplitude and time characteristics of the waveform shape.

Waveforms are diagrammatic only and rarely reflect what is actually going into the patient. Two factors influence the shape of the waveform and account for the difference between the illustrative waveform and the real. The first is the capacitive reactance property of tissue already discussed.[23] A load applied to a current, such as the resistance encountered in the body's tissues, will change the configuration or actual shape of the waveform. The actual waveform that is delivered when a load (resistance) is applied can be visualized on an oscilloscope. The second factor that determines the actual shape of the waveform is whether the equipment has constant-current or constant-voltage output.

Monophasic Waveform

A monophasic pulse has one phase. This pulse is unidirectional from the baseline carrying a positive or negative charge; therefore, like DC, one electrode is always positive and one is always negative. The polarity or chemical effects are not of the same magnitude as DC because pulsatile current flows for a shorter time period. The tissues are able to neutralize slightly between each pulse. The monophasic pulse is depicted in Figure 11-7.

There is often confusion differentiating between interrupted DC and pulsed monophasic current. These are two different current forms and cannot be referred to interchangeably. Interrupted DC is used for treatment of denervated muscle (EMS). Pulsatile current is unable to be used for this protocol owing to the small interruption in current between each pulse. Pulsed/pulsatile current is not the same as DC, which is continuous. The interruption makes the current less strong and incapable of accomplishing the same treatment goal. The continuous train of pulses is also not comparable to continuous DC for the same reason and therefore incapable of performing iontophoresis.

Those electrical stimulation units with the term high voltage **pulsed current** or "high volt" often cause significant confusion for clinicians owing to the presence of a polarity switch on the face of the units. These commercial units differ significantly and some are capable of delivering a monophasic pulse whereas others deliver a biphasic pulse that is unbalanced. Clinicians are encouraged to consult with the instruction manual to determine which type of "high volt" device they are using. Regardless of the type, both are pulsed and are still incapable of performing treatment interventions where DC is required.

Biphasic Waveform

A biphasic pulse is bidirectional with two phases. One phase deviates from the baseline in a positive direction and the other phase deviates in a negative direction; therefore, like AC, the electrodes continuously change their polarity.

Biphasic pulses can be subdivided into two types: (1) symmetrical biphasic and (2) asymmetrical biphasic. The phases of the *symmetrical biphasic pulse* are identical

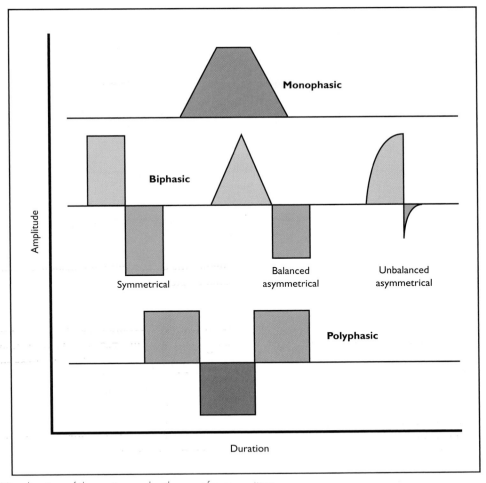

FIGURE 11-7 Visualization of the various pulsatile waveforms.

(see Fig. 11-7). The chemicals formed in one phase are neutralized by the reversal of current in the second phase. The charges of the two phases cancel each other out and there is a zero net charge (ZNC) across the baseline. No accumulation of positive or negative charge occurs. The variable muscle stimulation (VMS unit) and some battery-powered neuromuscular units produce this waveform.

A pulse is *asymmetrical biphasic* when the two phases are not identical. The asymmetrical biphasic pulse can be subdivided into (1) balanced and (2) unbalanced. When the charge of one phase is electrically equal to the charge of the other phase, the waveform is an asymmetrical *balanced* biphasic (see Fig. 11-7). The equal charges cancel each other out and a ZNC still exists across the baseline. A pulse is an asymmetrical *unbalanced* biphasic when the electrical charge of one phase is greater than the electrical charge of the other phase (see Fig. 11-7). The asymmetrical unbalanced biphasic pulse produces a net charge across the baseline with some residual charge in the tissues. This pulse is similar to the monophasic pulse in that there is accumulation of charge, but the electrochemical reactions are minimal because the pulse is biphasic.

Most commercial TENS units and some battery-powered neuromuscular stimulation units produce asymmetrical biphasic waveforms.

Polyphasic Waveform

Polyphasic means the pulse is composed of three or more phases (see Fig. 11-7). All polyphasic pulses are bursts. A burst is a finite series of pulses grouped together and delivered to the body as a single charge. A single pulse can be compared with the pull of a trigger on a gun. A single bullet is released. A burst is like the pull of a trigger on a machine gun. Many bullets are released at once. This is illustrated in Figure 11-8. The burst is perceived by the body as a single pulse. It behaves physiologically as a single pulse and has no physiological advantage over the single pulse.[16] The term "burst" is also synonymous with the terms "packet," "beat," and "envelope." Although all polyphasic pulses are bursts, not all bursts are polyphasic. A burst can also be a group of monophasic or biphasic pulses delivered as a single charge.

The modified or burst AC produced by the commercial interferential and Russian stimulators are examples of what may be referred to as a polyphasic pulse.

Phase Versus Pulse

The physiological effect of current on tissue is determined by the phase, not the pulse parameters. The monophasic pulse has only one phase. The phase characteristics therefore describe the whole pulse.

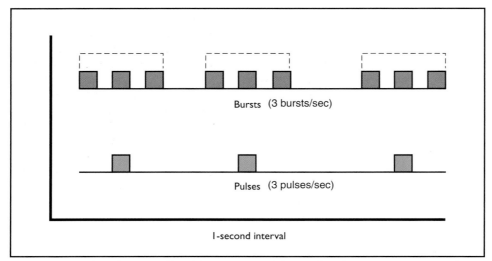

FIGURE 11-8 The burst and single pulse. Example of three bursts and three pulses delivered in a 1-second time interval. Each burst comprises three monophasic pulses in this illustration.

The biphasic pulse has two individual phases. The terms "phase" and "pulse" are not the same. The description of one phase is sufficient in the symmetrical biphasic pulse since the phases are equal. The characteristic of each phase needs to be identified in the asymmetrical biphasic pulse, especially if it is unbalanced in cases in which the charges are not equal.

Waveform Comfort

Many studies have investigated the comfort levels of different waveforms during electrical stimulation.[9,24-28] The symmetrical biphasic waveform is cited as preferred more often. In a comparison among symmetrical biphasic, asymmetrical balanced biphasic, monophasic, and polyphasic waveforms, the biphasic waveforms were most preferred.[9] Between the two biphasics, symmetrical biphasic was preferred with stimulation of large muscles while there was no preference between the two in small muscle stimulation.[9] One conclusion drawn from many of the studies is that there is a variety in preference in a small subgroup of patients. Therefore, if one waveform is not tolerated, another should be tried before abandoning electrical stimulation as a treatment intervention. Preference for different types of electrical stimulation can also vary in different muscle groups within the same person. Clinicians need to be mindful of the positive potential outcome but also remember that patients do not understand the rationale in many instances and may need encouragement to adhere to the treatment regimen.

Waveform Selection

All waveforms are basically effective for activating peripheral nerves, but one consideration on selection should be the waveform's ability to activate nerves with minimum electrical charge. The symmetrical biphasic waveform meets that qualification without the potential skin reactions that may occur with a monophasic waveform.[29] Some treatment protocols may dictate the waveform selection. The requirement of specific electrochemical effects

in treatment, as in wound healing, precludes the use of the biphasic waveforms. Monophasic waveforms would be the appropriate choice. It was also found that while symmetrical biphasic is preferred on large and small muscles, when used with stimulation of small muscles, it is not discrete in its recruitment and there is overflow.[9] Therefore, asymmetrical balanced biphasic may be a better choice with small muscles. Monophasic and symmetrical biphasic waveforms were found to generate muscle contractions with greater torque than polyphasic waveforms and they were also less fatiguing.[30]

BEFORE YOU BEGIN

Remember that the selected waveform of the stimulus will affect:

- Patient comfort
- Fatigue
- Chemical or polarity effects

AMPLITUDE

Peak amplitude (*peak current, peak voltage*) is the maximum current or voltage delivered in one phase of a pulse. It is the magnitude or intensity of the stimulus and it is one factor determining strength of stimulation. It is also one of three criteria necessary for depolarization: *the stimulus must be strong enough*. Peak amplitude describes the maximum amplitude of the monophasic pulse but refers only to the maximum amplitude of one phase of the biphasic pulse.

Peak-to-peak amplitude denotes the maximum current or voltage amplitude over the two phases of biphasic pulses. Peak-to-peak amplitude does not indicate the strength of the pulse because it does not reflect the difference in electrical charge between the positive and negative phases. The peak amplitude of each phase must be compared to determine differences in electrical strength between phases.

RMS (root-mean-square) voltage or current describes the average strength of the biphasic pulse. It takes into consideration the opposite charges of the phases. Peak amplitude and peak-to-peak amplitude are shown in Figure 11-9.

Peak amplitude is measured in current (milliamperes or microamperes) or voltage (volts) depending on the electrical stimulation unit. The amplitude is read on either a milliamp meter or a volt meter. The amplitude control on stimulator units is labeled intensity. Table 11-4 provides many of the synonyms that are commonly used for electrical stimulation devices.

Current and voltage are directly related as defined by Ohm's law. A machine with a high-voltage output is capable of producing a high peak current.[16] Most commercial units are low voltage (0 to 100 V), except for the high-voltage units, which have a maximum output of 500 V.

Peak amplitude is associated with depth of current penetration.[17] Higher peak amplitudes penetrate deeper into tissue. The electrical conductivity of the tissues under the electrode determines how deep this penetration will be. A high-voltage output generating a high peak amplitude will have no more penetration than a low-voltage output device if the tissues under the electrodes are composed of adipose and bone, which are not good electrical conductors.

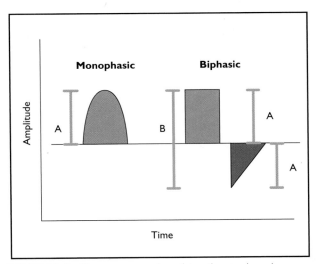

FIGURE 11-9 Characteristics describing the single pulse. (A) Peak amplitude. (B) Peak-to-peak amplitude.

Electrical stimulation produces three excitatory responses: (1) sensory, (2) motor, and (3) pain.[31] The peak amplitude influences the response of tissue to electrical stimulation. Low peak amplitudes may fail to excite tissue, whereas high peak amplitudes may cause pain and not produce the intended response. The level of current necessary to excite a nerve fiber is inversely proportional to the fiber's diameter.[17] The larger-diameter nerve offers less resistance because of its greater cross-sectional area. The larger sensory fibers are recruited before small pain fibers in "ideal" conditions. The anatomical location of the nerve fiber to the electrode is a factor with electrical stimulation.[22] Sensory fibers will generally fire first with the sensation of tingling, prickling, or pins and needles. Sensory fibers are smaller and have a higher threshold than do motor fibers but are usually more superficial and closer to the electrode. Selective discrimination of each excitatory response occurs as amplitude or intensity is increased slowly over time recruiting first sensory, then motor, and finally pain. When amplitude is increased rapidly, all nerve fibers meet threshold simultaneously and the immediate response is pain, usually described as a sharp burning sensation that is easily located. Let's Find Out, at the end of this chapter, illustrates these concepts.

Four clinical levels of stimulation are possible with electrical stimulation devices. They are commonly referred to in terms of the responses that are accomplished: (1) subsensory, (2) sensory, (3) motor, and (4) noxious or uncomfortable levels of sensation. Table 11-5 provides a listing of the different types of stimulation levels and the most commonly associated sensations and/or fiber types associated with them. The choice of stimulus level depends primarily on the treatment goal. A training period may be necessary for the patient to achieve the target stimulus strength necessary for treatment.

WHY DO I NEED TO KNOW ABOUT...

PEAK AMPLITUDE

Peak amplitude, which is adjustable, refers to:

- Tissue excitability (criteria for an action potential)
- Strength of stimulus
- Discrimination between excitatory responses for innervated and denervated tissues

TABLE 11-4 | Electrical Synonyms and Their "Translations"

Amplitude	Intensity	mAmps	Amps	Voltage	Current
Frequency	How many?	Hertz (Hz)	Rate	Cycles per second (cps)	
Pulse Duration	How long?	sec	Seconds	Pulse width (misnomer since time has no "width")	
Reciprocal	Alternating (a then b)		One channel is on and then the other is on while the first one is off		
Simultaneous	Both channels are either on or off together		Co-contraction		

TABLE 11-5 | Clinical Levels of Stimulation

Subsensory:	No nerve fiber activation
	No sensory awareness
Sensory:	Nonnoxious paresthesias
	Tingling, prickling, or pins and needles
	Cutaneous *A-beta* nerve fiber activation
Motor:	Strong paresthesias
	Muscle contraction
	A-alpha nerve fiber activation
Noxious:	Strong, uncomfortable paresthesias
	Strong muscle contraction
	Sharp or burning pain sensation
	A-delta and *C fiber* activation

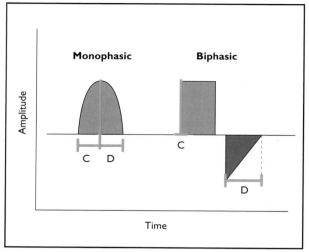

FIGURE 11-10 Characteristics describing the single pulse. (C) Rise time. (D) Decay time.

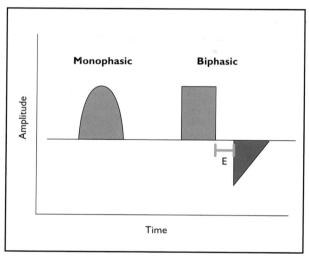

FIGURE 11-11 Characteristics describing the single pulse. (E) Intrapulse interval.

RISE TIME AND DECAY TIME

The **rise time** is the time it takes for the amplitude of the pulse to increase from zero to peak amplitude. The rate of rise directly affects the ability to excite nervous tissue,[17] and it is the second criterion necessary for depolarization: *the stimulus must be fast enough.* Nerve membranes accommodate or adapt to slow introductions of current over time (slow rise time) with an automatic rise in threshold. The membrane has time to adjust to the voltage change, and a greater stimulus is then needed to cause depolarization (excitation). Increasing amplitude can compensate for waveforms with slow rates of rise. Denervated muscle does not exhibit accommodation and can be selectively excited by current forms with slow rates of rise.[17]

Decay time is the time it takes for the peak amplitude to decrease back down to zero and defines the terminal end of the phase. Rise and decay times are fixed by the pulse shape. Figure 11-10 depicts these parameters.

INTRAPULSE INTERVAL

The **intrapulse interval** (*interphase interval*) defines the time period between the end of one phase and the beginning of the second phase of one pulse when peak amplitude drops to the baseline (Fig. 11-11). It is measured in microseconds and usually fixed by the manufacturer. A monophasic pulse does not have an intrapulse interval since it has only one phase.

It has been reported that when the anodal (positive) phase immediately follows the cathodal (negative) phase, the excitation caused by the stimulating cathode phase is depressed and may reverse.[32] Greater peak amplitude is then required for excitation. The introduction of an intrapulse interval abolishes this effect of the anodal phase and decreases the amount of amplitude needed to evoke excitation.[32] There is some discrepancy in the literature concerning the length of the intrapulse interval needed to abolish the anodal effect.[26,32]

BEFORE YOU BEGIN

Remember that rise time relates to:
- Tissue excitability (criteria for depolarization)
- Accommodation or adaptation of the tissue

DURATION

Phase duration is the time period extending from the beginning to the end of one *phase* of a pulse. Pulse duration is the time interval between the beginning and end of all the phases of the *pulse*, including the intrapulse interval. Phase duration is the third criterion for depolarization: *the stimulus must be long enough.* The terms phase and pulse duration are synonymous in the monophasic pulse. The pulse duration of a biphasic pulse includes the *duration of phase 1 + intrapulse interval + duration of phase 2*. Phase and pulse durations are measured in microseconds and are illustrated in Figure 11-12.

The strength (*amplitude*) and time (*duration*) of current determine tissue excitability. This is the law of excitation.[3] The strength-duration curve (SDC) demonstrates the inverse relationship between these two variables. As phase duration increases, less peak amplitude is required to achieve the desired physiological response (Fig. 11-13). There is a minimum stimulus duration below which no amplitude of stimulus can cause excitation and a minimum amplitude below which no duration can cause excitation.[17] Nerve and muscle membranes function as capacitors, meaning that they have the ability to store charge. Their membranes are capable of absorbing a certain amount of charge before reaching their excitation threshold. The minimum duration

necessary to excite muscle is longer than that of a nerve because muscle membranes have greater capacitance levels than nerve membranes.[17]

If you think of a capacitor as a container that can be filled with a liquid, and charge as the liquid, you can continue to add more and more liquid to the container until it is filled. However, once it is full, if you add more, whatever is added will spill out. The same holds true for current being added to tissues that are electrically conductive but have capacitive loads. The capacitive load must be reached before excitation will take place.

BEFORE YOU BEGIN

Remember that . . .

Intrapulse interval refers to the time in between the end of one phase and the beginning of the second phase and affects:

- Excitation of the tissues that you are attempting to stimulate
- Fatigue of muscle
- Chemical or polar effects, and may be adjustable

Phase duration, like peak amplitude, is associated with discrimination between the excitatory responses. Each excitable tissue has its own SDC. Discrimination, therefore selectivity, is greatest between the different nerve fibers at the shortest durations. The ability to discriminate between the different fibers decreases as phase durations increase,[17] as shown in Figure 11-14. Shorter durations excite the large sensory afferents, whereas the longer durations are necessary to excite the smaller A-delta and C fibers.[22,33,34] Stimulus durations between 20 and 200 microseconds are effective for discrimination.[16] Discrimination ability is lost at phase durations exceeding 1,000 microseconds (1 millisecond).[35]

Phase duration affects the comfort level of the stimulation. The comfort level of the stimulation often decreases as

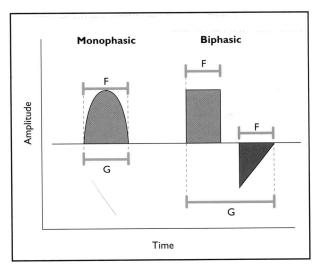

FIGURE 11-12 Characteristics describing the single pulse. (F) Phase duration. (G) Pulse duration.

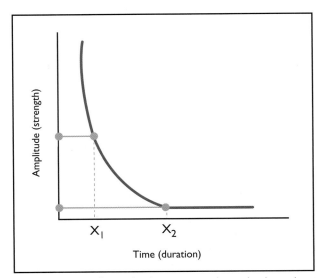

FIGURE 11-13 Relationship between peak amplitude and phase duration as defined by the strength-duration curve (SDC). Note the different amplitude requirements at durations (X_1) and (X_2). Less current amplitude is required to achieve threshold as phase duration increases.

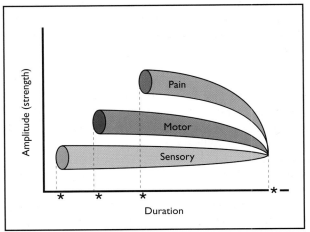

FIGURE 11-14 Discrimination of the excitatory responses in electrical stimulation. As the phase duration increases, the ability to selectively discriminate between the activation of sensory, motor, and pain nerve fibers decreases, and a point is reached at which all the excitatory responses are evoked at the same time.

the duration increases. No optimal phase duration has been defined for surface electrodes. Several studies have indicated that 50 to 1,000 microseconds (μsec) may be within an optimal range with 300 microseconds being the most comfortable duration compared 50- and 1,000-microsecond durations.[9,24,26]

The magnitude of chemical changes in the tissue is directly proportional to the phase duration. Increased chemical effects occur as the phase duration increases, which makes the pulse more closely resemble a more continuous on time rather than a pulsed waveform.

WHY DO I NEED TO KNOW ABOUT...

PHASE DURATION

Phase duration relates to the time of the phases and affects (Box 11-1):

- Tissue excitability (criteria for depolarization)
- Strength of stimulus
- Patient comfort
- Amount of chemical effect
- Impedance
- Discrimination between excitatory responses

BOX 11-1 | Intensity Versus Pulse Duration

Phase duration has been described as something that also describes the strength of the stimulus, but how can that be true? Wasn't that what intensity was supposed to be? They both are, but for different reasons and here's a practical way of thinking about them. They are both represented on the strength duration curve (SDC) on different axes with the intensity represented vertically and duration horizontally. So think about the square footage that one might find in a skyscraper in a large city as compared with a single-story building that consumes a full city block. Is it possible that they both have the same space capacity? **YES, they DO!** Take a look:

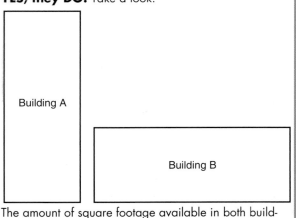

The amount of square footage available in both buildings is the same but distributed differently. The same would occur with a short duration but high intensity pulse duration versus long pulse duration and a low intensity waveform of electrical stimulation. The amount of charge would be the same but it would have been delivered in a different manner to the body.

Short pulse and phase durations are associated with decreased impedance and better conductivity of current into the tissue.[16] Remember that the goal with any form of electrical stimulation is to have the current enter into the tissue, so the easier that occurs, the better! If the current meets excessive resistance at the skin, then it will be:

- Difficult for it to pass into the underlying tissues to accomplish any therapeutic treatment goal
- More likely for it to be uncomfortable for the patient.

Phase duration can be fixed by the manufacturer or a variable control on the stimulation device. Variable phase durations permit custom fitting of the strength and duration of the current to the patient.

CHARGE

Phase charge is the amount of electrical energy delivered to the tissue with each phase of each pulse which can be measured in micro coulombs per second (μC/sec). It is quantity of charge defined by amplitude and duration. Charge is represented by the area of the phase. Pulse charge is the sum of all the phase charges in the pulse. The phase charge equals the pulse charge in a monophasic pulse. Phase charge is illustrated in Figure 11-15.

Phase charge reflects the capable strength of the electrical stimulation unit. Machines are classified as weak, moderate, or powerful depending on the maximum phase charge that the unit is capable of producing. The phase charge of the unit may be as weak as 12 mC or as powerful as 40 mC. Adequate phase charge determines tissue excitability. Excessive phase charge results in tissue damage.

BEFORE YOU BEGIN

Remember that . . .

Phase charge relates to:

- Strength of the stimulus or intensity
- The potential for issue damage dependent on values of other parameters (duration)

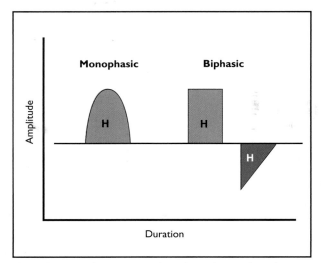

FIGURE 11-15 Characteristic describing the single pulse. (H) Phase charge.

The amount of charge necessary to evoke the three excitatory responses decreases as pulse and phase durations decrease.[36] This may be the result of reduced impedance at shorter pulse or phase durations lowering the charge needed for excitation.[16]

DESCRIBING THE PULSE TRAIN

All of the parameters related to the single pulse have been discussed. These characteristics are summarized in Figure 11-16. This section details the characteristics describing a series of pulses or the *pulse train*.

INTERPULSE AND INTERBURST INTERVALS

The interpulse interval is the time period extending from the end of one pulse to the beginning of the next pulse and is measured in milliseconds (msec). Bursts are separated by an interburst interval. The interburst interval is shorter than the interpulse interval because each burst contains more phases (Fig. 11-17). The interpulse interval decreases as phase or pulse durations increase (Fig. 11-18). Most stimulators produce relatively short pulse durations with long interpulse intervals. The interpulse interval, like the intrapulse interval, represents an interruption of current and results in less electrical stimulation fatigue. However, again like the intrapulse interval, there is no relaxation because the absence of current is too brief.[35] Any parameter decreasing the interpulse interval will increase the time of current flow and increase fatigue to electrical stimulation.

One reason the effects of polarity are minimized with pulsatile current is because of the intrapulse and interpulse intervals. Even though they are of extremely brief microseconds and milliseconds, respectively, they both shorten the period of time during which the current is on. The tissues have time to neutralize the chemical effects between phases or pulses and there is less residual electrical charge buildup in the tissues.

BEFORE YOU BEGIN

Remember that . . .

Interpulse interval relates to:
- Fatigue
- Chemical or polar effects in the underlying tissues dependent on values of other parameters

FREQUENCY

The **frequency**, which often is referred to as pulses per second (pps) or pulse rate, is the number of pulses delivered to the body in 1 second. The body responds to the number of pulses, not the number of phases. A single monophasic, biphasic, or polyphasic pulse is counted as one pulse by the body. Carrier frequency is the base frequency of the AC sine wave produced before it is modified and delivered to the patient at a different frequency.

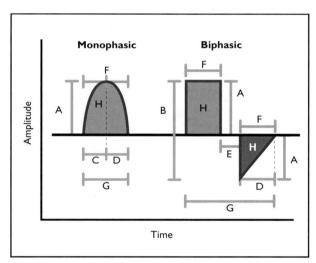

FIGURE 11-16 Summary of the characteristics describing the single pulse. **(A)** Peak amplitude. **(B)** Peak-to-peak amplitude. **(C)** Rise time. **(D)** Decay time. **(E)** Intrapulse interval. **(F)** Phase duration. **(G)** Pulse duration. **(H)** Phase charge.

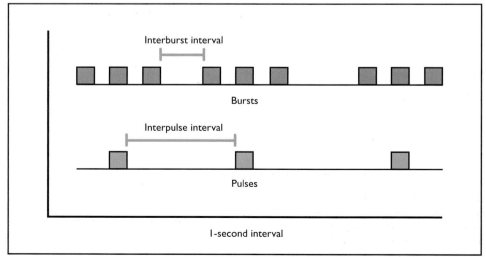

FIGURE 11-17 Characteristics describing the pulse train. The interburst and interpulse intervals. The interburst interval is shorter because the duration of the burst is longer than that of the pulse.

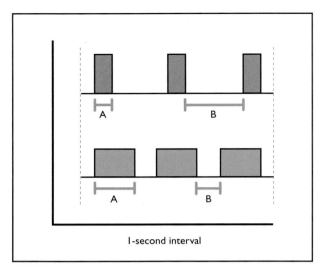

FIGURE 11-18 Relationship between (A) phase duration and (B) the interpulse interval. The interpulse interval shortens as phase duration increases.

The frequency of AC is expressed in hertz (Hz) or cycles per second (cps). Burst frequency is the number of *bursts per second*. Fatigue is greater at higher frequencies because the interpulse interval shortens (Fig. 11-19).

Whereas peak amplitude defines the intensity of the muscle response, frequency defines the quality of the muscle response dictating a twitch or tetanic contraction. A **twitch** response indicates that at least one motor unit is responding to the stimulus, producing a non-functional muscle contraction. A **tetanic muscle contraction** is a more functional representation wherein more motor units contract together in a meaningful way. Muscle response changes from twitch to tetany as frequency increases. The critical fusion frequency represents the point where the muscle twitch converts to a tetanic contraction.

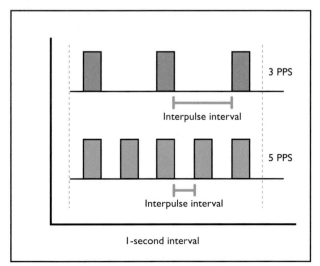

FIGURE 11-19 Characteristics describing the pulse train. Pulse frequency. The length of the interpulse interval decreases as frequency increases.

Impedance is influenced by frequency. The capacitive reactance characteristic of tissue is inversely proportional to frequency.[37] Impedance will decrease as frequency increases.

Electrical stimulators are often referred to as low-, medium-, or high-frequency units, the low and medium frequencies having the ability to stimulate excitable tissue. Unfortunately, the classification of electrical stimulators into low and medium frequency has just resulted in confusion. Essentially all therapeutic electrical stimulation machines are low frequency. The medium-frequency machines use a medium carrier frequency of AC that is delivered to the patient as a low-frequency current in the form of bursts. A carrier frequency of 2,500 Hz has been found to be more comfortable than stimulation with 1,000 or 5,000 Hz.[25]

Frequency is a variable control on electrical stimulators and is usually labeled as pulse rate. A frequency range of 1 to 120 pps is sufficient for most therapeutic treatment goals.[35] Purposeful fused muscle contractions occur at frequencies from 15 to 50 pps.[38] It has been found that stimulation at 50 pps is more comfortable than 35 pps.[9] Large-diameter nerves have higher firing rates than small-diameter nerves. Bioelectric investigations are providing some insight into the most appropriate frequency ranges for affecting both excitable and nonexcitable tissues. A frequency window has been postulated suggesting that cells may be receptive to certain frequencies and unresponsive to others,[39] an important concept for tissue and bone healing.

BEFORE YOU BEGIN

Remember that . . .

Frequency, which is adjustable, affects the:

- Fatigue
- Quality of muscle contraction
- Activation of fiber types
- Impedance

DUTY CYCLE

Perhaps one of the more confusing concepts that shouldn't be, is that of the duty cycle. The **duty cycle** of an electrical stimulation unit represents the on-and-off time and whether or not there is a ratio between them when there is more than one channel on the electrical stimulation unit. "On" time is the period of time the current is delivered to the patient. "Off" time is the period of time current flow stops. Both times are measured in seconds and are shown in Figure 11-20. The current must be on for at least 1 second and off for at least 1 second to be a true interruption of current with relaxation. Intrapulse, interpulse, and interburst intervals are much shorter than 1 second and therefore do not result in a true relaxation.

On time versus *off time* can be expressed as a ratio. If the current is on for 5 seconds and off for 20 seconds, the ratio is 1:4. Duty cycle is the percentage of time that the current is actually on. It represents the *on time* divided *by the sum*

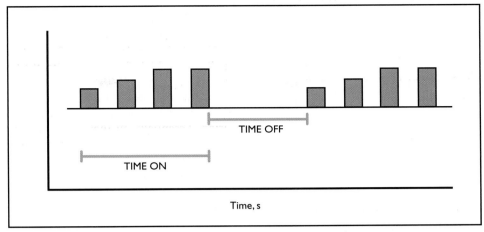

FIGURE 11-20 Characteristics describing the pulse train. On time/off time (duty cycle).

of on and off time expressed as a percentage. In the example above, the duty cycle would be 20%. The duty cycle must be known to calculate total stimulation time. Using the same example, if 5 minutes of contracting time was necessary, the total treatment time would have to be 25 minutes.

Muscle contractions generated by electrical stimulation are more fatiguing than those generated by the nervous system. The on-off time ratio plays an important role in circumventing muscle fatigue during stimulation. If the off time is longer relative to the on time, there will be less fatigue.

BEFORE YOU BEGIN

Remember that . . .

Duty cycle, which is adjustable, affects fatigue and ramp times affect patient comfort and the smoothness of the muscle contraction.

RAMP TIME

Ramp time is the increase in amplitude to peak of the *pulse train*. It is how long it takes for the current to go from zero to peak amplitude and how long it takes for the current to

go from peak amplitude back down to zero (Fig. 11-21). Ramp time is not synonymous with rise time. Rise time describes the change in amplitude in a single pulse. Ramp time describes the change in amplitude of the pulse train over a specific time period of current flow. *Ramp up* is an increase in amplitude over time. *Ramp down* is a decrease in amplitude over time. Both ramp times are measured in seconds.

Ramp time may be fixed or variable, depending on the stimulator. There may be one ramp feature, usually ramp up, or none at all. When variable, the adjustable range is generally 1 to 8 seconds.

Ramp time is associated with the comfort of stimulation, and a 2-second ramp is often adequate.[38] The ramp-up feature allows for more normal motor recruitment and smoother muscle contraction with slow buildup of current to peak amplitude. The ramp-down feature can increase patient comfort. The ramps are analogous to on ramps and off ramps on a highway. When attempting to merge onto a highway, there is an on ramp to allow the driver to accelerate up to the speed of the traffic on the roadway and an off ramp to permit the driver to adjust when exiting. An 8- to 10-second ramp-up is recommended when applying

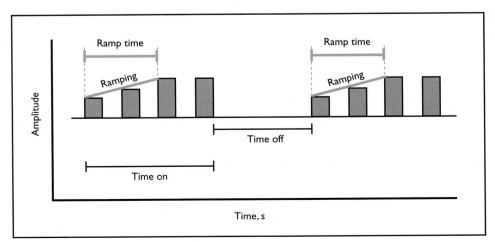

FIGURE 11-21 Characteristics describing the pulse train. Ramp time.

electrical stimulation to the antagonist of a spastic muscle.[38] Quick stretch and activation of the 1A afferents in the spastic muscle is then avoided.

The ramp time is added to the on time to ensure that peak contraction time is long enough. If a 10-second peak muscle contraction is desired with a 2-second ramp-up, the total on time is 12 seconds.

TOTAL CURRENT

Total current (average current) is the amount of current delivered to the tissue per second and is measured in milliamperes (mAmps or mA). Total current is very closely related to phase charge. Total current *equals* phase charge *times* number of phases *times* pulses per second.[16]

Total current determines safety of treatment and magnitude of the physiological effect. Tissue damage is the result of thermal and electrochemical effects in the tissue and both are a function of total current.[40] Heat dissipation is generally not a problem with surface stimulation.[40] Tissues can be harmed if the total current is excessive and there will be no physiological response if total current is too low. Most machines function within safe limits, but there are several commercial units with high total current outputs, such as interferential and Russian stimulation.

Any parameter increasing the strength of the current stimulus or decreasing the length of the interpulse interval will increase the total amount of current to the patient. *Peak amplitude*, *pulse frequency*, and *phase duration*

are all directly proportional to total current, as shown in Figure 11-22. Changes in peak amplitude and phase duration affect the strength of the pulse charge. Changes in phase duration and pulse frequency affect the length of the interpulse interval.

Total current is related to electrode size. A safe range of total current to the patient is considered to be 1 to 4 mA/cm² electrode area.[41] The lowest level of stimulation producing the desired response is the current level best used. Small electrodes should not be used with machines capable of delivering high total current. The strength of current is too concentrated and could cause tissue damage in the form of a burn.

MODULATION

Modulation refers to the ability of the electrical stimulation units being able to vary one or more of the electrical parameters over time while delivering the stimulus. This prevents adaptation to the current. If the underlying tissues adapt to the current, the effectiveness of the electrical stimulation may decrease, so adding modulation may help decrease that possibility. The single pulse or pulse train can be modulated. Amplitude and duration can be modulated in the pulse. Examples of modulation in the pulse train include frequency modulation, ramp time, on-off time, and bursting.

Amplitude, phase or pulse duration, and frequency can be modulated individually or in combination. Figure 11-23 illustrates the intermittent modulations of these parameters.

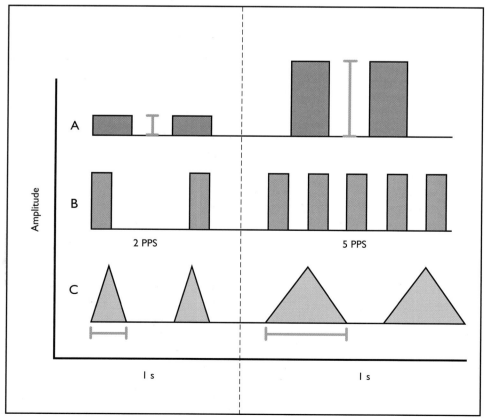

FIGURE 11-22 Total current can be increased by increasing **(A)** peak amplitude, **(B)** pulse frequency, and/or **(C)** phase duration.

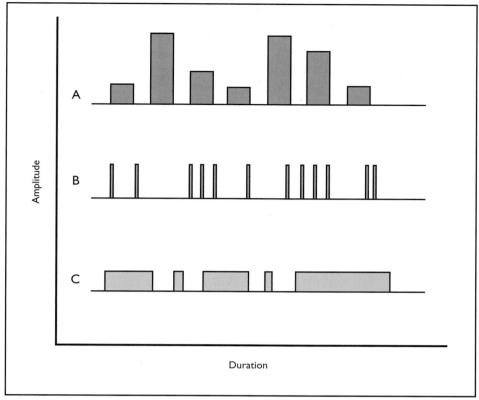

FIGURE 11-23 Modulation of current: (A) peak amplitude, (B) pulse frequency, and (C) phase duration.

WHY DO I NEED TO KNOW ABOUT...

TOTAL CURRENT

Total current will affect:

- Patient comfort
- Magnitude of the potential physiological effect
- Tissue damage dependent on the values of other parameters and
- Modulation, which can be adjusted, to help decrease adaptation to the sensation

Sweep is a term used by manufacturers to denote sequential modulation of pulse frequency. This feature gives the option of a constant sequential modulation (sweep) of the entire available frequency range or portions of it.

Ramping is the sequential modulation of phase charge by changing the phase duration or amplitude. Ramp time has been discussed and it is an example of amplitude modulation.

Current can be delivered continuously or interrupted. The ability of the machine to do both is an important feature for versatility of treatment. On continuous mode, the current is delivered without interruption for the length of the treatment. On interrupted mode, the current ceases for specific periods of time of at least 1 second. The on-off time controls are used to set the periods of time. The interrupted mode can be set to activate all channels of the unit at the same time (simultaneous) or alternate between two channels (reciprocate).

THE BIG PICTURE

Each electrical parameter dictates a specific response in the body and intimately relates to many other parameters. The pulse and current variables form a delicate web of cause and effect, and it is important to choose the optimal parameters for treatment. The clinician who understands the basic concepts of electricity, terminology, relationships between electrical parameters, and effect on body tissue will be able to execute treatment confidently, safely, and effectively.

Delivery of Electrical Stimulation

An electrical stimulation unit must be assessed in terms of its electrical features as "yes, effective to accomplish the goal" or "no, lacking the necessary features for this treatment goal or protocol."

Delivery of electrical stimulation can be either from a household-powered source (wall plug) clinical stimulator or a portable battery-operated stimulator. The battery-operated unit was found to be as effective as the wall-plug powered stimulator for generating contractions providing the parameters of intensity were available.[30] The current or voltage, depending on stimulator output, is converted from the power source current into the appropriate therapeutic current waveforms. Oscillator circuits within the machine allow independent control of the different treatment variables such as frequency, phase duration, and duty cycle.

Electrical stimulation is delivered to the body through electrodes. A lead wire connects the generator to the electrode. Electrodes are capable of two distinct functions. They can apply a stimulating current to the body tissue to excite, or they can record and detect the presence of an electrical signal in the body. The principles of electrode use and placement are discussed in detail in Chapter 12.

The electrical current can be introduced through transcutaneous electrodes in contact with the skin or through subcutaneous electrodes. The subcutaneous electrode is invasive and can be inserted through the skin via a wire or needle electrode percutaneously or surgically implanted in excitable tissue.[42] The percutaneous method is often used to assess the patient's response and reactions to the electrical stimulation prior to implantation.

MUSCLE AND NERVE PHYSIOLOGY

An understanding of the physiological basis of nerve and muscle stimulation is essential for safe and effective delivery of electrical stimulation. The reader may find it helpful to review these concepts in more detail. Table 11-6 outlines the major concepts and important key terms.

MOTOR UNIT RECRUITMENT

There are several differences between a central nervous system generated muscle contraction (active) and one generated by an electrical stimulation unit (passive). The torque output or strength of a muscle contraction is determined by the number of motor units recruited. When a muscle is contracted by the central nervous system, small motor units are recruited first assuring development of smooth and gradual tension. Small motor units are usually made up of type I muscle fibers and tend to be fatigue resistant. The first motor units to be recruited can then sustain the longest contraction. Large motor units are recruited as contraction strength increases. The order of motor unit recruitment is reversed with electrical stimulation. Large, superficial motor units are recruited first and these are usually made up of fatigable type II muscle fibers.

TABLE 11-6 | Muscle and Nerve Excitation: Concepts to Review

- Resting membrane potential
- Action potential generation and propagation
- Nerve and muscle structure
- Synaptic structure and function
- Classification of peripheral nerves
- Muscle fiber type and recruitment pattern
- Muscle excitation and contraction
- Structure of the motor unit
- Motor unit recruitment

Key Terms: absolute and relative refractory periods, all or none phenomenon, accommodation, adaptation, saltatory conduction, nodes of Ranvier, orthodromic and antidromic conduction, sliding filament theory, size principle of recruitment

---

Another difference between the central nervous system and electrical stimulation generated muscle contraction is the firing pattern of the motor units. During a voluntary contraction, motor units are activated asynchronously, constantly turning on and off in an alternate fashion. Asynchronous firing is highly energy efficient, delaying the onset of fatigue, and helps maintain smooth, steady muscle tension. There is no asynchronous firing in electrical stimulation. The motor units that meet stimulus threshold fire and continue to fire until the electrical stimulus stops. This is called synchronous recruitment and, unlike asynchronous muscle contractions, is very fatiguing to the muscle.

A third difference between central nervous system and electrical stimulation generated action potentials is the direction of propagation. In the central nervous system, the action potential moves away from the nerve cell body in an ortho-dromic direction. When a muscle contraction is caused by an electrical stimulus, there is the generation of an action potential in two directions rather than just one, which is what occurs normally. So not only do we see an ortho-dromic action potential, but we also see an anti-dromic action potential back toward the cell body from the stimulus site.

The combination of reversed recruitment order, synchronous recruitment, and bidirectional propagation of the action potential makes electrical stimulation very inefficient. Therefore, to avoid unnecessary fatigue, careful choice of stimulus parameters, such as frequency and on-off time, is important when designing neuromuscular stimulation programs.

MEMBRANE EXCITABILITY

As previously discussed, there are three criteria for depolarization: the stimulus must be *strong enough* (amplitude), *long enough* (duration), and *fast enough* (rise time).

The resistive and capacitive reactance properties of nerve and muscle membranes allow these tissues to oppose current flow and store an electrical charge. If the membrane resistance is multiplied by its capacitance, it yields a value known as the time constant. The time constant sets the rate at which a charge across the membrane is altered by an electrical stimulus. The time constant of a membrane represents the minimum time that a stimulus must be applied before depolarization will occur.

If the duration of the stimulus that is applied is infinitely long, which is defined as 300 milliseconds, the minimum current amplitude that will produce excitation is called **rheobase**. If the rheobase intensity is doubled, the amount of time (pulse duration) that current must flow to achieve excitation is called chronaxie. If one gradually decreases the stimulus duration below 300 milliseconds and records the minimum intensity of stimulation required to generate a threshold response, a curve can be plotted representing the tissue's excitability, which is the strength duration curve (SDC) discussed earlier in this chapter.

ACCOMMODATION

There are conditions under which a nerve cell will not generate an action potential even in the presence of what would normally be considered a threshold stimulus. These conditions include subthreshold depolarization of the nerve prior to delivery of a threshold stimulus or presenting the nerve with a stimulus that has a slowly rising intensity (slow rise time). These situations raise the threshold of the nerve cell so that it now takes a supra-threshold (extremely high) stimulus to elicit an action potential. This property is called **accommodation**, which is unique to nerve cells. The ability of muscle cells to accommodate is minimal. In addition to meeting certain minimal excitation requirements of the nerve, the current must reach its maximum intensity rapidly in order to avoid the effects of accommodation; otherwise, the stimulus will be ineffective in generating an action potential.

IONTOPHORESIS

Medications or drugs may be introduced into the body by a variety of means including enteral (swallowing) or **parenteral** (injection) routes or through passive absorption through the skin (transcutaneously) over extended periods of time. The routes bypass the liver, which is referred to as **hepatic** circulation, thus avoiding a major site of potential degradation.[43] Mechanisms of parenteral drug delivery include injection, passive transcutaneous delivery, and the use of electrorepulsive forces (iontophoresis) or mechanical (phonophoresis). Iontophoretic delivery is desirable for drugs that

- Demonstrate significant hepatic metabolism
- Require constant plasma levels
- Are being used for topical or local transcutaneous tissue effects

Phonophoretic delivery may also achieve the some of the previously stated goals. We now review the biophysical and cellular composition of the skin (**integument**) as related to transcutaneous drug delivery, as well as the currently accepted mechanism(s) by which drugs transcutaneously permeate the skin under passive, iontophoretic conditions. The iontophoretic devices and electrodes currently available within the United States for human use are also discussed. Finally, the experimental and clinical evidence supporting iontophoretic application in rehabilitation is examined.

Patient Perspective

"You mean I don't have to have a shot, I can have the medication go through that pad?"

Remember that your patient does not understand what you are about to do. A simple explanation using a magnet as an example, describing how like poles on a magnet repel each other, might help the patient to understand how the charge of the medication will be repelled by the electrode into his or her body. This explanation will also help you to reassure yourself that you are applying the medication under the correct polarity during iontophoresis.

Patients' Frequently Asked Questions

1. What will this feel like?
2. Can I take all my medications this way?
3. If you turn it up higher, will it be better for me?
4. Shouldn't I feel something like I do with the other electrical stimulation devices?
5. Is it safe to touch that while it is on?

Integumentary System: Our Skin

MORPHOLOGY AND FUNCTION

The integument is the largest organ of the body and consists of two main layers. The epidermis is the superficial **avascular** layer, meaning that it does not have its own blood supply; the dermis is a deeper vascularized layer, and the basal lamina separates the two (Fig. 11-24). The epidermis consists of five layers. The deepest layer, stratum basale, is a single layer of cells that continuously divide and differentiate as one "daughter cell" randomly migrates to the surface. The most superficial layer, stratum corneum, represents the most differentiated cells, and is composed of about 10 to 15 layers of these flattened cornified cells (corneocytes). The total thickness of skin is about 2 to 3 mm, but the thickness of stratum corneum is only about 10 to 15 mm. Most of the epidermal mass is concentrated in the stratum corneum. The stratum corneum is the major barrier to both environmental and infectious insults. This protection is afforded by the differentiation that occurs as the cells migrate from the stratum basale to the stratum corneum.

The cells migrating upward from the stratum basale layer differentiate and their cellular metabolism decreases as they move away from their source of oxygen and nourishment. During this superficial migration and differentiation, the cells synthesize intracellular keratin and extrude lipids. These lipids constitute this extracellular lamellar matrix and are composed of ceramides, cholesterol, and free fatty acids.[44] **Ceramides** are found in high concentrations within the cell membranes of cells. They are one of the component lipids, or fats that make up one of the major lipids in the double layer of fats of the cell membrane. The cells maintain attachment to each other via **adherens junctions**, which are the protein complexes that occur at cell–cell junctions in epithelial tissues (desmosomes). This intracellular keratinization and extracellular lipid secretion provide the

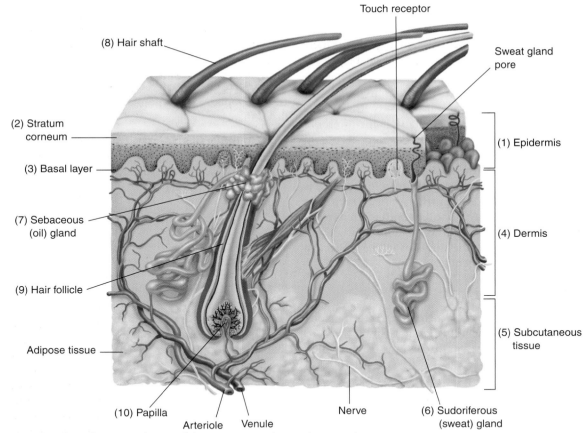

FIGURE 11-24 Three-dimensional view of the integument (skin) with appendages.
(From Gylys, BA, and Wedding, ME: Medical Terminology Systems: A Body Systems Approach, ed 5. Philadelphia: FA Davis, 2005, with permission.)

"bricks and motor" barrier of the stratum corneum. Movement of molecules into the body requires a tortuous passage through either the **aqueous** or hydropzzhobic channels of the stratum corneum (Fig. 11-25). *Aqueous* simply means "watery" and hydrophobic is used to describe things that are incapable of dissolving in water indicating that molecules either select a watery or non-watery pathway.

The basal lamina is an irregular surface that separates the avascular epidermis from the underlying vascularized dermis. The **dermis** is also referred to as the sensitive connective tissue layer of the skin.

The lamina contains an interconnecting network of collagen and glycoproteins that assists in anchoring the epidermis to the underlying dermis. In addition, the laminar

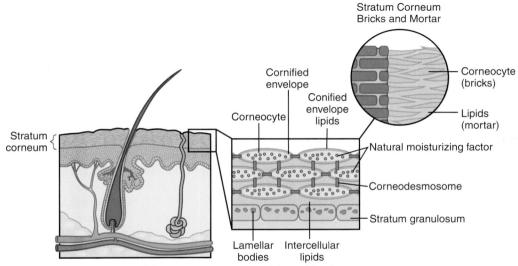

FIGURE 11-25 Cellular representation of the stratum corneum and the cell-lipid matrix.

surfaces increase the overall surface area for nutrient and oxygen diffusion into the epidermis.

The dermis is separated into two main regions: the more superficial papillary layer and the deeper reticular layer. The papillary layer lies directly underneath the basil lamina, the extracellular matrix providing continuity and structural support between the epidermis and deeper structures. The reticular layer is the major component of the dermis. The ground substance, collagen/elastin network provides the turgor to the integument. **Elastin** is the main component that provides the elastic properties to the fibers. This **turgor** that is referred to represents the tension produced by the fluid content within the tissues and is accomplished by the collagen and elastin proteins restricting the expansion when the sugar precursors attract water, much the same way thread wound around a sponge in water restricts the sponge's expansion. This ground substance also promotes the **plasticity** of the skin, or its ability to change and regain shape.

The integument or skin is responsible for several non-barrier functions. The integument synthesizes vitamin D_3 from cholesterol using ultraviolet radiation and protects tissue from this same electromagnetic radiation by synthesizing melanin. Melanin is described earlier in this text. Finally, the integument has an immune-regulatory role in cutaneous antigen recognition and a biometabolism role in processing cutaneously absorbed molecules, those molecules absorbed through the skin.

WHY DO I NEED TO KNOW ABOUT...
HYDRATION

Hydration is a key component to the healing process. Without moisture, cells cannot migrate.

The vasculature for the integument is divided into two major plexuses. The superficial plexus is located between the papillary and reticular layers of the dermis, and the deeper vascular plexus is located between the reticular layer of the dermis and subcutaneous tissue. These vascular plexuses are involved in nutritional blood flow for the integument and thermoregulation of core body temperature. The epidermis itself is avascular, meaning that it has no specific blood supply of its own. Nerve innervations located within the dermis also provide the nervous system with information via various afferent chemical, thermal, and sensory receptors. Finally, the integument has different appendages that originate or penetrate through the dermis to the epidermis. These appendages include hair follicles and sweat glands. These glands are involved in thermoregulation or temperature regulation, and the production and release of scent recognition in other nonhuman vertebrates.

ELECTRICAL PROPERTIES OF THE SKIN

The role and mechanism(s) of the stratum corneum as the high resistance layer to the flow of electric current and a significant component in skin impedance have been extensively reviewed elsewhere.[45–48] The stratum corneum forms the high electric resistance layer and is a significant component in skin impedance.[49] The high resistance of this layer in turn is due in part to its lower water content (about 20%) compared with the normal physiological level (about 70%). The charge the skin maintains in an electric field is dependent on the pH of the solution. At a pH greater than 4, the skin maintains a negative charge when placed in an electric field, and at a pH lower than 3, the charge of the skin is positive. Thus, at the normal pH of the skin, a negative charge is present. This pH (3 to 4) about which the change in charge occurs is called the isoelectric point and is similar isoelectric point of keratin in the stratum corneum layer.[50] Biological tissues such as skin also have a capacitance, an ability to store electrical charge, and are thus electrical capacitors. If you are in doubt about this, think about the last time that you walked across a wool rug and then touched something that was metal. If you got a "shock" it was actually your body's way of discharging the charge that you had built up from the carpet.

When an electric circuit contains both capacitive and resistant elements, the circuit is said to be reactive. The equivalent circuit model for the skin is that of a resistor parallel to a resistor and a capacitor.[49] A reactive circuit demonstrates impedance. The impedance represents the total electrical opposition of the circuit to the passage of a current. The human skin has an impedance to an alternating current of low frequency, but this impedance decreases as frequency of the alternating electric current is increased.[51] Owing to variations in skin impedance, the current intensity of voltage-regulated stimulators cannot be easily controlled; thus, most manufacturers use current regulated stimulators.[52] The loss of skin impedance with application of current may be the result of a re-orientation of molecules along the ion transport pathways, such as the possible realignment of lipid molecules in hair follicles and sweat glands.[53] Also, application of current will lead to an increase in the local ion concentration, which will result in reduced impedance.[54] Thus, application of electrical current reduces skin impedance. This reduction may account for part of the enhanced transcutaneous drug delivery by application of an electrical current. The current-voltage relationship in skin is nonlinear.[55,56] The hydration status of the skin significantly influences this relationship, with higher hydration resulting in reduced impedance. Finally, temperature also affects the impedance of the skin, with reduced impedance at increasing cutaneous temperatures.[57]

WHY DO I NEED TO KNOW ABOUT...
IMPROVING CONDUCTANCE

If your goal is to improve conductance (which is the opposite of impedance) then you have a few choices:

- Heat the skin before applying electrical stimulation.
- Make sure that the skin is hydrated before applying electrical stimulation.
- Apply a comfortable level of electrical stimulation prior to the "treatment level" to help decrease impedance levels.

Transcutaneous Transport

TRANSCUTANEOUS DRUG PENETRATION

As previously described, the stratum corneum acts as a barrier that minimizes transepidermal water loss. It is also the principal barrier to transcutaneous drug delivery. The transcutaneous delivery of small molecules can easily be compared with molecular diffusion through a barrier. Based on theoretical models, drugs can diffuse through the stratum corneum via a transepidermal route or transappendageal route.[45,47,58,59] Transepidermal drug delivery through the stratum corneum may occur within the lipid-rich lamellar matrix between the cells (intercellular route) or through both the transcellular route (protein-filled intracellular and intercellular domains) (Fig. 11-26). The transappendageal shunt pathway normally contributes little to no passive transcutaneous drug delivery, due to the small fraction of the total human skin surface made up by these structures.[47,59]

The more aqueous the channels within the intercellular lamellar matrix, the more likely it is for the potential pathway for passive transcutaneous delivery of hydrophilic drugs to take place. However, hair follicles and sweat ducts can interfere and act as diffusion "shunts" for ionic molecules during iontophoretic transport.

PASSIVE DRUG DELIVERY

Passive drug delivery methods are used for both local and systemic indications. A broad spectrum of drugs may be delivered by passive delivery and range from assistance to quit smoking (nicotine) to motion sickness (scopolamine). Thus, cutaneous absorption of a variety of drugs exists. Passive intracutaneous and transcutaneous delivery of anti-inflammatory drugs have been documented in both animal and human investigations.[60–63] Passive delivery of piroxacam, a nonsteroidal anti-inflammatory drug (NSAID), into the musculature under the application site has been

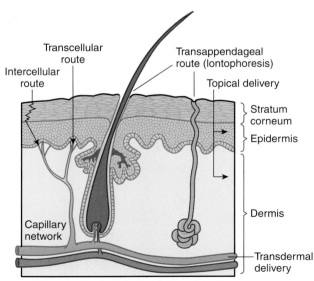

FIGURE 11-26 Schematic representation of the potential pathways for intracutaneous and transcutaneous drug delivery.

reported.[60] However, other investigations examining a variety of analgesics have reported that maximal depth of local tissue penetration during passive delivery, which is not attributable to systemic vasculature, occurs at the fascia to superficial muscle interface.[64–66] The consensus of these investigations is that maximal depth of delivery of these drugs is at best the superficial musculature, with deeper tissue penetration being dependent on systemic vascular absorption and redistribution.

WHY DO I NEED TO KNOW ABOUT...
TRANSCUTANEOUS TRANSPORT
- The longer a topical agent is applied to the skin, the greater is the potential for it to be absorbed passively.
- The electrical stimulation is not the only cause for the delivery of the medication during iontophoresis.

Finally, under clinical conditions the duration of application to achieve this tissue delivery is measured from one-half day to multiple days.[60,62,63] Thus, passive delivery for localized decrease of pain and dysfunction associated with musculoskeletal inflammation is achievable only after a prolonged period of application.

IONTOPHORETIC ENHANCEMENT

A history of iontophoresis and the broad potential of pharmaceutics that may be transcutaneously delivered has been previously reviewed.[47,48] Topical, or transcutaneous, delivery of drugs, that is, drug delivery into or through the skin, can be assisted by electrical energy. The mechanism(s) involved may be iontophoresis, electro-osmosis, or electroporation.[45,47] Electro-osmosis is a phenomenon that accompanies iontophoresis and will be discussed in conjunction with iontophoresis.

Iontophoresis implies the use of small amounts of physiologically acceptable electric current to deliver drugs into the body. The technique has the potential to enhance transcutaneous permeation of both ionic (charged)[64–68] and nonionic (uncharged)[69–70] compounds several-fold over passive delivery. With iontophoresis, an electrode of the same polarity as the charge on the drug drives the drug into the skin by electrostatic repulsion (Fig. 11-27).

Lidocaine, which is a cationic drug that carries a positive charge, would use the anode or positive electrode for charge-charge repulsion to be delivered into the body. In contrast, dexamethasone phosphate, which is an anionic drug and negatively charged, would need to use the cathode or negative electrode for delivery. Iontophoresis may be used for systemic or localized drug delivery and provides a programmed delivery, as drug transport is proportional to the electric current used to "push" or apply it. Patient adherence to therapy will also improve, and the dose may be adjusted to account for interpatient variability by adjusting the current.

Hair follicles and sweat glands within the skin make up only 0.1% of the surface area and represent pores within the skin with different radii, polarity, and charge

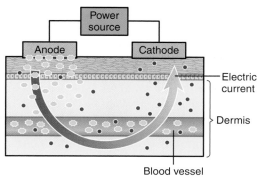

FIGURE 11-27 Iontophoretic concept using charge-charge repulsion to deliver drugs from both the anode "A" (positive electrode) and cathode (negative electrode) "B." Cationic drugs such as lidocaine (L+) would be delivered from the anode. Anionic drugs such as dexamethasone phosphate (D−) would be delivered from the cathode.

concentrations.[47] As such, these pores may restrict transcutaneous permeation of compounds larger than the pore or of the opposite polarity.[68] Evidence suggests that iontophoresis transcutaneously delivers drugs through these pores, and these pores account for the previously discussed transappendageal shunt pathway[71,72] (see Fig. 11-27).

BEFORE YOU BEGIN

- You must know the polarity electrodes *and* of the medication that you are going to apply.
- You must solicit patient allergies from the patient to ensure his or her safety.
- You must document that you asked the patient about allergies and that he or she denied having a known specific allergy to the medication that is about to be administered if that was the patient's response to your question.

During iontophoresis, the greatest concentration of ionized substances is expected to move into regions of the skin either where the skin is damaged or along the sweat glands and hair follicles. In these areas, the resistance of the skin to permeation of the drug is least. Iontophoresis may also stimulate pore formation in regions not associated with appendages.[73,74] The extracellular lipid domain and transcellular transport contribute little to hydrophilic drug transcutaneous iontophoretic transport.[73–76] The opening of the pores during iontophoresis is time dependent, as is the closing following the iontophoretic process.[59,77,78] The time required for the opening and closing of these pores depends upon the duration of current applied and the current density. Since augmented passive drug delivery continues following termination of the applied current, iontophoretic applicators (electrodes) should remain in place to maximize the amount of drug delivered transcutaneously. In conclusion, the iontophoretic pore pathway model is intercellular and aqueous in nature, with transcutaneous drug transport delayed after the initiation and continuing after the termination of iontophoresis.

If a voltage difference is applied across a charged porous membrane such as the skin, bulk fluid flow or volume flow, electro-osmosis, occurs in the same direction as flow of counter-ions. The term "ionto-hydrokinesis" was used in early literature to describe this water transport during iontophoresis.[79] This flow is not diffusion and involves a motion of the fluid without concentration gradients.[80] The counter-ions are usually cations and electro-osmotic flow occurs from anode or positive electrode to the cathode or negative electrode. The major cation transported through epidermis is Na^+. Thus, the skin, and the stratum corneum in particular, is a permselective membrane with negative charge at physiological pH.[50,81] Electro-osmosis enhances the flux of positively charged (cationic) drugs from the anode, while hindering drug flux of negatively charged (anionic) drugs or neutral drugs being delivered from the cathode. In such cases for either neutral or negatively charged drugs, transcutaneous delivery from the cathode may actually increase after the current is stopped.[70] Finally, the predicted contribution of electro-osmotic flow to total drug flux during iontophoresis depends upon additional drug-formulation and skin-related variables, which have been reviewed elsewhere.[47]

The biophysical parameters for electrical enhancement of transcutaneous delivery, in realistic terms, constitute a rather complex area with a large number of operating variables.

Instrumentation and Application of Iontophoresis

Manufacturers market iontophoretic devices for a variety of clinical uses from hydrosis in cystic fibrosis detection to systemic delivery of opiate analgesics. The U.S. Food and Drug Administration (FDA) is responsible for both testing and regulating medical equipment that is used on humans in the United States. There is a lengthy process that any manufacturer must undergo to prove that their device is safe and effective before it can be marketed. One of the first steps involves gaining pre-market approval and then being ranked into different types of classifications based upon the degree of potential risk to human life. Iontophoresis kits have been classified by the FDA as Class III devices.[82] However, they have not undergone the clinical trials because they were marketed prior to 1976. Most were cleared under the 510(k) pre-market approval process that applies to grandfathered Class III devices. The iontophoretic power sources will be discussed followed by the drug delivery electrode applicators.

WHY DO I NEED TO KNOW ABOUT...

FDA RATINGS

Whenever applying a medical device to a patient, it is important to know what the status of that device is at the FDA. This will provide insight into the body of knowledge regarding the application of the treatment intervention.

IONTOPHORETIC POWER SOURCES

Current iontophoretic systems are a combination of battery-dependent stimulators, used to provide either pre-programmed or programmable electric current for a specified time dosage, and two electrodes. The drug applicator electrode may be selected as either the anode or the cathode. The second electrode is present only to complete the electrical circuit. The patient is also incorporated into the electrical circuit. The completed electrical circuit includes the drug delivery electrode, the patient, and the non-treatment electrode. The electrical waveform for iontophoretic devices is direct current (DC). Variations in skin impedance result in the current intensity of voltage-regulated iontophoretic devices as demonstrating inter-subject variability. This results in a variable time duration required to deliver a single iontophoretic dosage with different patients, or within the same patient as two different time points. The iontophoretic dosage is expressed in Box 11-2.

In addition, current through the tissue has been proposed as the most significant iontophoretic parameter.[47] Constant current devices adjust the voltage based on the skin impedance of the patient so that the current stays constant. In the event of poor electrode contact, manufacturers of constant current devices have incorporated automatic

---

BOX 11-2 | Dosage Calculation of Milliamp Minutes

Calculation of milliamp-minutes is based on the following formula:

Dosage (mA*min) = Current (mA) × time (minutes)

---

shutdowns should the voltage reach predetermined levels. This safety feature is to prevent electrical burns at the electrode sites.

BEFORE YOU BEGIN

Know what the desired amount of dosage in mA*min is, and base your intensity on the patient sensation and time available, remembering that longer treatment times may be better.

Several manufacturers market iontophoretic devices in the United States for the rehabilitation medicine profession. Some of these manufacturers include IOMED, Empi, Life-Tech, and Birch Point Medica. The annual market for iontophoresis is about $20 million for physical therapy.[82] The first four companies market external palm-sized current-controlled devices in which the iontophoretic dosage may be programmed for each patient. These current-controlled devices are connected to separate electrodes for transcutaneous drug delivery. In contrast, Birch Point Medical Inc. uses a voltage-controlled self-contained unit with the battery and electrodes designed into a single, larger figure-of-eight bandage. The current amplitude range for all marketed iontophoretic devices is between 0 to 4 mA (Table 11-7). The iontophoretic dosage (mA*min) delivered is programmable in with the Empi, Iomed, and Life-Tech devices. The iontophoretic dosage for the Birch Point Medical device is not programmable and is set at the factory at 40 or 80 mA*min. A mA-min is determined by multiplying the number of mA (intensity) by the number of minutes that the current is delivered. For example, 40 mA*min = 4 mA and a 10-minute treatment time. As the Birch Point Medical device is voltage controlled, the treatment duration

---

TABLE 11-7 | Parameters for the Commercially Available Iontophoretic Power Sources

MANUFACTURER	AMPERAGE RANGE (MA)	MAXIMUM DOSAGE (MA*MIN)	CHANNELS	POLARITY
Dupel *EMPI* *St. Paul, MN*	0–4	160	2	+ or −
Phoresor II Auto *IOMED* *Salt Lake City, UT*	0–4	80	1	+ or −
Iontophor PM/DX	0–4	N.C.	1	+ or −
Microphor (*Check*) *Life-Tech* *Houston, TX*	0.5–4	80	1	+ or −
Iontopatch *Birch Point Medical, Inc.* *Oakdale, MN*	0.1 *	40 or 80 fixed	1	+ or −

The abbreviations are as follows: polarity, cathode (−) or anode (+). Voltage-dependent device and the current (*) vary depending upon patient's impedance, with the range on a 20 mA-minute dosage 0.05 to 0.16 mA. N.C. no maximum dosage limits with the power source.

for a single iontophoretic dosage may vary between patients, or for the same patient at two different times (see Table 11-7). When a 20 mA*min dosage was conducted with the Birch Point Medical device, the current varied from 0.05 to 0.16 mA, and the treatment duration would vary from 2.1 to 6.7 hours. Thus, when iontophoresis is conducted in the clinic, where time commitments for treatment are constrained, current-controlled iontophoretic devices are dominant. However, the Birch Point Medical device is designed for the patient to wear after leaving the clinic. Finally, each device contains circuitry unique from those of other manufacturers. For example, the Phoresor II Auto system requires the setting of dose and current from which it calculates the treatment duration required. In contrast, the DUPEL device is a dual-channel system where the user can set the dosage and current levels for each channel independently.

ELECTRODE DESIGNS

Initial clinical investigations with iontophoresis used gauze or paper towels saturated with the drug.[83],[84] The electric current generator was attached to these electrodes containing the drug with alligator clips. Alternatively, other investigators had their patients place the treatment site in a basin containing the drug solution. One electrode from the electric current generator was attached to the side of the basin, if metal, or placed at the bottom of the container within the solution but not in contact with the skin of the patient.[85],[86] The second electrode was attached to the patient away from the basin so as to complete the electric circuit. Later commercial electrodes consisted of simple plastic bubbles that acted as fluid reservoirs.[87]

Commercially available electrode designs differ among manufacturers (Table 11-8). The general design for most electrodes is depicted in Figure 11-28. In general, the electrode design consists of an adhesive backing which allows the electrode to adhere firmly to the skin of the patient. An electrically conductive layer is added to this backing to evenly distribute the electric current over the electrode surface area. The conductor composition may be carbon or other conductor and varies by manufacturer. The drug reservoir consists of a substance that holds the drug solution during iontophoresis. The composition of this layer varies between manufacturers, but typically consists of absorptive-type materials (see Table 11-8). Finally, several manufacturers use an additional outer layer that is in contact with the skin. This last layer serves to stabilize the underlying layers of the electrode and/or act as a wicking layer to absorb the applied drug solution. Empi has taken this concept further by separating the drug delivery electrode into a bilayer design that is described in greater detail later. The exception to the above electrode design is IOMED, which uses a polymerized gel (Hydrogel), either alone or within a sponge matrix, as a drug reservoir. A Hydrogel formulation provides a conductive base, easier application, and uniform current distribution at the treatment site.

Appropriate choice of electrodes is a factor that is critical to successful iontophoretic delivery of a drug.[47] The electrode material determines the electrochemistry

TABLE 11-8 | Commercially Available Electrodes

MANUFACTURER	SIZES	DRUG RESERVOIR COMPOSITION	BUFFER SYSTEM
B.L.U.E. ‡ Upper Lower *EMPI* *St. Paul, MN*	4	Cotton Flannel Polyurethane Foam	Ion Exchange Resin
Trans-Q	2	Hydrogel	Ag/AgCl
Trans-Q E	2	Hydrogel/Sponge	Ag/AgCl

Iogel
    IOMED
    Salt Lake City, UT
	3	Hydrogel/Sponge	Ag/AgCl

DynaPak Life-Tech *Houston, TX*	7	Cotton/Rayon	0.9% Saline* 0.5% NaHPO$_4$–*
Iontopatch *Birch Point Medical, Inc.* *Oakdale, MN*	1	Polypropylene Cathode: AgCl/Ag	Anode: Zn/Zn++

The abbreviations are as follows: Ag/AgCl: silver/silver-chloride electrode, Zn: Zinc; * optional buffer addition; ‡ B.L.U.E.: Bilayer Ultra Electrode. The cathode is the negative electrode and the anode is the positive electrode.

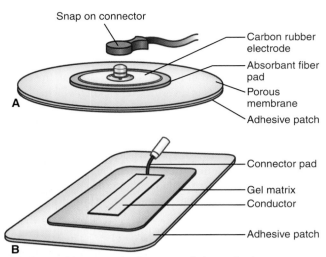

FIGURE 11-28 General schematics of electrode designs for fiber-based **(A)** and hydrogel-based **(B)** iontophoretic electrodes.

occurring at the electrodes. Electrical current must be transferred from the electronic environment, that is, the wires, to the ionic environment, that is, the electrode aqueous solution and the body. Unless suitable mechanisms are used, iontophoresis is accompanied by electrolysis of water. This electrolysis results in a change in the pH within both the electrode and at the electrode-skin interface as follows:

$$2\,H_2O \rightarrow 4\,H^+ + O_2 + 4\,e^- \text{ (anode) } \textit{decrease pH (acid)}$$

Oxidation of water at the anode results in the production of hydrogen ion (H⁺) and a decrease in pH.

$$2\,H_2O + 2\,e^- \rightarrow H_2 + 2\,OH^- \text{ (cathode) } \textit{increase pH}$$
$$\textit{(alkaline)}$$

Reduction of water at the cathode results in the formation of hydroxyl ion (OH⁻) and an increase in pH. This pH change may initiate chemical irritation of the skin, or alter the skin conductivity of the electric current. In addition, both H⁺ and OH⁻ are mobile in the iontophoretic electric field, competing with the ionized drug to carry the current, and ultimately decreasing the transport of the drug into the underlying tissues. A pH-induced drug degradation may also occur at the electrode, decreasing the efficiency of iontophoretic drug delivery.

To avoid these pH changes in the electrode and in the skin at the application site, buffering agents may be used (see Table 11-8). Minimizing pH changes at the electrode may also be accomplished by polymeric ion exchange resins,[46] such as those used by EMPI in the Bilayer Ultra Electrode (BLUE) design (see Table 11-8).

Empi has developed a bilayer drug reservoir electrode with the immobile polymeric resin impregnated into the upper fiber-type layer (BLUE). The lower layer acts as a hydrophilic matrix to absorb and retain the drug solution.

No iontophoresis electrode design is capable of delivering all drugs under every potential condition. Thus, the electrode designs and commercial availability may limit their clinical use for prolong periods or result in suboptimal iontophoretic

delivery with some drugs. The use of saturated gauze or paper towels may result in a nonhomogeneous electric field due to unequal saturation of these applicators with the solution. Such unequal saturation results in higher electric current density through the parts of the towel or gauze that is wetter. This problem may also exist with current marketed iontophoretic electrodes if they are not filled with the solution volume recommended by the manufacturer. The use of a basin to iontophorese the drug removes this high current density problem. However, not all body parts are amenable to being placed in a basin containing the drug solution. In addition, the volume required to fill the basin results in an excessive waste of the drug solution, as the solution will be disposed of following the iontophoresis. The alligator clips that attached the electric current generator also may result in a high electric current density where the clip is attached to the gauze or towel. Marketed electrodes use a dispersal layer to evenly apply the electrical current over the entire surface area of the electrode applicator and through the remaining layers of the electrode. The absence of buffers in the electrode matrix may result in a pH change at both the anode and cathode.

However, a recent investigation examined pH changes in commercially available electrodes at various iontophoretic dosages, and with the cathode as the delivery electrode.[89] With an iontophoretic dosage less than 40 mA-min, no statistically significant pH changes were noted in the non-buffered, buffered, or sacrificial electrode designs. When the iontophoretic dosage was 80 mA*min, there was an increase in the pH of the non-buffered electrode design. These results would suggest that clinical iontophoretic dosages of 40 mA*min or less could be safely conducted in non-buffered electrode designs.

WHY DO I NEED TO KNOW ABOUT...
pH CHANGES
- A pH change at the cathode and the anode may result in minor skin irritation under the electrodes following the treatment intervention.
- Owing to this minor skin irritation, it is advisable to use a moisturizing lotion on the skin after treatment.

BEFORE YOU BEGIN
Ask the patient whether he or she is allergic to the drug that is about to be administered. If there is an allergy, *do not* administer the drug. It is *not* appropriate to assume that the question has been asked previously!

Iontophoretic drug delivery is also proportional to the applied current.[90] In general, 0.5 mA/cm² is often stated to be the maximum current density that should be used on humans.[47] The charge, size, and structure of the drug will influence its potential to be an iontophoresis candidate. Ideal candidates for iontophoresis should be water-soluble, potent drugs that exist in their salt form with high charge density.[91,92] In an iontophoretic formulation, a relative increase in drug concentration compared with other ions will typically result in higher iontophoretic delivery.[93,94] In contrast, an increase in formulation viscosity may decrease the iontophoretic drug flux by hindering the mobility of the drug.[94,95] The pH of the solution will also determine whether the drug is charged or the ratio of the charged and uncharged species.[76] Thus, iontophoretic drug delivery is dependent upon electrode design, drug formulation and charge, and the barrier characteristics of the skin. If the skin is fragile, it will be sensitive to iontophoresis.

APPLICATION GUIDELINES

Based on the previous discussions of the basic concepts of iontophoresis, specific methods should be used during application.

1. The clinician should determine the treatment area and the size of the drug delivery electrode for the application. The electrode should be large enough to cover the treatment area, but not so small that the electrical current density exceeds the 0.5 mA/cm².
2. The clinician should saturate the delivery electrode with the drug solution. This results in the entire surface area of the delivery electrode transferring the current, and minimizes the potential that the localized current density exceeds 0.5 mA/cm². In addition, complete contact between the electrodes and the surface of the skin will also minimize localized high current densities.
3. The clinician should determine the polarity of the drug that was prescribed by the patient's physician to be used for the specific treatment, and whether the drug is an anion or cation when ionized. The drug must be ionized at a pH used for iontophoretic application so that charge-charge repulsion will assist with the transcutaneous delivery. In addition, the clinician should attempt to use a drug solution that has the fewest competing ions to that of the drug.

Once charge of the drug is determined, the appropriate electrode from the battery source should be attached to the delivery electrode, the cathode for anionic drugs and the anode for cationic drugs. Finally, the drug delivery site and the return electrode site should be thoroughly cleaned with an alcohol solution. This removes oils and the uppermost cells from the stratum corneum, the main barrier to iontophoretic drug delivery, and ultimately enhances iontophoretic drug delivery. The placement of the delivery and return electrodes should be according to the manufacturer. In general, the minimal distance between the two electrodes should be 2 cm, or approximately 1 inch. Closer placement of the electrodes may result in a "short circuit current" across the stratum corneum surface without penetration of the electrical current into the deeper tissues. The removal of the drug delivery electrode following the iontophoretic treatment may be determined by the clinician on an individual patient basis. The potential for further drug delivery exists even after the battery source is removed. However, no controlled investigations have been conducted to determine if this additional application has any positive or negative effects on the treatment outcomes.

Experimental and Clinical Iontophoresis of Anti-Inflammatory Drugs

EXPERIMENTAL IONTOPHORESIS OF ANTI-INFLAMMATORY DRUGS

Various pharmacological agents have been iontophoresed to achieve both localized and systemic delivery, and have been reviewed extensively elsewhere.[47,48] Within rehabilitation medicine, the major use of iontophoresis is for the localized delivery of anti-inflammatory drugs. However, clinical investigations documenting the positive outcomes for this procedure are inconsistent. This may be due to the absence of pharmacokinetic data on experimental iontophoresis that is performed under conditions that parallel the clinic. Pharmacokinetics is the examination of the mechanism of absorption, distribution, and elimination of drugs in the body. Pharmacokinetic research examining iontophoresis to prevent local inflammation has used both **steroidal anti-inflammatory drugs** (SAIDs) and NSAIDs. The former are anti-inflammatory drugs derived from cholesterol and classified as glucocorticoids.[96] NSAIDS are a chemically diverse group of drugs that inhibit the production of prostaglandin-type compounds.[97]

Dexamethasone phosphate is an anionic prodrug from the SAID class. The prodrug dexamethasone phosphate is converted to the active form of the drug, dexamethasone, within the tissues.[98] The initial and most commonly cited pharmacokinetic analysis of dexamethasone phosphate iontophoresis in a single rhesus monkey calculated a 26% loss from the from the applicator electrode, supposedly into the underlying tissue. Post-iontophoretic drug penetration was documented down to submuscular tissues and intra-articular spaces. Once converted to dexamethasone, the negative charge is absent from the drug. However, the iontophoretic parameters used in this initial investigation do not parallel current clinical use of dexamethasone phosphate iontophoresis. The delivery electrode was the anode, theoretical constructs suggest the cathode as the appropriate electrode, the dosage exceeded most clinical dosages at 100 mA*min (Table 11-9), chloride ions were present in solution and should decrease the drug delivery efficiency, and the current density (at 0.94 mA/cm²) exceeded the previously specified safety limit (of 0.5 mA/cm²). Finally, the drug pharmacokinetics were indirectly measured by radioactivity. Subsequent in vitro research has established that optimal parameters for dexamethasone phosphate iontophoresis are from the cathode, and without competing anions such as chloride in solution.[99,100] In addition, investigators[101] have proposed that during iontophoresis dexamethasone phosphate, and other drugs, carry the ionic current from the delivery electrode into the epidermis. Here smaller more highly mobile and numerous competing ions such as Cl⁻, for dexamethasone phosphate, carry the ionic current to the other electrode in the circuit. The dexamethasone phosphate is "dropped off" in a depot in the epidermis. Deeper tissue penetration by the drug is

TABLE 11-9 | Clinical Iontophoresis of Glucocorticoids in Musculoskeletal Dysfunction

DYSFUNCTION	IONTO POLARITY	PARAMETERS DOSAGE (MA*MIN)	PHARMACOLOGICAL AGENT	RX	OUTCOME
Musculoskeletal Inflammation	Anode	85	Dex/Lido	1–3	Subjective Pain Relief[127]
Musculoskeletal Inflammation	?	45	Dex/Lido	4	Subjective & Objective Improvements[128]
Musculoskeletal Dysfunction	Anode & Cathode	3–7	Kenacort-A	11	56% Subjects Pain Relief[129]
Infrapatellar Tendinitis	?	40–80	Dex/Lido	6	Subjective & Objective Improvements[130]
Carpal Tunnel Syndrome	?	40–45	Dex/Lido	3	58% Subjective & Objective Improvements[131]
Rheumatic Knee	Cathode	80	Dex	3	Subjective Improvement Only[78]
Plantar Fasciitis	Cathode	40	Dex	6	Enhanced Rehabilitation[79]
TMJ Dysfunction	Cathode	40	Dex/Lido	3	Conflicting Results[80,81]

Abbreviations: **Dex**: Dexamethasone; **Dex/Lido**: Dexamethasone and Lidocaine; **Kenacort-A**: Triamcinolone-acetonide; **Ionto**: Iontophoresis; **Rx**: Number of Treatments; **TMJ**: Temporomandibular Joint

Sources:

78- Li, Ghanem, Peck, et al

79- Gudeman, Eisele, Heidt, et al

80- Reid, Dionne, Sicard, Rosenbaum, et al

81- Schiffman, Braun, and Lindgren

127- Harris

128- Bertolucci

129- Chantraine, Ludy, and Berger

130- Pellecchia, Hamel, and Behnke

131- Banta

dependent upon passive diffusion and removal by the vasculature.

Pharmacological support exists for the concept that vasodilation at the iontophoretic site decreases localized drug delivery and increases systemic absorption, whereas vasoconstriction at the iontophoretic site has the opposite effect.[102–104] Glucocorticoids, such as dexamethasone phosphate, have a vasoconstrictive effect on the human cutaneous vasculature.[62] This vasoconstriction is not observed during 40 mA-min conventional cathodic iontophoresis, at 3 mA, due to the galvanic induced erythema, but is observed following a similar cathodic iontophoresis dosage using low current (0.05 to 0.1 mA).[101] Thus, further increases in localized dexamethasone phosphate delivery may occur if iontophoretic current densities that do not cause erythema at the application site are used.

Dexamethasone phosphate was not measurable in the local venous vasculature in humans during or following 40 or 80 mA*min cathodic iontophoresis of dexamethasone phosphate at the forearm.[106]

The pharmacokinetics of anionic NSAIDs have also been examined.[48] Although the iontophoretic transport between dexamethasone phosphate and NSAIDs and their pharmacokinetics post-iontophoresis are not identical, relevant general constructs concerning the iontophoresis of anionic anti-inflammatory drugs for localized delivery may be derived. However, many newer investigations examining transcutaneous iontophoretic delivery of NSAIDs use iontophoretic parameters not clinically available. Therefore, the clinical value of these investigations is questionable and will not be discussed. Iontophoresis of several different NSAIDs under clinically relevant parameters is optimal from the cathode, and tissue penetration under the application site appears to be down to the fascia-superficial muscle interface.[64,108–110] An initial pharmacokinetic conclusion from several of the in vivo iontophoretic investigations using the NSAID ketoprofen was that higher current densities, 0.28 compared with 0.14 mA/cm^2, resulted in greater drug delivery for the same 160 mA-min dosage.[48,108,109] However, subsequent re-evaluation of the results suggest that the higher current density resulted in greater iontophoresis induced erythema and increased absorption of this NSAID from the application site into the systemic vasculature. This is based upon evidence that ketoprofen efficiently redistributes from the interstitial space under the iontophoretic site into the local vasculature and that iontophoretic currents in the range of 0.5 mA/cm^2 stimulate localized erythema.[111–113] Several investigations also documented a time requirement for transcutaneous transport of ketoprofen.[108,109,111,112] The time delay between initiation of iontophoresis with ketoprofen and presence in the local vasculature is due to the permeation of the drug across the epidermis. A similar time delay for transcutaneous permeation of dexa-methasone phosphate may also occur. Glucocorticoids such as dexamethasone do not have extensive extravascular binding, and drug delivered to the interstitial space should redistribute quickly into the local vascular compartment.[96] However, for dexamethasone phosphate the precise time requirement for an iontophoresis treatment in order to obtain transcutaneous transport is at present undocumented. Finally, as with the dexamethasone phosphate iontophoretic investigation,[107] following an 160 mA*min cathodic iontophoresis of ketoprofen no drug was detectable in the articular space.[114]

The pharmacokinetics for iontophoresis of SAIDs and NSAIDs has been examined. What is still uncertain is the local tissue depth at which SAIDs and NSAIDs are delivered by the iontophoresis, and to what extent the systemic vasculature delivers these drugs to the deeper tissues.

CLINICAL IONTOPHORESIS OF ANTI-INFLAMMATORY DRUGS

Clinically, in the United States, the majority of iontophoresis in rehabilitation medicine uses dexamethasone phosphate. In a placebo-controlled investigation the capability of iontophoresis to prevent experimentally induced delayed onset muscle soreness (DOMS) in 18 female subjects was examined.[115] The subjects were exposed to quadriceps eccentric exercise. Lidocaine/dexamethasone phosphate anodic iontophoresis, at a dosage of 65 mA*min, was administered 24 hours later, and final assessment was conducted 48 hours post exercise. Muscle function assessments and patient perception of soreness were conducted every day during the following 3-day trial. Although the iontophoresis-treated group demonstrated significant improvement in the subjective assessment of muscle soreness, none of the objective muscle function tests were different between the groups.

A major application of iontophoresis within rehabilitation medicine is the treatment of acute musculoskeletal inflammation. The clinical investigations examining glucocorticoid iontophoresis as a treatment for these dysfunctions, the iontophoretic parameters, pharmacological agent used, and the clinical outcomes are reviewed in Table 11-9. As may be observed from the table, the polarity of the drug delivery electrode is absent from a number of the publications. This void would make replication of these studies difficult. In addition, several of the investigations used drug solutions with competing ions to the dexamethasone phosphate. These competing ions would be Cl$^-$ from the lidocaine, as the lidocaine is formulated as a chloride salt. The presence of Cl$^-$ would result in suboptimal transcutaneous dexamethasone phosphate. The majority of investigations in Table 11-9 found improvements in both subjective and objective outcomes. However, one investigation found only an improvement in the subjective outcome, but not the objective outcome.[116] Another significant clinical observation is from an investigation treating plantar fasciitis.[117] Patients in the experimental group received dexamethasone phosphate iontophoresis in addition to the regular physical therapy regimen. The patients in the control group received placebo iontophoresis with the same physical therapy regimen. The iontophoretic group demonstrated an enhanced rate of rehabilitation. However, at the 1-month follow-up, both groups demonstrated equivalent clinical scores. These results suggest that dexamethasone phosphate iontophoresis in certain musculoskeletal dysfunction may enhance the rate of rehabilitation, but may not ultimately affect the long-term outcome. Only one musculoskeletal pathophysiology has been examined in two separate investigations. Temporomandibular joint (TMJ) dysfunction was examined by two investigations using similar dexamethasone phosphate iontophoretic protocols.[108,109] One investigation documented positive outcomes from the treatments,[119] whereas the other found no significant difference between the treatment and placebo groups.[118]

Finally, physical therapists are being requested to use iontophoresis for conservative nonsurgical treatment of Peyronie's disease.[120] However, when conducted in accordance with the literature, this is polypharmacy treatment, and should be conducted in close association with a pharmacist for formulary services. From the published controlled investigations several iontophoretic and pharmaceutical parameters are available. The anode is used for the drug delivery electrode, and is a result of the other drugs co-iontophoresed with dexamethasone phosphate. The iontophoretic dosage varies between 60 to 100 mA*min, and the number of treatments varies both between investigations and between patients with a range of 3 to 53. The other drugs co-iontophoresed with dexamethasone phosphate again vary between investigations but may include verapamil, lidocaine, and orgotein. The clinical value of this iontophoretic procedure will await further clinical examination.

In aggregate, clinical investigations suggest that dexamethasone phosphate iontophoresis may result in improved objective and/or subjective clinical outcomes in variety of musculoskeletal dysfunctions. However, inter-investigation variability makes comparisons difficult, and basic pharmacokinetic and pharmacodynamic mechanisms remain unexplained. Finally, insufficient experimental evidence exists to determine the precise depth of subcutaneous tissue delivery following iontophoresis of anionic anti-inflammatory drugs or which drugs provide the greatest potential for transcutaneous permeation by iontophoresis.

Reported Adverse Responses From Iontophoresis

Adverse reactions reported by the patients during and after iontophoresis have been related to the procedure. These adverse effects include first-degree burn, transient erythema at the drug delivery electrode, metallic taste when iontophoresis was used on the face, and one of the following during iontophoresis: tingling, burning, stinging, or a pulling sensation.[46,121,122] Additional reports of shock to patients have been documented as a result of abruptly turning the device off while the patient is still connected to the device circuit.[122] Finally, one clinical study documented contact dermatitis in a patient following iontophoresis of 5-fluorouracil at both the site of application and a distant site.[123] This last report suggests a systemic reaction as the result of a drug iontophoresed for local application.

Use of Electrical Stimulation

APTA's *Guide to Physical Therapist Practice*[8] categorizes electrical stimulation under the procedural intervention Electro-therapeutic Modalities. This intervention has application across multiple practice patterns and is a valuable adjunct therapy in the treatment of musculoskeletal, neuromuscular, and integumentary system problems. The general indications, contraindications, and precautions are discussed in this section.

INDICATIONS

Electricity can be applied to the body to treat (clinical stimulation) or to diagnose (nerve conduction velocity studies). Electricity from the body can be recorded to treat (biofeedback) or to diagnose (electromyography). Many indications are addressed in the section on therapeutic goals.

Electrotherapy has been long associated with pain management, muscle strengthening, and stimulation of denervated muscle. It also has a place in wound care, fracture healing, promotion of circulation, and edema management. It has been used to increase joint ROM, deliver medications through the skin (iontophoresis), replace orthotics, reduce muscle guarding and spasticity, and reduce scoliosis.

CONTRAINDICATIONS

The contraindications of electrical stimulation are relatively few. Pregnancy should be considered a contraindication even when applied to an area distant from the abdomen. Pain management with electrical current during labor is occasionally used.

Electrical current can interfere with the functioning of a pacemaker. A demand pacemaker senses the heart activity and responds accordingly. A pulse from an external stimulator could deceive a demand pacemaker into suppressing needed rhythms or creating abnormal rhythms.[38] Fixed pacemakers could be affected by signals through the leads.

Electrical stimulation should not be used in the presence of other electrical implanted stimulators, in patients with cardiac arrhythmic instability, or in cases with cardiac conduction disturbances. A stable cardiac patient with a history of angina or myocardial infarction may receive electrical stimulation, but electrodes must be placed cautiously avoiding current flow across midline in the chest area. The patient should be monitored with an ECG initially and then closely monitored during treatment. Some therapists do not apply electrical stimulation to a patient with cardiac disease, whether stable or not.

Cancer is treated as a contraindication because of the risk of metastasis. This contraindication is sometimes waived in favor of the pain relief when patients are in advanced stages.

Stimulation should not be performed adjacent to or distal to an area of thrombophlebitis or phlebothrombosis because of risk of emboli. Many therapists treat these conditions as totally contraindicated for an electrical stimulation treatment.

Electrical stimulation should not be used in the presence of active tuberculosis. It should not be done over the carotid sinus or in areas of active hemorrhage.

PRECAUTIONS

Electrical stimulation should be used cautiously in the presence of obesity. Fat is an electrical insulator and stimulation is generally not well tolerated. Greater-than-normal current levels are often required to achieve the desired physiological effect.[38]

Caution should be exercised in areas of absent or diminished sensation. Areas of abnormal impedance should be avoided. Electrical currents can exacerbate eczema, psoriasis, acne, and dermatitis and can spread infections.[19] Patients including those with diabetes with thin fragile skin could be at risk for breakdown.

Peripheral neuropathies may prevent generation of muscle contractions at stimulation levels that are comfortable and safe.[38] Areas of denervation will not respond to any form of current other than DC.

In the presence of metal, either internal or external fixation devices, electrodes should be positioned with the metal well outside the pathway of current.

The patient should be cleared for active exercise in protocols requiring motor levels of stimulation. Care should be taken that the force of contraction is within a tolerated and permitted range of motion.[38]

Judgment is necessary to determine if electrical stimulation should be applied to any patient who is unable to follow instructions or provide feedback to the therapist. The treatment must be closely supervised if the decision is made to deliver the electrical stimulation.

Stimulation to patients with spinal cord injury may enhance an episode of dysreflexia.[38]

Electrical Safety
Equipment and User

Electrical shock is the response of the body to any electrical exposure that places the person within the circuit. This statement has just described treatment with electrical stimulation. The clinician must be aware of the potential dangers of applying electrical current and the measures ensuring safe treatment.

The magnitude of electrical shock depends on the amount of current (amperes) forced into the body. Currents between 100 and 200 mA are lethal.[124] Physiological reactions to current intensities follow a progression of sensation, muscle contraction, fibrillation, defibrillation, and burns.[125] Electrical shock is first perceived as a faint tingling by sensory nerves around 1 mA, but current levels as low as several microamperes have been perceived by the finger tips.[126] Let-go current is the maximum current level allowing the voluntary release of the current source and emphasizes the danger of AC over DC. The motor response to DC is a twitch, whereas AC causes a holding or tetanizing contraction. The ability to *let go* may be lost at current levels of AC around 20 mA.[126] This value increases with pulsatile currents. The intrapulse and interpulse intervals provide current interruptions. Breathing can become labored at 20 mA of AC and cease before 75 mA.[124] Uncoordinated twitching of the heart's ventricles (ventricular fibrillation) occurs at levels greater than 80 mA.[42] The heart will maintain a sustained contraction (ventricular defibrillation) at 6 Å (6,000 mA) and return to normal rhythm if exposure to current at that level is of short duration.[127] Burns occur at current levels above 12 Å.

Electrical shock is either *macroshock* or *microshock*. Macroshock is a perceptible current at levels of greater than or equal to 1 mA.[42] It occurs when current is introduced to the body through the skin and enters the body cavity. Microshock is below perceptible range and results from exposure to currents below 1 mA applied directly to the myocardium.[42] The current bypasses skin and enters the heart directly through cardiac catheter tips or myocardial electrodes. Pacemakers can be very susceptible to microshock through the pacemaker wires. The upper safety limit margin of current passing directly to the heart is 10 mA.[126]

As discussed earlier in the chapter, body tissues offer resistance to the passage of current. Skin resistance protects internal organs from shock and determines how much current enters. This resistance varies between people and varies within the individual depending on point of contact and skin hydration. Dry skin offers around 500,000 V of resistance, whereas moist skin offers approximately 1,000 V.[124] This protective resistance is bypassed when an invasive electrode is used, but the use of this type of electrode is not common practice clinically.

Electric power is delivered to the machine through the ends of two wires having an electrical potential of 115 V between them. The *live* (hot) wire has the high electrical potential. The *neutral* wire has 0 potential and connects to the ground. The term "ground" refers to anything with an electrical connection to the earth. Earth is an inexhaustible source of electrons and is capable of accepting or donating large quantities of charge.[128] Generally,

current flows from the live wire through the electrical unit back to the neutral wire and then to earth.[18] An exchange occurs between charged bodies and earth. A positively charged body will take electrons and a negatively charged body will give electrons to earth. Current flows. Grounded means there is no difference in potential between the conductor and earth, so current will not flow.

One potential clinical hazard is direct contact with the live wire circuit through a frayed power cord or an outlet problem.[126] Another possible hazard, earth shock, results from an indirect connection made between the live wire and the ground.[18] The live wire, possibly because of faulty or old insulation, makes contact inside of the machine with its casing. A person touching the casing and standing on the ground draws this current and completes a circuit between the live wire and the ground. Newer machines are now usually cased in plastic or other insulating material. Earth shock can also result from a phenomenon called leakage or *stray* current. It is an inherent flow of a small amount of current from the live circuit along an insulating surface such as the casing or accessories. Electric shocks can also result from contact with grounded objects such as water pipes, damp floor, and radiators during electrical treatments.

Earth shock can be avoided by a grounding wire that provides the path of least resistance from the machine casing to earth. The grounding wire, normally not conducting current, triggers a fuse on the live wire when electrical problems cause current to flow through it. This stops current flow and alerts the operator to a problem. A polarized outlet and three-pronged plug provide this grounding circuit. The outlet receptacle has three slots, a small rectangular one for the live wire connection, a larger rectangular one for the neutral wire connection, and a round opening for the ground wire connection. This protective round pin is longer than the rectangular prongs, assuring that the ground wire is the first wire connected to the circuit and the last unplugged.[19]

Failure of the grounding wire to be connected in the building to a ground source or breaking of the ground wire in the receptacle can go undetected, creating a potential hazard. The electrical system is believed to be safe when in actuality the grounding circuit is non-functional. A ground fault interrupter (GFI) is a sensor shutting down the electrical circuit when it senses changes in electrical potentials, impedance, or an increase in normal leakage current levels.

Preventive maintenance is necessary to assure electrical safety in the treatment area. New equipment purchased should have the Underwriters Laboratory (UL) approval seal, assuring the maximum degree of safety.[128] Table 11-10 outlines other safety guidelines that should be observed in the clinic. Electrical safety comes with awareness and knowledge. The clinician should always read the manufacturer's manual and be sure that he or she understands the limitations of the unit as well as its safety features.

TABLE 11-10 | Electrical Safety in the Clinic

- Replacement of standard outlets with ground fault interrupters (GFI).

- Replacement of plugs with hospital-grade Underwriters Laboratory (UL) plugs with green dot.
- Yearly maintenance checks of all electrical equipment by biomedical engineer.
- Dated inspection sticker affixed to all electrical units.

- Unplug equipment not in use.

- Disconnect machines from outlet receptacles by plug, not cord.
- Frequently check the integrity of plugs, cords, and electrical stimulation leads for fraying or disruptions.
- Report loose-gripping connections between plug and outlet receptacles.

- Never use extension cords.

- Never use cheater adapters allowing three-pronged plugs to be used in receptacles made for two-pronged plugs only.
- Do not use electrical equipment near objects or environments that draw current.

- Post sign notifying usage of equipment that may interfere with pacemakers.

- These reduce the chance of dangerous power surges affecting patient safety.
- The UL seal indicates that the plug is safe for use and grounded to protect patient safety.
- All electrical medical equipment that will be used with patients needs to be maintained annually! Biomedical engineers are specifically trained to perform safety checks on equipment that is intended to be used on humans.
- If something is not in use, unplug it to protect it from power surges that could potentially damage the safety mechanisms built into the system.
- Plugs, not power cords, are built to be pulled from the wall receptacle.
- If a power cord is frayed, it could potentially be a source of an unanticipated electrical short.
- Loose connections may result in electrical shorts, which may result in a fire hazard.
- Extension cords may not be capable of handling the amount of current that the electrical stimulator requires, which could then lead to a safety hazard.
- Three-pronged plugs are grounded for safety. Do *not* remove safety elements from treatment interventions with patients!
- Using electrical equipment in an environment where current can be altered means that the parameters may vary without knowledge of the clinician.
- Pacemakers could potentially pick up transient electromagnetic energy that may alter their function.

Patient Factors
Patient Education

The public is familiar with electricity and the potential for shock and electrocution. Many patients may be initially fearful of treatment. A patient may be anxious or reluctant to place his or her foot in a tub of water containing two electrodes.

The key to successful treatment is patient education and cooperation. The questions concerning patient education that must be posed are *what* and *how much*. It has been shown that information can sometimes increase and develop stressful feelings that might not have been present ordinarily.[129] Two types of coping styles are identified. There are those people who seek information to get through an aversive event and there are those people who would rather not know anything. Patients treated according to their coping style exhibited increased tolerance levels to electrical stimulation.[129]

Certain safety instructions are necessary. Information that must be given includes the sensation of treatment and instructions concerning touching of controls, changing body position, and calling the therapist when there is a problem or change in sensation. Informational material includes the goal and expected outcome of treatment, number of expected treatment sessions, and the treatment time. Patients using the unit at home require more detailed instructions on how the unit works, application of electrodes, purpose and consequence of dial adjustments, how to protect the skin and inspect area before and after treatment, and under what circumstances to discontinue treatment. Written instructions should be given, especially diagrams of electrode placement.[130]

Patient Perspective

Remember that patients have had virtually no experience with electrical stimulation and there will be questions. Patients will need to know that it is safe, that you have felt it, and what to expect when they feel it. The patient may not let you adjust the intensity to a high enough level to produce a motor response during the first visit. You will need to establish a level of trust with the patient before he or she will let you accomplish this. It is also important to remember that positive reinforcement is very helpful to the patient who is not quite sure what to expect when he or she feels a muscle contract with electrical stimulation.

Patients' Frequently Asked Questions

1. **Is it safe to use electrical stimulation during an electrical storm?**
2. **Will I be "electrocuted" by the stimulator?**
3. **What is the difference between the stimulators that are used in the clinic and a defibrillator?**
4. **How long will the sensation of the stimulator continue after treatment?**

Equipment Positioning

Electrical stimulation delivered by a line-powered unit (versus battery unit) should be administered in a predetermined area within the clinical setting where appropriate outlets (GFIs) have been installed. Electrical equipment generates heat and should be well ventilated. Equipment should not be placed next to water pipes, radiators, or other sources that may draw current, creating a shock hazard. The machine should be situated close to the wall outlet to avoid tension on the cord and possible tripping over cords. Positioning of the electrical stimulation unit must allow easy access to the therapist for adjustment of controls as well as avoiding excessive tension on lead wires or a situation where the patient is able to adjust parameters without supervision. The patient should be informed as to which dial controls the amplitude and how to turn it down. The current interruption switch should be easily accessed.

Skin Inspection

The intensity of stimulation is guided by the patient's response and tolerance level. A sensory assessment of the treatment area is essential to establish patient reliability. The skin must be carefully inspected before electrodes are applied. Skin tone and color should be assessed for indications of circulatory impairment and fragility that could result in breakdown or tissue damage. The skin should be examined for conditions affecting skin impedance such as edema, ischemia, scars, skin lesions, and abrasions. Areas of abnormally high impedance require increased current levels for penetration. Areas of abnormally low impedance draw current and increase total current in a small area. Tissue damage could result from either situation. Abrasions and open areas that cannot be insulated with petroleum jelly should not be treated unless the treatment objective is wound healing.

Patient Positioning

The basic tenets of positioning are patient comfort and accessibility to the treatment area. There are several considerations specific to electrical stimulation. Positioning should permit enough slack in lead wires from machine to electrodes so that connections will not disengage during treatment. Firm contact and securing of electrodes will influence choice of position. Some placement sites may require the patient's body weight on the electrodes. The patient must be in a position to use a call button or disengage the machine if a problem arises.

The Treatment

A training period may be necessary with electrical stimulation, and required stimulation levels may not be achieved during the first session. Patient anxiety can sometimes be relieved by allowing the patient control of increasing the amplitude dial.

Muscle contraction time can be limited to 5- to 7-second peaks with low-level repetitions of 10 to 15 contractions the first treatment to prevent initial soreness. On and off times have a high ratio initially (1:4; 1:5) but are reduced in subsequent treatments with conditioning. Please keep in mind that these ratios must be spelled out in terms of the number of seconds of On time and Off time for documentation purposes to decrease the potential for confusion. An On time of 2 seconds and Off time of 8 seconds does fit into the 1:4 ratio but it is not the same as 10 seconds On and 40 seconds Off which would also fit into that ratio.

The patient should be asked if he or she feels tingling in all areas of the electrode. The electrode could be secured improperly or losing its conductivity if the answer is no. If the patient is not feeling any sensation at all as amplitude is increased past a point where sensory fibers should fire, stop immediately and drop the amplitude control back down to zero before making any adjustments. Most contemporary machines have reset controls to protect against high levels of current surging into the patient when machines are energized with current levels up. These types of controls require that amplitude dials be clicked off prior to increasing the amplitude. Never increase amplitude during the off phase of the current cycle.

Clinical judgment must be exercised as to when a treatment should be discontinued because of physical or mental intolerance, preventing the safe achievement of intended goals.

The electrical stimulation treatment can be divided into *pretreatment*, *delivery*, *post-treatment*, and *documentation*. Patient comfort, tolerance, and safety are priorities. The manufacturer's instruction manual must be carefully read, understood, and followed. The following general guidelines will only assist with sequencing the treatment.

PRETREATMENT

1. Machine wires and electrode check (inspection dates should be periodically checked) is performed.
2. Patient education is given.
3. Machine is plugged into the wall outlet.
4. Turn the machine power switch on.
5. Patient is positioned.
6. Skin in treatment area is inspected; gross assessment of sensation is made.
7. Electrical stimulation machine is positioned.
8. Electrode placement sites are determined.
9. Treatment area is cleaned; electrodes are prepared and secured.
10. Preset parameters on machine area adjusted such as frequency, phase duration, delivery mode (interrupted or continuous), on-off time, ramp, and choice of polarity, treatment timer.
11. Make sure amplitude dials are set on zero.

DELIVERY

1. Increase amplitude to stimulation level but always within patient's tolerance.
2. Ask patient *what he or she feels* and *where he or she feels. it.*
3. Adjust any parameters requiring modification
4. Stay with patient for several minutes to monitor reaction, tolerance, and appropriate amplitude level.
5. Continue to monitor patient reaction and tolerance periodically through treatment.

POST-TREATMENT

1. Turn amplitude to zero.
2. Remove electrodes.
3. Turn machine power off.
4. Inspect treatment area.
5. Note all variables set for treatment and document.
6. Unplug unit from wall receptacle.

DOCUMENTATION

Documentation must be thorough and inclusive. Notes must stand up under close scrutiny in this age of liability and reimbursement. The written note ensures consistent replication of treatment; is a written record describing the patient's physical state, reactions, and progress; validates treatment success or failure to determine effectiveness; and justifies treatment for appropriate reimbursement.

The general elements of the electrotherapy note include the problem, therapeutic goal, type of application (e.g., ESTR), skin status, electrode technique, electrode size, number and placement of electrodes, commercial stimulation unit used, electrical parameters of treatment, treatment time, and response to treatment.

Give specific settings for all parameters adjusted. Documented parameters may include, but are not limited to the following:

- Location of treatment area, side of body
- Duration of treatment
- Delivery mode (continuous, interrupted)
- Therapeutic stimulation level (subsensory, sensory, motor, noxious)
- Current type (AC, DC, pulsed)
- Waveform (monophasic, biphasic, polyphasic)
- Polarity of active electrode (monophasic waveforms)
- Frequency (pps, burst frequency, carrier frequency)
- On-off/ramp times

A thorough note, reflecting all of the parameters, is essential for the first treatment. Changes in parameters and patient response will suffice for subsequent notes.

Clinical Decision-Making

Clinical decision-making is an ongoing process during patient/client management. In electrical stimulation, decisions may range from "*the choice to use electrical stimulation*" to "*the determination of the current parameters.*" Figure 11-29 outlines the components of the clinical decision-making process with electrical stimulation.

Summary

Throughout this chapter, electrical stimulation has been discussed with the hope that there is an understanding of basic concepts, terminology, and the underlying physiology so that the learner will be able to differentiate between them and make sound decisions regarding their application for patient treatment interventions. Electrical stimulation can sometimes be one of the most frightening forms of treatment that a patient receives unless the clinician clearly understands what he or she is applying and how to make it comfortable for the patient. Those skills come from a real sense of knowing what the parameters of electrical stimulation are and how to adjust them, explain the relationship of their adjustment to what the patient will feel, and, ultimately, accomplish a treatment goal.

If DC is selected, electrical stimulation can be used to deliver medication across the skin for specific localized effects to the underlying tissues. However, if the wrong polarity is selected for the treatment electrode, nothing will cross into the patient. The application of DC and all other forms of electrical stimulation relies first upon the learner having a thorough understanding of the mechanics behind what they are using. When attempting to use DC, the same polarity must be used for the active electrode if the ultimate goal is the delivery of a medication via iontophoreses. It is also imperative that the clinician ask the patient whether or not he or she is allergic to the medication and document the patient's positive or negative response.

Electrical stimulation is a modality that is capable of helping clinicians to accomplish several treatment goals. All it takes is a thorough understanding of the devices and some basic understanding of Ohm's law. The primary role that the skin plays is one of protection, preventing the passage of current into the body. Once a clinician has a good understanding of how to manage skin resistance, then using electrical stimulation can facilitate the accomplishment of treatment goals.

Electrical Stimulation Clinical Decision Making Tree

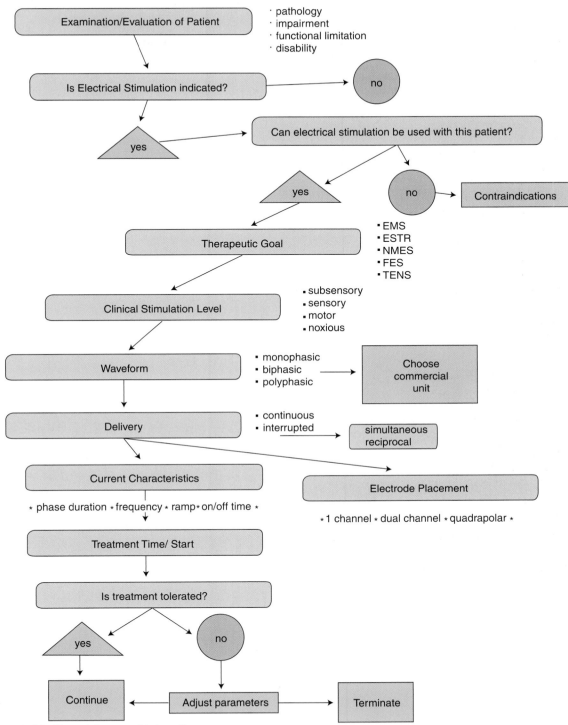

FIGURE 11-29 Clinical Decision-Making Tree.

Review Questions

1. Which of the following definitions best fits DC?
   a. It is the continuous monophasic interrupted flow of charged particles ceasing for at least 1 second, resulting in a net charge
   b. It is the continuous monophasic uninterrupted flow of charged particles ceasing for at least 1 second, resulting in a net charge
   c. It is the continuous monophasic uninterrupted flow of charged particles, resulting in a net charge
   d. It is the continuous monophasic interrupted flow of charged particles, resulting in a net charge

2. Which of the following definitions best fits AC?
   a. It is the continuous biphasic uninterrupted flow of charged particles, resulting in no net charge
   b. It is the continuous biphasic uninterrupted flow of charged particles ceasing for at least 1 second, resulting in a net charge
   c. It is the continuous biphasic interrupted flow of charged particles ceasing for at least 1 second, resulting in a net charge
   d. It is the continuous biphasic interrupted flow of charged particles ceasing for at least 1 second, resulting in no net charge

3. Which of the following definitions best fits PC?
   a. It is the continuous biphasic interrupted flow of charged particles ceasing for at least 1 second, which may result in a net charge
   b. It is biphasic or monophasic interrupted flow of charged particles ceasing for at least 1 second, which may result in a net charge
   c. It is biphasic or monophasic uninterrupted flow of charged particles ceasing for at least 1 second, resulting in a net charge
   d. It is the continuous monophasic interrupted flow of charged particles ceasing for at least 1 second, resulting in no net charge

4. Which of the following statements is most accurate regarding the application of iontophoresis?
   a. The treatment electrode must be the same polarity as any medication that is being delivered to the patient
   b. The dispersive electrode must be the same polarity as any medication that is being delivered to the patient
   c. The patient must be informed that he or she will need to expect to tolerate discomfort with the electrical stimulation with iontophoresis
   d. It is not necessary to ask patients if they are allergic to iontophoretic medications since they have been prescribed these by their physician

5. You are adjusting the electrical stimulation unit on a patient and she reports that what she is feeling is a thumping sensation but you wanted it to feel smooth and tingling. Which parameter would you need to adjust to make the sensation feel more like a tingling sensation?
   a. The pulse duration
   b. The intensity
   c. The polarity
   d. The frequency

DISCUSSION QUESTIONS

1. How does Ohm's law relate to constant current and constant voltage outputs? Why would it potentially be important to know about the equipment that is being used?

2. Identify the three types of current and describe how they differ in structure and usage.

3. What are the differences between the different waveforms in terms of structure, chemical effects, and usage?

4. What are the differences between (a) ramp and rise time; (b) intrapulse, interpulse, and off time; (c) pulse and burst; and (d) phase charge and total current?

5. What are the indications, contraindications, and precautions for the use of electrical stimulation and why are they so listed?

6. What are the differences between sensory, motor, and pain fiber activation in terms of sensation, recruitment order, and the relationship of their strength duration curves?

7. How does a central nervous system generated contraction differ from one generated by electrical stimulation?

8. What can be done to reduce fatigue when using electrical stimulation to elicit a muscle contraction?

REFERENCES

1. Watkins, A: A Manual of Electrotherapy. Lea & Febiger, Philadelphia, 1962.
2. American Physical Therapy Association: Electrotherapeutic Terminology in Physical Therapy. Section on Clinical Electrophysiology, 2001, Alexandria, VA.
3. Geddes, L: A short history of the electrical stimulation of excitable tissue. Physiologist (Suppl) 27:S-1, 1984.
4. Licht, S: History of electrodiagnosis. In Licht, S (ed): Electrodiagnosis and Electromyography, ed 3. Elizabeth Licht, New Haven, CT, 1971.
5. Licht, S: History of electrotherapy. In Stillwell, G (ed): Therapeutic Electricity and Ultraviolet Radiation, ed 3. William and Wilkins, Baltimore/London, 1983.
6. Marcello, P: The Ambiguous Frog: The Galvani-Volta Controversy on Animal Electricity, translated by Mandelbaum. Princeton University Press, Princeton, NJ, 1992.
7. McNeal, D: 2000 Years of electrical stimulation. In Hambrect, T, and Reswick, J (eds): Functional Electrical Stimulation: Application in Neural Prosthesis, Vol 3. Marcel Dekker, New York, 1977.
8. American Physical Therapy Association: Guide to Physical Therapist Practice. 2001: American Physical Therapy Association, Alexandria, VA.
9. Baker, L, et al: Effects of waveform on comfort during neuromuscular electrical stimulation. Clin Orthop Rel Res (233):75, 1988.
10. Bleese, P, et al: Implanted cardiac pacemakers: Clinical experience and evaluation. Med Progr Technol 1:69, 1972.
11. Ko, W: Instrumentation for neuromuscular stimulation. In Hambrect, T (ed): Functional Electrical Stimulation: Application in Neural Prosthesis. Marcel Dekker, New York, 1977.
12. Nashold, B, Somjen, G, and Friedman, H: The effects of stimulating the dorsal columns of man. Med Progr Technol 1:89, 1972.
13. Shealy, C: Electrical control of the nervous system. Med Progr Technol 2:71, 1974.
14. Mills, P, Deakin, M, and Kiff, E: Percutaneous electrical stimulation for ano-rectal incontinence. Physiotherapy 76:433, 1990.
15. Shelly, T: Implanted stimulators for the control of urinary incontinence: the physicians and patients standpoint. Med Progr Technol 1:82, 1972.
16. Ward, AR: Electrical stimulation using kilohertz-frequency alternating current. Phys Ther 89:181, 2009.
17. Binder, S: Applications of low- and high-voltage electrotherapeutic currents. In Wolf, S (ed): Electrotherapy. Churchill Livingstone, Edinburgh, Scotland, 1981.
18. Forster, A, and Palastanga, N: Clayton's Electrotherapy: Theory and Practice, ed 8. Bailliere Tindall Books, London, 1981.
19. Wadsworth, J, and Chanmugam, A: Electrophysical Agents in Physiotherapy: Therapeutic and Diagnostic Use, ed 2. Science Press, Marrickville, Australia, 1983.
20. Rutkove, SB: Electrical Impedance Myography: Background, Current State, and Future Directions. Muscle Nerve 40(6):936–946, 2009.
21. Kahn, A, and Maveus, T: Technical aspects of electrical stimulation devices. Med Progr Technol 1:58, 1972.
22. Kukulka, C: Principles of neuromuscular excitation. In Gersh, M (ed): Electrotherapy in Rehabilitation. FA Davis, Philadelphia, 1992.
23. Patterson, R: Instrumentation for electrotherapy. In Stillwell, G (ed): Therapeutic Electricity and Ultraviolet Radiation. Williams & Wilkins, Baltimore, 1983.
24. Gracanin, F, and Trnkoxzy, A: Optimal stimulation parameters for minimum pain in the chronic situation of innervated muscle. Arch Phys Med Rehabil 56:243, 1975.
25. Baker, L, et al: Effect of carrier frequency on comfort with medium frequency electrical stimulation (abstract). Phys Ther 69:373, 1979.
26. Bowman, B, and Baker, L: Effects of waveform parameters on comfort during transcutaneous neuromuscular electrical stimulation. Ann Biomed Eng 13:59, 1985.
27. Delitto, A, and Rose, S: Comparative comfort of three waveforms used in electrically eliciting quadriceps femoris muscle contraction. Phys Ther 66:1704, 1986.
28. Baker, L, et al: Waveform and comfort of electrical stimulation in the upper extremity (abstract). Phys Ther 69(372), 1989.
29. Kantor, G, et al: The effects of selected stimulus waveforms on pulse and phase characteristics at sensory and motor thresholds. Phys Ther 74:951, 1994.
30. Laufer, Y, et al: Quadriceps Femoris muscle torques and fatigue generated by neuromuscular electrical stimulation with three different waveforms. Phys Ther 7:1307, 2001.
31. Alon, G: High voltage stimulation: Effects of electrode size on basic excitatory responses. Phys Ther 65(890), 1985.
32. Honert, C, and Mortimer, J: The response to the myelinated nerve fiber to short duration biphasic stimulating currents. Ann Biomed Eng 7(117), 1979.
33. Li, C, and Bak, A: Excitability characteristics of the A and C fibers in a peripheral nerve. Exp Neurol 50:67, 1976
34. Howson, D: Peripheral neural excitability: Implications for transcutaneous nerve stimulation. Phys Ther 58:1467, 1978.
35. Alon, G: Northeast Seminars: Electrosynthesis (lab course). Course Publication, 1993.
36. Alon, G: High voltage stimulation: Effects of electrode size on basic excitatory responses. Phys Ther 66:890, 1985.
37. Reilly, J: Electrical Stimulation and Electropathology. Cambridge University Press, Cambridge, 1992.
38. Benton, L, et al: Functional Electrical Stimulation: A Practical Guide, ed 2. Ranchos Los Amigos Rehabilitation Engineering Center, Downy, CA, 1981.
39. Charman, R: Cellular reception and emission of electromagnetic signals. Physiotherapy 76(509), 1990.
40. Crago, P, et al: The choice of pulse duration for chronic electrical stimulation via surface, nerve and intramuscular electrodes. Ann Biomed Eng 2:252, 1974.
41. Ray, C, and Maurer, D: A review of neural stimulator system components useful in pain alleviation. Med Progr Technol 2:121, 1974.
42. Polasek, KH, Hoyen, HA, Keith, MW, Kirsch, RF, and Tyler, DJ: Stimulation stability and selectivity of chronically implanted multicontact nerve cuff electrodes in the human upper extremity. IEEE Trans Neural Syst Rehab Eng 17:5, 2009.

43. Benet, LZ, Kroetz, DL, and Sheiner, LB: Pharmacokinetics: the dynamics of drug absorption, distribution, and elimination. In Hardman, J, and Limbird, L (eds): Goodman and Gilman's: The Pharmacological Basis of Therapeutics, ed 9. McGraw-Hill, New York, 1996, pp 3–28.

44. Fartasch, M: The nature of the epidermal barrier: Structural aspects. Adv Drug Del Rev 18:273–282, 1996.

45. Riviere, JE, and Heit, MC: Electrically-assisted transdermal drug delivery. Pharm Res 14:687–697, 1997.

46. Prausnitz, MR: The effect of pulsed electrical protocols on skin damage, sensation and pain. Proc Int Symp Control Rel Bioact Mater 25–26, 1997.

47. Banga, AJ: Electrically-Assisted Transdermal and Topical Drug Delivery. Taylor and Francis, London, 1998.

48. Banga, AK, and Panus, PC: Clinical applications of iontophoretic devices in rehabilitation medicine. Crit Rev Phys Rehab Med 10:147–179, 1998.

49. Yamamoto, T, and Yamamoto, Y: Electrical properties of the epidermal stratum corneum. Med Biol Eng 14:151–158, 1976.

50. Lin, RY, Ou, YC, and Chen, WY: The role of electroosmotic flow on in vitro transdermal iontophoresis. J Control Release 43:23–33, 1997.

51. Plutchik, R, and Hirsch, HR: Skin impedance and phase angle as a function of frequency and current. Science 141:927–928, 1963.

52. Boxtel, AV: Skin resistance during square-wave electrical pulses of 1 to 10 mA. Med Biol Eng Comput 15:679–687, 1977.

53. Kalia, YN, and Guy, RH: The electrical characteristics of human skin in vivo. Pharm. Res. 12:1605–1613, 1995.

54. Burnette, RR, and Bagniefski, TM: Influence of constant current iontophoresis on the impedance and passive Na+ permeability of excised nude mouse skin. J Pharm Sci 77:492–497, 1988.

55. Kasting, GB, and Bowman, LA: DC electrical properties of frozen, excised human skin. Pharm Res 7:134–143, 1990.

56. Kasting, GB, and Bowman, LA: Electrical analysis of fresh, excised human skin: A comparison with frozen skin. Pharm Res 7:1141–1146, 1990.

57. Oh, SY, Leung, L, Bommannan, D, et al: Effect of current, ionic strength and temperature on the electrical properties of skin. J Control Release 27:115–125, 1993.

58. Roberts, MS: Targeted drug delivery to the skin and deeper tissues: Role of physiology, solute structure and disease. Clin Exp Pharmacol Physiol 24:874–879, 1997.

59. Prausnitz, MR: Reversible skin permeabilization for transdermal delivery of macromolecules. Crit Rev Ther Drug Carrier Syst 14:455–483, 1997.

60. McNeill, SC, Potts, RO, and Francoeur, ML: Local enhanced topical delivery (LETD) of drugs: does it truly exist? Pharm Res 9:1422–1427, 1992.

61. Radermacher, J, Jentsch, D, Scholl, MA, et al: Diclofenac concentrations in synovial fluid and plasma after cutaneous application in inflammatory and degenerative joint disease. Br J Clin Pharmacol 31:537–541, 1991.

62. Vickers, CFH: Existence of reservoir in the stratum corneum. Exp Proof Arch Dermatol 88:72–75, 1963.

63. Grahame, R: Transdermal non-steroidal anti-inflammatory agents. Br J Clin Pract 49:33–35, 1995.

64. Singh, P, and Roberts, MS: Iontophoretic transdermal delivery of salicylic acid and lidocaine to local subcutaneous structures. J Pharm Sci 82:127–131, 1993.

64. Singh, P, and Roberts, MS: Deep tissue penetration of bases and steroids after dermal application in rat. J Pharm Pharmacol 46:956–964, 1994.

66. Singh, P, and Roberts, MS: Skin permeability and local tissue concentrations of nonsteroidal anti-inflammatory drugs after topical application. J Pharmacol Exp Ther 268:144–151, 1994.

67. Green, P: Iontophoretic Transdermal Drug Delivery: A New Commercially Feasible Technology. Hotel International, Basel, Switzerland, October 17–18 (Organized by A. K. Banga and P. Green through Technomic Publishing), 1996.

68. Singh, P, Anliker, M, Smith, GA, et al: Transdermal iontophoresis and solute penetration across excised human skin. J Pharm Sci 84:1342–1346, 1995.

69. Li, SK, Ghanem, AH, Peck, KD, et al: Iontophoretic transport across a synthetic membrane and human epidermal membrane: A study of the effects of permeant charge. J Pharm Sci 86: 680–689, 1997.

70. Kim, A, Green, PG, Rao, G, et al: Convective solvent flow across the skin during iontophoresis. Pharm Res 10:1315–1320, 1993.

71. Burnette, RR, and Ongpipattanakul, B: Characterization of the pore transport properties and tissue alteration of excised human skin during iontophoresis. J Pharm Sci 77:132–137, 1988.

72. Turner, NG, and Guy, RH: Iontophoretic transport pathways: Dependence on penetrant physicochemical properties. J Pharm Sci 86:1385–1389, 1997.

73. Menon, GK, and Elias, PM: Morphologic basis for a porepathway in mammalian stratum corneum. Skin Pharmacol 10:235–246, 1997.

74. Craane Van Hinsberg, IW, Verhoef, JC, Spies, F, et al: Electroperturbation of the human skin barrier in vitro: II. Effects on stratum corneum lipid ordering and ultrastructure. Microsc Res Tech 37:200–213, 1997.

75. Hinsberg, WHMC, Verhoef, JC, Bax, LJ, et al: Role of appendages in skin resistance and iontophoretic peptide flux: Human versus snake skin. Pharm Res 12:1506–1512, 1995.

76. Cullander, C: What are the pathways of iontophoretic current flow through mammalian skin? Adv Drug Del Rev 9:119–135, 1992.

77. Turner, NG, Kalia, YN, and Guy, RH: The effect of current on skin barrier function in vivo: Recovery kinetics postiontophoresis. Pharm Res 14: 1252–1257, 1997.

78. Li, SK, Ghanem, AH, Peck, KD, et al: Characterization of the transport pathways induced during low to moderate voltage iontophoresis in human epidermal membrane. J Pharm Sci 87: 40–48, 1998.

79. Gangarosa, LP, Park, N, Wiggins, CA, et al: Increased penetration of non-electrolytes into mouse skin during iontophoretic water transport (iontohydrokinesis). J Pharmacol Exp Ther 212: 377–381, 1980.

80. Pikal, MJ: The role of electroosmotic flow in transdermal iontophoresis. Adv Drug Del Rev 9:201–237, 1992.

81. Burnette, RR, and Ongpipattanakul, B: Characterization of the permaselective properties of excised human skin during iontophoresis. J Pharm Sci 76:765–773, 1987.

82. Gwynne, P: Companies developing more uses for iontophoresis. Scientist 11:1, 1997.

83. Kahn, J: Acetic acid iontophoresis for calcium deposits. Phys Ther 57: 658–659, 1977.

84. Kahn, J: A case report: lithium iontophoresis for gouty arthritis. J Orthop Sports Phys Ther 4:113–114, 1982.

85. LaForest, NT, and Cofrancesco, C: Antibiotic iontophoresis in the treatment of ear chondritis. Phys Ther 58:32–34, 1978.

86. Saggini, R, Zoppi, M, Vecchiet, F, et al: Comparison of electromotive drug administration with ketorolac or with placebo in patients with pain from rheumatic disease: A double-masked study. Clin Ther 18:1169–1174, 1996.

87. Wieder, DL: Treatment of traumatic myositis ossificans with acetic acid iontophoresis. Phys Ther 72:133–137, 1992.

88. Johnson, MTV, and Lee, NH, inventors; Empi, assignee. PH buffered electrodes for medical iontophoresis. 4(973):303. 1990. (Patent Application)

89. Guffey, JS, Rutherford, MJ, Payne, W, et al: Skin pH changes associated with iontophoresis. J Orthop Sports Phys Ther 29: 656–660, 1999.

90. Phipps, JB, Padmanabhan, RV, and Lattin, GA: Iontophoretic delivery of model inorganic and drug ions. J Pharm Sci 78: 365–369, 1989.

91. Gangarosa, LP, Park, NH, Fong, BC, et al: Conductivity of drugs used for iontophoresis. J Pharm Sci 67:1439–1443, 1978.

92. Lattin, GA, Padmanabhan, RV, and Phipps, JB: Electronic control of iontophoretic drug delivery. Ann N Y Acad Sci 618:450–464, 1991.

93. Miller, LL, and Smith, GA: Iontophoretic transport of acetate and carboxylate ions through hairless mouse skin: cation exchange membrane model. Int J Pharm 49:15–22, 1989.

94. Thysman, S, Preat, V, and Roland, M: Factors affecting iontophoretic mobility of metoprolol. J Pharm Sci 81:670–675, 1992.

95. Chu, DL, Chiou, HJ, and Wang, DP: Characterization of transdermal delivery of nefopam hydrochloride under iontophoresis. Drug Dev Ind Pharm 20:2775–2785, 1994.

96. Schimmer, B, and Parker, K: Adrenocorticotropic hormone; adrenocortical steroids and their synthetic analogs; inhibitors of the synthesis and actions of adrenocortical hormones. In Hardman, J, and Limbird, L (eds): Goodman and Gilman's The Pharmacological Basis of Therapeutics, ed 9. McGraw-Hill, New York, 1996, pp 1459–1485.

97. Insel, P: Analgesic-antipyretic and antiinflammatory agents and drugs employed in the treatment of gout. In Hardman, J, and Limbird, L (eds): Goodman and Gilman's The Pharmacological Basis of Therapeutics, ed 9. McGraw-Hill, New York, 1996, pp 617–658.

98. Glass, JM, Stephen, RL, and Jacobson, SC: The quantity and distribution of radiolabeled dexamethasone delivered to tissue by iontophoresis. Int J Derm 19:519–525, 1980.

99. Petelenz, TJ, Buttke, JA, Bonds, C, et al: Iontophoresis of dexamethasone: Laboratory studies. J Control Release 20:55–66, 1992.

100. Anderson, CR, Morris, RL, Boeh, SD, et al: Quantification of total dexamethasone phosphate delivery by iontophoresis. Int J Pharm Compound 7:115–159, 2003.

101. Anderson, CR, Morris, RL, Boeh, SD, et al: Effects of iontophoresis current magnitude and duration on dexamethasone deposition and localized drug retention. Phys Ther 83:161–170, 2003.

102. Riviere, JE, Monteiro Riviere, NA, and Inman, AO: Determination of lidocaine concentrations in skin after transdermal iontophoresis: effects of vasoactive drugs. Pharm Res 9:211–214, 1992.

103. Riviere, JE, Sage, B, and Williams, PL: Effects of vasoactive drugs on transdermal lidocaine iontophoresis. J Pharm Sci 80:615–620, 1991.

104. Singh, P, and Roberts, MS: Effects of vasoconstriction on dermal pharmacokinetics and local tissue distribution of compounds. J Pharm Sci 83:783–791, 1994.

105. Nowicki, KD, Hummer, CD, III, Heidt, RS, Jr, et al: Effects of iontophoretic versus injection administration of dexamethasone. Med Sci Sports Exerc 34:1294–1301, 2002.

106. Smutok, MA, Mayo, MF, Gabaree, CL, et al: Failure to detect dexamethasone phosphate in the local venous blood postcathodic Iontophoresis in humans. J Orthop Sports Phys Ther 32: 461–468, 2002.

107. Blackford, J, Doherty, TJ, Ferslew, KE, et al: Iontophoresis of dexamethasone phosphate into the equine tibiotarsal joint. J Vet Pharmacol Ther 23:229–236, 2000.

108. Panus, PC, Campbell, J, Kulkarni, SB, et al: Transdermal iontophoretic delivery of ketoprofen through human cadaver skin and in humans. J Control Release 44:113–121, 1997.

109. Panus, PC, Campbell, J, Kulkarni, B, et al: Effect of iontophoretic current and application time on transdermal delivery of ketoprofen in man. Pharm Sci 2:467–469, 1996.

110. Panus, PC, Ferslew, KE, Tober-Meyer, B, et al: Ketoprofen tissue permeation in swine following cathodic iontophoresis. Phys Ther 79:40–49, 1999.

111. Tashiro, Y, Kato, Y, Hayakawa, E, et al: Iontophoretic transdermal delivery of ketoprofen: novel method for the evaluation of plasma drug concentration in cutaneous vein. Biol Pharm Bull 23:632–636, 2000.

112. Tashiro, Y, Kato, Y, Hayakawa, E, et al: Iontophoretic transdermal delivery of ketoprofen: effect of iontophoresis on drug transfer from skin to cutaneous blood. Biol Pharm Bull 23:1486–1490, 2000.

113. Grossmann, M, Jamieson, MJ, Kellogg, DL Jr, et al: The effect of iontophoresis on the cutaneous vasculature: Evidence for current-induced hyperemia. Microvasc Res 50:444–452, 1995.

114. Eastman, T, Panus, PC, Honnas, CM, et al: Cathodic iontophoresis of ketoprofen over the equine middle carpal joint. Equine Vet J 33:614–616, 2001.

115. Hasson, SM, Wible, CL, Reich, M, et al: Dexamethasone iontophoresis: Effect on delayed muscle soreness and muscle function. Can J Sport Sci 17:8–13, 1992.

116. Li, LC, Scudds, RA, Heck, CS, et al: The efficacy of dexamethasone iontophoresis for the treatment of rheumatoid arthritic knees: A pilot study. Arthritis Care Res 9:126–132, 1996.

117. Gudeman, SD, Eisele, SA, Heidt, RS, Jr, et al: Treatment of plantar fasciitis by iontophoresis of 0.4% dexamethasone. A randomized, double-blind, placebo-controlled study. Am J Sports Med 25:312–316, 1997.

118. Reid, KI, Dionne, RA, Sicard Rosenbaum, L, et al: Evaluation of iontophoretically applied dexamethasone for painful pathologic temporomandibular joints. Oral Surg Oral Med Oral Pathol 77:605–609, 1994.

119. Schiffman, EL, Braun, BL, and Lindgren, BR: Temporo_man_dibular joint iontophoresis: A double-blind randomized clinical trial. J Orofac Pain 10:157–165, 1996.

120. Riedl, CR, Plas, E, Engelhardt, P, et al: Iontophoresis for treatment of Peyronie's disease. J Urol 163:95–99, 2000.

121. Lener, EV, Bucalo, BD, Kist, DA, et al: Topical anesthetic agents in dermatologic surgery. A review. Dermatol Surg 23:673–683, 1997.

122. Lesions and shocks during iontophoresis. Health Devices 26:123–125, 1997.

123. Anderson, LL, Welch, ML, and Grabski, WJ: Allergic contact dermatitis and reactivation phenomenon from iontophoresis of 5-fluorouracil. J Am Acad Dermatol 36:478–479, 1997.

124. Clinic Notes: The fatal current. Phys Ther 46:968, 1966.

125. Sances, A, et al: Electrical injuries. Surg Gynecol Obstet 149:97, 1979.

126. Berger, W: Electrical shock hazards in the physical therapy department. Clin Management 5:24, 1994.

127. Bruner, J, and Leonard, P: Electricity, Safety and the Patient. Year Book Medical Publishers, Chicago, 1989.

128. Buban, P, and Schmitt, M: Technical Electricity and Electronics, ed 2. McGraw-Hill, New York, 1977.

129. Delitto, A, et al: A study of discomfort with electrical stimulation. Phys Ther 72:11, 1992.

130. Lampe, G: Introduction to the use of transcutaneous electrical nerve stimulation. Phys Ther 72:11, 1978.

LET'S FIND OUT

Lab Activity: Foundations of Electrical Stimulation

Purpose
This lab activity is designed to familiarize students/learners with the common terminology associated with electrical stimulation devices. There is a wide variety of adjustable parameters and often several names for the same parameter. Students/learners will be guided through a familiarization process with the devices, and then they will apply electrodes to each other and adjust individual parameters.

This lab activity is not intended to demonstrate specific electrode placement sites for the accomplishment of therapeutic goals. It is an informal practice session and is intended to foster a minimal comfort level with electrical stimulation devices.

Equipment
electrical stimulation devices (portable
and clinical models with
adjustable parameters)
1 pair large electrodes
1 pair small electrodes
conductive interface samples (e.g., self-adhering, sponge, gel) for each pair of electrodes
straps to secure electrodes

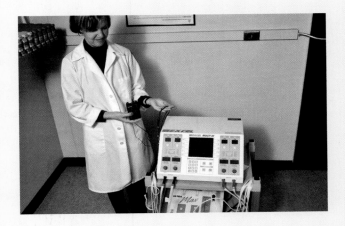

FIGURE 11-30 Clinician holding a portable electrical stimulator in her hand while standing next to a clinical stimulator.

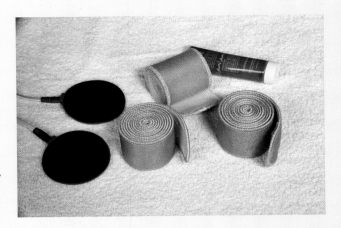

FIGURE 11-31 Electrodes, straps, and electrically conductive gel that can be used on the electrodes to promote conductivity.

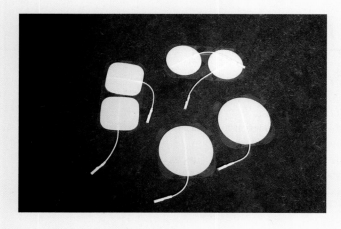

FIGURE 11-32 Three different sizes of self-adhering reusable electrodes.

Precautions and Why

Precaution	Why?
Unstable fracture	If electrical stimulation is used for a motor response, this fracture is a contraindication. However, if no motor response is elicited, electrical stimulation can be considered safe.
Decreased sensation	If the desired response is dependent on sensation, then electrical stimulation may be useless. However, if the desired response relies on a motor response, then the application may be considered safe.
	If the application involves the transmission of ions through the skin, the patient must be able to report sensation to avoid an adverse response.
Impaired cognitive ability	If the desired response is dependent on sensation, then electrical stimulation may be useless. However, if the desired response relies on a motor response, then the application may be considered safe.
	If the application involves the transmission of ions through the skin, the patient must be able to report sensation to avoid an adverse response.
Pregnancy	If the application is after the first trimester, there is little risk to the fetus or the patient. Electrical stimulation has been safely used for analgesia during labor and delivery, but it may interfere with fetal monitors.
Heart problems (suspected or diagnosed)	Vital signs should be closely monitored before, during, and after treatment for potential changes.
Documented evidence of epilepsy, cerebral vascular accident, or reversible ischemic neurological deficit	Patients should be monitored carefully when electrical stimulation is used in the cervical region. Possible adverse responses may include temporary change in cognitive status, headache, vertigo, and other neurological signs.
Recent surgical procedure	A muscle contraction may cause a disruption in the healing process.
Pacemaker	Electrical stimulation devices may interfere with the electrical demands of the pacemaker (dependent upon the type of pacemaker and more common with demand pacemakers).

Contraindications and Why

Contraindication	Why?
Pregnancy (first trimester)	There are no data to indicate the level of safety for the fetus with the application of electrical stimulation during the first trimester of pregnancy.
Over the carotid sinus	If the circulation to the brain were altered, there could be adverse effects.
Malignancies	Most application techniques have the potential to produce an increase in circulation to the area. The possibility exists that electrical stimulation over or in proximity to cancerous lesions may enhance the development of metastasis.

Lab Activities: Orientation to Electrical Stimulation Equipment

1. Select an electrical stimulator and identify and record the following information.

Name of Stimulator:
Manufacturer:
No. of Lead Wires:
No. of Available Channels:

Identify the controls on your stimulator. Other words may be used to identify these controls; circle those that you find on the unit that you examine. (**Not all stimulators will have all of these controls.**)

Rate; Hz

Frequency	Rate, PPS, (Hertz), CPS, Carrier, Burst
Intensity	mAmp, V
On/Off Times	Ratios, 10/10, 10/50
Pulse Duration	Pulse width
Reciprocal	Simultaneous, alternating
Other	

3. Inspect the electrodes that you will use and record your observations. (Are they cracked, shiny, uniformly covered? How many electrodes attach to the lead wire?)

Observations: _____

_____

Number of electrodes per lead wire? _____

4. There are several common forms of lead wires and electrodes used in the clinic. For electrical stimulation to take place, there must be at least two electrodes in contact with a conductive interface and the patient. These two electrodes must be from one channel of the stimulator. Circle which of the following types of lead/pin setups you have on the stimulator that you selected (Figs. 11-33 and 11-34).

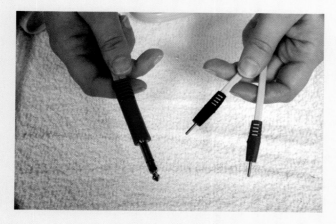

FIGURE 11-33 The proximal end of a lead wire with a stereo jack and the distal end with pin leads.

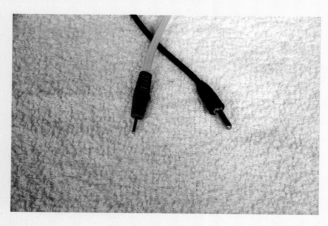

FIGURE 11-34 Compare the size of a pin lead on the left with a banana pin on the right.

- 1, 2, or more stereo jacks
- 1, 2, or more single-lead jacks
- Bifurcated lead (split lead with 2 pins)
- Pin leads (small diameter, nonadjustable)
- Banana pins (larger diameter, adjustable)
- Other (describe)

_____

_____

5. Plug the leads into your electrodes so that no metal shows from the pins (Figs. 11-35 and 11-36).

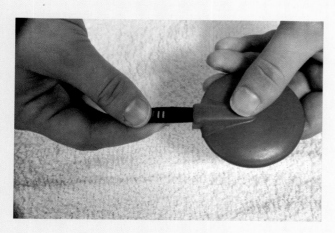

FIGURE 11-35 Lead wire and pin that has been inserted into an electrode.

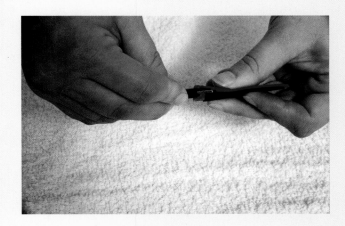

FIGURE 11-36 The pin from the lead wire must be fully engaged in the electrode to reach the conductive aspect of the electrode.

Orientation to the Sensations and Responses of Electrical Stimulation Parameters

Select a classmate/patient to receive electrical stimulation to his or her forearm. The area should be assessed for sensation and any abnormalities such as scars or excessively dry skin or hair, which may alter the conductivity of the skin.

Clinical models start with these steps:

- Check the power cable for any fraying or loose wires (Fig. 11-37).
- Plug the stimulator into the wall outlet.
- Turn on the power to the stimulator.

Portable models start with these steps:

- Turn all outputs to zero.
- Plug the leads that you will be using into the stimulator.

Everyone continue here:

- Prepare the electrodes for attachment to the patient (e.g., wet sponges, spread gel, peel off plastic).
- Attach the electrodes to the patient (one over the wrist extensor muscle belly, one on the distal extent of the muscle belly).
- Set the following parameters:

Treatment time	10 minutes
Frequency	100 Hz (or highest available setting for that unit)
Pulse Duration	200 µsec pulse duration
On Time	Continuous on time

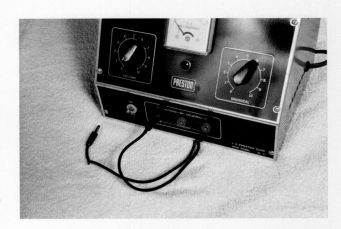

FIGURE 11-37 A frayed lead wire. A lead wire in this condition is considered unsafe for use.

1. Gradually increase the intensity and record the amount needed for the patient to first start feeling something.
2. Ask the patient to describe the sensation, and record his or her response.

Setting the Intensity

Intensity required to feel something
How did your patient describe it?

1. Increase the intensity until the sensation is strong but tolerable and record it. How high was it in comparison to the initial setting?
2. After 5 minutes, ask the patient to describe how the sensation has changed and record his or her response.

What was the intensity level when it was "strong but tolerable"
How much higher is it than initial level?
How has sensation changed after 5 min?

Continue with the following steps.
- Decrease the intensity to zero.
- Disconnect the electrodes from the patient.
- Turn off the power to the stimulator.
- Repeat this exercise until everyone in your group has had a chance to be both the clinician and the patient.
- Select another stimulator and familiarize yourself with the controls, leads, and electrodes.

What Effect Do the Parameters Have on Sensation?
Set the following parameters:

Treatment time	15 minutes
Frequency	1 Hz
Pulse duration	200 µsec pulse duration
On/Off time	Continuous on time

Attach the electrodes to the same sites as described previously.
1. Gradually increase the intensity and record the amount needed for the patient to first start feeling something.
2. Ask the patient to describe the sensation, and record his or her response.

What was the intensity required to feel something
How did your patient describe it?

1. Increase the intensity until the sensation is strong but tolerable and record it. How high was it in comparison to the initial setting?
2. After 5 minutes, ask the patient to describe how the sensation has changed and record his or her response.

Intensity level when "strong but tolerable"
How much higher is it than initial level?
How has sensation changed after 5 min?

Repeat the following steps:

- Decrease the intensity to zero.
- Disconnect the electrodes from the patient.
- Turn off the power to the stimulator.
- Repeat this exercise until everyone in your group has had a chance to be both the clinician and the patient.
- Select another stimulator and familiarize yourself with the controls, leads, and electrodes.

Changing a New Parameter

Gradually increase the frequency. Ask the patient how the sensation changes and record his or her response.

1. Increase the frequency to 50 Hz and record your observations.

How did increasing the frequency change
   the sensation? _____

What happened when the frequency reached
   50 Hz? How did it feel or what occurred? _____

2. Decrease the intensity to zero, disconnect the electrodes from the patient, and turn off the power to the stimulator.

Mapping Your Personal Strength Duration Curve

Fill in the following chart with the data that you have collected. (Intensity is on the vertical axis, and pulse duration is on the horizontal axis.)

- Use dots for tingling sensation.
- Use triangles for contraction.
- Use squares for sharp pain (Fig. 11-38).

Personal Strength Duration Curve

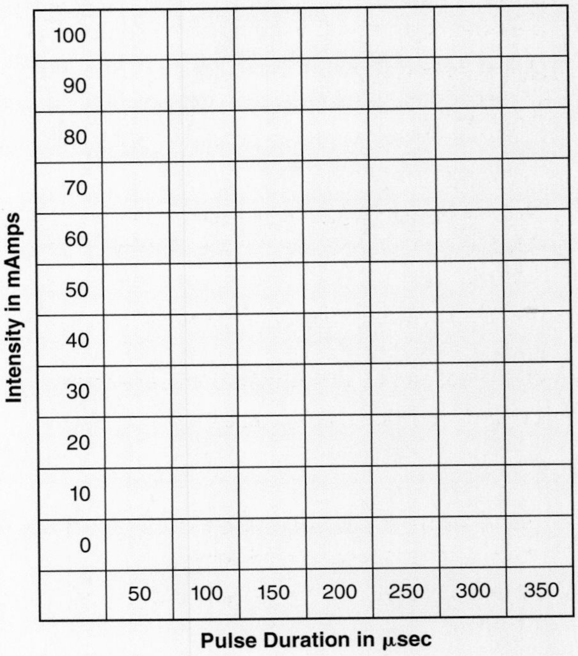

FIGURE 11-38 Personal strength duration curve.

Lab Questions

1. What terms were used to describe frequency?
2. Which frequency produced a "buzzing" sensation?
3. Which frequency produced a "thumping" sensation?
4. What were the terms used to describe pulse duration?
5. What happened when the sensory level of intensity was increased above initial sensation?
6. Why was there a specific sequence for powering up and powering down the stimulators?
7. What would happen if an electrode fell off during treatment? What would the patient feel?
8. If you were treating a patient with electrical stimulation and you were using a portable unit that had adjustable parameters, what would you do if the intensity were turned up as high as possible and the patient still did not feel the stimulus?
9. From your "Personal Strength Duration Curve," answer the following questions based on the information you collected:

   - Which of the sensations required the least amount of intensity to elicit?
   - Which of the sensations required the shortest pulse duration to elicit?
   - What would it mean if a patient started to have a twitching type contraction?
   - What would the minimum pulse duration be, and how high would the intensity be, and what would the frequency be?

10. When turning off an electrical stimulator, what controls should be returned to zero and why?
11. What controls may be left alone when turning off an electrical stimulator?
12. If you were adjusting the intensity and the patient reported that he or she felt the current very strongly, just after you started to increase it, what would be the possible explanations for this?
13. You are increasing the intensity on a unit, and after increasing it to the maximum level, the patient still reports that he or she feels little or no sensation. What are the possible causes and remedies?
14. You are setting up an electrical stimulation unit and while adjusting the unit, the patient reports that he or she is feeling a throbbing sensation under the electrodes. What would be the possible causes for this, and what would be the remedies?
15. If you had to explain the parameter terminology to a patient, what would you say that each of the controls represents in terms of the sensations that he or she will feel?
16. If a patient reports to you that he or she feels a sharp, knife-like sensation underneath the electrodes, what would be the potential causes and remedies for this?
17. What would you tell a patient to potentially expect when you are adjusting the intensity of the stimulus to a motor level?

CHAPTER 12

Electrodes and Lead Wires: Material and Care

Barbara J. Behrens, PTA, MS

Learning Outcomes

Following the successful completion of this chapter, the learner will be able to:

- Differentiate between the various types of electrodes that are available, citing advantages and disadvantages to their application for various treatment goals.
- Describe the components and care of the electrode interface to improve conduction.
- Demonstrate the lead wire inspection process that takes place prior to the application of various forms of therapeutic electrical stimulation to a patient to maintain patient safety.
- Outline the process of electrode selection and placement for the accomplishment of therapeutic treatment goals.
- Demonstrate the foundation problem-solving skills to rule out whether or not a "problem" with an electrical stimulation application is due to the electrodes, the lead wires, the patient, or the electrical stimulator.

Key Terms

Active
Bifurcator
Bipolar
Channel
Circuit
Conductive
Dispersive

Electrode
Electrode interface
Jack
Leads
Lead wire
Longitudinal
Monopolar

Parallel
Percutaneous
Pin
Quadripolar
Target area
Transcutaneous

"A mistake is simply another way of doing things." —Katharine Graham

Patient Perspective

"Will I be electrocuted by what you are doing?"

Clinical electrical stimulation involves the passing of current through the skin via electrodes. An **electrode** is used either to deliver electric current or to record electrical activity of muscle, such as in electromyography (EMG). The delivery of current is accomplished through a system of electrically **conductive** elements.[1] Current will be able to travel from point A to point B if several things are in place including an energy source and a pathway that is capable of carrying or conducting that current. This chapter focuses on the pathway, which includes the lead wire, two or more electrodes per **circuit**, a conductive substance, which is referred to as the **electrode interface**, and the patient. Each of these components will affect the amount of electrical charge delivered to the patient. The influence of each of the components will either facilitate the flow of current, if the resistance is low, or inhibit the flow of current, if the resistance within the system is too high. Refer to previous chapter for a review of resistance and current flow.

Electrodes represent the "instrument" for current delivery from an electrical stimulation generator. **Leads** or **lead wires** connect the electrodes to the stimulator. Each lead has both a **jack** and a **pin** to interconnect the electrode to the lead and the lead to the stimulator.[1] Jacks represent the point of connection at the base of a lead wire into the stimulator, so this portion is usually bulkier than the other end of the lead wire, which might divide into two smaller wires with **pin tips**. Each of these components is discussed in terms of the structures themselves, their possible configurations, and appropriate handling techniques.

Electrodes vary in shape, size, and flexibility to fit the needs of the therapeutic application of the electrical current to the patient. An electrode is made of an electrically conductive material that is housed or covered in a nonelectrically conductive material. The purpose of the housing material is to inhibit the delivery of electrical energy to either the patient or the clinician so that if either touches the back of the electrode, no charge would be delivered unexpectedly.

Patient Perspective (continued)

Remember that your patient is curious about what you are doing with electrical stimulation. Some of the terms might be familiar, such as "stereo jack" or "lead wire," but he or she will not know what you are going to do or why. Another key thing to remember is that you are deliberately moistening the electrodes, yet your patient may be fearful of the combination of water and electricity. It is the responsibility of the clinician to properly inform the patient about the rationale behind the tasks that are involved.

Patients' Frequently Asked Questions

1. Do you use tap water or distilled water? Why?
2. Why do you use water?
3. Will I be electrocuted by what you are doing?
4. Where will I feel that, and what will it feel like?
5. Why are you doing that to me?
6. Have you ever had this done to you?

Types of Electrodes

METAL PLATE ELECTRODES

Early electrodes were composed of metal plates such as tin, steel, aluminum, and zinc, which are good electrical conductors for therapeutic stimulation. The electrode was usually contained within a rubber casing with only one surface exposed to the patient. The interface between the metal electrode and skin was accomplished through a sponge or felt pad moistened with tap water. This served to reduce the skin–electrode impedance, because tap water is a good conductor of electricity. Distilled water should not be used; it contains no free ions, which are required for the transmission of electrical current,[1] and therefore would not be electrically conductive (Fig. 12-1).

WHY DO I NEED TO KNOW ABOUT...
APPLICATION OF ELECTRODES

You will be applying electrodes to patients and need to be familiar with the terminology and the purpose to be successful.

Disadvantages of metal plate electrode systems include the following:

- Metal plates may not be flexible enough to maintain adequate contact with certain body parts.
- These electrodes may be difficult to secure comfortably to the patient.
- There are few sizes of these electrodes, making specific treatment goals for smaller treatment areas difficult to accomplish.

CARBON-IMPREGNATED RUBBER ELECTRODES

Electrodes composed of rubber, silicon, and polymer have mostly replaced the older metal plate electrodes and are typically used with clinical devices. Carbon-impregnated silicon rubber electrodes are commonly used in many clinics. They are backed with a nonconductive material to prevent unintentional current delivery. These electrodes are available in many shapes and sizes, and they can be trimmed or fitted to different locations of the body (Fig. 12-2).

Carbon-impregnated silicon rubber electrodes should be replaced when necessary. They degrade over time, resulting in nonuniformity of current delivery, or the presence of "hot spots." Hot spots represent those areas of the electrode that continue to maintain their conductivity while other

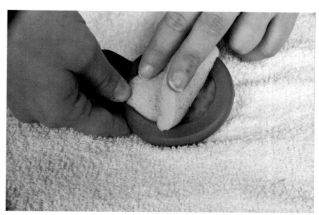

FIGURE 12-1 Metal plate electrode. The metal surface of the electrode is covered by a sponge that would be soaked in water. The left-hand corner of the sponge is folded back to reveal the metal plate. The electrode is encased in a nonelectrically conductive rubber cover.

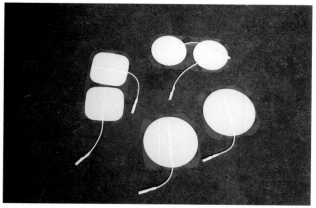

FIGURE 12-2 Several different sizes of self-adhering electrodes that have a mesh of electrically conductive material woven into them. This photograph depicts other self-adhering electrodes with smaller conductive surface areas and also illustrates the flexibility of the mesh electrodes. The mesh electrodes easily conform to irregular body surfaces.

areas of the surface no longer conduct electrical energy. The result is analogous to 10 cars trying to merge onto an uncrowded highway versus those same 10 cars trying to merge onto a crowded highway. The 10 cars will enter the crowded highway, but if time were a factor, the amount of resistance that they would face in meeting their goal would be significantly higher when the traffic was heavy or the window to merge was smaller. Carbon rubber electrodes should be rinsed off and dried after each use. Replace these electrodes every 12 months to ensure good conductivity. Again, if the goal is to have current pass through the electrodes, then they must be taken care of to maintain their conductivity.

SELF-ADHERING SINGLE-USE OR REUSABLE ELECTRODES

Self-adhering single-use or reusable electrodes are composed of other flexible conductors such as foil or metal mesh, conductive Karaya, or synthetic gel layered with an adhesive surface (see Fig. 12-2). The advantage of these electrodes is convenience of application. No strapping or taping is necessary to secure the electrodes to the patient.

Clinicians should carefully read the manufacturer's suggestions before using these electrodes. Because of the potential for cross-contamination, use of a package of electrodes for each patient is prudent. The package can be marked with the patient's name and identification number so that they will be used only for a given patient.

CONSIDERATIONS FOR ELECTRODE SELECTION

There are advantages and disadvantages with each type of electrode, including self-adhering electrodes. Often, the impedance of these electrodes is significantly higher than that of other electrode systems, resulting in reductions in potential current outputs of the stimulation device. These limitations may make it difficult or impossible to accomplish the desired clinical goal with a given stimulator, if the output of the stimulator is not sufficient to overcome the resistance of the electrodes.

The resistance of the electrode, which is listed in ohms, should be as low as possible when significant motor levels of stimulation are required. If the desired effect is a comfortable nonmotor level of stimulation, the impedance value of the electrodes is not as critical to success. If the impedance value of the electrodes is high, then the stimulator will need to overcome that value before the current is delivered to the patient. This may result in higher output levels of stimulation, which may be uncomfortable to the patient. The package of the electrodes may indicate the ohms of resistance, which will be lower with larger electrodes and higher with smaller electrodes.

LET'S THINK ABOUT IT...

Why would the resistance be lower with larger electrodes than with smaller electrodes?
Suppose your goal was to be able to enter a building and you had two options to choose from, a porthole-sized opening and a full-size doorway. Which one would be easier for you to pass through?

The method of current delivery into the electrode will also affect the uniformity of the current delivery from the electrode. Some self-adhering electrodes have a metal wire that inserts into the center of a conductive-adhesive or adherent surface. The current delivery at the point of attachment of the wire to the surface will be relatively higher than the current delivery to the periphery of that electrode. This may result in a hot spot at which the wire connects to the surface of the electrode. Optimally, the conductive surface of the electrode will have "uniform" conductivity. This potential for uniformity of conductivity is enhanced through foil or mesh surfaces within the electrode to spread out the delivered current.

BEFORE YOU BEGIN

Ask yourself what types of electrodes are available and which ones would be the most economical and appropriate for the patient you are treating. Not all clinics will have individual single-patient reusable electrodes. The insurance coverage for some patients does not permit this type of expense, so reusable carbon-impregnated rubber electrodes may need to be used.

ELECTRODE SIZE AND CURRENT DENSITY

Current density describes the amount of current concentrated under an electrode. It is a measure of the quantity of charged ions moving through a specific cross-sectional area of body tissue.

Electrode surface area is inversely related to total current flow. The same total current flow passing through large and small electrodes would result in lower current density under the larger electrode. The total current would be distributed over a larger surface area. Conversely, the smaller electrode would be delivering a high-current density because of its smaller surface area. Therapeutic electrical stimulation involves the active or stimulating electrode, the one that exhibits the greater current density, and the dispersive or inactive electrode, which delivers less current density. Electrodes should be appropriately sized for the desired result. If, for example, the treatment goal involved a motor response of one of the forearm muscles, an electrode that was 3 inches in diameter would produce a great amount of overflow of current into the surrounding muscles. This overflow would be due to the excessive size of the electrode in comparison to the small size of the muscles in the treatment area. Figure 12-3 illustrates the response of oversized electrodes applied in the forearm with an unbalanced current density.

It would be more appropriate to use a small electrode that more closely approximates the size of the target tissue, such as a 1.5-inch diameter electrode (see Fig. 12-3). The reverse is also true. If the treatment goal involved a tetanic contraction of the rectus femoris, then the electrode size that would afford the greatest comfort would probably be 3 inches in diameter or greater. Smaller electrodes may provide too great a current density, but not enough current flow to elicit a tetanic contraction (Fig. 12-4).

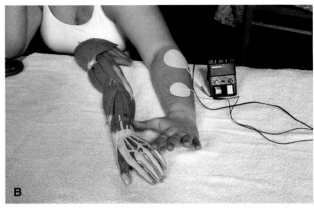

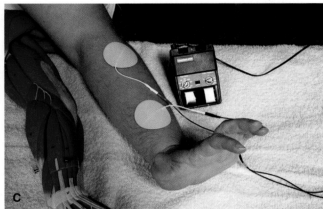

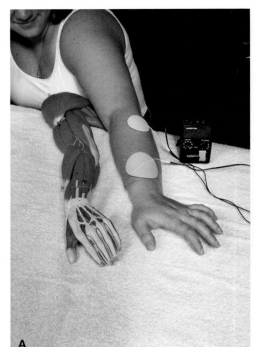

FIGURE 12-3 Each of the photographs depicts identical electrode placement sites with identical electrical stimulation parameters. The goal for the stimulation was wrist extension. However, in **A**, the distal electrode is larger than the proximal electrode, causing ulnar deviation. In **B**, the proximal electrode is larger than the distal electrode, causing radial deviation. In **C**, wrist flexion is accomplished this time with equally sized electrodes.

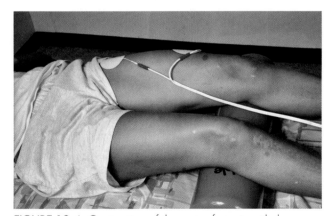

FIGURE 12-4 Contraction of the rectus femoris with the use of electrical stimulation delivered through two 3-inch-round electrodes placed on the muscle.

COUPLING MEDIA AND ATTACHMENT

Surface stimulation electrodes require the use of a coupling medium. This medium can be tap water via soaked sponges, or an electrically conductive gel. The coupling medium reduces the impedance at the interface between the electrode and the skin. This results in less current amplitude needed to produce the desired effects of stimulation.[2,3]

WHY DO I NEED TO KNOW ABOUT...
ELECTRODE SIZE
Remember that Ohm's law states that the delivered energy is directly related to the amount of resistance encountered. If you use small electrodes, the resistance will be higher and the sensation potentially more uncomfortable, which may make it very difficult to accomplish a treatment goal.

Pliability of the electrode to conform to the body part is necessary. Rigid metal electrodes do not conform well to contoured anatomical regions. Poor conformity can also result in hot-spot delivery of the electrical energy. In this case a high concentration of electrical energy over a small area, for example, the "hot spot," is a factor of not having the entire conductive surface of the electrode in contact with the patient's skin. Patient responses indicative of this would be noticeable after several minutes of treatment: the patient might have moved, he or she now feels a prickling sensation (hot spot) and is afraid to move back to the original position. To remedy this, the concentration of the energy will diminish if the patient returns to the original position, because the uniformity of the contact between the electrode and the patient will have been restored. It is often difficult to convince a patient that if he or she leans back on the electrode that is causing the prickling sensation, then the degree of prickling will subside. Explanations for the phenomenon can reduce the patient's anxiety regarding the electrical stimulation and potentially offset increased muscle guarding as a result of that fear.

Caution should be exercised to make sure that the electrode interface has not dried out during the treatment. If so, repositioning the patient will not remedy his or her complaint, but rehydration of the electrode may do so. This is yet another reason to check on a patient after treatment with electrical stimulation has been initiated.

The electrode should conform to the anatomical region to obtain optimal stimulation. Electrode attachment methods to maximize surface contact include the use of straps, tape, or the selection initially of self-adhering electrodes.

STRAPS OR TAPE FOR THE ATTACHMENT OF ELECTRODES

Straps have been commercially manufactured to be easy to use, inexpensive, and versatile. Many of the commercially available straps have rubber-backed stretch "eyed" surfaces, with one end of the reversed side of the strap covered with hooks. These straps should be used to secure either the carbon-impregnated rubber electrodes or the metal plate electrodes. Proper use involves strapping circumferentially around the limb with sufficient pressure to maintain good uniform contact between the electrode and the patient's skin. The pressure should be centered so that the electrode remains flat against the surface of the skin; however, it shouldn't be so tight that it impairs circulation through the area. Once the strap is secured, it should be checked for positioning that may have changed slightly once the strap has been stretched. Straps come in a variety of lengths for different areas of the body and different strapping configurations (Fig. 12-5).

Tape can also be used to attach electrodes to the patient, and it has several distinct disadvantages. For example, it can be costly and patients may be allergic to the adhesive. If the electrodes are not properly cleaned after use, the adhesive may migrate to and collect on the conductive surface of the electrode. This decreases both the conductive surface area and increases the potential for skin irritation.

The jack plugs into the stimulator and is typically encased in hard plastic. The jack is the portion of the lead that is meant to be handled, and it is constructed to maintain its integrity even with multiple plugging and unplugging of the lead into and out of the stimulator. In order for the lead to be able to deliver electrical energy, the jack must be securely plugged into the stimulator so that there is no metal showing between the jack and its plug or receptacle. Each lead wire will usually have two electrodes attached to it by a metal tip that inserts into the electrode (Fig. 12-6). There are different types of electrode/lead wire configurations, such as the pin tip lead and the banana tip lead, which are attempts to standardize the lead–electrode interface and ease the attachment of the electrode to the lead for the clinician (Fig. 12-7). Regardless of the type of tip, it is prone to corrosion and should be cleaned regularly. Scheduled maintenance of the tips should prevent potential problems with current delivery. Steel wool can be used to clean a tip. Gentle rubbing with the steel wool should restore the shiny metal surface of the tip, which will maintain its conductivity.

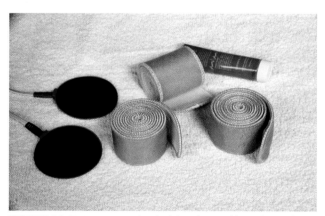

FIGURE 12-5 Straps used to hold carbon rubber electrodes with sponges or gel in place during treatment.

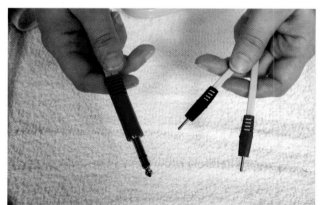

FIGURE 12-6 The lead wire to an electrical stimulation device connects to the device via a "stereo jack" and is divided into two leads, which are usually pin leads as pictured.

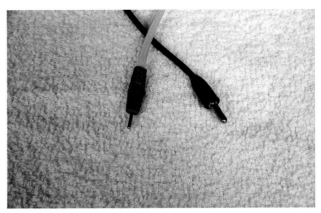

FIGURE 12-7 (A) "Pin" tip. (B) "Banana" tip. Banana tips are adjustable. If the tip no longer fits tightly in an electrode, then the sides of the tip may be spread apart slightly.

The tip can assist in the delivery of electrical energy only if it is in contact with the conductive surface of the electrode. There is a small housing that surrounds the tip opening within every electrode. The tip must be pushed as far as possible into the opening so that it does come in contact with the conductive surface of the electrode. There should be no metal showing between the plastic-coated pin housing and the electrode. Failure to insert the electrode properly will result in poor clinical results because current cannot be delivered to the patient (Figs. 12-8 and 12-9).

The U.S. Department of Health and Human Services, Food and Drug Administration (FDA), Center for Devices and Radiological Health regulates medical devices and their components to assure that they are safe. They do so by establishing performance standards that manufacturers must meet for various medical devices. Beginning in 1998, the first phase of a new performance standard was implemented that affected "patient transducer and electrode cables (including connectors). This standard required that all lead wires and patient cables must have a protected patient electrical connector.[4] Specific information is available from

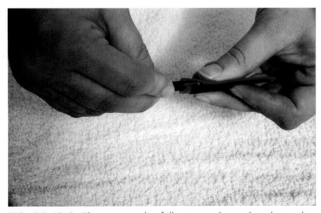

FIGURE 12-8 The tip must be fully inserted into the electrode so that the metal pin tip touches the conductive surface of the electrode. Failure to insert the pin into the electrode fully will result in poor current delivery to the electrode.

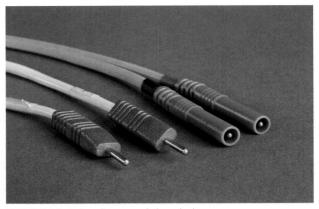

FIGURE 12-9 Lead wire with hooded pin tip.

the FDA Web site: http://www.fda.gov/MedicalDevices/DeviceRegulationandGuidance/ComplianceActivities/ucm106346.htm

WHY DO I NEED TO KNOW ABOUT...

TIP MAINTENANCE

Sometimes the reason that the current is not being perceived is as simple as the point of attachment to the electrode. *Before* checking to see if this is a problem, make sure that the unit is unplugged or turned off and the intensity is at *zero*.

Many electrical stimulation devices have multiple lead wires that have one stereo jack with two leads and pins for two electrodes. If the intended result is to cover a larger area and there are not any additional channels of electrodes available, then each lead may be "split" through the use of a bifurcator. A **bifurcator** is an attachment that fits on the pin of the lead wire and has two smaller leads coming off of it. Use of a bifurcator will split the output from that lead into the two electrodes attached to it, thereby decreasing the total amount of current flow through each independent electrode. (Current density is reduced or dispersed.) If a patient perceives too much sensation underneath one of the electrodes from a channel, then either the size of the electrode can be increased or a bifurcator can be used, which would then split the output delivered to that electrode.

Neither lead should be considered a ground but rather part of the electrical circuit. If there are not at least two points of contact between the electrical stimulation device and the patient, the patient will not have any electrical stimulation. A circuit has not been completed. Some older sources for electrical stimulation may use the term "ground"for the dispersive electrode, but this is a misnomer. Each electrical stimulation device will have its own set of peculiarities with respect to the management of leads. Examples of the channel setups and lead management can be found in Table 12-1. Potential causes and remedies for patient complaints of prickling or itching sensations underneath the electrodes are listed in Table 12-2.

TABLE 12-1 | Channel Setups and Lead Wire Management

TREATMENT GOAL	NO. OF LEADS AND ELECTRODES	MONOPOLAR	BIPOLAR	QUADRIPOLAR
Muscle (motor) stimulation	One lead per muscle with both electrodes on the same muscle, two leads if it is a larger muscle or if the device has more than one head		X	
Sensory stimulation	One or two leads depending upon the size of the area; use as many electrodes as possible for sensory stimulation			X
	One lead if only one lead and two electrodes fit into the treatment area		X	
	One lead with one electrode at the spinal nerve root and the other in the sensory area	X		
Delivery of medication	One lead and one electrode in the treatment area and the other more proximally placed on soft tissue	X		

TABLE 12-2 | Potential Causes and Remedies for Patient Complaints of Prickling or Itching Sensations Underneath the Electrodes

COMPLAINT	POTENTIAL CAUSE	REMEDY
Prickling or itching underneath the electrodes during treatment	The patient is moved off one of the electrodes during treatment.	Restoring contact with the electrode will restore the sensation; however, you may need to decrease the intensity of the unit first before a patient will let you do this.
	One of the electrodes is not making good contact.	Restoring contact with the electrode will restore the sensation; however, you may need to decrease the intensity of the unit first before a patient will let you do this.
	One of the electrodes has dried out.	Restoring the moisture necessary for good conduction can be as easy as rewetting the electrode.
	The patient has dry skin.	Restoring the moisture necessary for good conduction can be as easy as rewetting the electrode. If the patient has dry skin, his or her skin may absorb the moisture rapidly. Sponges may work better for these patients.
	The patient's skin is oily.	This patient may not be receiving the appropriate current density because of his or her own skin condition. Cleansing the skin with alcohol can remove the oil from the surface of the skin.
	The patient's skin is soiled under the surface of the electrode.	This patient may not be receiving the appropriate current density because of his or her own skin condition. Cleaning the skin with alcohol can remove the oil from the surface of the skin.
	The electrode is losing its conductivity.	The electrode may need to be replaced. The patient is *not* always the problem.
	A strap has come undone.	Restoring contact with the electrode will restore the sensation. You may need to resecure the straps. However, you may need to decrease the intensity of the unit first before a patient will let you do this.
	Water had dripped out from the sponge when the straps were applied.	Restoring the moisture necessary for good conduction can be as easy as rewetting the electrode. Restoring contact with the electrode will restore the sensation; however, you may need to decrease the intensity of the unit first before a patient will let you do this.

Transcutaneous and Percutaneous Electrodes

Electrodes that are applied to the surface of the skin are termed **transcutaneous** electrodes. Transcutaneous refers to the delivery of electrical energy or recording of electrical energy across the skin. **Percutaneous** electrodes are inserted into the skin. Percutaneous electrodes are commonly used for invasive EMG procedures, or they may be used for the application of electrical stimulation for patients with quadriplegia or paraplegia so that electrodes to stimulate muscles can be implanted permanently. Of the two types of electrodes, transcutaneous electrodes are more common in therapeutic delivery of electrical stimulation.

Terminology for Configurations of Electrode Setups

Electrodes can be oriented in **monopolar**, **bipolar**, and **quadripolar** manner, meaning one, two, or four electrodes in the treatment area, respectively. Placement across body tissues can be **longitudinal** and **parallel** to muscle fibers, as when stimulating the rectus femoris of the quadriceps muscle in the thigh to facilitate a stronger contraction. Alternatively the channels may be crisscrossed, as when administering electrical stimulation treatment for pain management when a muscle contraction is not the intended outcome. A **channel** is the term that refers to the electrodes that originate from one jack.

MONOPOLAR APPLICATION OF ELECTRODES

The monopolar technique involves a single electrode from a channel, usually smaller in size, placed over the treatment or **target area** called the **active** electrode. The greatest stimulation perception will be in the target tissue area. The larger **dispersive** electrode or second electrode is placed at a distance from the target electrode to complete the circuit. Its placement is usually over the nerve root supplying the target treatment area. The size differential between the electrodes ensures a greater current density in the treatment area (Fig. 12-10A).

BIPOLAR ELECTRODE SETUP

The bipolar electrode technique requires two electrodes from one channel within the target treatment area. They are usually of equal dimension and shape. Current flow through tissue is usually confined to the treatment area. When using the bipolar placement, the patient will experience an excitatory response and/or sensation under both electrodes. One can be smaller if the intention is a more effective activation of excitable tissues. This would be an appropriate electrode setup for eliciting a motor response.[5] One of the electrodes will be placed over the motor point, which is the area where it would take the least amount of current to elicit a muscle contraction, and the other electrode, which may be slightly larger, will be placed somewhere else over the muscle belly (Fig. 12-10B). Occasionally, a clinician may bifurcate or split the leads when a situation requires a larger target area, such as with a combination of back and lower extremity radiating pain. Bipolar techniques are well suited for stimulation of a large muscle.[6–10] Monopolar techniques are better suited for stimulation over a motor point or a wound.[11–14]

QUADRIPOLAR ELECTRODE PLACEMENT

The quadripolar method of electrode application involves electrodes from two or more channels, each lead with two electrodes. The electrodes can be positioned in a variety of configurations. Quadripolar electrode placement occurs with an interferential electrical stimulation device; however, it also occurs when there are four electrodes within the treatment area, regardless of the type of stimulator utilized to deliver the current.

Quadripolar electrode setups are often used to deliver the electrical stimulation to a larger area, such as in pain management techniques that rely on sensory stimulation of larger fibers for analgesia[15,16] (Fig. 12-11; see Fig. 12-10C, D).

WHY DO I NEED TO KNOW ABOUT...

PROPER TERMINOLOGY

The terminology for electrode setups is verbally communicated between clinicians. Knowing what is meant by the terms helps you to understand what other clinicians are referring to and decreases the confusion in an already terminology-laden intervention.

APPLICATION GUIDELINES

- Make sure that all connections are tight.
  - Stereo jack into the stimulator
  - Pin or banana into the electrode
  - Electrode interface onto the skin
- Make sure that electrode interfaces are moist.
  - Self-adhering
  - Sponges
- Gel must be electrically conductive.
- Water must *not* be distilled water as there are *no* ions present for the conduction of electrical current.
- Make sure that your patient does not move the electrodes once they are positioned.
- Make sure that your patient knows how to contact you if he or she needs to do so during treatment.

Care of Electrodes

Because electrodes represent the point of delivery of therapeutic electrical stimulation, the proper care for and cleaning of electrodes are essential. The impedance of

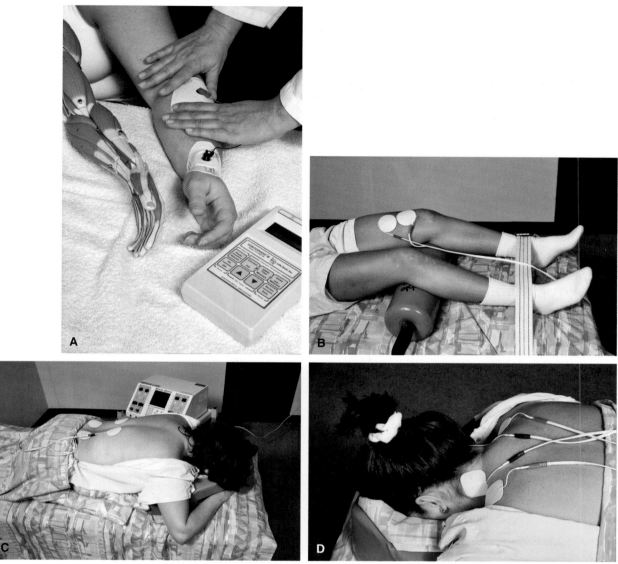

FIGURE 12-10 Various electrode setups. **(A)** Monopolor electrode placement setups with only one electrode from the channel in the target of treatment area. **(B)** A bipolar electrode setup, with both electrodes from the same channel in the target or treatment area. **(C)** A quadripolar treatment setup in the low back and **(D)** a dual bipolar setup for the cervical musculature.

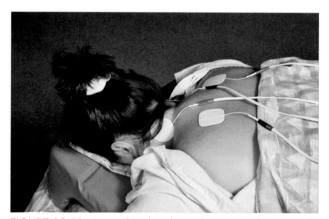

FIGURE 12-11 A quadripolar electrode setup in the cervical region to help provide analgesia and relieve muscle guarding as a secondary response to pain reduction.

carbon-impregnated silicon rubber electrodes can be significantly altered if the surface is allowed to dry or cake with gel. Carbon-impregnated silicone rubber electrodes can be easily cleaned in mild soap and warm water to remove gels. Cracking or polished appearance of the electrode surface may indicate that the surface is no longer uniformly conductive. This may result in the formation of spots of high current density on the electrode and poor current delivery. Harsh disinfectants can damage both carbon rubber and metal electrodes. Excessive alcohol use can cause carbon rubber electrodes to lose conductivity. An early sign of electrode wear is a stinging sensation under the electrodes. If there are cracks or uneven surfaces, the electrodes may need to be replaced.

Hot spots represent an increase in current concentration or current density within the electrode area, which could result in skin irritation. Patients who complain that they feel a biting or stinging sensation when receiving therapeutic current are probably describing an electrode with uneven conductivity. It is time to replace the electrode, or at least have it checked with an ohmmeter for resistance to determine whether use of the electrode should be continued.

If they are not cleaned on a regular basis, sponges soaked with water may be a source of potential cross-contamination from patient to patient. Germicidal soaps can be used to rinse through the electrodes before their application on a patient. Soap residue must be removed because soap acts as an insulator to the passage of electrical energy. It is usually easier, though, to replace the sponge electrodes with new ones.

Summary

Proper care and selection of electrodes could represent the success or failure of a treatment intervention with electrical stimulation. The electrodes, lead wires, and electrode interface must be appropriate for a treatment intervention to have a chance of being effective. If a patient is not feeling electrical stimulation where he or she is supposed to be feeling it because of an unpleasant sensation, clinicians must understand enough to know what to do to remedy the problem. This chapter provided a sampling of what to look for and what to do when problems arise. Familiarity with the equipment that is being used must include all of the peripherals, such as the lead wires and electrodes.

Review Questions

1. Which of the following would represent the greatest potential advantage of a self-adhering electrode over a carbon impregnated electrode?
   a. Ease of application
   b. Cost to the patient
   c. Possibility of cross-contamination
   d. Decreased impedance

2. What can you do to improve the electrode interface to enhance conduction?
   a. Use sandpaper to rough up the patient's skin
   b. Clean the patient's skin with a lotion-based cleanser
   c. Moisten the electrodes with water
   d. Replace the electrodes for each application

3. Which of the following would not be part of the process that takes place prior to the application of various forms of therapeutic electrical stimulation to a patient to maintain patient safety?
   a. Inspection of the lead wires
   b. Inspection of the electrodes
   c. Inspection of the power cord
   d. Confirm possession of electrical tape

4. Which of the following electrode configurations would be most appropriate for the accomplishment of a motor response in a specific superficial muscle?
   a. Quadripolar with two bifurcated channels crossing the muscle
   b. Monopolar with an active and dispersive electrode that is more than twice the size of the active electrode
   c. Monopolar with a dispersive and active electrode that is more than twice the size of the dispersive electrode
   d. Bipolar with one electrode over the motor point of the muscle

5. A patient whom you are treating with electrical stimulation has reported that he is intermittently feeling the sensation from the unit. Which of the following explanations would most likely be the cause for this if the unit had been set to function continuously without any Off time?
   a. One of the electrodes might have dried out and need to be re-hydrated
   b. One of the lead wires might have become disconnected and need to be re-connected
   c. One of the electrodes might have become detached from the lead wire and needs to be re-connected
   d. One of the lead wires might have a break in its continuity and needs to be replaced

CASE STUDY 1

Susan is an athletic trainer for the local community college women's field hockey team. She spends a great deal of time kneeling while taping the ankles of the team members. She fell down on her knees and has now been diagnosed with chondromalacia of the patella in both knees. There is marked weakness of the vastus medialis, edema superior to the patella, and a palpable painful crepitus in both knees when descending stairs.

The treatment goals include pain relief, edema reduction, and muscle strengthening. Electrical stimulation was applied in a quadripolar setup for each of Susan's knees, which initially felt "very comfortable." Susan is now complaining that it feels as though "ants are crawling around" on her knees.

- What probably happened, and what could be done to improve the situation?

DISCUSSION QUESTIONS

1. Of what significance is the choice of electrodes for a given patient?

2. If the patient complained of a prickling sensation underneath one of the electrodes, what would be the potential causes and potential remedies?

3. If a patient stated that he or she was not feeling the sensation underneath all of the electrodes, what might be the cause for this and what could you do?

4. Using terminology that a patient would understand, how would you explain electrical stimulation to him or her?

5. Your patient decides to lift up the corner of one of the electrodes; what would happen and why?

BIBLIOGRAPHY

Classic Titles in Electrical Stimulation

Baker, LL, et al: Electrical stimulation of wrist and fingers for hemiplegic patients. Phys Ther 59:1495, 1979.

Halstead, LS, et al: Relief of spasticity in SCT men and women using rectal probe electrostimulation. Paraplegia 31:715, 1993.

Kloth, LC, and Feedar, JA: Acceleration of wound healing with high voltage, monophasic, pulsed current. Phys Ther 68:503, 1988.

Melzack, R: Myofascial trigger points: Relation to acupuncture and mechanisms of pain. Arch Phys Med Rehabil 62:114, 1981.

Melzack, R, Stillwell, DM, and Fox, EJ: Trigger points and acupuncture points for pain: Correlations and implications. Pain 3:3, 1977.

Melzack, R, and Wall, DW: Pain mechanisms: A new theory. Science 150:971, 1965.

REFERENCES

1. Buban, P, Schmitt, ML, and Carter, CG, Jr: Electricity and Electronics Technology. Glencoe/McGraw-Hill, New York, 1999.
2. Nolan, MF: Conductive differences in electrodes used with transcutaneous electrical nerve stimulation devices. Phys Ther 71:746, 1991.
3. Lieber, RL, and Kelly, MJ: Factors influencing quadriceps femoris torque using transcutaneous neuromuscular electrical stimulation. Phys Ther 71:715, 1991.
4. U.S. Food and Drug Administration. Medical Devices. Retrieved from http://www.fda.gov/MedicalDevices/DeviceRegulationandGuidance/Compliance Activities/ucm106346.htm
5. Benton, LA, et al: Functional Electrical Stimulation—A Practical Clinical Guide, ed 2. Rancho Los Amigos Rehabilitation Engineering Center, Downey, CA, 1981, pp 34–36.
6. Snyder-Mackler, L, Delitto, A, Bailey, S, et al: Strength of the quadriceps femoris muscle and functional recovery after reconstruction of the anterior cruciate ligament. A prospective, randomized clinical trial of electrical stimulation. J Bone Joint Surg Am 77:1166–1173, 1995.
7. Fitzgerald, GK, Piva, SR, and Irrgang, JJ: A modified neuromuscular electrical stimulation protocol for quadriceps strength training following anterior cruciate ligament reconstruction. J Orthop Sports Phys Ther 33:492–501, 2003.
8. Snyder-Mackler, L, Ladin, Z, Schepsis, AA, et al: Electrical stimulation of the thigh muscle after reconstruction of the anterior cruciate ligament. Effects of electrically elicited contraction of the quadriceps femoris and hamstring muscle on gain and on strength of the thigh muscles. J Bone Joint Surg Am 73:1025–1036, 1991.
9. Lewek, M, Steven, J, and Snyder-Mackler, L: The use of electrical stimulation to increase quadriceps femoris force in an elderly patient following a total knee arthroplasty. Phys Ther 81: 1565–1571, 2001.
10. Gotlin, RS, Hershkowitz, S, Juris, PM, et al: Electrical stimulation effect on extensor lag and length of hospital stay after total knee arthroplasty. Arch Phys Med Rehabil 75:857–959, 1994.
11. Paternostro-Sluga, T, Fialka, C, Alacamliogiu, Y, et al: Neuromuscular electrical stimulation after anterior cruciate ligament surgery. Clin Orthog 368: 166–175, 1999.
12. McCulloch, JM, and Kloth, LC (eds): Wound Healing: Evidence-Based Management: Alternatives in Management, ed 4. FA Davis, Philadelphia, 2010.
13. Feedar, JA, et al: Chronic dermal ulcer healing enhanced with monophasic pulsed electrical stimulation, Phys Ther 71:639, 1991.
14. Feedar JA, Kloth, LC, and Gentzkow, GD: Chronic dermal ulcer healing enhanced with monophasic pulsed electrical stimulation. Phys Ther 71:639, 1991.
15. Fitzgerald, GK, and Newsome, D: Treatment of a large infected thoracic spine wound using high voltage pulsed monophasic current. Phys Ther 73:355, 1993.
16. Hurley, DA, Minder, PM, and McDunough, SM, et al: Interferential therapy electrode placement technique in acute low back pain: a preliminary investigation Arch Phys Med Rehabil 82:485–493, 2001.
17. Jarit, GJ, Mohr, KJ, Waller, R, et al: The effects of home interferential therapy on post-operative pain, edema, and range of motion of the knee. Clin J Sport Med 13:16–20, 2003.

LET'S FIND OUT

Self-Adhering Electrodes

A. Select two self-adhering electrodes of equal size. Plug the lead wires into the electrodes and into the stimulator. Set the stimulator with the following parameters:

Frequency: 120 Hz

Pulse Duration: Short (*lowest setting on the unit*)

Apply one electrode to your forearm over the muscle belly of the wrist extensors.

Apply the other electrode over the distal extent of the muscle belly, just proximal to the tendon (Fig. 12-12).

Slowly increase the intensity and record the sensation that is first perceived by your patient, along with the intensity setting that accomplished that sensation.

What did the sensation feel like?

What was the intensity to accomplish that sensation?

Turn the stimulator off and mark where the electrodes were placed on your patient.

B. Repeat the steps that you just completed in A, *but this time*, moisten the electrodes *first* with some water by:

Dipping your fingers in a cup of water

Rubbing your fingers over the surface of the electrodes

Apply one electrode to your forearm over the muscle belly of the wrist extensors.

Apply the other electrode over the distal extent of the muscle belly, just proximal to the tendon. (See Fig. 12-12.)

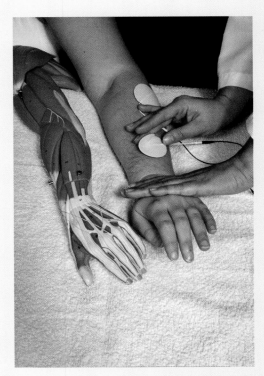

FIGURE 12-12 Electrode placement sites for wrist extensors using equally sized electrodes.

Slowly increase the intensity and record the sensation that is first perceived by your patient, along with the intensity setting that accomplished that sensation.

What did the sensation feel like?

What was the intensity to accomplish that sensation?

Turn the stimulator off and remove the electrodes from your patient. Replace the protective plastic over the surface of the electrodes.

Was there a difference between the intensity necessary to elicit a response once the electrodes were wet? Why or why not?

_____

_____

_____

_____

LET'S FIND OUT

Non–Self-Adhering Carbon Electrodes

Carbon electrodes have the advantage of being able to be used many times and tending to be cost effective. However, they do need to have an electrically conductive interface and do need to make good contact with the patient's skin to work effectively.

A. Select two of the carbon electrodes that are the same size as the self-adhering electrodes that you just used in the previous activity and corresponding sponges to fit them (Fig. 12-13). (There should be sponge extending beyond the border of the carbon electrode.)

B. Moisten the electrodes by fully submersing them in water and squeezing out the water so that some moisture remains, but not enough to leave a trail of dripping water under the sponge.

C. Secure the electrodes using the straps so that there is enough pressure to maintain even contact under the electrode but not so much pressure that circulation to the part is compromised (Fig. 12-14).

   Slowly increase the intensity and record the sensation that is first perceived by your patient, along with the intensity setting that accomplished that sensation.

What did the sensation feel like?

What was the intensity to accomplish that sensation?

   Was there a difference in the amount of intensity required to accomplish the same sensation with the carbon electrodes and sponges as with the self-adhering electrodes? Why or why not?

D. Select two of the carbon electrodes that are the same size as the self-adhering electrodes that you just used in the previous activity and this time cover the surface of the electrodes with electrically conductive gel before placing them on the surface of the skin.

E. Secure the electrodes with tape, but be sure that the patient is not allergic to the tape that you are using. It is also a good idea to be cautious with tape as some tape products stick so well to the integument that they may harm the skin when removed. In addition, the adhesive may be difficult to remove from the surface of the carbon electrode and sometimes migrates to to conductive surface of the electrode, which then decreases the current density of the conductive interface.

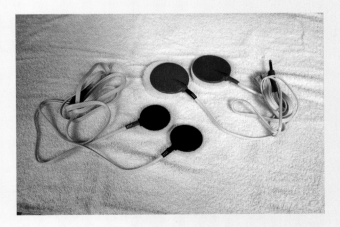

FIGURE 12-13 Sponge extends beyond the border of the carbon electrode.

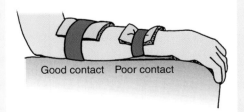

Good contact   Poor contact

FIGURE 12-14 Use of straps to secure carbon electrodes and sponges. It is important to make sure that there is enough pressure to maintain even contact under the electrode but not so much pressure that circulation to the part is compromised.

Slowly increase the intensity and record the sensation that is first perceived by your patient, along with the intensity setting that accomplished that sensation.

What did the sensation feel like?

What was the intensity to accomplish that sensation?

Was there a difference in the amount of intensity required to accomplish the same sensation with the carbon electrodes and electrically conductive gel as with the self-adhering electrodes or sponges? Why or why not?

Orientation to Current Density

A. You have been using two equally sized electrodes; set up a lead wire so that one electrode is less than half the size of the other electrode on that channel. Place the smaller electrode over the center of the muscle belly and the other electrode distal on the muscle belly (Fig. 12-15). *(You may use the forearm area again.)*

Gradually increase the intensity and record your patient's responses.

Does he or she feel the stimulation underneath both electrodes?

Is that stimulation equally perceived under both electrodes?

Gradually increase the intensity and record your patient's responses.

Does he or she feel the stimulation underneath both electrodes?

If not, which one is perceived as stronger, why?

B. Reverse the electrode setup that you are using. Move the smaller electrode to the distal extent of the muscle belly. Place the larger electrode over the center of the muscle belly (Fig. 12-16).

Gradually increase the intensity and record your patient's responses.

Does he or she feel the stimulation underneath both electrodes?

Is that stimulation equally perceived under both electrodes?

Gradually increase the intensity and record your patient's responses.

Does he or she feel the stimulation underneath both electrodes evenly?

If not, which one is perceived as stronger now, why?

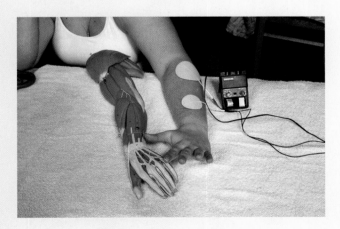

FIGURE 12-15 Electrode placement sites for wrist extensors using unequally sized electrodes with the proximal electrode larger than the distal electrode.

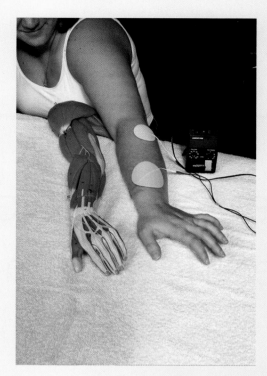

FIGURE 12-16 Electrode placement sites for wrist extensors using unequally sized electrodes with the proximal electrode smaller than the distal electrode.

CHAPTER 13

Neuromuscular Electrical Stimulation*

Joy C. Cohn, PT | Cecilia Mullin, PTA | Barbara J, Behrens, PTA, MS

Learning Outcomes

Following the successful completion of this chapter, the learner will be able to:

- Discuss the specific clinical applications for neuromuscular electrical stimulation (NMES) for strengthening and endurance, range of motion (ROM), facilitation of muscle function, management of muscle guarding, spasticity, edema reduction, and orthotic substitution.
- Discuss the factors that determine whether NMES would be appropriate for a patient.
- Discuss the clinical decision-making process for determining the effectiveness of the use of NMES and whether modifications should be made for that patient.

Key Terms

Amplitude
Balanced contraction
Duty cycle
Functional electrical stimulation (FES)
Intact peripheral nerve

Nerve conduction velocity (NCV)
Neuromuscular electrical stimulation (NMES)
Orthosis
Paretic

Partial denervation
Pulse duration
Ramp
Stimulation parameters

Chapter Outline

Identifying Appropriate Patients
Therapeutic Current Characteristics
    Waveforms
    Amplitude
    Pulse Duration
    Pulse Rate
    Timing Modulation Duty Cycle On-Off Ratio
    Ramp Modulation
General Guidelines for Clinical Applications
    Patient Positioning

    Electrodes
    Duration and Frequency of Intervention
Specific Clinical Applications
    Strengthening and Endurance
    Range of Motion
    Facilitation or Retraining of Muscle
Management of Muscle Guarding and Spasticity
    Edema Reduction
    Orthotic Substitution
    Partial Denervation

*The authors would like to thank Jean Scofield from Rancho Los Amigos for her assistance with photograph permission; Kathy Goodstein from Shriners Hospitals, Philadelphia Unit, for photography; Shriners Hospitals, Philadelphia Unit, Research Department for their support; and Elizabeth R. Gardner, MS, PT, NCS, Linda Baird-Jansen, MS, PT, Betsy Butterworth, PTA, Vicki Vanartsdalen, PTA, and Sophia Mullin Selgrath for their editorial recommendations. Most important, thanks to Andy, Alex, and Ellen for their understanding, love, and support.

"A good head and a good heart are always a formidable combination." —Nelson Mandela

Patient Perspective

"The stimulation seemed so scary when you suggested it but I can see the muscle working!"

The quotes that were selected for the start of this chapter reflect two important concepts that cannot be understated and must be kept in the forefront of every clinician's mind whenever working with electrical stimulation with a patient, especially when the treatment goal involves a muscle contraction. The first one is about having a good head and a good heart. The second one relates directly to the patient's initial reaction to what you are about to "do to them." This is a scary experience for virtually every patient. You might feel that way about it yourself when you feel your muscles contract without you initiating the contraction. That's what this chapter focuses on from both a theoretical and a clinical perspective.

The purposes of this chapter are to demonstrate the clinical use of surface electrical stimulation (ES) to accomplish a variety of therapeutic goals and to explore the guidelines for clinical decision-making and intervention selection.

Technological development of ES devices and the capability of these devices to treat a wider variety of patient diagnoses have progressed hand in hand to the present day, but not without confusion. To employ ES devices effectively, it is important to focus on the expected outcome. Although the technology for ES will continue to evolve over time, the goal of the treatment interventions will always be the reason that they were selected for use, and in many cases will probably remain the same.

This chapter considers the use of **neuromuscular electrical stimulation (NMES)** in physical therapy interventions. NMES is defined as "the use of electrical stimulation for activation of muscle through stimulation of the intact peripheral nerve."[1] **Functional electrical stimulation (FES)** and functional neuromuscular stimulation (FNS) are forms of NMES. They can be used as a substitute for an **orthosis** or external brace to activate muscle contractions in muscles that have impaired function (referred to as **paretic** or paralyzed muscles) to assist in functional activities such as standing or grasping an object. Other potential uses of electrical stimulation, such as wound healing, are covered in Chapter 14 of this text.

Identifying Appropriate Patients

NMES requires an intact, or at least partially intact, **peripheral nerve** to respond to the stimulation. The stimulus must reach the spinal cord so that the appropriate response to the stimulus can be expected. If the patient has a compromised "loop" then a different form of electrical stimulation that does not rely on the nerve would need to be applied. See Figure 13-1 for an example of an **intact peripheral nerve.**

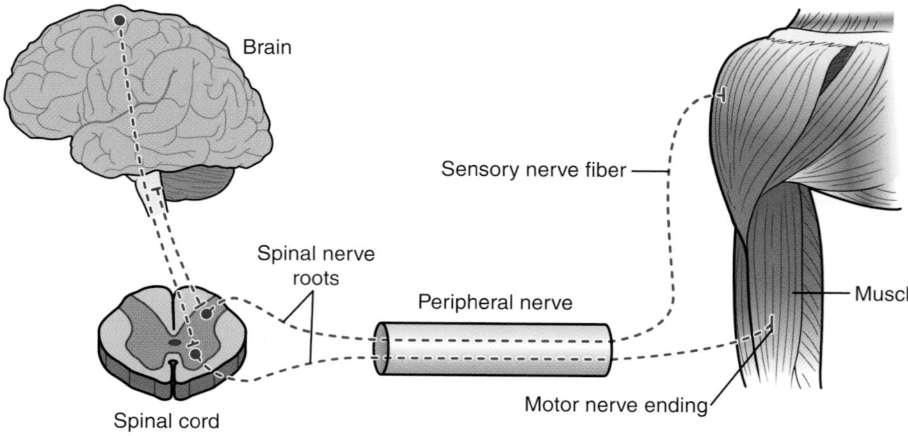

FIGURE 13-1 Intact peripheral nerve capable of perceiving sensory information and responding to that information after it is processed by the brain. This requires an intact "loop" within the spinal cord, brain, and peripheral nervous system.

A stimulated muscle contraction will always be generated via the innervating peripheral nerve, if intact. In the case of **partial denervation** because of a peripheral neuropathy of metabolic or neurological origin (e.g., diabetes or Guillain-Barré), it may not be possible to stimulate a contraction of any more strength than the patient is able to produce voluntarily as a result of diffuse denervation commonly associated with these diseases.

Electrical muscle stimulation (EMS) uses a pulsed monophasic waveform to activate denervated muscle directly. EMS is considered to be of questionable value[2] and so is not covered in this chapter. Innervation status, if in doubt, is determined via history, physical examination, and a strength-duration test (SD test), a **nerve conduction velocity** test **(NCV),** and/or an electromyographic (EMG) evaluation. These tests would be done to determine the viability of the nerve in conducting the electrical information that is necessary to cause a muscle contraction to take place. The NCV, specifically, records the amount of time for electrical energy to travel from "point A to point B." There is a questionable role for NMES in the presence of primary muscle disease such as muscular dystrophy. Further study is required.

There are a few contraindications to NMES.[3] The presence of a cardiac demand pacemaker is an absolute contraindication because of the possibility that the electrical current will interfere with the electronics of the pacemaker. Use of NMES with any other pacemaker should be undertaken with great caution, and the supervising physician should be contacted prior to use if ES is seen to be an essential part of the intervention plan. Precautions for NMES include the following[4,5] (Box 13-1):

- Older adult patients should be monitored closely for heart rate and blood pressure responses during initiation of a stimulation program to rule out unknown cardiac problems in response to exercise.
- The effect of NMES during pregnancy on the fetus is unknown. It may induce labor in a woman in her third trimester, and therefore should be avoided.
- Superficial metal (e.g., staples, pins, external fixation devices) will be a site of concentration for the current

---

BOX 13-1 | Contraindications to Electrical Stimulation

Absolute
- Presence of demand cardiac pacemaker

Relative
- Any other type of cardiac pacemaker
- Pregnancy in the third trimester
- Broken or irritated skin at electrode site

Precautions for Electrical Stimulation
- Older or cardiac patients monitor blood pressure and heart rate
- Superficial metal (i.e., staples, pins, external fixation)
- Absent or impaired skin sensation

---

delivered to the skin in the vicinity and can cause discomfort. Orthopedic metal implants (e.g., total hip replacement) are generally located too deep beneath the skin surface to be cause for concern.
- Absent or impaired skin sensation is not a contraindication but requires close monitoring of the skin response, careful choice of and application of electrodes, and, in general, use of biphasic and short-duration waveforms to avoid the potential tissue damage associated with direct current.

Therapeutic Current Characteristics

Individuals may respond negatively when first introduced to a stimulation program because of an innate fear of electricity or discomfort with stimulation. However, careful explanation of the goals of an intervention, gradual introduction of the stimulation amplitude, and readiness to consider a change in stimulation waveform or parameters can lead to success in most cases. This chapter contains a brief review of therapeutic interventions. The reader is urged to refer to Chapter 11 for a more detailed description of terminology.

The two main concerns in planning a program of NMES are

1. The quality of the stimulated muscle contraction
2. Patient comfort leading to cooperation with the intervention plan

Both are greatly affected by the **stimulation parameters.** The success of the intervention program is not based on the stimulator chosen; many different stimulators have been used effectively. It is knowledge of the features (i.e., parameters) of a particular stimulator that should most affect intervention planning (Box 13-2).

WAVEFORMS

Patient comfort has been investigated in many studies. Three studies of note investigated comparative comfort with differing waveforms. Delitto and Rose[6] found that there was no clear choice among three symmetrical biphasic waveforms, and that different preferences existed for different patients. In a comparison of symmetrical and asymmetrical biphasic waveforms, Bowman and Baker[7] found that normal female subjects preferred the symmetrical waveform when a large muscle group (quadriceps) was stimulated. But in another similar study,[8] it was found that when the target muscle groups were small (wrist flexors and extensors), normal subjects preferred an asymmetrical biphasic waveform. In a study comparing current frequencies with a symmetrical biphasic waveform,[9] the authors demonstrated a preference for higher frequencies when 30, 50, and 100 pulses per second (pps) were tested in stimulation of a tetanic contraction of the quadriceps muscle.

Different waveforms have also been investigated for the degree of torque and fatigue produced. In a study of quadriceps stimulation, monophasic and biphasic waveforms produced greater torque and less fatigue than polyphasic waveforms.[10]

AMPLITUDE

Current **amplitude** (intensity) must be gradually increased when first introducing a stimulation program to a patient. A patient will become comfortable with the sensation of stimulation within the first 15 minutes of gradually introduced stimulus amplitude, thereby becoming able to tolerate an increase in amplitude to achieve the desired muscle response. The desired muscle response can usually be accomplished within one or two sessions.

The quality of a stimulated muscle contraction is determined by a combination of many parameters, including stimulus amplitude, pulse duration, stimulus frequency, and duty cycle. Increasing the stimulus amplitude causes the recruitment of additional nerve fibers (e.g., smaller fibers and fibers farther from the electrode). This leads to increased force of the muscle contraction. There is a limit to the force increase observed once most of the muscle fibers have been recruited. Because most portable electrical stimulation devices use an arbitrary scale of 0 to 10 for the amplitude control, it is difficult to quantify the amount of current delivered to the patient, and the therapist must rely on the muscular response seen and the patient's sensory tolerance. The amplitude of current needed to achieve the desired response will also vary from patient to patient because of differences in resistance (impedance). In patients who are obese, it may not be possible to achieve the desired muscle response because the motor nerve may be too insulated by the intervening layer of adipose (fatty) tissue to allow sufficient stimulation without painful stimulation of the sensory nerves in the skin.

PULSE DURATION

The pulse duration has a corresponding relationship with stimulus amplitude. This relationship can be seen by examination of a strength duration curve. Short pulse durations (below 40 milliseconds) require much higher

---

BOX 13-2 | Current Characteristics to Consider in Planning a Treatment Intervention with Motor Levels of Electrical Stimulation

• Waveform	• Pulse rate
• Amplitude	• Duty cycle
• Pulse duration	• Ramp modulation

stimulus amplitudes. Higher stimulus amplitudes are necessary to elicit a motor response until pulse durations over 40 milliseconds are chosen. When the pulse duration is set between 40 and 500 milliseconds, an increase in amplitude between 15 and 40 mA (a relatively small range) will give you the full range of motor responses. Increasing the pulse duration above 500 milliseconds will not improve motor responses (Fig. 13-2).

One of the primary differences between stimulators lies in the pulse duration available for use. High-voltage pulsed-current stimulators have short and usually fixed-pulse durations (generally not above 200 milliseconds). Most other units appropriate for NMES have generally pulse durations between 20 and 500 milliseconds. Whether the pulse duration is adjustable varies from unit to unit. A unit that has pulse durations between 200 and 400 milliseconds will be more than adequate for NMES applications.

PULSE RATE

On many NMES units, the primary controls regulate amplitude and pulse rate (frequency). As pulse rate increases, the rate of motor nerve firing rises and the overlapping twitch response leads to a stronger contraction. However, there is a difference between voluntary and an electrically induced contraction. An electrically induced contraction results in reverse motor unit recruitment (large superficial motor units are usually recruited first) with synchronous activity of nerve and muscle fibers. This relationship causes action potentials of

nerve and muscle to be dependent on frequency; higher frequency leads to more rapid fatigue. To minimize fatigue, lower the pulse rate. Fused tetany can occur at frequencies as low as 12 pps, depending on the muscle.

TIMING MODULATION DUTY CYCLE ON-OFF RATIO

Another stimulus parameter that affects fatigue is the **duty cycle** or on-off ratio. Duty cycle is defined as "the ratio of on time to the total time of the trains of pulses or bursts."[11] Duty cycle is expressed as a percentage and calculated by dividing the on time by the total cycle time (on time + off time) and multiplying by 100. The on-off ratio is expressed in seconds and is calculated by dividing the on time by the off time. An example of a 1:3 ratio is where the on time is 4 seconds and the off time is 12 seconds (4/12 = 1:3).

The off time of the stimulation program represents the time during which a muscle is able to recover from the previous contraction and rest. Insufficient rest leads to rapid fatigue and limited success in achieving various intervention goals. The majority of clinical intervention paradigms utilize a 1:3 or 1:5 on-off ratio with the typical on time being 2 to 10 seconds. Total contractions for a typical 30-minute intervention session when a 1:5 on-off ratio is chosen are reduced by one-half. Knowledge of this fact should influence the length of the intervention session.[11] The on time chosen can often affect patient comfort as well. Because there is a range of on times from 2 to 10 seconds, documentation should

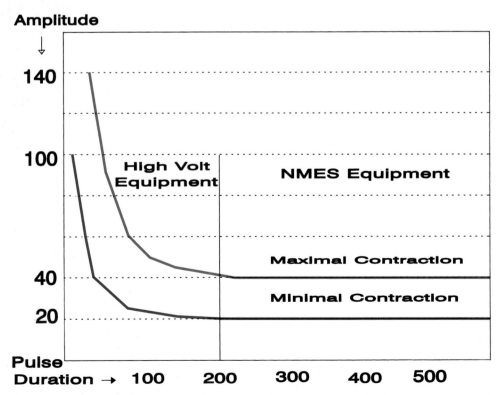

FIGURE 13-2 This annotated strength-duration curve demonstrates the inverse relationship between the amplitude of current and the pulse duration. The range of pulse duration available is one of the primary determinants of different classes of clinically available stimulation units.

include both the ratio and the actual on time. Patients generally find a contraction of 8 to 12 seconds in length to be very uncomfortable, sometimes likening it to a "charley horse" or cramp.

RAMP MODULATION

A **ramp** is another possible modulation of the therapeutic current chosen. The current is gradually increasing or decreasing with a plateau of stimulation.[13] The ramping of the current can be achieved by:

- A gradual increase of the amplitude, or
- Increase of pulse duration from zero to the maximum setting over a set time interval.

The perceived difference between a ramp of amplitude or pulse duration is "virtually indistinguishable"[13] and therefore is determined by the manufacturer in most devices and not often clearly identified for the user. The user must be aware that many devices include ramp time within the chosen on time. Therefore, to ensure that the stimulus reaches peak amplitude, the ramp time must be less than the on time. The usefulness of a ramp lies in the ability to grade the muscular response as it begins and ends with stimulation. Rarely do muscular movements occur abruptly. They are more commonly graded in intensity as the muscle fibers are recruited. This type of stimulated contraction is usually much more comfortable for a patient. A ramp-down of the stimulation allows a more controlled return of the limb to its resting position than would a sudden drop that occurs if the stimulation ends abruptly. When determining the on-off ratio of a stimulation program, the on time is considered to be only the time of the plateau of maximum stimulation and the off time should be set accordingly. In most clinical paradigms, a ramp of 2 seconds or less is sufficient. Ramps of greater than 2 seconds are generally chosen when there is a very high level of stimulation required or with a spastic muscle that is sensitive to a rapid stretch. Let's Find Out, Eliciting Motor Responses to Electrical Stimulation, at the end of this chapter is a short lab activity that will assist in your understanding the effects of frequency on motor levels of stimulation, electrode placement, and the sensations perceived to accomplish a motor level response.

General Guidelines for Clinical Applications

PATIENT POSITIONING

The patient should be positioned for comfort. A comfortable patient is best able to attend to the intervention program and can participate in reaching the therapeutic goals established. It is always worth the few extra minutes taken to achieve a comfortable starting position. Whenever possible, position a patient to allow him or her to see the results of a stimulated contraction. Visual feedback for the patient enhances sensory information and learning. Varying the patient's position during the course of an intervention will also enhance learning. For example, if the goal of an intervention is to achieve independent ankle dorsiflexion, the muscles for dorsiflexion

might be stimulated first in a supported long sitting position; progress to sitting with feet on the floor; and then progress to standing. Finally, the contraction could be timed to coincide with the correct phase of the gait cycle.

When stimulating weakened muscles, careful attention to limb position can take advantage of the length-tension relationship to enhance muscular performance. For example, a quadriceps contraction would be enhanced with stimulation if the patient were positioned semi-reclined with a bolster under the knee. In this position, the quadriceps is mildly stretched and more likely to achieve a visible limb movement.

The intervention program must take into account ROM limitations either imposed by a joint instability or dictated by a surgeon following a reconstruction. For example, in the early phase of rehabilitation following an anterior cruciate ligament reconstruction of the knee, patients may not actively or passively extend the knee beyond a position of 45° of flexion to avoid stressing the newly repaired ligament. Patients can safely perform stimulation augmented quadriceps and hamstring exercises by using isokinetic equipment, which allows for range limitations and/or locking the limb into fixed positions for isometric exercise (Fig. 13-3).

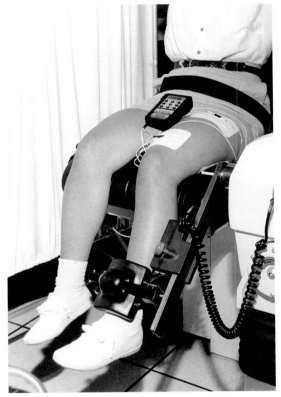

FIGURE 13-3 This patient setup illustrates how to exercise the quadriceps isometrically without endangering a recent anterior cruciate ligament repair. This setup can be used for isometric quadriceps contractions or co-contractions of the hamstrings and quadriceps. Note the carbon rubber electrodes secured by self-adhesive foam patches over the quadriceps muscle. Hamstring electrodes are not visible. (Ultra Stim model 650-01; Neuromedics, Inc., Clute, TX.)
(Photograph courtesy of Kathy Goodstein, Shriners Hospital, Philadelphia Unit.)

ELECTRODES

Three decisions must be made with regard to electrodes: type, size, and placement. These issues are discussed in Chapter 12.

A stimulated contraction will be most effective in meeting your goals if it closely approximates a normal contraction. In addition to the current modulations already discussed, it is important to attempt to achieve a **balanced contraction** to accomplish movement at the joint most affected by the electrically induced muscle contraction. For example, in stimulating the wrist extensors, the goal is extension of the wrist without excessive ulnar or radial deviation. A balanced contraction most closely approximates a functional movement in most cases and provides the patient with the best opportunity to reexperience normal movement. Careful electrode placement with a small electrode over the (small) target muscle and an asymmetrical biphasic waveform will offer the best chance of success.

DURATION AND FREQUENCY OF THE TREATMENT INTERVENTION

Clinical decision-making becomes most difficult when considering the duration and frequency of a treatment intervention. It is most dependent on the short-term goals, expected outcome, and patient response to the treatment intervention. Frequent re-assessment of the patient and his or her progress toward reaching the treatment goals will guide the decision to continue, change or discontinue this type of treatment intervention. The duration of a treatment intervention with NMES or FES will vary from as much as 6 weeks if the goal is muscle endurance, to as little as one session if the goal is muscle facilitation. A patient with an orthopedic injury and a normal nervous system will generally respond more quickly than patients with neurological disease or injury. This difference is the result of the injury or disease interfering with the ability of the loop to function properly and deliver the information efficiently to cause a muscle contraction. Remember, the goal of NMES and FES is that simple: to cause a muscle contraction. Anything that impairs, slows, or interrupts the information along the way will make it more difficult to accomplish that goal.

Specific Clinical Applications

STRENGTHENING AND ENDURANCE

The interest in using NMES to increase muscle strength was sparked after Russian athletes were observed being treated with ES during the 1976 Olympics. In 1977, a USSR physician, Dr. Kots, gave a series of lectures in Canada and made claims that ES with a "Russian current" stimulation protocol could lead to a 10% to 30% increase in muscular strength above what an athlete could achieve by conventional exercise regimens.[14] The Russian current he described has been investigated with mixed results. However, Kots's claims led to renewed interest in using other more familiar NMES devices and protocols to achieve strength gains in healthy normal individuals as well as patient populations with known musculoskeletal diagnoses.

Conventional exercise programs to increase strength are based on the overload principle of eliciting a small number of high-intensity contractions (at least 70% of a maximal contraction 3 to 10 repetitions or fewer) in a treatment session performed three to five times per week for 2 to 3 weeks. The same parameters of exercise apply when using NMES to augment strength in healthy and healthy-but-injured patient populations. There is compelling research evidence that NMES adds to the strength gains that normal individuals can achieve through conventional training programs alone.[15,16] However, in an intervention following limited traumatic or orthopedic injuries, NMES has been shown to lead to greater strength gains than those achieved with conventional exercise.[17-19]

Candidates for NMES can be any patients with multiple areas of weakness and deconditioning. These patients frequently benefit from a program that emphasizes endurance of the muscle or muscles of interest. This emphasis on endurance spotlights the other major function of a muscle, the ability to produce a force repetitively. Conventional endurance exercise programs consist of a decreased force of contraction and high repetitions (a Fair to Fair Plus contraction and a total of "30 to 60 minutes of stimulated contraction per day"[20]) in treatment intervention sessions five to seven times per week for 2 to 10 weeks. Several shorter sessions during the course of the day make the exercise programs more manageable, but the total time of cycled stimulation must take into account the total on time (in this instance, including the ramp time).

An example of a patient with a musculoskeletal injury could be a woman with a reconstruction of her anterior cruciate ligament (ACL) because of a skiing injury. This patient may not be allowed to fully extend her knee through an ROM against resistance in the early weeks of rehabilitation. One example of an intervention plan to enhance muscle performance could be as follows:

- Conventional exercise program to maintain right hip and ankle strength and overall aerobic capacity.
- NMES to increase isometric strength of the right quadriceps and hamstring muscles. Large rectangular electrodes should be used over large muscles like the quadriceps and hamstrings. Placing the proximal quadriceps electrode over the course of the femoral nerve near the femoral triangle will generally improve the muscular response.
- Ice to the right knee to control edema after exercise.

Results of studies using NMES have shown that superior isometric strengthening can be achieved in comparison to conventional isometric exercises.[20,21] The NMES program can be carried out in two ways: simultaneous stimulation of the quadriceps and hamstrings to achieve co-contraction with no net extension force or NMES to the quadriceps with the knee held in 45 degrees or more of flexion. In both instances, the use of an isokinetic machine to limit ROM and monitor the force produced by the stimulation program allows for safe exercise and quantitative information regarding improvement in force production (see Fig. 13-3).

If the hamstrings and quadriceps are both stimulated, the two channels of stimulation must be synchronized and balanced for comfort and force production. Stimulation of the quadriceps alone requires only one channel of stimulation. Amplitude is adjusted to achieve a maximally tolerated isometric contraction.

An example of a patient with a neurological deficit is a woman with a left middle cerebral artery infarct who had a flaccid right hemiplegia initially but progressed to walking with a straight cane and molded ankle-foot orthosis (MAFO) on the right leg. She is able to ambulate without the MAFO, but her ankle dorsiflexors on the right fatigue after ambulating 20 feet. A typical treatment intervention plan may include

- General conditioning exercises to improve overall fitness level
- Traditional strengthening exercises for all right lower extremity muscle groups
- Closed-chain exercises, including use of a biomechanical ankle platform
- NMES endurance program for the right ankle dorsiflexors

It is important to achieve a balanced response in the foot (Fig. 13-4) and an ankle with a neutral position relative to inversion and eversion without clawing or hyperextension of the toes (Fig. 13-5). Trimming a 2 × 2-inch electrode down to a 1-inch circle will increase the current density over the peroneal nerve proximally and usually improve the stimulated response. A portable NMES unit would be ideal to allow this patient to continue stimulation at home on a daily basis because endurance training requires an extended intervention protocol. See Box 13-3 for a suggested patient educational handout.

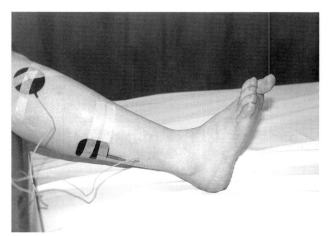

FIGURE 13-5 An unbalanced dorsiflexion response with excessive toe extension.

A meta-analysis from the Cochrane Library of the available published studies using NMES for quadriceps strengthening pre– and post–total knee replacement provided interesting findings. Patients were selected from the data for analysis. Only two studies met the selection criteria as being randomized controlled trials and controlled clinical trials despite searching in excess of seven databases. The meta-analysis objective was to "assess the effectiveness of NMES as a means of improving quadriceps strength before and after total knee replacement."[22] The results of the two studies identified for inclusion in the review found that there were no significant differences reported for maximum voluntary isometric torque or endurance between the NMES or control group. However, there was significantly better quadriceps muscle activation reported in the exercise and NMES group as compared with the exercise group alone. This difference was significant at the 6-week mark but not at the 12-week mark. Further study in this area is needed before any definitive statements can be made.[22] A subsequent randomized controlled trial with daily application of NMES to the quadriceps initiated 48 hours after total knee arthroplasty (TKA) found that improvements with NMES were still significant for several factors at 52 weeks after TKA.[23] (See Let's Find Out, Eliciting Motor Responses for Muscle Strengthening.)

RANGE OF MOTION

Methods to maintain ROM for some neurologically impaired and orthopedic patients are often taught to patients and their families. Passive ROM for neurologically impaired patients with mild spastic tone often has a good outcome. However, patients with moderate to severe spasticity tend to have difficulty making gains with passive ROM that may limit their daily functions. Patients with musculoskeletal impairments differ in that they have limited ROM as a result of immobilization of a muscle and/or a joint or pain.

A case example of a patient with a musculoskeletal impairment could include a male who has just had a cast removed because of a tibial fracture and is unable to fully

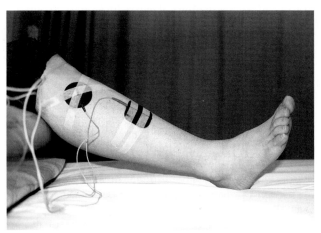

FIGURE 13-4 A balanced dorsiflexion response to NMES. Note electrode placement and extremity positioning.

BOX 13-3 | Educational Instructions for Home Use of Stimulator

Instructions for Home Use of Stimulator

1. Your treatment time is _____ minutes _____ times per day.
2. Your response to the treatment is dependent on your effort to adhere to the suggested program.

Preparing to Use the Stimulator

1. Clean the skin with mild soap and water in the area where you will place your electrodes.
2. Prepare your electrodes as instructed by your therapist and apply securely to the designated areas.
3. Connect the electrodes to the stimulator—be sure to insert all plugs completely so that there is no exposed metal.

Preparing to Exercise

1. Position yourself comfortably as instructed by your therapist.
2. Adjust the intensity control(s) until you experience a sensation and muscle response similar to your supervised exercise with your therapist.
3. Exercise for the length of time designated above.

Ending Your Exercise Session

1. Turn the intensity control(s) to off.
2. Disconnect all of the wires by pulling on the plugs. (Do not pull on the wires!)
3. Remove the electrodes and clean/store as instructed by your therapist.

Precautions for Stimulator Usage

- The stimulator is preprogrammed for your personal use only and should not be used on another part of your body or any other person. *(It is recommended that the patient also be given a diagram of electrode placement or preferably a photograph.)*
- Carefully inspect your skin in the electrode area before and after you apply the electrodes. Do not apply the electrodes to broken or irritated skin. Slight reddening of the skin under the electrodes is normal after stimulation. If you experience persistent skin irritation, stop using the stimulator until you see your therapist.
1. Do not bathe or shower while wearing the stimulator or electrodes.

Troubleshooting

No stimulation felt—
- Recheck all connections.
- Recheck electrode contact with skin.
- Recheck or replace batteries.

Stimulation uncomfortable—
- Recheck electrode contact with skin.
- Readjust intensity controls.
- Check skin under electrode for irritation.

Stimulation intermittent—
- Check wires for a break.
- Check connections.
- Check electrode contact with the skin.

extend his knee. An example of a treatment intervention plan is as follows:

- NMES of quadriceps muscle to achieve increased knee extension
- Home exercise program

It is important to avoid excessive knee joint compression when initiating this program to prevent increased joint irritation.

An example of a patient with a neurological deficit is a young woman with a closed head injury. The patient exhibits bilateral biceps brachii spasticity with elbow flexion contractures. An example of a treatment intervention plan is as follows:

- Serial casting
- NMES to the triceps muscle to restore elbow extension

In order not to limit her daily functions, such as self-feeding, the nondominant arm is treated first. The patient is casted in the available extension range, blocking flexion but not limiting extension while using NMES (Fig. 13-6). The time of ramp-up must be extended in this instance because of the spasticity present in the opposing muscle group. A ramp-up time of 6 to 8 seconds may be necessary to achieve a slow, effective stretch without increasing spasticity in the biceps by a quick stretch. Each week the serial cast should be removed and ROM measurements taken to document improvement. The serial cast is again applied in the available extension range, blocking flexion but not limiting extension to continue NMES sessions. In some instances a fabricated splint is preferred.

FACILITATION OR RETRAINING OF MUSCLE

Following a neurological injury or surgery (especially orthopedic surgery), a patient may have difficulty in initiating movement in a muscle group. This is especially the case if the patient has been unable to use the muscle for any length of time, leading to disuse atrophy, weakness, or pain. The central nervous system (CNS) relies heavily on the many forms of sensory feedback received to modulate performance. In the case of a neurological injury, that feedback can be greatly affected by sensory loss or distortion and/or change in available movement strategies and tone. In the case of surgery, the motor neuron pool can be directly inhibited by the pain efferents, and it has been suggested that cutting of a joint capsule during surgery can affect the normal proprioceptor activity.[21]

The desired response is a voluntary contraction that is enhanced by the NMES to increase CNS feedback and motor learning. Timing and coordination are crucial to the relearning of motor skills. Therefore, it is important that the NMES occurs at the correct time in the anticipated motor response. The timing of the stimulus must be controlled by the therapist or patient by use of an external trigger that is generally a foot or hand switch.

Sometimes the contraction must be initiated by NMES, but in other situations the stimulation is used to augment a weak voluntary response or to allow stabilization via stimulation of

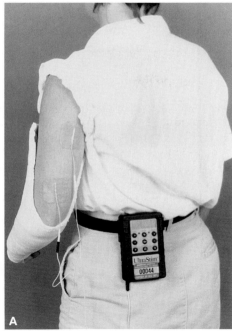

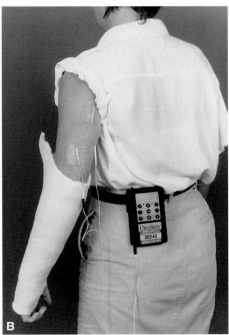

FIGURE 13-6 The "drop-out" cast required to achieve improved elbow extension range of motion. On the left side of the figure, elbow flexion is blocked by the front of the cast. On the right side of the figure, elbow extension is stimulated with the electrode placements illustrated to gain additional extension range. (Ultra Stim model 650-01; Neuromedics, Inc., Clute, TX; Pals Reusable Neurostimulation Electrodes, Axelgaard Mfg. Co., Ltd, Fallbrook, CA.)
(Photograph courtesy of Kathy Goodstein, Shriners Hospital, Philadelphia Unit.)

a related muscle group. This type of NMES program is not generally used by patients independently, but it represents a powerful adjunct for the therapist during an intervention session. Facilitation, to be most effective, requires patient cooperation and timing of stimulation within functional tasks.

An example to emphasize these concepts is a female who is status post a left total knee replacement (TKR). In attempting to teach the woman quadriceps isometric exercises, the treating clinician acknowledges that despite a strong effort, the patient is unable to activate her quadriceps effectively. One example of an intervention plan is as follows:

- NMES to facilitate quadriceps activity
- Conventional exercises to maintain ipsilateral hip and ankle strength and prevent circulatory stasis
- Protected weight-bearing and gait training with appropriate assistive device when indicated
- Ice to the left knee to control edema after exercise

The location of the distal electrode over the quadriceps may have to be modified if staples are still present at the incision site because electrical current can concentrate around superficial metal and cause pain. The distal electrode should be moved more proximally (leaving a gap of at least 1 inch between the electrode and staples) so that the staples are not within the main current path. An alternative is to use an asymmetrical biphasic waveform and place one electrode posteriorly on the hamstrings. This should ensure a comfortable stimulus for the patient. If not, NMES should be reconsidered, if needed, once the staples are removed. Close observations of the incision site are called for with an intervention to ensure that there is not excessive pull on a healing incision. A decrease in the amplitude may still be effective in giving a sensory cue for a quadriceps contraction. It is expected that this type of facilitation will be needed for only a short period of time because this patient has a normal CNS requiring possibly only one or two sessions of 15 to 20 minutes each before the patient is able to continue strengthening exercises on her own.

An example of a patient with a neurological deficit is a woman who had a left middle cerebral artery thrombosis 3 months prior to her initial examination. She has returned for additional therapy because she states that she has begun to move the fingers of her right hand. As part of a complete evaluation, it is found that she can actively flex and extend her fingers (although not through a complete range), but she cannot actively extend and stabilize the wrist, limiting her ability to produce a functional grasp. One example of an intervention plan is as follows:

- Conventional rehabilitation to maximize motor learning for functional independence
- NMES to facilitate voluntary movement in right wrist extensors
- Functional training in conjunction with NMES as appropriate

It is important to cue this patient visually so that she can receive visual, kinesthetic, and cutaneous feedback and coordinate stimulation with volitional prehension activities.

The wrist and finger muscles are very close in the forearm and careful placement can include or eliminate activity in the fingers as desired. Balanced wrist extension without excessive ulnar or radial deviation is optimal. Trimming electrodes to small patches can help limit spread of the stimulus to other muscles. Also, carefully consider the path of the current between the electrode placements to limit spread of stimulation. This patient has an abnormal CNS and may have increased difficulty in recruiting some muscle groups, although the electrically stimulated response in this group can approach the torque achieved in an unimpaired muscle group.[24] Therefore, she may require more experience with NMES to be capable of activating her wrist extensors independently and appropriately and can then achieve close to normal torque. The intervention time could be as limited as 15 to 20 minutes per session, but the duration of the treatment intervention might be as long as a week or two, especially if an effort is made to vary the motor learning experience by attempting functional activities such as grasp and release or different upper extremity positioning during wrist extension activation. If a patient is not successful with a trial of NMES because of her evolving neurological status, it may be appropriate to try again at another time in the course of her treatment intervention (see Let's Find Out, Experiencing Functional Electrical Stimulation for Activities of Daily Living).

Management of Muscle Guarding and Spasticity

NMES is widely used to address pain by reducing the tension in a muscle in spasm because of injury. However, if the mechanism of improvement is not clear, high-frequency stimulation can lead to rapid muscle fatigue in a constantly active muscle. It is possible to break the so-called pain-spasm-pain cycle with relief of pain for up to several hours post-intervention. This allows one to improve ROM and treat the particular areas of injury effectively.

In a patient with neurological impairment, stimulating a spastic muscle causes relaxation similar to that of a muscle in spasm; however, the relaxation period is brief because of the continued underlying abnormality in the CNS. During this brief relaxation period, the extremity can be repositioned to allow casting or bracing to be applied effectively.

An example of a patient with musculoskeletal impairments is a secretary who has been spending hours upon hours at the computer and has neck pain with muscle spasms of the right upper trapezius and rhomboids and limited rotation and forward flexion of the cervical spine with pain upon movement. When evaluated, the patient demonstrates acute muscle guarding with limited rotation and forward flexion because of pain with movement. One example of an intervention plan is as follows:

- Pulsed current (see Fig. 13-7 for an example of this application) to trapezius muscles
- Heat or ice is frequently used in conjunction with stimulation
- Home exercise program
- Patient education on sitting posture

This patient might benefit from either a bipolar or monopolar electrode placement (see Chapter 12). Documentation of the time frame of pain relief after a treatment intervention will assist in determining the necessity to continue the electrical stimulation intervention.

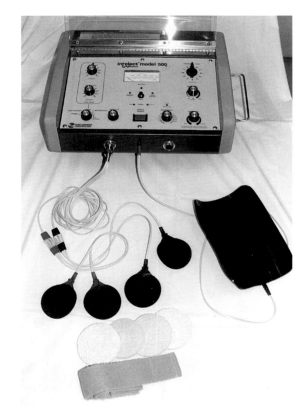

FIGURE 13-7 This unit illustrates the available adjustable parameters and electrode selection with one version of a clinical High Volt Pulsed Current Stimulation Unit. *(Intelect model 500; Chattanooga Corp, Chattanooga, TN.)*

(See Let's Find Out, Reduction of Muscle Guarding Using Three Different Electrical Stimulation Setups.)

EDEMA REDUCTION

Acute edema develops because of trauma to the blood vessels with leakage of blood cells and plasma proteins into the interstitial space. These blood components are negatively charged and, when exposed to a negative polarity, they are repelled from the area.[25] As a result the excess fluid, because of its attachment to the negatively charged proteins, is also shifted from the area.[26] Chronic edema requires venous and lymphatic drainage that is enhanced by cyclic muscle contractions. Treatment of edema (both chronic and acute) typically includes ice application or cool water immersion, elevation, and compression. NMES can be an effective adjunct to these standard interventions because the cyclical muscle pumping is achieved, which is what is required for chronic edema and venous and lymphatic drainage.

An example of a patient with edema is a construction worker who sustained a crush injury to the left hand 3 days ago. There were no fractures, but the patient has severe edema with limited ROM. An example of a treatment intervention plan is as follows:

- NMES to the hand with the injured hand elevated
- Elevation for exercising and rest
- Active ROM exercises as tolerated

Electrodes would be placed over the volar and dorsum of the hand with the hand in elevation. The reduction of edema will be most effective if the muscles within the hand (the intrinsics) contract, so the active electrode should be moved to maximize the intrinsic activity. The current should be adjusted to elicit a brief but effective contraction of the local muscles (frequency of 20 to 50 pps). Continuation of an intervention is based on edema reduction.

ORTHOTIC SUBSTITUTION

The ability to activate innervated but inactive, paretic, or paralyzed muscle has proved to be an effective replacement for orthotics in the management of deformity, or to assist purposeful movement. Beginning in the 1960s, a great deal of research took place with what has come to be called functional electrical stimulation, or FES. This continuing research explores many areas, including the restoration of standing and ambulation in patients who are paraplegic (Fig. 13-8), a dorsiflexion assist for patients with hemiplegia, and surface stimulation to substitute for bracing in patients with idiopathic scoliosis.[27-29] Many of the functional activities in which FES offers promise are complex activities (such as walking) requiring multiple channels of stimulation and feedback to allow the stimulation to be modulated to meet varying conditions. These crude systems are experimental presently.

Electrical stimulation to activate the ankle dorsiflexors in the swing phase of the gait cycle is widely used in the clinic because of the repetitive, rarely varying nature of the movement (Fig.13-9). The system requires a portable electrical stimulator with an external switch under the heel and one channel of stimulation (Fig. 13-10). The stimulation is activated by the heel rising off the floor at the end of stance leading to stimulation of the ankle dorsiflexors to allow toe clearance during swing.

Because of the repetitive nature of the muscular activity necessary to achieve long-term substitution for orthotics,

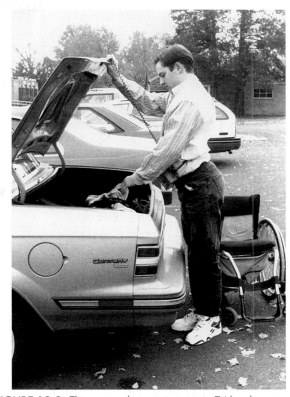

FIGURE 13-8 This research participant is a T4-level paraplegic who is pictured using an experimental, multichannel neuro-muscular stimulator (worn at his waist) to achieve standing without bracing.
(Photograph courtesy of Kathy Goodstein, Shriners Hospitals, Philadelphia Unit.)

any clinical application of NMES as an orthotic substitute first requires the development of muscular endurance described earlier in this chapter. Baker and associates[29] have clearly described an FES program to address shoulder subluxation, which can accompany the flaccid paralysis of a cerebrovascular accident.

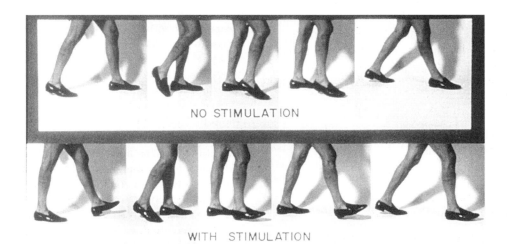

NO STIMULATION

WITH STIMULATION

FIGURE 13-9 This is a comparison of the swing phase of the right lower extremity with and without the aid of timed NMES. The patient seen here had experimental implanted electrodes instead of the clinically used surface electrodes.
(From Los Amigos Research and Education Institute, Downey, CA, with permission.)

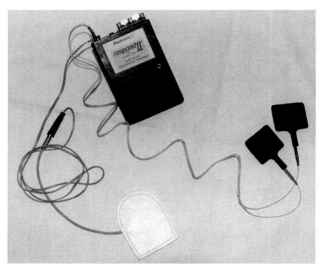

FIGURE 13-10 This unit is a commonly available portable unit for NMES with two channels of stimulation and an optional external heel switch to time the stimulated contraction with the gait cycle.
(Respond II FES Unit, Model 90003108; Medtronic Corp., San Diego, CA.).

PARTIAL DENERVATION

NMES can be effective in retraining a muscle that is recovering its innervation following a peripheral nerve injury. The re-innervation process following a nerve injury is slow, unpredictable, and seldom complete. The degree of expected function is difficult to predict and depends on many factors, including the

- Degree of atrophy
- Mechanism and extent of the nerve injury
- Time since the injury

With the paresis or paralysis associated with a peripheral nerve injury comes a "disconnection" of the CNS to the particular muscle(s).

With re-innervation, many patients find that they are no longer able to activate the muscle without the sensory cues associated with NMES: cutaneous, kinesthetic, and visual. The otherwise normal CNS readily accommodates allowing the patient to begin to reconnect and initiate movement. In addition the muscle strength can increase, usually within only a few sessions. It is difficult, however, to predict the muscular response achievable, given limited knowledge of the innervation status.

An example of a patient with partial denervation is a man who experienced a peroneal nerve injury during a right TKR 9 months ago. The patient has needed an ankle-foot orthosis (AFO) on the right because of a footdrop since surgery, and he is unable to actively dorsiflex the right ankle. According to the results of an EMG, the tibialis anterior muscle is re-innervating; however, the patient is unable to perform a volitional contraction. An example of a treatment intervention plan is as follows:

- NMES to reeducate re-innervating muscle
- Conventional strengthening exercises if patient learns to contract voluntarily

- Gait training with externally triggered NMES if appropriate to progress to ambulation without the AFO

In the presence of partial denervation, the motor point placement is difficult to predict with motor points moving more distally in most instances.[31,32] A stimulus with a longer pulse duration is preferable in the presence of partial denervation. The patient may have to be followed monthly or quarterly to assess re-innervation status until a Fair Minus or Fair contraction can be generated volitionally. Re-innervation is difficult to predict and requires frequent reexamination.

Safety Considerations

EQUIPMENT

It is the clinician's responsibility to ensure the safety and proper operation of all equipment. Inspection of equipment before use is an important safety measure that should be implemented as routine. A professional inspection of equipment should be scheduled yearly with a sticker clearly showing the date of the last inspection.

Every piece of equipment comes with an operating manual. Take the time to read the manual, which should be readily available. Equipment should never be operated if the user is not thoroughly familiar with its operation. Although the clinician's safety is an important factor when using electrical equipment, the patient's safety is obviously paramount. Refer to Chapter 11 for details on safety conditions.

PATIENT FACTORS

Medical History

It is recommended that before a treatment intervention with NMES or FES the patient should be questioned relative to the indications and contraindications of the modality being used. At the time of the examination, the patient may have forgotten to mention a possible problem or may have developed a problem that could make the application of the modality questionable. Thus, it is good practice to interview the patient prior to all interventions.

Skin Condition and Sensation

A visual inspection of the area to be treated will identify both normal and abnormal skin conditions. Normal findings may include birthmarks or other skin discolorations that will remain after an intervention is given. Observations should be clearly documented in the patient's medical chart to inform other therapists who may provide the intervention and to enable the treating therapist to identify any change in skin conditions that may result from an intervention.

After an intervention, the stimulated skin area may be pink as a result of an increase in the superficial blood flow that results from a treatment intervention. These changes should resolve within 30 to 60 minutes following the treatment. If the area remains quite red and/or color changes do not resolve, an electrical burn may have occurred and the patient must be treated immediately with the appropriate first aid. *(If there is a burn, an incident report must be completed to document the event consistent with the policies of the facility where the patient is being treated and medical personnel must be informed so that the burn can be treated appropriately.)* Maintenance of a good interface between the electrode and the patient by using an adequate amount of gel, complete contact of the electrode with the skin, and adequate fixation will prevent tissue damage.

Your communication with and observation of the patient and the area being treated are critical. Careful selection of waveform, pulse duration, and electrodes will prevent tissue damage from stimulation electrodes.

Cognitive Issues

Cognition, psychological abilities, and neuromuscular performance are interdependent. Impairment of cognition may be identified during the examination and relayed to you, or you may identify cognitive impairment through your careful observations and communication skills with the patient. Cognitive impairments include a decreased ability to learn or understand instructions or an inability to translate instructions into expected outcomes. Clear and concise communication is essential. The use of visual and tactile cues will be beneficial. Demonstration and palpating a normal muscular contraction on an unaffected body part may be one way to explain the goal of muscle reeducation clearly. Remember that most patients do not have medical backgrounds. The use of laypersons' terms to describe procedures is important.

Cognitive dysfunction can be incorrectly translated to poor motivation. Clinicians must continuously encourage and reinforce positive results throughout the treatment intervention. Patient understanding can be determined by asking the patient to repeat the instructions, the process, and the expected outcomes. Most important, help the patient understand *why* the intervention is needed and *how* it will relate to his or her everyday activities.

Lack of cognition does not prohibit the use of electrical stimulation. Electrical stimulation has been found to be very effective in decreasing spasticity and improving ROM in patients who are comatose.[33] Careful observation is mandatory for safety in this application.

Patient Education

EXPECTED OUTCOMES

Expected outcomes are directly related to the patient's education and understanding before, during, and after an intervention. Patients must understand the reason for the intervention, the process of the intervention, and the outcomes and benefits of the intervention. Explaining the rationale for treatment interventions will allow the patient the opportunity to communicate his or her needs, which then can be incorporated into the overall treatment intervention plan. The reason for the treatment intervention is usually identified or most understood in functional terms. Electrical stimulation for muscle reeducation to the quadriceps may benefit the patient in transfers or ambulation potential. It is important to communicate the expected outcome and not provide false hope to the patient.

Explaining procedures used during the treatment intervention process and the expected sensations will reduce the patient's fears and anxieties. Education and understanding of these procedures and sensations will allow the patient to better communicate and give the therapist feedback with which to maximize the treatment intervention.

Proper education of the expected outcomes and benefits is crucial. Clinicians must understand these outcomes prior to the initiation of a treatment intervention and appropriately use them with each patient. Electrical stimulation has many uses in physical therapy as was previously discussed. Electrical stimulation may be used for muscle relaxation as in the case of spasticity. Achievement of this relaxation may assist antagonist muscles to function, or improve mobility through increased ROM. Muscle reeducation is commonly seen with the use of electrical stimulation. Increased strength and utilization of extremities are often seen as volitional control is redeveloped. Reduction of edema through the utilization of electrical stimulation can also enhance ROM and use of extremities in all facets of activities of daily living.

Clinical Decision-Making

EVALUATING INTERVENTION EFFECTIVENESS AND MODIFYING THE INTERVENTION

Goals should be realistically and reliably achieved. A thorough understanding of the application of electrotherapy is very important to its use, especially because it is not a modality that is readily understood by many physicians or insurance companies, much less the patients who will experience it. It is equally important to be able to assess the outcome of the treatment intervention once initiated. It is impossible to do so without timely, appropriate, and reliable measurements of the patient's physical status before, during, and after the treatment intervention. On a daily basis, it is important to assess skin integrity, patient's response to the last treatment intervention, and any complaints of discomfort or change in symptoms.

DOCUMENTING A TREATMENT INTERVENTION WITH NMES

At examination and subsequent regular reexaminations, other measurements of status are made. Although the issue of reliability of clinical measurements is beyond the scope of this chapter, certain types of measurement have been accepted as generally reliable. Isokinetic examinations of strength are frequently used and in many cases have been shown to be very reliable for the examination of strength and endurance.[33] Active and passive ROM measurements are very useful in documenting progress in contracture management and motor control. It is frequently important to measure both active and passive ROM. In the examination of edema and hypertrophy, girth measurements at reproducible landmarks with a nonstretch measuring tape are frequently used. Volumetric measurements of the amount of water displaced by a limb are also reliable though rarely used. Accurate descriptions of gait or movement patterns and measurement of the temporal aspects of gait with a stopwatch are all useful, and when available, videotaping of the patient's performance is especially helpful.

The use of NMES to address the wide variety of patient scenarios presented in this chapter requires a familiarity with the equipment available in your facility and the characteristics of the available waveforms and stimulation parameters available with that equipment. Portable equipment in general will be less powerful, have fewer adjustable parameters, and can be more prone to damage. Clinical models will be potentially more versatile (for applications such as iontophoresis and wound healing, which are beyond the scope of this chapter), but less portable and more powerful, with a greater likelihood of causing tissue damage.

As stated previously, patient comfort is of primary importance because a treatment intervention that cannot be tolerated is an ineffective treatment. It is very important for the patient to be monitored closely during the initial treatment intervention sessions to assess comfort and whether a change in parameters should be considered.

Summary

In this chapter, the application of NMES as a clinical modality has been briefly reviewed. Understanding the rationale for using NMES when making clinical decisions for your patients will ultimately be reflected in their progress. This broad topic merits additional study through further reading.

Review Questions

1. Which of the following parameters on an electrical stimulator would be considered essential if your treatment goal was muscle strengthening?
   a. Frequency
   b. Pulse duration
   c. Intensity
   d. On/off times

2. Which of the following features or parameters on an NMES unit would be most helpful in differentiating between your ability to use it for range of motion (ROM), facilitation of muscle function, management of muscle guarding, edema reduction, or orthotic substitution?
   a. Portability
   b. Potential output intensity
   c. Flexibility within pulse duration settings
   d. Flexibility within on/off time settings

3. Which of the following features or parameters on an NMES unit would differentiate it from others and make it possible for use with both denervated and fully innervated patients for muscle reeducation and orthotic substitution?
   a. Potential output intensity
   b. Flexibility within pulse duration settings up to continuous
   c. Flexibility within on-off time settings
   d. A polarity setting that is adjustable

4. While you are working with a patient for the facilitation of muscle function, she complains of a prickling sensation under the electrode on her VMO. Which of the following is the most likely cause for this type of complaint and appropriate remedy?
   a. She's fatigued and needs to rest before resuming the activity
   b. She's feeling the effects of the electrode drying out and it needs to be rehydrated to reduce the impedance
   c. She's faking it. If she feels something you wouldn't be using NMES to facilitate a muscle contraction.
   d. The intensity needs to be higher. What she is reporting is the first sensation just before the appropriate level is perceived by the patient.

5. One of the "temps" who is filling in for a clinician who is out on maternity leave has set up a patient who has been receiving electrical stimulation to assist in the reduction of edema in her lower leg. You overhear the "temp" instructing the patient what should be felt during the treatment. Which of the following would be *incorrect* for this treatment goal?
   a. Let me know when you start to feel something. I've supported your leg so that it is elevated above your heart, which is how you should rest it whenever possible.
   b. Once you have started to feel something I will be increasing the intensity a little higher so that we can start to see a muscle contraction. Work with that. It will only be on for a couple of seconds but it will help pump some of the fluid back out of the area.
   c. Let me know when you start to feel something. Once you have started to feel something, I will be decreasing the intensity a little so that it's not so strong. I've supported your leg so that it is elevated above your heart, which is how you should rest it whenever possible.
   d. This should feel comfortable but I also need to see a contraction of the muscle. It will be off and on and I would like you to work with it.

CASE STUDY

Keith is an avid downhill skier who fell during a training run in preparation for an upcoming event. He tore his ACL and had it repaired, which is what brought him into the physical therapy department this afternoon. The PT evaluated him and found that although there are some limitations in his ROM as a result of the surgery, his primary complaint is weakness in the knee with the quadriceps significantly atrophied on the R as compared with the L, which was not injured. He is highly motivated and, at age 24, has to be cautioned not to overdo things.

- Would Keith potentially benefit from home use of NMES for muscle strengthening? Why or why not? Please support your response.

- Would Keith potentially benefit from use of clinical NMES for muscle strengthening? Why or why not? Please support your response.
- Once able to do so, what electrode placement sites could potentially be used for a patient who had undergone an ACL repair and needed quadriceps strengthening?
  - What parameters would you select to accomplish muscle strengthening for this type of patient?
  - Do you foresee any potential problems with Keith? Why or why not? What might they be if you answered yes?

DISCUSSION QUESTIONS

1. What are the sensory and motor effects of altering current, amplitude, and pulse duration?

2. When stimulating a patient, what is the importance of the current path?

3. If a patient has external metal on his or her skin such as staples, can electrical stimulation be used, and why should your placement of the electrodes be carefully considered?

4. When stimulating the ankle, should you be concerned with deviations such as inversion and eversion? What can you do to address these deviations produced by the electrical stimulation?

5. What size surface electrode would you choose when stimulating the gluteus maximus, and why is the size of the surface electrode important?

BIBLIOGRAPHY

An essential reference is Electrotherapeutic Terminology in Physical Therapy Revision 2000, which is available from the American Physical Therapy Association at their Web site: www.apta.org.

REFERENCES

1. Electrotherapeutic Terminology in Physical Therapy. Section on Clinical Electrophysiology: American Physical Therapy Association, Alexandria, VA, 1990, p 29.
2. Nelson, RM, and Currier, DP: Clinical Electrotherapy. Appleton and Lange, Norwalk, CT, 1987, p 110.
3. Baker, LL, et al: Neuromuscular Electrical Stimulation: A Practical Clinical Guide, ed 3. Los Amigos Research and Education Institute, Downey, CA, 1993, p 73.
4. Baker, LL, et al: Neuromuscular Electrical Stimulation: A Practical Clinical Guide, ed 3. Los Amigos Research and Education Institute, Downey, CA, 1993, p 75.
5. Snyder-Mackler, L, and Robinson, AJ: Clinical Electro_physiology—Electrotherapy and Electrophysiologic Testing. Williams & Wilkins, Baltimore, 1989, p 131.
6. Delitto, A, and Rose, SJ: Comparative comfort of three waveforms used in electrically eliciting quadriceps femoris muscle contractions. Phys Ther 66:1704, 1986.
7. Bowman, BR, and Baker, LL: Effects of waveform parameters on comfort during transcutaneous neuromuscular electrical stimulation. Ann Biomed Eng 13:59, 1974.
8. Baker, LL, Bowan, BR, and McNeal, DR: Effects of waveform on comfort during neuromuscular electrical stimulation. Clin Orthop Related Res 233:75, 1988.
9. McNeal, DR, et al: Subject preference for pulse frequency with cutaneous stimulation of the quadriceps. Proc Rehabil Eng Soc North Am 9:273, 1986.
10. Laufer, Y, Ries, JD, Leininger, PM, and Alon, G: Quadriceps femoris muscle torques and fatigue generated by neuromuscular electrical stimulation with three different waveforms. Phys Ther 81:1307–1316, 2001.
11. Electrotherapeutic Terminology in Physical Therapy. Section on Clinical Electrophysiology: American Physical Therapy Association, Alexandria, VA, 1990, p 25.

12. Baker, LL, et al: Neuromuscular Electrical Stimulation: A Practical Clinical Guide, ed 3. Los Amigos Research and Education Institute, Downey, CA, 1993, p 87.
13. Electrotherapeutic Terminology in Physical Therapy. Section on Clinical Electrophysiology: American Physical Therapy Association, Alexandria, VA, 1990, p 21.
14. Ward, AR, and Shkuratova, N: Russian Electrical Stimulation: The Early Experiments. Phys Ther 82:1019–1030, 2003.
15. Currier, DP, and Mann, R: Muscular strength development by electrical stimulation in healthy individuals. Phys Ther 63:915, 1983.
16. Robinson, AJ, and Snyder-Mackler, L (eds): Clinical Electro_physiology—Electrotherapy and Electrophysiologic Testing, ed 2. Williams & Wilkins, Baltimore, 1995, pp 129–130.
17. Delitto, A, et al: Electrically elicited co-contraction of thigh musculature after anterior cruciate ligament surgery. Phys Ther 68:45, 1988.
18. Selkowitz, DM: Improvement in isometric strength of the quadriceps femoris muscle after training with electrical stimulation. Phys Ther 6:186, 1985.
19. Lewek, M, Stevens, J, and Snyder-Mackler, L: The use of electrical stimulation to increase quadriceps femoris muscle force in an elderly patient following total knee arthroplasty. Phys Ther 81:1565–1571. 2001.
20. Baker, LL, et al: Neuromuscular Electrical Stimulation: A Practical Clinical Guide, ed 3. Los Amigos Research and Education Institute, Downey, CA, 1993, p 51.
21. Draper, V, and Ballard, L: Electrical stimulation versus electromyographic biofeedback in the recovery of quadriceps femoris muscle function following anterior cruciate ligament surgery. Phys Ther 71:455, 1991.
22. Monaghan, B, Caulfield, B, O'Mathuna, DP: Cochrane Abstracts: Surface neuromuscular electrical stimulation for quadriceps strengthening pre and post total knee replacement. Abstracts assessed as up to date 01/07/2008.The Cochrane Library 2012.
23. Stevens-Lapsley, JE, Balter, JE, Wolfe, P, Eckhoff, DG, and Kohrt WM: Early neuromuscular stimulation to improve quadriceps muscle strength after total knee arthroplasty: a randomized controlled trial. Phys Ther 92:210, 2012.
24. Landau, WM, and Sahrmann, SA: Preservation of directly stimulated muscle strength in hemiplegia due to stroke. Arch Neurol 59:1453–1457, 2002.
25. Sawyer, P (ed): Biophysical Mechanisms in Homeostasis and Intravascular Thrombosis. Appleton-Century-Crofts, New York, 1965.

26. Nelson, RM, and Currier, DP: Clinical Electrotherapy. Appleton and Lange, Norwalk, CT, 1987, p 176.
27. Phillips, CA: Functional electrical stimulation and lower extremity bracing for ambulation exercise of the spinal cord injured individual: A medically prescribed system. Phys Ther 69:842, 1989.
28. Baker, LL: Neuromuscular electrical stimulation in the restoration of purposeful limb movements. In Wolf, SL (ed): Clinics in Physical Therapy—Electrotherapy. Churchill Livingstone, New York, 1981, p 25.
29. Eckerson, LF, and Axelgaard, J: Lateral electrical surface stimulation as an alternative to bracing in the treatment of idiopathic scoliosis. Phys Ther 64:483, 1984.
30. Baker, LL, and Parker, K: Neuromuscular electrical stimulation of the muscles surrounding the shoulder. Phys Ther 66:1930, 1986.
31. Richardson, AT, and Wynn-Parry, CB: The theory and practice of electrodiagnosis. Ann Phys Med 4:3, 1957.
32. Wynn-Parry, CB: Strength duration curves. In Licht, S (ed): Electrodiagnosis and Electromyography, ed 2. Elizabeth Licht, 1961, p 241.
33. Baker, LL, Parker, K, and Sanderson, D: Neuromuscular electrical stimulation for the head injured patient. Phys Ther 63:1967, 1983.
34. Farrell, M, and Richards, JG: Analysis of the reliability and validity of the kinetic communicator exercise device. Med Sci Sports Exer 18:44, 1986.

LET'S FIND OUT

Lab Activity: Eliciting Motor Responses to Electrical Stimulation

Equipment
Clinical and portable electrical stimulation units with adjustable parameters:
  pulse duration
  frequency
  intensity
  ramps
  electrodes and lead wires appropriate for the electrical stimulation units
See Figures 13-11 and 13-12.

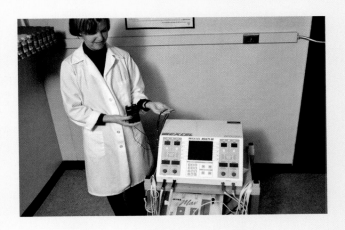

FIGURE 13-11 Clinician standing holding a portable model of an electrical stimulation unit in her hand. She is standing next to a clinical model of an electrical stimulation unit with multiple channels of stimulation that is "line operated," meaning that the unit plugs into the wall for power.

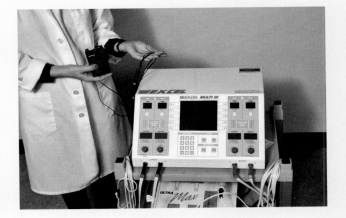

FIGURE 13-12 Both the clinical and portable models of electrical stimulation units but upon closer inspection, it is clear that the sizes of the lead wires for the two units are different and would not be interchangeable.

Precautions and Why

Precautions	Why
In the presence of an unstable fracture	If the electrical stimulation is used for a motor response, this is a contraindication. However, if no motor response is elicited, electrical stimulation can be considered safe.
Over an area with decreased sensation	If the desired response is dependent upon sensation, then electrical stimulation may be useless. However, if the desired response relies on a motor response, then the application may be considered safe. If the application involves the transmission of ions across the skin, then the patient must be able to report sensation to protect him or her from an adverse response.
When the patient has decreased cognitive ability	If the desired response is dependent upon sensation, then electrical stimulation may be useless. However, if the desired response relies on a motor response, then the application may be considered safe. If the application involves the transmission of ions across the skin, then the patient must be able to report sensation to protect him or her from an adverse response.
During pregnancy	Safety of powered muscle stimulators for use during pregnancy has not been established. If the application is after the first trimester, this should be used with caution. Electrical stimulation has been safely for analgesia used during labor and delivery, but it may interfere with fetal monitors.
Patients with documented evidence of epilepsy, cerebral vascular accident (CVA), or reversible ischemic neurological deficit	These patients should be monitored carefully when electrical stimulation is used in the cervical region for possible adverse responses.

Contraindications	Why
During the first trimester of pregnancy	There are no data to indicate the level of safety for the fetus with the application of electrical stimulation during the first trimester of pregnancy.
Over the carotid sinus	There would be potential problem if the circulation to the brain were altered.
In the presence of a pacemaker	Electrical stimulation devices could potentially interfere with the electrical demands of the pacemaker.
Over or in proximity to a malignancy	Most application techniques with electrical stimulation involve the potential for an increase in circulation to the area. The possibility exists that the electrical stimulation may enhance the development of a metastasis.
Over or around the carotid sinus	Sustained muscle contraction of the cervical muscles surrounding the carotid sinus may impair circulation to the brain.
In the presence of a thrombus	If a muscle contraction is elicited in the extremity with a thrombus, the possibility of dislodging the thrombus increases.

Lab Activities: Dorsi and Plantar Flexors of the Ankle

1. Select a classmate/patient for electrical stimulation to elicit a motor response in his or her calf. Position your patient as if he or she had an acutely sprained edematous ankle (Fig. 13-13).

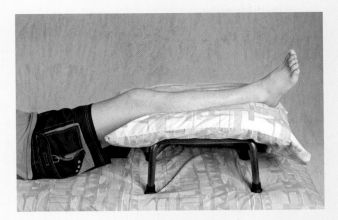

FIGURE 13-13 Patient positioning for an acutely sprained edematous ankle.

Determine where the electrodes should be placed to elicit muscle contractions in the tibialis anterior (Fig. 13-14).

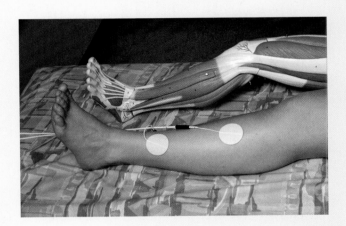

FIGURE 13-14 Electrode placement sites to elicit muscle contraction in the tibialis anterior.

2. Select a stimulator capable of producing levels of stimulation that elicit a tetanic muscle contraction. Preset the following parameters:

Pulse duration	200 μs or more
Pulse rate	50 Hz
On-off times	10/10 (Adjustable in seconds)
Reciprocal stimulation	Yes

3. Prepare and apply the electrodes that you have selected. They should be appropriately sized relative to the sizes of the muscles that you will be stimulating.

Remember that electrode size influences the ease of eliciting a comfortable muscle contraction. Large electrodes have generally lower resistance levels, which translates into lower intensities necessary to elicit a muscle contraction. *(Try eliciting a contraction with small electrodes and then with electrodes twice that size.)*

How much more intensity was necessary to elicit a muscle contraction than was necessary for the patient to report that a stimulus was felt?	Intensity for a sensory response = Intensity for a motor response = Difference =
What happens to the *quality* of the contraction as you slowly increase the frequency up to 80 pps *(during the on times)*?	Contraction quality
What happens to the quality of the contraction as you slowly decrease the frequency down to 10 pps *(during the on times)*?	Contraction quality
What was the "optimal frequency" for the muscles that you were stimulating?	Optimal frequency

LET'S FIND OUT

Vastus Medialis and Rectus Femoris

1. Electrical stimulation has been used successfully for the enhancement of an isometric muscle contraction. It is one of the tools used in a comprehensive treatment plan for postoperative recovery for several orthopedic procedures. The key components of this form of stimulation include the isolation of the muscle group and the stabilization of the joint that the muscle acts upon.

2. Select a classmate/patient for electrical stimulation to the vastus medialis and the rectus femoris (Fig. 13-15). Position your patient so that he or she is supported in about 20° of knee flexion and no joint motion is permitted. (You may use a commercial dynamometer to stabilize the joint isometrically or devise some other means to stabilize the joint.)

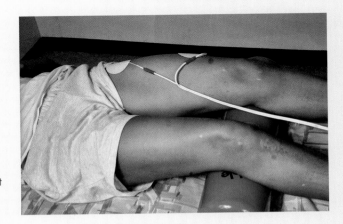

FIGURE 13-15 Patient who is positioned so that she is supported in about 20° of knee flexion and no joint motion is permitted.

3. Set up the stimulator that you have selected so that you will be able to elicit strong muscle contractions. Identify electrode placement sites for both muscles, and apply the electrodes securely, one channel for each muscle (Figs. 13-16 and 13-17).

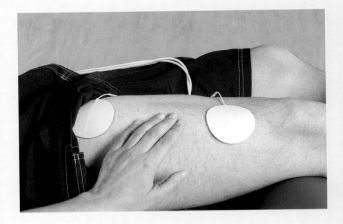

FIGURE 13-16 Electrode placement for the rectus femoris.

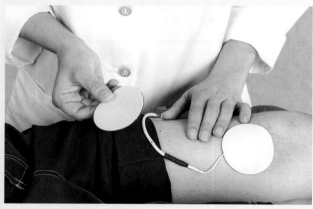

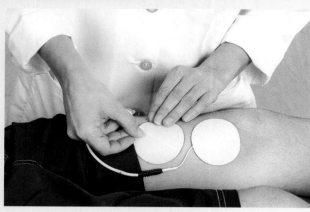

FIGURE 13-17 Electrode placement for vastus medialis.

4. Slowly increase the intensity of the stimulus until a strong muscle contraction is elicited.

What should the patient feel?

What would make the stimulus more comfortable for your patient?

Try one of *your* potential solutions for comfort. Does it make a difference?

How much intensity can your patient tolerate?

What is the optimal frequency for a tetanic contraction for this patient?

What would the rationale be for a 10-second on time and 50-second off time?

Does the quality of the muscle contraction that you are eliciting change with successive contractions? If yes, how?

What happens to the sensation of the stimulation if the patient *contracts* with the stimulation?

Try other options that you believe may make the stimulus more tolerable for your patient. Observe the responses. What was the "best" setup or option for your patient?

LET'S FIND OUT

Lab Activity: Experiencing Functional Electrical Stimulation for ADLs

Reduction of Shoulder Subluxation

Electrical stimulation has been used to augment muscle function in a wide variety of areas, including urinary incontinence, shoulder subluxations, footdrop during gate, and standing stability for the patient population with paraplegia. One of the common elements to these applications is the development of portable intelligent technology that is capable of producing the necessary parameters when the patient needs them and in a way that does not actually interfere with a patient's ability to perform the activity itself. For example, the technology has been in existence for years to elicit a muscle contraction with electrical stimulation; however, a 6-foot power cord was usually necessary to provide the power source of stimulation. Devices are now much more portable and accessible for patients than they ever have been.

1. Select a classmate/patient for electrical stimulation to his or her middle deltoid and supraspinatus. You will be adjusting the parameters so that you can elicit a tetanic muscle contraction to help reduce a subluxation of the humoral head (Figs. 13-18 and 13-19).

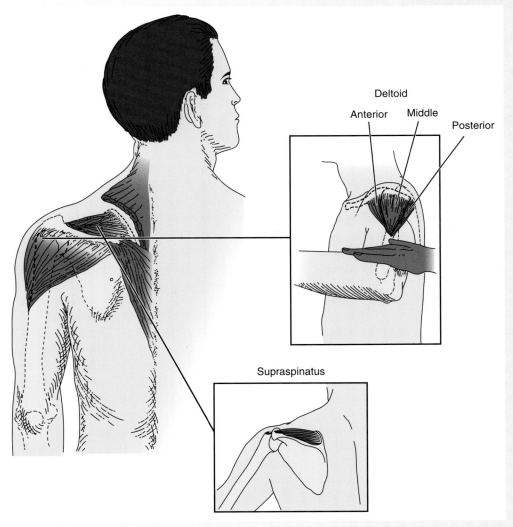

FIGURE 13-18 Supraspinatus and middle deltoid showing the humeral head underneath.

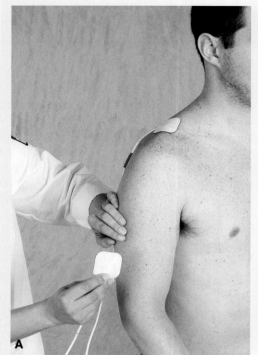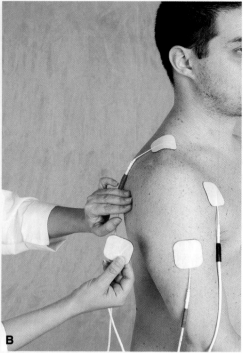

FIGURE 13-19 Electrode placement sites to elicit responses from both the supraspinatus and middle deltoid to approximate the humoral head. (left)A, Anterior view; (right)B, posterior view.

2. Position your patient so that he or she will be able to see what you are doing.

3. Teach the patient the electrode placement sites that he or she will need to use and how to assess success in eliciting the desired response.

4. Familiarize yourself and the patient with the portable stimulator that you will be using.

   Teach your patient how to inspect the treatment area and the unit, care for and apply the electrodes, and adjust the intensity controls.

5. Determine the appropriate on-off timing for your patient and whether or not on ramps are functional for this patient. Turn the unit on, and have the patient set the intensity level.

   a. Why do you think that you were instructed to teach the patient so much during this lab activity?

   b. How much more time did it take to complete the instruction?

   c. What parameters did you use?

      • Frequency
      • Pulse duration
      • On-off times
      • Ramps

   d. Which is more important, a specific intensity reading or a specific response? Why?

   _____

   _____

   _____

LET'S FIND OUT

Lab Activity: Reduction of Muscle Guarding Using Three Different Electrical Stimulation Setups

Whenever an injury occurs to soft tissue, one of the natural responses that takes place is muscle guarding, which acts to protect the area from further movement or injury. Muscle guarding impedes the circulation to the area and promotes metabolite retention. This may increase pain perception owing to the sensitization of the nociceptors by the presence of metabolic by-products. *Reduction in muscle guarding is a therapeutic technique used to help with pain reduction.*

1. Select a classmate/patient for electrical stimulation to the upper trapezius muscles bilaterally. Position your patient so that he or she is comfortable and the upper trapezii are in a resting position. If your patient has some palpable muscle tightness, assess the degree of tightness and tenderness to palpation (Figs. 13-20 and 13-21).

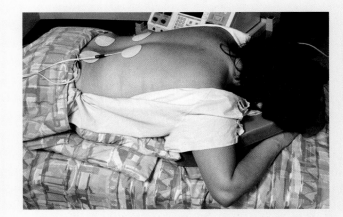

FIGURE 13-20 Patient positioning so that he or she is comfortable and the upper trapezii are in a resting position.

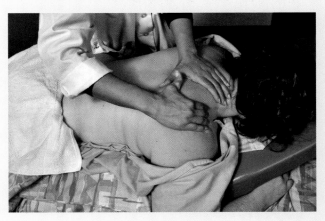

FIGURE 13-21 Palpation to the upper trapezii to determine the presence of increased palpable tightness or fibrous nodules.

2. Identify the parameters that you will need to elicit a tetanic muscle contraction and select the electrodes that you will be using. Apply the electrodes in each of the following setup configurations: crossed, horizontal, and vertical (Figs. 13-22, 13-23, and 13-24).

   a. First try each of the setups with reciprocal on-off times and 3-second on ramps. Which was the most comfortable for your patient?

   _____

   b. Then choose a simultaneous on time for each of the setups. Was there a difference in the sensation for any of the three setups? Why or why not? Which is more comfortable, using on ramps or not using them? Why?

   _____

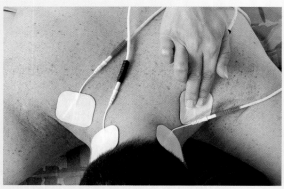

FIGURE 13-22 Electrode placement sites for bilateral upper traps with a crossed setup.

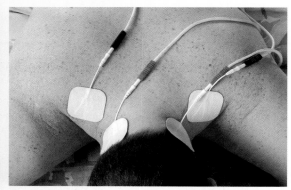

FIGURE 13-23 Electrode placement sites for bilateral upper traps with a horizontal setup.

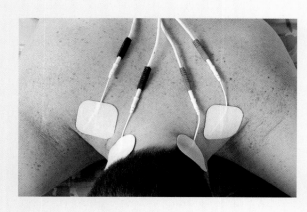

FIGURE 13-24 Electrode placement sites for bilateral upper traps with a vertical and parallel setup.

c. If your goal was to decrease muscle guarding, specifically in the upper trapezius muscles bilaterally, which setup would be the most logical for accomplishing your goal?

_____

d. If your goal was to decrease the muscle's ability to maintain a contraction, what parameters would you adjust and what would be your rationale for adjusting them? .

_____

e. If your patient for this exercise had palpable muscle tightness before you applied the stimulation, reassess the tightness. Was there a noticeable change to you? To the patient?

_____

Patient Scenarios

Read through the patient scenarios, and determine the following:

- Whether or not electrical stimulation would be indicated and your rationale for your response
- What the parameters for stimulation should be for the patient if electrical stimulation is indicated
- Where the electrode placement sites should be
- What additional considerations there might be for a patient to be considered a good candidate for electrical stimulation
- Whether the electrical stimulation should be applied clinically or at home and why
  A. Mary is a 55-year-old woman who has been admitted to the rehabilitation hospital subsequent to an unsuccessful attempt to reduce the effects of arteriosclerosis in her carotid arteries. She has had bilateral cerebrovascular accidents (CVAs) as a result of the procedures performed. She is otherwise healthy, with no previous medical complications. She has been referred for physical therapy to see whether electrical stimulation can be used to reduce the subluxation of her right shoulder. She is alternately expressively and receptively aphasic and has limited manual dexterity skills. At

present, she is nonambulatory because of balance difficulties and an inability to use her upper extremities for support with assistive devices.

B. Joe is a 48-year-old shoemaker who has been referred to the physical therapy department subsequent to a CVA. At present, he has flexor spasticity in his right upper extremity, and he has foot-drop on the right. His goal is ambulation without the short leg brace that he has been ambulating with for the last 3 months since the CVA.

C. Cynthia is a legal secretary who has been referred to the physical therapy department subsequent to injuries that she sustained in an automobile accident 3 days ago. She has a cervical strain with pronounced muscle guarding throughout the cervical spine, shown by limitations in active ROM in all directions. She also is scheduled to have a medial meniscectomy next week. Her physician and employer are concerned about her ability to return to work after the knee surgery and want her to be as prepared as she can be preoperatively to ensure a prompt return to work. (She is an aerobics instructor at night and a long-distance bicycle racer, with a race in 2 months.)

D. Mike is an athletic trainer for the track team of a local high school. He has been referred to physical therapy for edema reduction for his left ankle, which has now been sprained a total of six times in the past 3 years. His attempts at icing the joint have not been successful in reducing the edema. He has lateral instability and marked weakness in the ankle invertors and evertors on the left. Mike is well motivated and has no other medical complications.

Documentation

Documentation of treatments rendered with electrical stimulation involves the recording of the treatment goal for which the stimulation was applied and the outcome. Documentation of electrode placement sites, parameters, or stimulator used would be necessary only if there were some significant trial-and-error period before optimal results were achieved and if there were some unusual techniques used to accomplish the results. For example, if a patient had tendon transplant surgery, it would be important to know where the electrode placement sites were located. Once the goal is identified, the parameters to accomplish the goal and the electrode placement sites necessary should be fairly obvious to other clinicians who may be reading the documentation to duplicate the treatment rendered.

Select two of the patients whom you applied modalities to during the laboratory exercise and write a progress note that includes each patient's subjective complaints, the objective information that you recorded, the physical agent that was applied and manner of application, the response to the applied physical agent, and your assessment.

Lab Questions

1. What was the optimal frequency to accomplish a tetanic contraction?
   - How did your optimal frequency compare with those of your classmates?
   - Of what significance is an optimal frequency?
   - What were some of the common factors for the applications of electrical stimulation performed during this lab activity?
2. If you had two stimulators to choose from, and one had a maximum pulse duration of 100 msec and the other stimulator had a maximum pulse duration of 200 msec, which one would require a lower intensity to elicit a tetanic muscle contraction? Why?
3. Of what potential value are on ramps?
4. Why is it more difficult to adjust parameters other than the intensity on portable functional electrical stimulators?
5. What do you think would be the most significant barriers to the successful use of functional electrical stimulation for gait? How would you potentially overcome them?
6. What objective measures could you employ to ensure that the level of electrical stimulation consistently elicited the same level of muscle contraction response?
7. Describe the necessary parameters for electrical stimulation to maintain muscle strength.

Frequency	
Pulse duration	
On-off times	
Treatment time	
Level of intensity required	

CHAPTER 14

Electrical Stimulation for Tissue Repair

Ute H. Breese, PT, MEd, OCS | *Peter C. Panus, PT, PhD*
Elizabeth Buchanan, PT | *Barbara J. Behrens, PTA, MS*

Learning Outcomes

Following the successful completion of this chapter, the learner will be able to:

- Describe the use of electrical stimulation for tissue repair.
- Outline the proposed mechanisms of healing of human tissue.
- Discuss the classifications of wounds.
- Discuss the electrical potentials of normal and injured tissues.
- Review the findings for the use of electrical stimulation in tissue repair.
- Outline the application of electrical stimulation to promote tissue repair.

Key Terms

Antimicrobial
Arterial insufficiency
Autolytic débridement
Chemotaxis
Current of injury

Galvanotaxis
Hemostasis
Macrophages
Plethysmography
Polyarteritis nodosa

Polymorphonuclear cells
Transepithelial potential difference
Venous insufficiency

Chapter Outline

> *"Physical therapy . . . . The science of healing. The art of caring."* —*American Physical Therapy Association*

Patient Perspective
"Is it really doing something if I don't feel anything?"

The use of electrical stimulation as a therapeutic intervention has its beginning in the 1700s. Work during this time included the discovery of direct current by Luigi Galvani in 1791, the invention of the alternating current induction motor by Nikola Tesla in 1882, and demonstration of the **current of injury** by Carlo Matteucci in the 1800s. This current of injury is the production of an electrical current by injured tissue and is believed to activate the body's healing response to the wounded tissue.[1-3]

Electrical stimulation for wounds has been defined as "the use of a capacitive coupled electrical circuit to transfer energy to a wound."[4] A complete description of electrical stimulation devices, terminology, and definitions is beyond the scope of this chapter; for greater detail, the reader is advised to consult additional sources of information and previous chapters in this text.

Although electrical stimulation has been used to promote healing of bone and other musculoskeletal injuries, this chapter focuses on how electrical stimulation has been used in the healing process of wounds. The first part of this chapter reviews the cascade of wound repair and then centers on the proposed mechanisms by which electrical stimulation may affect tissue repair. The next part of the chapter discusses the some of the conclusions of research studies on the effectiveness of electrical stimulation in healing wounds. The final part of the chapter reviews the literature on the protocols for clinical procedures using electrical stimulation for tissue healing. While stimulation parameters and mechanisms of tissue healing have yet to be completely defined, the underlying conclusion of many studies is that electrical stimulation may be of benefit in tissue repair.[2,5-15]

Patient Perspective

Remember, your patient will be very cautious and curious about what you are going to do. It is important to explain thoroughly what you are going to do and what would be reasonable for your patient to expect. This type of application is very new to most patients and some might be skeptical about the potential benefits. Explain them to your patients.

Patient Comments

The wound seems to be healing a lot better since starting the electrical stimulation.

Cascade of Injury Repair: How Do Wounds Heal?

The healing model that is discussed in this section is that of an acute full-thickness integumentary wound. Chronic full-thickness wounds are thought to heal by a similar process, but these wounds may be hindered in their progression toward healing owing to various factors that are yet to be fully identified.[4] For a more detailed discussion, the reader is referred to wound care texts such as McCulloch and Kloth's *Wound Healing Evidence-Based Management*, now in its fourth edition. Luther Kloth, who was a professor at

Marquette University for many years, and continues to be an active voice in the section on Clinical Electrophysiology and Wound Care and field of physical therapy, has been credited by some as one of the most influential figures in the United States for advancing research and reimbursement for electrical stimulation for wound healing. His research in the late 1980s was considered groundbreaking in this area.[11]

When damaged, wound tissue generally heals by following three phases of repair that coincide and overlap to some extent (Fig. 14-1). The following description characterizes the three phases.[4,16,17]

When the integument is damaged, an inflammatory process occurs that allows the body to seal off the area, prevent the spread of a potential infectious process, and stop the bleeding of tissues. This process lasts for 3 to 7 days[4] and is defined as the inflammatory phase. In this phase **hemostasis** occurs during the first hours, meaning that localized blood flow through blood vessels stops. Vasoconstriction is followed by a localized vasodilation and arrival of different types of cells, including **polymorphonuclear cells** and macrophages. Polymorphonuclear cells make up a group of white blood cells that have what appear to be multi-lobed nuclei. **Macrophages** are cells that are part of our immune system that aid in the destruction of foreign bacteria and viruses. The process of migration of these cells to the site of injury by way of a chemical signal is called **chemotaxis**.[18] These cells help rid the injury site of the associated tissue debris or pathogenic organisms.[16] When the wound is clean, the second phase of injury repair may begin.

The second phase is termed the proliferative phase, characterized by several events, including the formation of new blood vessels (angiogenesis or neovascularization) and the production of an extracellular matrix to fill the defect within the tissues. The matrix repair occurs through the formation

WHY DO I NEED TO KNOW ABOUT...

INFLAMMATION

Inflammation is an important step in the healing process that must take place in preparation for tissue repair. If inflammation is not permitted to occur, then the underlying tissues are not ready for healing to take place. The cells that are needed to prepare the area have not been signaled into the area!

of granulation tissue that acts as the foundation for scar tissue development.[19] The main cell involved in this process is the fibroblast. Another event that occurs during the proliferative phase is that of wound contraction. Wound contraction consists of myofibroblast activity within the wound bed that pulls the edges of the wound together.[17] In addition, throughout the first two phases of healing, and especially in the second phase, epithelial cells regenerate and migrate from the margin to the center of the wound.[19]

LET'S THINK ABOUT IT...

When you were a child, you probably fell and skinned your knee on more than one occasion. If you did, you probably noticed that once the bleeding stopped, your knee developed a scab that helped to protect the area. (If you didn't skin your knee, you probably injured another bony prominence with a similar outcome.)

After a couple of days, the scab might have started to itch or appear pink around the edges as the wound margin was contracting. The pink that appeared around the edges was fresh granulation tissue. If you think about it, you actually observed your first examples of wound healing when you were a child!

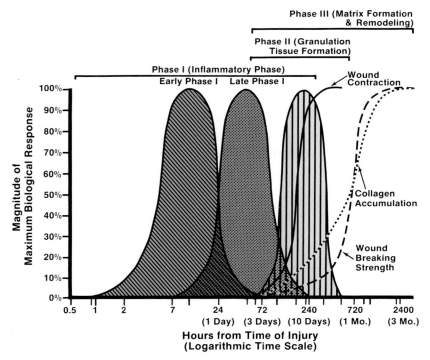

FIGURE 14-1 The Phases of healing and relative time.
(Reprinted with permission: In McCulloch, JM, and Kloth, LC [eds]: Wound Healing Evidence-Based Management, ed 4. FA Davis, Philadelphia, 2010, p 9.)

WHY DO I NEED TO KNOW ABOUT...

WOUND HEALING

The newly formed tissue will appear pink, representing angiogenesis. The wound will contract, which will limit motion if mobility of the surrounding tissue is not maintained.

If you think back to the example of the skinned knee, at some point you broke the scab by bending your knee too far. However, that was relative to the scab that was limiting your motion. If you didn't break the scab, you wouldn't have been able to do what children do, which at the time probably included riding a bicycle, running, and playing soccer and kickball. Placing the knee through the motions that it needed to go through for it to be functional for you at that time was what needed to happen so that you could heal properly.

The third phase is the remodeling phase. This process can last for as long as 2 years following wound closure.[17] In this phase, the amount of collagen in the healing tissue increases, and there is a gradual conversion from type III collagen to type I collagen.[16] During the remodeling phase, the initial highly disorganized and weak scar is transformed into a more organized and stronger scar, with progression from a raised and reddened scar to a thinner, less bulky, and more elastic scar.[4,16,17,20]

Electrical Stimulation for Tissue Repair: What Are the Findings?

There are many theories concerning how electrical stimulation can promote the healing of tissues. Some of the main concepts and proposed mechanisms of healing are described in this section, but it is important to note that definitive explanations for the effect of electrical stimulation on healing tissues have yet to be fully defined.

THE CURRENT OF INJURY

Injured tissue has been found to produce a measurable "current of injury."[21-23] This current applies to the presence of the skin battery potential, in which negative potentials exist in the stratum corneum with respect to the underlying dermis.[24] Normally, intact skin creates a barrier that results in a **transepithelial potential difference** (TEPD) between the dermis and epidermis of the skin. This TEPD voltage across an epithelium is the sum of the membrane potentials for the outer and inner cell membranes. In various diagnoses the TEPD is increased, making it a potential diagnostic tool for those disorders. The TEPD is believed to be produced by the sodium (Na^+) ion pump.[23,25] When the skin is damaged, the difference in potential is believed to be the source of the current of injury that occurs as a result of an interruption in the barrier,[22] and a lateral voltage gradient exists in the skin at the edge of the wound[23,26] (Fig. 14-2). A flow of current with a positive polarity occurs within the wound.[22,23]

This current has been suggested as a trigger to wound healing[1-3] and also appears to be associated with the moist wound-healing process.[3] Experimental research has shown that wounds that are permitted to dry cease demonstrating a post-wounding current of injury, while wounds that are kept moist maintain a post-wounding current of injury.[23] The value of the moist wound healing process has been described,[17,27,28] and the association between the current of injury and the moist wound-healing process has been proposed as one reason why the rate of healing in dry wounds is reduced compared with moist wounds.[4,25] Further support for the beneficial effect of the current of injury is supported by an experimental study in which transepithelial sodium transport was inhibited, resulting in a reduced current of injury and reduced wound healing.[29]

Scientists have suggested that the application of electrical stimulation influences the current of injury and the lateral electric field that exists in areas of skin disruption.[22] Electrical stimulation may mimic the body's own bioelectric currents, and thus "jump-start," re-initiate, or facilitate the wound-healing process,[4,24,25,30] although the actual contribution of the Na^+ current of injury to wound healing has not been determined.[16]

The positive wound potential is believed to serve as an indicator of healing: When the wound closes over, the positive potential disappears.[22] However, an experimental study has reported changes in the polarity of wounds in guinea pigs as healing progresses.[21] In this study, the current within the wound was initially positive during the first 3 to 4 days following injury, and then became negative during the subsequent days of healing. This finding is of interest in view of electrical stimulation protocols in which

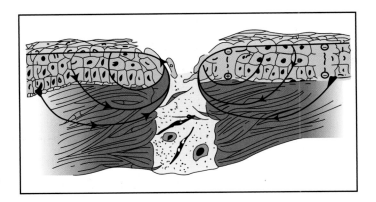

FIGURE 14-2 The "current of injury" flows out from the wound, and returns to the battery via the sodium ion pump.
(Reprinted from Clinics in Dermatology, Vol. 2, L.F. Jaffe and J.W. Vanable, Electric Fields and Wound Healing, 34–44, 1984, with permission from Elsevier.)

the polarity of the treatment electrode is alternated during the healing process. Several clinical studies have used such protocols,[2,7,8,14,31] whereas others have used the same polarity for the treatment electrode throughout the study's duration.[9,10]

GALVANOTAXIS

Galvanotaxis describes the process in which cells possessing a positive or negative charge are attracted to an electric field of opposite polarity.[16] As a result, the positively or negatively charged cells that normally respond to injury may be attracted to the positive or negative pole of the stimulating electrode, depending on the cell's polarity.[16,17,30] This concept is supported by the findings of several in vitro studies in which the cells involved in tissue repair were found to be preferentially attracted to one pole of the stimulating electrode.[32,33] Neutrophils are attracted to the positive pole of the stimulating electrode at pH 8.0 to pH 6.8, and to the negative pole at pH 4.9.[32] Macrophages are attracted to the positive pole,[33] whereas fibroblasts have maximum stimulation of protein and DNA synthesis when in proximity to the negative pole.[34] Isolated epidermal cells, cell clusters, and cell sheets migrate toward the negative pole in DC electric fields of 0.5 to 15 V/cm.[35] However, basic science research results show enhanced epithelialization of partial thickness wounds by a regimen of an initial day of negative polarity followed by 7 days of positive polarity using monophasic pulsed current.[36] These results were found in comparison with other regimens consisting of only negative polarity; only positive polarity; or daily alternating negative and positive polarities. Results from another study, using high-voltage monophasic pulsed current, suggested a higher rate of epithelialization (compared with a control group) in dermal wounds stimulated using a regimen of 3 days' negative polarity followed by 4 days' positive polarity of the treatment electrode.[37]

ANTIMICROBIAL EFFECTS

Electrical stimulation has been demonstrated to have a bacteriostatic or bacteriocidal effect on various pathogenic organisms that are commonly found to infect wounds.[38–43] Caution is recommended in applying the results of these studies to predict the effectiveness of electrical stimulation on pathogenic organisms in the clinical treatment of wounds. This is because of the difficulties inherent in applying the results of in vitro studies[38–41,43] to predict in vivo behavior, and in the use of studies with acute wounds in animals[42] to predict the behavior of chronic wounds in humans.

WHY DO I NEED TO KNOW ABOUT...
GALVANOTAXIS

Using the information from these studies, the theory of galvanotaxis may be used as a basis for the selection of polarity in the treatment electrode.[16]

Studies vary in the type of electrical stimulation used. The use of electrical stimulation as an antimicrobial, something that kills or inhibits the growth of microorganisms such as bacteria, fungi, or protozoans, has been demonstrated with the use of microamperage direct current,[38,41,42] milliamperage direct current,[39] and high-voltage pulsed current.[38,41,42] However, the range of high voltages such as those found to be effective with high-voltage pulsed current are unlikely to be well tolerated if applied clinically.[16,40]

The effects of electrical stimulation against pathogenic organisms may be affected by factors such as electrode polarity and electrode composition. The cathode (−) is associated with antimicrobial effects against *Pseudomonas aeruginosa*,[42] whereas both the anode (+) and the cathode (−) are associated with action against *Staphylococcus aureus*.[38–40,43] Electrode composition may also be an important factor; one study[38] demonstrated that electrodes consisting of silver wire showed superior antimicrobial effects when compared with stainless steel, platinum, or gold wire electrodes while using anodal stimulation in the 0.4 to 4.0 microampere range.

For clinical application, these studies indicate there may be a possible antimicrobial effect with the use of low-intensity direct current, although further research is needed in this area.

EFFECTS ON BLOOD FLOW

One of the proposed mechanisms by which electrical stimulation is believed to accelerate wound repair is by enhancing blood circulation. In studies of electrical stimulation and blood flow, various assessment measures have been used to determine blood flow including skin temperatures,[44–46] transcutaneous oxygen ($TcPO_2$) levels,[47–51] venous occlusion plethysmography,[52,53] photoplethysmography,[54] ultrasonic Doppler flowmetry,[55,56] and laser Doppler flowmetry or imaging.[57–60] **Plethysmography** is a test used to measure changes in blood flow or air volume in different parts of the body. Comparison of study results is difficult owing to the differences in the outcome measures, as well as in methodologies, electrode placement sites, study populations, and other factors.

Electrical stimulation using alternating square wave pulses at 80 Hz was found to increase blood flow in ischemic skin flaps.[59] Blood flow was also noted to increase with the application of low-frequency transcutaneous electrical nerve stimulation (TENS) to the forearms of healthy volunteers[58] and to the lower legs of nine healthy female volunteers.[60] However, there was great individual variation in the latter study[60] results, with two individuals showing marked responses, and the rest demonstrating less obvious responses. Another study[57] using low-frequency TENS was found to increase blood flow in chronic leg ulcers and in the intact skin surrounding the ulcer. In this study, the electrical stimulation unit delivered constant biphasic square wave pulses at 2 Hz, and electrodes were placed 5 cm proximal, and 5 cm distal, to the ulcer.

Several other studies have reported changes in blood flow associated with the use of electrical stimulation. Studies using motor level stimuli have reported increases in blood flow[52,53,55] or no effect on blood flow.[56] In contrast with these studies, which primarily assessed the effect of electrical stimulation on blood flow in the same extremity in which the electrodes were placed, another study[44] assessed the effect of electrical stimulation on blood flow in all four extremities. This study found that motor level stimuli, using stimulation of a distant point (electrodes were placed on one hand), resulted in a skin temperature rise in the extremities. In contrast, a study that used sensory level stimuli with pulsed galvanic stimulation over arterial blood vessels in the upper extremity was found to have no effect on blood flow.[54]

The circulatory system allows oxygen and nutrients to reach tissues,[61] and sufficient oxygen is required for all phases of wound healing.[4] Diminished oxygen levels, as determined by $TcPO_2$ levels, show a trend of being associated with the presence of pressure ulcers in individuals with spinal cord injury.[62] In addition, low $TcPO_2$ levels have been tied to a reduced potential for the ability of ulcers to heal.[4,16] The use of electrical stimulation has been associated with increases in $TcPO_2$ levels in individuals with spinal cord injury,[50] normal adults,[47] and individuals with diabetes.[47,48,51] However, at least one other study has shown conflicting results when assessing the effect of electrical stimulation on $TcPO_2$ levels in individuals with diabetes.[49] In this study, cathodal high-voltage pulsed current was applied to the foot or leg at the most distal site where the 5.07 Semmes Weinstein monofilament could be felt. $TcPO_2$ levels were found to decline following treatment. However, the study authors reported there was a subgroup of patients that had increased skin blood flow in response to electrical stimulation, and suggested the need for further research.

Several studies have examined the effect of electrical stimulation on skin temperatures. Wong and Jette[46] found that the use of TENS over acupuncture points in the forearm and hands was associated with decreases in index finger skin temperature in healthy subjects. Scudds et al[45] found that high- and low-frequency TENS had no effect on finger skin temperature in asymptomatic subjects, while high-intensity, low-frequency TENS was associated with a rise in mean hand temperature as measured by infrared thermography. As noted previously, a study by Kaada[44] reported that the use of low-frequency TENS on the hands of individuals with Raynaud's phenomenon or diabetic polyneuropathy was associated with an increase in skin temperatures in the extremities.

Some researchers have suggested that skin temperature is not a reliable measure of skin blood flow,[54,60] and newer, more precise methods such as laser Doppler imaging are suggested.[60] Support for this concept is seen in a study that assessed the effect of TENS on cutaneous blood flow.[58] This study concluded that low-frequency TENS applied to the skin overlying the median nerve resulted in significant increases in blood perfusion as measured by laser Doppler flowmetry, while concurrent measures of skin temperature were found to have no significant changes. Other discrepancies have been noted in which skin temperatures were

found to have little or no relationship with photoplethysmography,[54] laser Doppler imaging,[57,60] or laser Doppler flowmetry.[58] Researchers have suggested that the laser Doppler technique may be a more sensitive measure of microcirculation in the skin.[60]

Other study findings for the effect of electrical stimulation on blood flow suggest that results may be affected by factors such as the electrode placement sites,[63] the presence of impaired peripheral perfusion,[51] the use of motor level versus sensory level stimuli,[47] the stimulation frequency,[52,55,58,60] and, as noted previously, the outcome measure that is used. Further research in this area would be beneficial.

EFFECTS ON NECROTIC OR DEVITALIZED TISSUE

A suggested use for electrical stimulation is to facilitate **autolytic débridement**, which is the process by which the body attempts to shed devitalized tissue by the use of moisture via the galvanotaxis theory.[30] Using the theory of galvanotaxis, a treatment electrode of positive polarity is placed over the wound to attract the negatively charged neutrophils and macrophages to promote autolysis.[30] Conversely, autolytic débridement may be supported by the use of polar effects to produce an alkaline pH to soften up or solubilize the necrotic wound tissue.[16] Production of an alkaline pH is more likely to occur with the use of cathodal direct current, as compared with the use of pulsed currents.[16]

Electrical stimulation for autolytic débridement of necrotic tissue is supported by observations in two studies, although no randomized controlled studies that have specifically examined this effect have been found. In one study,[2] the wounds of 30 hospital inpatients were treated with 2 hours of electrical stimulation twice daily using low-intensity direct current. Negative polarity was used for the first 3 days, then positive polarity until the wound healed or a plateau in healing was reached. All wounds were débrided prior to admission to the study. However, only the treated wounds did not require any further débridement during the duration of the study. In another, more recent study[10] 42 chronic leg ulcers of varying etiologies were treated with cathodal (−) high-voltage pulsed current or sham treatments. These wounds were also débrided, primarily on a single occasion for removal of excess callus from foot ulcers during a 1- to 2-week period of conventional wound care at the initiation of the study. Only the treated ulcers showed improvement based on scores using the Photographic Wound Assessment Tool (PWAT), and these improvements were attributed to the loss of necrotic tissue and an increase in granulation tissue.

Does Electrical Stimulation Work?

In 1994, the Agency for Health Care Policy and Research[64] recommended that clinicians "consider a course of treatment with electrotherapy for Stage III and IV pressure ulcers that have proved unresponsive to conventional therapy. Electrical stimulation may also be useful for recalcitrant

Stage II ulcers." The strength of evidence rating was assessed at a "B" rating, indicating that "results of two or more controlled clinical trials on pressure ulcers in humans provide support, or when appropriate, results of two or more controlled trials in an animal model provide indirect support."[64]

Clinical studies have reported beneficial results associated with the use of electrical stimulation in the healing of wounds,[2,5-13,15] although at least two recent reviews have concluded that there were difficulties in reaching conclusions[65] or insufficient reliable evidence[66] about the effectiveness of electrical stimulation. The first of these publications was a critical review of electrical stimulation for pressure ulcers. The study authors determined that conclusive results could not be drawn for the efficacy of electric currents in relation to wound healing, and that further study using clinical trials are needed. The second was a technology assessment that was published in 2001, and included a review of 16 randomized controlled trials (RCTs) that examined effectiveness of electrical therapies on chronic wounds. The conclusions of this study were that there was "insufficient reliable evidence to draw conclusions about the contribution of . . . electrotherapy . . . to chronic wound healing."[65] The study also concluded that electrotherapy for the treatment of pressure sores was one of the most promising physical therapies for further investigation.

Two meta-analyses of electrical stimulation and tissue healing have recently been published.[67,68] Gardner et al[68] reviewed studies that included ulcer or periulcer electrical stimulation of chronic wounds in human subjects. Chronic wounds were defined as pressure ulcers, venous ulcers, arterial ulcers, or neuropathic ulcers. For inclusion in the meta-analysis, the studies had to report quantitative data of baseline and post-treatment wound size, or the percent of wound healing per week. Results of this meta-analysis showed the rate of healing per week to be 22% for the electrical stimulation samples, and 9% for control samples. The electrical stimulation healing rate represents an increase of 144% over the control rate. The authors stated that study findings supported "the merits of electrical stimulation for treating chronic wounds." The study authors also called for additional research to examine factors such as the optimal-dose response and factors related to the electrical stimulation device or wound.

The second meta-analysis[67] reviewed the results of RCTs for the effect of electrical or electromagnetic field stimulation on musculoskeletal tissues that included both bone and soft tissues. Twenty-nine RCTs were identified for soft tissues and joint; 16 of these studies used end points that were sufficient for calculation of a combined effect in the meta-analysis. The overall statistical analysis for the 16 studies demonstrated support for the effectiveness of electrical stimulation. In interpreting this information, clinicians should note that less than half of these studies used electrical stimulation to treat wounds, while the rest used electrical stimulation or electromagnetic field stimulation to treat wounds or other musculoskeletal disorders. The authors also noted that while the results of this meta-analysis did not constitute conclusive evidence that electrical stimulation has specific effects on health, the statistically significant results of the pooled data could not be ignored.

The Centers for Medicare & Medicaid Services (CMS) issued a decision of coverage of electrical stimulation for chronic wounds in July 2002.[69] This decision of coverage was limited to chronic wounds such as Stage III and Stage IV pressure ulcers, arterial ulcers, diabetic ulcers, and venous stasis ulcers. The decision was based on a systematic review of published clinical trials and input from a number of sources, including the American Physical Therapy Association, the Emergency Care Research Institute, the Association for the Advancement of Wound Care, the Agency for Health Care Policy and Research, and the Medical and Surgical Procedures Panel of the Medicare Coverage Advisory Committee.

WHY DO I NEED TO KNOW ABOUT...
CURRENT TRENDS IN HEALTH CARE POLICY

Without reimbursement for electrical stimulation for chronic wounds and pressure ulcers, these beneficial physical therapy treatment interventions would no longer be used.

CURRENT TYPE: DOES IT MATTER WHICH TYPE IS USED?

Various types of electromedical currents exist and have been classified by the section on Clinical Electrophysiology and Wound Care of the American Physical Therapy Association (Fig. 14-3). Researchers have reported beneficial results with the use of low-intensity direct current (Fig. 14-4),[2,14,31,70] pulsed current,[5-11,13,15] and alternating current.[12] Further differentiation between the different pulsed current characteristics shows beneficial results with the use of low-voltage monophasic pulsed current (for an example of this current type, see Fig. 14-5),[7,8] high-voltage monophasic pulsed current (for an example of this current type, see Fig. 14-6),[9-11] and low-voltage asymmetric biphasic pulsed current (for examples of this current type, see Figs. 14-7 and 14-8).[5,6,13] The asymmetric biphasic pulsed current waveform, in studies by Baker and colleagues,[7,8] was found superior to a symmetric biphasic pulsed current waveform when wounds were differentiated into those demonstrating "good responses" among ulcers in patients with spinal cord injury,[6] and into those requiring more than 8 days of treatment among ulcers in patients with diabetes.[5] Both studies had three stimulation groups (asymmetric biphasic stimulation; symmetric biphasic stimulation; micro-current stimulation) and a control group. Significantly improved healing rates were found for the asymmetric biphasic waveform when compared with the micro-current or control group in the first study, and when compared with the combined results from the micro-current and control groups in the latter study. The study by Stefanovska and colleagues[13] concluded that an asymmetric biphasic pulsed current waveform seemed to be more effective than low-density direct current but that

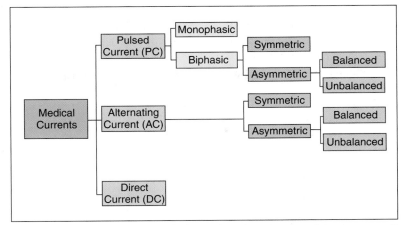

FIGURE 14-3 Classification of Electrical Currents, Clinical Electrophysiology Section of the American Physical Therapy Association (2001). With this classification model, the various types of pulsed current that are used with the majority of electrical stimulation devices have been classified under the heading of "pulsed current." Pulsed currents are actually a subdivision of the
main two types of current, alternating current and direct current. The separate and additional classification for "pulsed current"
is intended to ease the interpretation of the various types of electromedical currents that exist.
*(Reprinted with permission from Kloth, LC: Electrical stimulation for wound healing. In McCulloch, JM, and Kloth, LC [eds]: Wound Healing Evidence-Based
Management, ed 4. FA Davis, Philadelphia, 2010, p 464.)*

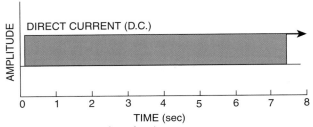

FIGURE 14-4 Waveform for direct current.
*(Reprinted with permission from Kloth, LC: Electrical stimulation for wound heal-
ing. In McCulloch, JM, and Kloth, LC [eds]: Wound Healing Evidence-Based
Management, ed 4. FA Davis, Philadelphia, 2010, p 464.)*

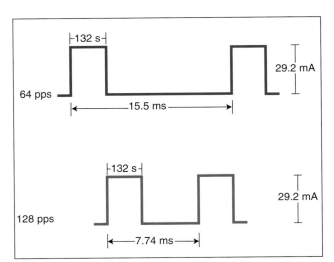

FIGURE 14-5 Low-voltage monophasic pulsed current waveform used in the study by Feedar et al.
*(Reprinted with permission from Feedar, JA, Kloth, LC, and Gentzkow, GD:
Chronic dermal ulcer healing enhanced with monophasic pulsed electrical
stimulation. Phys Ther 71:639–149, 1991.)*

comparisons regarding the size of the difference were premature. The current type used in a study by Wood et al[15]
is reported as a pulsed low-intensity direct current. However, according to the electrotherapeutic terminology
adopted by the Clinical Electrophysiology section of the
American Physical Therapy Association in 1991,[71] the
stimulation characteristics reported in the study by Wood
et al may be classified as low-voltage, monophasic pulsed
current.[16] Review of these studies demonstrates that various electrical stimulation current types have been reported
as beneficial in enhancing the healing of chronic wounds.

Does Polarity Matter?

Treatment protocols that use concepts such as galvanotaxis, enhancement of the current of injury, and potential
bacteriocidal effects may incorporate the use of polar effects. The use of currents that are capable of producing
polar effects may be a factor in facilitating a healing response. Researchers have reported findings suggesting that
wounds possess a specific polarity, usually positive, although an experimental study with wounds in guinea pigs
has reported changes in the polarity of wounds, from positive to negative, as healing progresses.[21] Researchers have
questioned whether such shifts in potential are related to
the healing process.[26]

Studies have reported beneficial effects on tissue healing
for the use of currents capable of introducing polar effects.[2,5–14,31] Polar effects may be introduced to tissues by
a variety of current types, including monophasic and unbalanced or asymmetric biphasic waveforms. The potential
for polar effects may be further modified by the selection
of continuous versus pulsed current, the use of a specific
polarity for the treatment electrode, and by varying the
treatment electrode polarity during the episode of care.

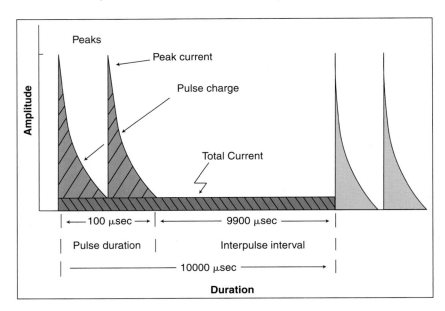

FIGURE 14-6 High-voltage monophasic pulsed current waveform.
(Reprinted with permission from (Reprinted with permission from Kloth, LC: Electrical stimulation for wound healing. In McCulloch, JM and Kloth, LC [eds]: Wound Healing Evidence-Based Management, ed 4. FA Davis, Philadelphia, 2010, p 464

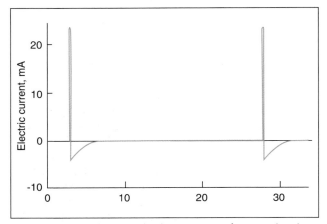

FIGURE 14-7 Biphasic, pulsed current waveform used in the study by Stefanovska et al.[13]
(Reprinted with permission from Stefanovska, A, Vodovnik, L, Benko, H, and Turk, R: Treatment of chronic wounds by means of electric and electromagnetic fields. Part 2. Value of FES parameters for pressure sore treatment. Med Biol Eng Comput 31:213–220, 1993.)

rates of wound closure with positive alternating with negative currents on 3-day cycles. Several clinical studies have reported successful results for tissue healing using protocols in which the treatment electrode polarity was changed throughout the healing process.[2,7,11,14,31]

The results from these studies suggest that polar effects may be an important factor in the healing process. Further support for this concept may be noted in the results of studies by Baker and colleagues, who found the use of an asymmetrical biphasic waveform superior to a symmetric biphasic waveform.[5,6] The asymmetric waveform may have allowed chemical changes in the tissues as a result of the charge asymmetry. These chemical changes would then account for the enhanced healing of the asymmetric waveform.

Electrode Placement: Which Protocol Is Best?

Electrode placement can vary, and methods include the direct technique and the periwound technique.[17] Studies have reported beneficial effects for both the direct technique[2,7,9–11] and the periwound technique.[5,6,13] The direct technique used in these studies is with placement of the stimulating electrode directly over the wound, with a dispersive electrode located on intact skin peripheral to the wound. This method has also been described as a monopolar technique.[4] The periwound technique used in these

Experimental evidence exists for beneficial effects with the use of electrical stimulation protocols in which treatment electrode polarity is varied during the episode of care. In basic science research, one study[36] found that the use of negative polarity for one day followed by the use of positive polarity on subsequent days resulted in the highest percentage of wounds healed. Another study[72] found increased

	A	B	MC
Amplitude	Below contraction	Below contraction	4 mA
Phase duration(s)	100	300	10
Frequency (pps)	50	50	1
On:off times(s)	7:7	7:7	7:7
Waveform	⎍___⌐	⎍⌐	⎍⌐

FIGURE 14-8 Group A illustrates the asymmetric biphasic waveform used in studies by Baker et al.[5,6]
(Reprinted with permission from Baker, LL, Chambers, R, DeMuth, SK, and Villar, F: Effects of electrical stimulation on wound healing in patients with diabetic ulcers. Diabetes Care 20:405–412, 1997.)

studies is with placement of two electrodes on intact skin surrounding the wound. This method has also been described as a bipolar technique.[4] In general, research studies have reported the use of the periwound technique with asymmetric biphasic pulsed current types[5,6,13] and the direct technique with low-intensity direct current[2] or monophasic pulsed current types.[7,9–11] Exceptions include the study by Wood et al,[15] which used pulsed low-intensity direct current with the application of electrodes at opposite sides of the wound on clinical normal skin. This study, however, did not report on the type of electrode that was used. Another exception is a study by Lundeberg et al,[12] in which alternating current was used with application of stimulation outside the ulcer surface area.

Finally, another type of electrode arrangement that has been used includes the use of a Dacron silver mesh sock and sleeve electrode system to deliver high-voltage monophasic pulsed current as an adjunct to healing diabetic foot ulcers.[73] Researchers assessing the use of this system in providing eight hours of stimulation nightly found enhanced wound healing when study results were stratified according to patient compliance.

Of interest to clinicians is the decision memorandum by the CMS, in which electrical stimulation is defined as "the application of electrical current through electrodes placed directly on the skin in close proximity to the wound."[69]

Indications

Various categorizations have been provided for integument wounds by previous authors. Four main categories that have been reported to be treated with electrical stimulation are wounds as a result of pressure (decubitus), venous insufficiency, arterial insufficiency, or diabetes mellitus.[10,16,68,74] The present discussion will provide a brief review of potential pathophysiologies that may result in wounds from these categories.

Pressure ulcers (wounds) result from application of external force sufficient to exceed capillary filling pressure interrupting blood flow.[75] These individuals include patients with spinal injury, and patients immobilized in critical or extended care facilities, or following hip fracture. Wounds resulting from **venous insufficiency** are a hallmark of stasis dermatitis in the lower extremities.[75] These wounds are the result of impaired venous outflow, venous insufficiency, and occur in patients with preexisting conditions such as venous thrombosis or incompetence of the valves within the veins, that is, varicose veins. Wounds due to **arterial insufficiency** result from an interruption of blood flow into the tissues. The pathophysiological etiologies responsible for these wounds are more diversified. These wounds may occur as a result of vasculitis in patients with **polyarteritis nodosa**, which is a serious blood vessel disease in which small- and medium-size arteries become swollen and damaged, no longer able to carry oxygenated blood to organs and tissues. It occurs when certain immune cells attack the affected arteries. Arterial insufficiency wounds may also result from peripheral vascular disorders such as atherosclerotic occlusive disease or thrombo-angiitis obliterans (inflammatory occlusive peripheral vascular disease).[75] Alternatively, arterial insufficiency may be a manifestation of rheumatic disorders such as systemic lupus erythematosus or rheumatoid arthritis.[76] Integument wounds resulting from diabetes mellitus are complex in origin, resulting from peripheral neuropathy and/or dysfunction of both the large and small arteries.[77] These wounds occur commonly on the planter surface of the foot, but may also appear on the dorsal surface or at other locations, and result from loss of sensation due to peripheral neuropathy and decreased blood flow due to arterial damage. Finally, although not commonly classified in one of the four previous categories, integument wounds resulting from increased sympathetic activity also occur. Raynaud's disease/phenomenon results in intense vasoconstriction of the digits of the upper and occasionally lower extremities.[75] Multiple etiologies exist for this disorder, varying from idiopathic to previous mechanical or thermal injury at the site. Electrical stimulation increases localized blood flow to the ischemic digits.[44,78] Thus, integument wounds may result from multiple pathophysiologies.

Contraindications and Precautions

Very few actual contraindications exist in regard to electrical stimulation for tissue repair. The majority of situations result in precautions with regard to the electric stimulation due to the anatomic location of the wound. Several contraindications are based on empirical assessment. The U.S. Food and Drug Administration (FDA) has issued a statement of contraindication concerning application of TENS devices for both patients with synchronous (demand) cardiac pacemakers, and application of these devices over the carotid sinus.[79] Although the FDA statement concerns transcutaneous electrical stimulation for pain relief, any transcutaneous electrical stimulator with a varying electric field may fall under the ruling. The logic for the contraindication in patients with demand cardiac pacemakers is that a changing electric field of the TENS may interfere with the performance of the cardiac pacemaker. Literature supporting TENS interference with demand cardiac pacemakers is contradictory. Several investigations have documented placement of TENS for pain relief in both the axial and appendicular regions of the body without interference of the cardiac pacemaker.[80,81] In contrast, a case report of two patients documented cardiac pacemaker dysfunction in patients receiving TENS for pain relief.[82] Stimulation of the carotid sinus may result in the patient feeling dizzy or a vasovagal response, and stimulation of other structures in the anterior of the neck, such as the larynx may result in laryngeal spasm and asphyxiation.[16] Other areas considered to be contraindications to the use of electrical stimulation include those overlying vital organs or nerves, such as the heart.[83] In addition, transcerebral or transcranial application of electrical muscle stimulator (EMS) devices is contraindicated.[84]

Various types of skin lesions, such as basal cell carcinoma, squamous cell carcinoma, or melanoma at the application site, may all be contraindications. This contraindication exists for both the presence of one of these neoplasia, or previous documentation of the neoplasia at the application site. Electrical stimulation of these neoplastic cells may result in further mitogenic or growth activity,[16] or increased blood flow to the tissue may assist in the neoplastic metastasis. Other types of skin lesions may be considered contraindications to the application of electrical stimulation devices if the underlying etiology, such as thrombophlebitis, prevents the use of electrical stimulation.[84]

Various characteristics, such as an infection in the bone (osteomyelitis) beneath the integument wound, have also been described as a contraindication to electrical stimulation of the wound. The explanation for this contraindication is that premature closing of the integument may result in an abscess formation.[4,16] In addition, increased blood flow to the tissue as a result of electrical stimulation may result in septicemia or bacteremia. Septicemia is a serious infection in the bloodstream that may travel to different parts of the body because of its location in the bloodstream; bacteremia refers to bacterium in the bloodstream, which could potentially travel as well. Actively bleeding wounds are another example of described contraindications to the use of electrical stimulation.[17]

The presence of metal ions from antimicrobial medications[4] or metallic implants in the underlying tissue may pose a contraindication. Direct electrical currents may drive metal ions from antimicrobial medications into the tissues. Alternatively, electrical stimulation with biphasic or pulsed monophasic waveforms may result in inappropriate heating of metal ions or metallic implants damaging the surrounding tissue. Treatment of wounds in the lumbar or lower abdominal region in pregnant women should also be considered a contraindication. Although no documentation exists that transcutaneous currents at these energy levels are sufficient, the potential for mutagenic effects on the fetus in utero exist.

Several subpopulations of patients may be included in those in whom caution should be utilized when applying electrical stimulation for tissue repair. Treatment of wounds in the cranium or upper cervical area with electrical stimulation should be considered judiciously, and the treatment monitored closely. Additional precautions should be taken in these treatments if the patient has documented evidence of epilepsy, cerebrovascular accident (CVA), or reversible ischemic neurological deficit. Electrical stimulation of this region in these patients may initiate an epileptic event or alter cerebral blood flow, exacerbating CVA or reversible ischemic neurological deficit. Finally, although a patient who is insensate at the wound site may be considered a contraindication to application of electrical stimulation for tissue repair, the application of electrical stimulation at this wound site is considered appropriate. Because of the lack of sensation or insensate condition of the wound site, precaution should be used in establishing the initial electrical stimulation parameters. Several different types of patients may present insensate at the wound site, including patients with pressure ulcers resulting from spinal injury or diabetic wounds.

Adverse Site Responses

Several adverse responses may also occur at the application site. During application of the electric current the patient may complain of an unpleasant buzzing or tingling. This response is both amplitude dependent and frequency dependent. In addition, if the electrode surface area is insufficient for the electrical amplitude or there is an uneven distribution of current density, a local overheating or hyperthermic reaction may occur that results in a thermal burn. One study has reported a single instance of bleeding at the ulcer site associated with the use of pulsed current.[85] Finally, contact dermatitis may occur at the application site resulting from components of the electrode. Any of the components of the electrode may initiate this response. The contact dermatitis may be expressed by two distinctly different inflammatory processes: irritant and allergic dermatitis.[86] Irritant dermatitis is a non–immune mediated response and is a result of the direct action of the irritant on the skin. In contrast, allergic dermatitis represents a type IV delayed cell-mediated immune hypersensitivity response. The clinician may differentiate these two responses. In irritant dermatitis, the cutaneous response is directly proportional to the amount of the irritant applied. In contrast, in allergic dermatitis, only minute quantities are necessary to elicit an overt response. Repeated dermal exposures to compounds initiating irritant dermatitis may eventually result in allergic dermal responses.

Treatment Considerations

To date, electrical stimulation devices for wound healing have not been approved or received premarket approval by the FDA.[83] Safety and effectiveness of the devices must be demonstrated in order to obtain premarket approval.[83] At this time, the only FDA-approved indication for the use of electrical stimulation, as related to the previous discussion on potential mechanisms of action in wound care, is in the promotion of increased local blood flow.[4,87,88] Other FDA-approved indications for the use of electrical stimulation may include muscle reeducation, maintaining or increasing range of motion, pain suppression, and prevention of disuse atrophy.[4,88] Electrical stimulation for patients with wounds is used as an off-label indication.[87] Clinicians are advised to consider this information when selecting a protocol with electrical stimulation and to review all appropriate guidelines as part of the decision-making process. Further sources of information on this topic may be found elsewhere.[4,87,88]

APPLICATION

The use of two application techniques are considered in this chapter: (1) the direct technique (as used with high-voltage monophasic pulsed current—active electrode placed on the wound bed, with dispersive electrode located 15 to 20 cm distant to the wound), and (2) the periwound technique (as used with alternating or asymmetric biphasic pulsed current—electrodes placed adjacent to the wound bed on intact skin). In comparison with the direct technique, several additional considerations may apply to the use of the periwound technique. The periwound technique may result in less current density within the wound.[6] The periwound technique, as applied with both electrodes over skin with normal innervation, may be more advantageous when attempting to activate sensory nerves in the skin.[6] In addition, other advantages for the periwound technique include less potential for disturbance of the wound bed, and a reduced chance of cross-contamination between the wound and the electrode.[6] Finally, while indirect application methods of wound care (such as ultrasound to periulcer skin) may require minimal specialized training, the use of direct techniques with application of the modality directly to the wound bed are considered to require more advanced specialized training for the proper use of equipment and techniques.[89]

With each technique, clinicians should be aware that charge dosage, current density, and depth of penetration may vary when changes occur in stimulation parameters, electrode size, electrode arrangement, and specific wound characteristics. Since patients with wounds may have impaired sensation at the wound itself (depending on depth of the wound), and in the skin surrounding the wound, these factors should be among those considered when selecting treatment parameters and stimulation intensity.

Stimulation parameters have been proposed for the use of electrical stimulation in tissue healing for wound care. Kloth[16] has described formulas for calculating electrical charge dosages for low- and high-voltage pulsed current electrical simulation. A dosage range of 250 to 500 mC/sec has been found to be a shared quality among several studies.[16] Another stimulation parameter is that of charge density, or the amount of electrical charge per unit of a cross-sectional area of an electrode.[16] This value relates to electrode size; for example, the larger the size of the electrode, the smaller is the charge current density.[4] Absolute charge density transfer is obtained by multiplying the average spatial current density by the effective duty cycle and by the total duration of treatment.[90] Reich[90] suggested, based on an observed trend in several studies, that an absolute charge density transfer of 0.1 to 2.0 C/cm² may be effective in enhancing healing. Reich encouraged that further research be done in this area.

Many protocols call for the use of intensity (amplitude) that is at sub-motor levels. For patients with impaired sensation, caution should be used to confirm the use of sub-motor intensities and to prevent the use of excessive current intensities.[17] Finally, while selecting the stimulus intensity using the direct technique, clinicians should recall that the wound lacks skin and impedance is lower than the surrounding tissues.[91]

Direct Technique

The direct technique is used in high-voltage monophasic pulsed current research studies.[9-11] With this technique, the electrode may be placed directly on the wound, using saline-moistened sterile gauze. The moistened gauze is placed within the wound bed following wound irrigation or débridement as needed. The treatment electrode is placed over the moistened gauze. Treatment electrode types have consisted of metalline gauze,[10] carbon electrode, or aluminum foil.[9] Metalline gauze electrodes, as used in the study by Houghton et al,[10] are sterile, single-use electrodes. Carbon electrodes require a cleaning process with an approved disinfectant,[4,17] while aluminum foil electrodes are disposed of following a single application.[17] The treatment electrode is secured in place over the wound, while the dispersive electrode is placed on intact skin (Figs. 14-9 and 14-10). Dispersive electrode placement has been described as 15 cm distant to the wound,[11] 20 cm proximal to the wound,[10] or on the medial thigh as used in a study for healing of pressure ulcers in patients with spinal cord injury.[9] Dispersive electrode size has not always been reported; one study used a size of 20 × 25 cm,[9] whereas Kloth[16] recommends for dispersive electrode size to be similar to the wound surface area.

Periwound Technique

The periwound technique is used in asymmetrical biphasic pulsed current research studies.[5,6,13] With this technique, two electrodes are placed on intact skin adjacent to the wound. Electrode types have consisted of self-adhesive skin electrodes[13] or carbon rubber electrodes.[5,6] In studies that have specified electrode location, placement is generally proximal and distal to the wound (Fig. 14-11), although medial and lateral placement has been used for ulcers in region of the coccyx.[6]

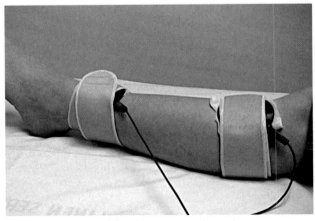

FIGURE 14-9 Use of the direct monopolar technique using carbon rubber electrodes. With this technique, one electrode is placed over saline-moistened gauze over the wound, and a dispersive electrode is placed 15 to 20 cm away on intact skin.

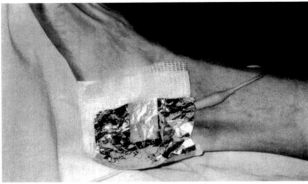

FIGURE 14-10 Aluminum foil electrode with alligator clip. With the direct monopolar technique, one electrode is placed over saline-moistened gauze over the wound, and a dispersive electrode is placed over 15 to 20 cm away on intact skin. *(Reprinted with permission from Sussman, C, and Byl, NN: Electrical stimulation for wound healing. In Sussman, C, and Bates-Jensen, BM [eds]: Wound Care, ed 2. Aspen, Gaithersburg, MD, 2001, p 527.)*

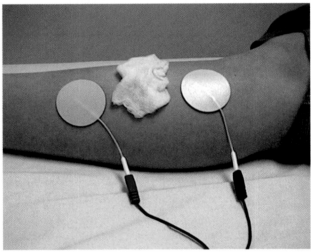

FIGURE 14-11 Use of the indirect bipolar technique with proximal/distal (6:00 and 12:00) placement of self-adhesive electrodes. The gauze pad represents the location of the wound. With this technique, electrodes are placed on intact skin adjacent to the wound.

Application Check List

- Determine whether treatment with electrical stimulation is appropriate and decide upon the desired treatment parameters (equipment and current type, the type of technique to be used).
  - This may be in part determined by the equipment available in your practice setting. Make sure that the specific parameters are recorded so that treatment protocols can be repeated as needed with the SAME piece of equipment.
- Prior to each treatment, assess the wound, periwound, and wound drainage characteristics.
  - Documenting the progress of the wound with photographs of the healing process is excellent if such a system is available in your setting.

- Provide patient instructions. Explain the procedure/equipment to be used and describe the anticipated effects of treatment (see patient instruction section later in this chapter).
- Check electrical stimulation equipment to be sure it is intact and functioning properly.
- After checking to be sure the electrical stimulation unit is not turned on and the intensity control is in the off position, apply electrical stimulation electrodes (application techniques will differ depending upon whether the direct or periwound technique is used).

Direct Technique

The checklist for the direct technique follows:

- Prepare wound.
- Ensure that the wound is free of any metallic substances or petrolatum products.
- Determine the desired polarity of the treatment electrode.
- Apply saline-moistened sterile gauze to the wound, followed by application of the treatment electrode.
- Select dispersive electrode of size similar to wound surface area.
- Apply dispersive electrode 15 to 20 cm from the wound on intact skin.

Periwound Technique

The checklist for the periwound technique follows:

- Prepare wound.
- Ensure that the wound is free of any metallic substances or petrolatum products.
- Apply treatment electrodes on intact skin near the edges of the wound. See Box 14-1 for specific electrode application parameters.
- Set the electrical stimulation parameters (Boxes 14-1 and 14-2).
- When ready, turn on the electrical stimulation unit and gradually increase intensity until the desired range is reached.
- For initial treatments, use lower dosage parameters in order to assess skin tolerance before full protocol dosage parameters are used.
- Ensure that the patient is comfortable, and provide the patient with a call light or bell.
- Recheck with the patient during the treatment session to determine the patient's continued comfort and tolerance to treatment.
- When treatment is concluded, decrease intensity to the off position, remove electrodes, and follow the appropriate disinfection or disposal procedures. Check the wound/periwound and the skin under the electrodes for any signs of allergic reaction or thermal injury. Clean electrode wires with an approved disinfectant.
- Document the treatment performed.

In an alternative to the electrical stimulation parameters described in Box 14-2, a recent study[10] used the following parameters: pulse frequency at 100 Hz, peak intensity 150 V, pulse duration of 100 microseconds, and treatment duration of 45 minutes for 3 days a week. Negative polarity

---

BOX 14-1 | Electrical Stimulation Parameters: Asymmetric Biphasic Pulsed Current or Alternating Current

Following is a summary of research protocols for the use of asymmetric biphasic pulsed currents or alternating pulsed currents.

- *Asymmetric Biphasic Current*—Research protocol for pressure ulcers and diabetic ulcers.[5,6] *Pulse frequency and duration*—50 pps, 100 msec phase duration, 7:7 on-off time (sec). *Stimulus intensity*—below contraction level. *Treatment duration*—30 minute treatment sessions, totaling 30 to 90 minutes daily, 5 days per week. *Electrode configuration*—carbon rubber electrodes of similar size placed on intact skin less than 1 cm from edge of the wound. Electrodes typically placed proximal and distal to the ulcer, but medial and lateral placement was used for ulcers in the region of the coccyx. The electrode whose polarity was negative during the leading phase of the waveform was placed proximal to the wound. *Electrode size*[6]—dependent on wound size and location, sizes ranged from 2.5 × 2.5 cm to 5 × 10 cm.
- *Asymmetric Biphasic Current*—Research protocol for pressure ulcers.[13] *Pulse frequency and duration*—40 Hz, 0.25 milliseconds pulse duration, 4 second stimulation trains rhythmically alternated with pauses of the same duration. *Stimulus intensity*—tetanic contractions produced, generally at 15 to 25 mA. *Treatment duration*—2 hours daily. *Electrode configuration*—two self-adhesive skin electrodes placed on healthy skin at the edge of the wound. *Electrode size*—adjusted to wound size, average size was 30 ± 10 cm² each.
- *Alternating Constant Current Square Wave Pulses* (with inference of an asymmetrical unbalanced wave)—Research protocol for diabetic leg ulcers due to venous stasis.[12] *Pulse frequency and duration*—80 Hz, alternating constant current with pulse width 1 millisecond. *Stimulus intensity*—intensity-evoking paresthesia. *Treatment duration*—20 minutes twice daily. *Electrode configuration*—stimulation applied just outside the ulcer surface area. Polarity of treatment electrode was changed after each treatment. *Electrode size*—treatment electrode was 4 × 6 cm.

BOX 14-2 | High-Voltage Monophasic Pulsed Current

The following description summarizes the electrical stimulation parameters described by Kloth[16] using a high-voltage electrical stimulation device as an example:

- *Voltage 75 to 150 V*
- *Pulse frequency* of 100 pps
- *Treatment duration* of 60 minutes, 7 days per week
- *Polarity* of the wound treatment electrode is varied according to the wound phase or the clinical needs of the wound.

Please see Kloth[16] for further information regarding polarity of the wound treatment electrode. While this protocol suggests varying the treatment electrode polarity during the episode of care, two studies using high-voltage pulsed current[9,10] have used protocols in which the treatment electrode was maintained at negative polarity throughout the duration of the study.

PATIENT INSTRUCTIONS

- Explain that research findings have supported the use of electrical stimulation as an effective adjunctive therapy for chronic wounds that have not shown signs of healing during the past 30 days.
- As indicated, relate that studies have shown that chronic wounds similar to the patient's wound have responded favorably to the use of electrical stimulation.
- Describe the anticipated effect of electrical stimulation on the healing of the patient's wound, including advantages/disadvantages and potential adverse effects.
- Discuss the equipment to be used and indications/contraindications for the use of the equipment. Explain the specific procedure. Include any directions or guidelines suitable to the patient's participation in the treatment.
- Explain the measures that will be used to help determine whether the treatment is effective.
- Describe the duration of each treatment session and for the overall episode of care.
- Explain that treatment will be performed with the patient's consent. The treatment is not expected to produce any discomfort, but the patient may experience a tingling sensation under the electrodes in areas of intact sensation.
- Advise the patient not to disturb or remove the electrodes during the treatment session.
- Advise the patient to continue to follow other recommendations for the treatment of his or her wound.
- Ask the patient to use the call light or bell if any discomfort is experienced or if any questions arise during the treatment session.

of the treatment electrode was maintained throughout the 4-week study. This study assessed the effect of high-voltage pulsed current for treatment of chronic vascular leg ulcers. Study results indicated that high-voltage pulsed current reduced wound surface area to approximately one-half the initial wound size, and that this effect was over two times greater than that seen with wounds treated with sham electrical stimulation unit.

Summary

Our skin is our body's largest organ, but it's also one of the organs that we take for granted unless we have an opening or a wound. That's when we start to realize just how important it is as a primary defense system against infection, fluid loss, and maintaining homeostasis.

Human tissue repair is a fascinating topic area that we are just beginning to understand. The use of electrical stimulation to "jump-start" the healing process is something that although well documented in the literature, still needs further research to become more widely accepted and practiced. It is important to our success as clinicians to be able to effectively communicate with our patients and our peers about the potential benefits that this modality can have in such a profound way for those who have pressure ulcers for which little else has been effective.

Review Questions

1. Which of the following forms of electrical stimulation has been used effectively for tissue repair with human tissues?
   a. NMES
   b. IFC
   c. HVPC
   d. TENS

2. What is meant by the term "current of injury"?
   a. Injured tissue produces an electrical current that is different from the surrounding current potentials
   b. Tissues become injured when electrical stimulation is applied and produce a current of injury that can be measured
   c. Matching the action potential of the current of injured tissues can balance and heal that tissue
   d. Using the opposite action potential of the current of injury for an injured area will promote tissue healing

3. What is the rationale behind promoting mobility during the various stages of wound healing?
   a. There is none; the tissue will not heal unless it is immobilized
   b. Alignment of the collagen fibers will be based upon function if mobility is permitted during the remodeling phase
   c. Tissue repair will be enhanced as a result of constant re-injury and repair that will be caused by motions taking place throughout the injured area
   d. Angiogenesis will not occur unless motion accompanies healing

4. What would be the appropriate application of electrical stimulation to promote autolytic débridement for tissue repair?
   a. Placement of the negative electrode over the wound to attract the positively charged neutrophils and macrophages to promote autolysis
   b. Placement of the negative electrode over the wound to attract the negatively charged neutrophils and macrophages to promote autolysis
   c. Placement of the positive electrode over the wound to attract the positively charged neutrophils and macrophages to promote autolysis
   d. Placement of the positive electrode over the wound to attract the negatively charged neutrophils and macrophages to promote autolysis

5. Which of the following techniques is most accurate regarding the application of HVPC for wound healing?
   a. Use a periwound technique with electrodes placed adjacent to the wound bed on intact skin
   b. Use a direct technique with electrodes placed adjacent to the wound bed on intact skin
   c. Use a periwound technique with the active electrode placed on the wound bed, with dispersive electrode located 15 to 20 cm distant to the wound
   d. Use a direct technique with the active electrode placed on the wound bed, with dispersive electrode located 15 to 20 cm distant to the wound

CASE STUDY 1

The following case study is characteristic of a patient needing electrical stimulation for a nonhealing ulcer.

Patient's age: 71
Initial assessment
Reason for referral

The patient came to physical therapy secondary to a left dorsal foot ulcer that would not heal. Patient reported undergoing orthopedic surgery on the left foot 3 months prior to initial physical therapy evaluation and development of a blood blister post-surgery. Patient reported the wound continued to break down. The patient received home health nursing for several weeks with no significant progress. Patient stated previous ulcer care had consisted of cleaning the wound with Betadine at home and applying a topical antibiotic ointment with a gauze dressing.

Medical History

No history of diabetes, heart disease, or vascular insufficiency reported.

Wound Assessment

The wound had irregular borders measuring 3.0 cm at the widest point and 4.5 cm in length. There was no undermining or tunneling of the wound. The wound had a partial thickness skin loss with a moderate amount of exudate. The wound bed consisted of approximately 30% red granulated tissue and approximately 70% yellow necrotic adherent tissue. There was also erythema surrounding the wound and moderate edema of his *left* lower extremity.

Signs of Vascular Insufficiency

Signs of venous insufficiency included hair loss on the foot, erythema surrounding the wound, and edema of the *left* lower extremity.

Treatment

Each treatment consisted of saline cleansing and selective débridement prior to electrical stimulation.

Electrical stimulation using high-voltage pulsed current was initiated on the third visit (1.5 weeks post start of care) with the following parameters: (–) polarity of the treatment electrode was primarily used throughout treatment episode with a few occasions of (+) polarity. Treatment duration was 25 to 30 minutes with frequency of 5 times a week for 3 weeks. Treatment was then decreased to 3 times a week for 2 weeks, for a total of 20 treatments.

Electrical stimulation was discontinued after 5.5 weeks secondary to a fully granulated wound base with lack of necrotic tissue and signs of increased epithelialization. Wound size had decreased approximately 40% to 50%.

In addition to electrical stimulation, wound dressings consisted of a petrolatum-impregnated gauze for 3 visits, enzymatic débridement ointment for 7 visits, then progressed to alginate dressing for 9 visits. Dressing change to alginate dressing was secondary to the presence of greater than 70% granulated tissue in the wound bed. Once granulation tissue exceeded 95%, dressing was changed to petrolatum-impregnated gauze with a four-layer bandaging system to promote edema control.

Outcomes

In 4.5 weeks, the wound measured 2.0 cm in width and 3.2 cm in length, and had greater than 95% granulation tissue.

In 6 weeks, the wound decreased in size by 40% to 50%.

At 11 weeks, the patient was discharged secondary to a clean wound base and being independent with home dressing care. The patient was scheduled to follow up with the physician.

CASE STUDY 2

Joan is a vivacious 67-year-old woman who has been referred to physical therapy because of the presence of a longstanding ulcer on her right calcaneus. She had previously been treated in an inpatient setting for treatment of a hip fracture that has since healed. She had led an active lifestyle that included swimming, dancing, and sightseeing as the leader of her retirement group.

Following recovery from her hip fracture, her lifestyle has changed specifically because of the development of the calcaneal ulcer that has now remained open for 2 months and measures approximately 4 cm across at the widest point. She reports that she received home care nursing without significant progress. Joan has no significant medical history.

Questions

1. Assuming that Joan would be a good candidate for electrical stimulation to help improve the possibility of accomplishing wound closure, what parameters would you select and why?
2. Where would you place your electrodes and why?
3. What instructions would you give to Joan?

Continued

CASE STUDY 2—cont'd

4. Approximately how long would you expect it to take before you see any changes in the condition of the wound and what are you basing your response on?
5. What would those changes that you mentioned be?
6. What medical conditions that Joan does *not* have would have complicated this scenario?

7. What resources could you consult to find out more information about how to proceed with the application techniques for electrical stimulation for wound and tissue repair?

DISCUSSION QUESTIONS

1. What is the "current of injury"?

2. How may the galvanotaxis theory be used in the treatment of wounds?

3. What are the types of ES current associated with increases in blood flow?

4. How can I find out what type of waveform an ES device supplies?

5. For an infected wound, what are two ways in which the use of ES may promote antimicrobial action?

6. What are the direct monopolar and indirect bipolar techniques for ES treatment of wounds?

7. What are the advantages of each technique?

BIBLIOGRAPHY

Additional Sourceswww.apta.org Section on Clinical Electrotherapy and Wound Care
www.cms.hhs.gov Centers for Medicare and Medicaid Services.
www.hookedonevidence.org Hooked on Evidence a resource data base established by the American Physical Therapy Association.

Databases
American Physical Therapy Association. Available at http://www.apta.org/(Guide to Physical Therapist Practice, ed 2. Phys Ther 81[1], 2001).
APTA Online Courses (text based) (No. 2: Wound Healing and Management; No. 8: Clinical Electrotherapy: Physiology and Basic Concepts). Available at http://www.apta.org/
Centers for Medicare and Medicaid Services. Available at http://www.cms.hhs.gov/
Centers for Medicare and Medicaid Services. Electrostimulation for wounds: Decision memorandum (CAG-00068N). Centers for Medicare and Medicaid Services, 2002. Available at http://www.cms.hhs.gov/ncdr/memo.asp?id=27 Accessed November 25, 2003.
CINAHL—Cumulative Index of Nursing and Allied Health Literature. Available at http://www.cinahl.com/
The Cochrane Library. Available at http://www.update-software.com/cochrane/
MEDLINE/PubMed: reference source for biomedical journals. Available at http://www.ncbi.nlm.nih.gov/entrez/query.fcgi

REFERENCES

1. Becker, RO: The electrical control of growth processes. Med Times 95:657–669, 1967.
2. Carley, PJ, and Wainapel, SF: Electrotherapy for acceleration of wound healing: low intensity direct current. Arch Phys Med Rehabil 66:443–446, 1985.
3. Weiss, DS, Kirsner, R, and Eaglstein, WH: Electrical stimulation and wound healing. Arch Dermatol 126:222–225, 1990.
4. Sussman, C, and Byl, NN: Electrical stimulation for wound healing. In Sussman, C, and Bates-Jensen, BM (eds): Wound Care, ed 2. Aspen , Gaithersburg, MD, 2001, pp 497–545.
5. Baker, LL, Chambers, R, DeMuth, SK, et al: Effects of electrical stimulation on wound healing in patients with diabetic ulcers. Diabetes Care 20:405–412, 1997.
6. Baker, LL, Rubayi, S, Villar, F, et al: Effect of electrical stimulation waveform on healing of ulcers in human beings with spinal cord injury. Wound Rep Regul 4:21–28, 1996.
7. Feedar, JA, Kloth, LC, and Gentzkow, GD: Chronic dermal ulcer healing enhanced with monophasic pulsed electrical stimulation. Phys Ther 71:639–649, 1991.
8. Gentzkow, GD, Pollack, SV, Kloth, LC, et al: Improved healing of pressure ulcers using Dermapulse, a new electrical stimulation device. Wounds 3:158–170, 1991.
9. Griffin, JW, Tooms, RE, Mendius, RA, et al: Efficacy of high voltage pulsed current for healing of pressure ulcers in patients with spinal cord injury. Phys Ther 71:433–442, 1991, discussion 442–444.
10. Houghton, PE, Kincaid, CB, Lovell, M, et al: Effect of electrical stimulation on chronic leg ulcer size and appearance. Phys Ther 83:17–28, 2003.
11. Kloth, LC, and Feedar, JA: Acceleration of wound healing with high voltage, monophasic, pulsed current. Phys Ther 68:503–508, 1988.
12. Lundeberg, TC, Eriksson, SV, and Malm, M: Electrical nerve stimulation improves healing of diabetic ulcers. Ann Plast Surg 29:328–331, 1992.
13. Stefanovska, A, Vodovnik, L, Benko, H, et al: Treatment of chronic wounds by means of electric and electromagnetic fields. Part 2. Value of FES parameters for pressure sore treatment. Med Biol Eng Comput 31:213–220, 1993.
14. Wolcott, LE, Wheeler, PC, Hardwicke, HM, et al: Accelerated healing of skin ulcer by electrotherapy: preliminary clinical results. South Med J 62:795–801, 1969.
15. Wood, JM, Evans, PE, III, Schallreuter, KU, et al: A multicenter study on the use of pulsed low-intensity direct current for healing chronic stage II and stage III decubitus ulcers. Arch Dermatol 129:999–1009, 1993.
16. Kloth, LC, and Zhao, M: Endogenous and exogenous electrical fields for wound healing. In McCulloch, JM, and Kloth, LC (eds): Wound Healing Evidence Based Management, ed 4. FA Davis, Philadelphia, 2010, pp 450–513.
17. Myers, BA: Electrotherapeutic modalities, physical agents, and mechanical modalities. In Myers, BA (ed): Wound Management: Principles and Practice. Prentice-Hall, Upper Saddle River, NJ, 2004, pp 152–183.
18. Sommer, C: Immunity and inflammation. In Porth, CM (ed): Pathophysiology: Concepts of Altered Health States, ed 6. Lippincott Williams & Wilkins, Philadelphia, 2002, pp 331–355.
19. Porth, CM: Cellular adaptation, injury, and death and wound healing. In Porth, CM (ed): Pathophysiology: Concepts of Altered Health States, ed 6. Lippincott Williams & Wilkins, Philadelphia, 2002, pp 95–113.
20. Gogia, PP: Physiology of wound healing. In Gogia, PP (ed): Clinical Wound Management. SLACK , Thorofare, NJ, 1995, pp 1–12.
21. Burr, HS, Harvey, SC, and Taffel, M: Bio-electric correlates of wound healing. Yale J Biol Med 103–107, 1938.
22. Cunliffe-Barnes, TC: Healing rate of human skin determined by measurement of the electrical potential of experimental abrasions: a study of treatment with petrolatum and with petrolatum containing yeast and liver extracts. Am J Surg 69:82–88, 1945.
23. Jaffe, LF, and Vanable, JW, Jr: Electric fields and wound healing. Clin Dermatol 2:34–44, 1984.

24. Foulds, IS, and Barker, AT: Human skin battery potentials and their possible role in wound healing. Br J Dermatol 109: 515–522, 1983.

25. Borgens, RB, Vanable, JW, Jr, and Jaffe, LF: Bioelectricity and regeneration: large currents leave the stumps of regenerating newt limbs. Proc Natl Acad Sci U S A 74:4528–4532, 1977.

26. Lee, RC, Canaday, DJ, and Doong, H: A review of the biophysical basis for the clinical application of electric fields in softtissue repair. J Burn Care Rehabil 14:319–335, 1993.

27. Kerstein, MD: Moist wound healing: the clinical perspective. Ostomy Wound Manage 41:37S–44S, 1995, discussion 45S.

28. Ovington, LG: Dressings and ajunctive therapies: AHCPR guidelines revisited. Ostomy Wound Manage 45:94S–106S, 1999, quiz 107S–108S.

29. Rajnicek, AM, Stump, RF, and Robinson, KR: An endogenous sodium current may mediate wound healing in Xenopus neurulae. Dev Biol 128:290–299, 1988.

30. Kloth, LC, and McCulloch, JM: Promotion of wound healing with electrical stimulation. Adv Wound Care 9:42–45, 1996.

31. Gault, WR, and Gatens, PF, Jr: Use of low intensity direct current in management of ischemic skin ulcers. Phys Ther 56:265–269, 1976.

32. Fukushima, K, Senda, N, Inui, H, et al: Studies on galvanotaxis of leukocytes. Med J Osaka Univ 4:195–208, 1953.

33. Orida, N, and Feldman, JD: Directional protrusive pseudopodial activity and motility in macrophages induced by extracellular electric fields. Cell Motil 2:243–255, 1982.

34. Bourguignon, GJ, and Bourguignon, LY: Electric stimulation of protein and DNA synthesis in human fibroblasts. FASEB J 1: 398–402, 1987.

35. Cooper, MS, and Schliwa, M: Electrical and ionic controls of tissue cell locomotion in DC electric fields. J Neurosci Res 13: 223–244, 1985.

36. Mertz, PM, Davis, SC, Cazzaniga, AL, et al: Electrical stimulation: acceleration of soft tissue repair by varying the polarity. Wounds 5:153–159, 1993.

37. Brown, M, McDonnell, M, and Menton, DN: Polarity effects on wound healing using electrical stimulation in rabbits. Arch Phys Med Rehabil 70:624–627, 1989;

38. Barranco, SD, Spadaro, JA, Berger, TJ, et al: In vitro effect of weak direct current on Staphylococcus aureus. Clin Orthop 100: 250–255, 1974.

39. Guffey, JS, and Asmussen, MD: In vitro bactericidal effects of high voltage pulsed current versus direct current against Staphylococcus aureus. J Clin Electrophysiol 1:5–9, 1989.

40. Kincaid, CB, and Lavoie, KH: Inhibition of bacterial growth in vitro following stimulation with high voltage, monophasic, pulsed current. Phys Ther 69: 651–655, 1989.

41. Laatsch, LJ, Ong, PC, and Kloth, LC: In vitro effects of two silver electrodes on select wound pathogens. J Clin Electrophysiol 7:10–15, 1995.

42. Rowley, BA, McKenna, JM, Chase, GR, et al: The influence of electrical current on an infecting microorganism in wounds. Ann N Y Acad Sci 238:543–551, 1974.

43. Szuminsky, NJ, Albers, AC, Unger, P, et al: Effect of narrow, pulsed high voltages on bacterial viability. Phys Ther 74: 660–667, 1994.

44. Kaada, B: Vasodilation induced by transcutaneous nerve stimulation in peripheral ischemia (Raynaud's phenomenon and diabetic polyneuropathy). Eur Heart J 3:303–314, 1982.

45. Scudds, RJ, Helewa, A, and Scudds, RA: The effects of transcutaneous electrical nerve stimulation on skin temperature in asymptomatic subjects. Phys Ther 75:621–628, 1995.

46. Wong, RA, and Jette, DU: Changes in sympathetic tone associated with different forms of transcutaneous electrical nerve stimulation in healthy subjects. Phys Ther 64:478–482, 1984.

47. Baker, LL, Chambers, R, Merchant, L, et al: The effects of electrical stimulation on cutaneous oxygen supply in normal older adults and diabetic patients. Abstract. Phys Ther 66:749, 1986.

48. Dodgen, PW, Johnson, BW, Baker, LL, et al: The effects of electrical stimulation on cutaneous oxygen supply in diabetic older adults. Abstract. Phys Ther 67:793, 1987.

49. Gilcreast, DM, Stotts, NA, Froelicher, ES, et al: Effect of electrical stimulation on foot skin perfusion in persons with or at risk for diabetic foot ulcers. Wound Repair Regen 6:434–441, 1998.

50. Mawson, AR, Siddiqui, FH, Connolly, BJ, et al: Effect of high voltage pulsed galvanic stimulation on sacral transcutaneous oxygen tension levels in the spinal cord injured. Paraplegia 31:311–319, 1993.

51. Peters, EJ, Armstrong, DG, Wunderlich, RP, et al: The benefit of electrical stimulation to enhance perfusion in persons with diabetes mellitus. J Foot Ankle Surg 37:396–400, 1998, discussion 447–448.

52. Heath, ME, and Gibbs, SB: High-voltage pulsed galvanic stimulation: effects of frequency of current on blood flow in the human calf muscle. Clin Sci (Lond) 82:607–613, 1992.

53. Miller, BF, Gruben, KG, and Morgan, BJ: Circulatory responses to voluntary and electrically induced muscle contractions in humans. Phys Ther 80:53–60, 2000.

54. Hecker, B, Carron, H, and Schwartz, DP: Pulsed galvanic stimulation: effects of current frequency and polarity on blood flow in healthy subjects. Arch Phys Med Rehabil 66:369–371, 1985.

55. Tracy, JE, Currier, DP, and Threlkeld, AJ: Comparison of selected pulse frequencies from two different electrical stimulators on blood flow in healthy subjects. Phys Ther 68:1526–1532, 1988.

56. Walker, DC, Currier, DP, and Threlkeld, AJ: Effects of high voltage pulsed electrical stimulation on blood flow. Phys Ther 68: 481–485, 1988.

57. Cosmo, P, Svensson, H, Bornmyr, S, et al: Effects of transcutaneous nerve stimulation on the microcirculation in chronic leg ulcers. Scand J Plast Reconstr Surg Hand Surg 34:61–64, 2000.

58. Cramp, AF, Gilsenan, C, Lowe, AS, et al: The effect of high- and low-frequency transcutaneous electrical nerve stimulation upon cutaneous blood flow and skin temperature in healthy subjects. Clin Physiol 20:150–157, 2000.

59. Lundeberg, T, Kjartansson, J, and Samuelsson, U: Effect of electrical nerve stimulation on healing of ischaemic skin flaps. Lancet 2:712–714, 1988.

60. Wikstrom, SO, Svedman, P, Svensson, H, et al: Effect of trans-cutaneous nerve stimulation on microcirculation in intact skin and blister wounds in healthy volunteers. Scand J Plast Reconstr Surg Hand Surg 33:195–201, 1999.

61. Porth, CM: Control of the circulation. In Porth, CM (ed): Pathophysiology: Concepts of Altered Health States, ed 6. Lippincott Williams & Wilkins, Philadelphia, 2002, pp 399–428.

62. Mawson, AR, Siddiqui, FH, Connolly, BJ, et al: Sacral transcutaneous oxygen tension levels in the spinal cord injured: risk factors for pressure ulcers? Arch Phys Med Rehabil 74:745–751, 1993.

63. Cramp, AF, Noble, JG, Lowe, AS, et al: Transcutaneous electrical nerve stimulation (TENS): the effect of electrode placement upon cutaneous blood flow and skin temperature. Acupunct Electrother Res 26:25–37, 2001.

64. Bergstrom, N, Bennett, MA, Carlson, CE, et al. Pressure ulcer treatment. Clinical practice guideline. Quick reference guide for clinicians, No. 15. Rockville, MD: U.S. Department of Health and Human Services, Public Health Service, Agency for Health Care Policy and Research. AHCPR Pub. No. 95-0653. Dec. 1994.

65. Sheffet, A, Cytryn, AS, and Louria, DB: Applying electric and electromagnetic energy as adjuvant treatment for pressure ulcers: a critical review. Ostomy Wound Manage 46:28–33, 36–40, 42–44, 2000.

66. Collum, N, Nelson, EA, Flemming, K, et al: Systematic reviews of wound care management: (5) beds; (6) compression; (7) laser therapy, therapeutic ultrasound, electrotherapy and electromagnetic therapy. Health Technol Assess 5, 2001.

67. Akai, M, and Hayashi, K: Effect of electrical stimulation on musculoskeletal systems: a meta-analysis of controlled clinical trials. Bioelectromagnetics 23:132–143, 2002.

68. Gardner, SE, Frantz, RA, and Schmidt, FL: Effect of electrical stimulation on chronic wound healing: A meta-analysis. Wound Repair Regen 7:495–503, 1999.

69. Centers for Medicare and Medicaid Services: Electrostimulation for Wounds: Decision Memorandum (#CAG-00068N), 2002; accessed December 6, 2003. Web site: http://www.cms.hhs.gov/mcd/index

70. Assimacopoulos, D: Low intensity negative electric current in the treatment of ulcers of the leg due to chronic venous insufficiency. Preliminary report of three cases. Am J Surg 115: 683–687, 1968.

71. American Physical Therapy Association: Electrotherapeutic Terminology in Physical Therapy: Section on Clinical Electro_physiology. Author, Alexandria, VA, 1990.

72. Stromberg, BV: Effects of electrical currents on wound contraction. Ann Plast Surg 21:121–123, 1988.

73. Peters, EJ, Lavery, LA, Armstrong, DG, et al: Electric stimulation as an adjunct to heal diabetic foot ulcers: A randomized clinical trial. Arch Phys Med Rehabil 82:721–725, 2001.

74. Tunis, S, Shuren, J, Ballantine, L, et al: Medicare Coverage Policy—NCDS: Electrostimulation for Wounds. July 23, 2002. Web Page.

75. Porth, CM: Alterations in blood flow in the systemic circulation. In Porth, CM (ed): Pathophysiology: Concepts of Altered Health States, ed 6. Lippincott Williams & Wilkins, Philadelphia, 2002, pp 429–458.

76. Bancroft, DA, and Pigg, JS: Alterations in skeletal function: Rheumatic disorders. In Porth, CM (ed): Pathophysiology: Concepts of Altered Health States, ed 6. Lippincott Williams & Wilkins, Philadelphia, 2002, pp 1367–1390.

77. Guven, S, Kuenzi, JA, and Matfin, G: Diabetes mellitus. In Porth, CM (ed): Pathophysiology: Concepts of Altered Health States, ed 6. Lippincott Williams & Wilkins, Philadelphia, 2002, pp 925–952.

78. Kaada, B: Systemic sclerosis: successful treatment of ulcerations, pain, Raynaud's phenomenon, calcinosis, and dysphagia by transcutaneous nerve stimulation. A case report. Acupunct Electrother Res 9:31–44, 1984.

79. Food and Drug Administration Guidelines for Electromedical Devices. 1975.

80. Rasmussen, MJ, Hayes, DL, Vlietstra, RE, et al: Can transcutaneous electrical nerve stimulation be safely used in patients with permanent cardiac pacemakers? Mayo Clin Proc 63:443–445, 1988.

81. Shade, SK: Use of transcutaneous electrical nerve stimulation for a patient with a cardiac pacemaker. A case report. Phys Ther 65:206–208, 1985.

82. Chen, D, Philip, M, Philip, PA, et al: Cardiac pacemaker inhibition by transcutaneous electrical nerve stimulation. Arch Phys Med Rehabil 71:27–30, 1990.

83. Ojingwa, JC, and Isseroff, RR: Electrical stimulation of wound healing. J Investig Dermatol 36:1–12, 2002.

84. American Physical Therapy Association: Clinical Electrotherapy: Physiology and Basic Concepts, APTA Continuing Ed Series No. 8. 2003. Accessed November 25, 2003. Web site: http://www.apta.org

85. Mulder, GD: Treatment of open-skin wounds with electric stimulation. Arch Phys Med Rehabil 72:375–377, 1991.

86. Cohen, DE, and Rice, RH: Toxic responses of the skin. In Klasssen, CD (ed): Casarett and Doull's Toxicology: The Basic Science of Poisons, ed 6. McGraw-Hill, Medical Publishing Division, New York, 2001, pp 653–672.

87. Kloth, LC: The APTA electrical stimulation lawsuit and its aftermath. American Physical Therapy Association. Adv Wound Care 12:472–475, 1999.

88. Unger, PG: Update on high-voltage pulsed current research and application. Top Geriatr Rehabil 16:35–46, 2000.

89. Houghton, PE, and Campbell, KE: Choosing an adjunctive therapy for the treatment of chronic wounds. Ostomy Wound Manage 45:43–52, 1999.

90. Reich, JD, and Tarjan, PP: Electrical stimulation of skin. Int J Dermatol 29:395–400, 1990.

91. Mehreteab, TA: Clinical Uses of Electrical Stimulation. Appleton & Lange, Norwalk, CT, 1994, pp 283–293.

92. Kirsner, RS, and Bogensberger, G: The normal process of healing. In Kloth, LC, and McCulloch, JM (eds): Wound Healing Alternatives in Management, ed 3. FA Davis, Philadelphia, 2002, pp 3–34.

93. Nelson, RM, and Currier, DP (eds): Clinical Electrotherapy. Norwalk, CT, Appleton & Lange, 1987.

LET'S FIND OUT

Purpose

This exercise provides learners with the opportunity to review tissue response concepts that may have been presented previously in other courses.

Objectives

- To familiarize the learner with the specific terminology of electrical stimulation
  - Polarity
    - Cathode
    - Aanode
- To familiarize the learner with the effects that can commonly be associated with each of the poles
- To familiarize the learner with the potential responses that a patient might experience in response to the application of electrical stimulation for tissue repair and that could include
  - Pain
  - Altered sensation
  - Edema (swelling)
  - Loss of function

Precaution	Why?
Over an area with decreased sensation	If the application involves the transmission of ions across the skin, then the patient must be able to report sensation to protect him or her from an adverse response.
When the patient has decreased cognitive ability	If the application involves the transmission of ions across the skin, then the patient must be able to report sensation to protect him or her from an adverse response.
During pregnancy	If the application is after the first trimester, then there is little risk to the fetus or the patient. This should be used with caution. Electrical stimulation has been safely used for analgesia during labor and delivery, but it may interfere with fetal monitors.
Patients with documented evidence of epilepsy, cerebral vascular accident, or reversible ischemic neurological deficit	These patients should be monitored carefully when electrical stimulation is used in the cervical region for possible adverse response.
Patients with suspected or diagnosed heart problems	Caution should be used to monitor the patient's response and the patient's vital signs should be closely monitored before, during, and after treatment for potential changes.
Following recent surgical procedures	If a muscle contraction occurs, it may cause a disruption in the healing process.

Contraindications

Contraindications	Why
Over the carotid sinus	There could be a potential problem if the circulation to the brain were altered.
In the presence of a pacemaker	Electrical stimulation devices could potentially interfere with the electrical demands of the pacemaker.
The presence of metal ions from antimicrobial medications or metallic implants	Direct electrical currents may drive metal ions from antimicrobial medications into the tissues. Pulsed waveforms may result in tissue heating, which also might be inappropriate.
During the first trimester of pregnancy	There are no data to indicate the level of safety for the fetus with the application of electrical stimulation during the first trimester of pregnancy.
Over or in proximity to cancerous lesions	Most application techniques with electrical stimulation involve the potential for an increase in circulation to the area. The possibility exists that the electrical stimulation may enhance the development of the metastasis.

Lab Questions and Activities
Polarity
1. Look up the responses of tissues under an anode and cathode in several sources and develop a composite description that encompasses all of the sources. Your response should be in terms that a patient would be able to comprehend; in other words, you need to be able to explain what you are doing with the device to a patient, not a colleague.

Describe tissue responses under the anode.

_____

_____

_____

Describe tissue responses under the cathode.

_____

_____

_____

Composite Descriptions
1. What are the principal differences between using the anode and using the cathode for electrical stimulation?

_____

_____

_____

When would you select the cathode?

_____

_____

_____

When would you select the anode?

_____

_____

_____

2. How could this potentially be useful information for you as a clinician?

_____

_____

_____

Infection

1. Review your definitions for infection. How would the presence of an infection potentially limit healing or a return to function?

_____

_____

2. Would the presence of an infection alter your selection of the polarity of your active electrode? Why or why not?

_____

_____

3. When could electrical stimulation potentially be used to promote wound healing?

_____

_____

4. Of what potential benefit would the addition of electrical stimulation for tissue repair be to the healing process?

_____

_____

CHAPTER 15

Pain Management With Electrical Stimulation

Barbara J. Behrens PTA, MS | Kathleen M. Kenna, PT

Learning Outcomes

Following the completion of this chapter, the learner will be able to:

- Discuss the concepts of pain management in contrast to pain relief.
- Outline the procedures for the use of electrical stimulation to promote analgesia.
- Explain the concepts of endogenous mechanisms for pain management.
- Discuss the clinical decision-making involved for determining the appropriate parameters for electrical stimulation to accomplish pain relief.
- Discuss appropriate documentation for the use of electrical stimulation to promote analgesia.
- Compare clinical and patient options for pain management with electrical stimulation.
- Describe electrode placement site selection guidelines for pain management.
- Apply TENS to a patient for pain management and instruct a patient in the self-application and self-adjustment of a TENS unit.
- Apply electrical stimulation with a clinical electrical stimulation device to accomplish sensory analgesia.

Key Terms

Analgesia
Anesthesia
Endogenous

Noxious
Opiates
Pain management

Paresthesia
Transcutaneous

"The greatest evil is physical pain." —St. Augustine

Patient Perspective
"Is that really supposed to do something? All I feel is tingling, no pain."

People experience pain in different ways dependent upon the cause. Their ability to express it or deal with it is based on a multitude of factors that has only been complicated in recent times by the concept of multitasking and compartmentalizing our daily lives. Society today expects everyone to accomplish a great deal within very little time, ignoring the fact that we are human beings and not machines. We recognize that if you overwork a machine, it will break down but somehow do not make that connection when it comes to ourselves. This unfortunately puts the expression of pain as a symptom very low on a priority list until that pain has escalated into something quite serious. That should not be the case, since pain is one of the cardinal signs of inflammation and it most often does signal that something has been injured. Early management of the cause of the pain can often lead to a faster recovery. Fortunately, there are many different ways that pain can be effectively managed, and one of them includes electrical stimulation.

Pain is a sensation that has both physical and psychological components. As discussed in Chapter 2, it has been studied and numerous instruments have been developed in an attempt to capture its extent. The capturing of these types of data has been a perpetual battle, in part because the individual experiencing the discomfort is really the only one who knows how much discomfort he or she is experiencing. The individual is also the only one to know how this level of discomfort is affecting his or her life.

Numerous physical agents have had a positive impact on decreasing the level of discomfort perceived by the patient. Electrical stimulation is one of those physical agents that has been used successfully for more than 50 years to provide sensory stimulation and to block or "gate" the painful stimulation from reaching the brain. This served as the foundation for Melzack and Wall's Gate Control Theory for pain relief and subsequent work.[1]

Pain commonly brings people to seek therapeutic interventions to relieve it. Clinicians have many different types of physical agents to choose from to effectively manage the patient's underlying pathology, symptoms, and associated dysfunctions. Thermal and mechanical agents have been presented in this text as tools to address a variety of patient problems. In this chapter, the use of electrical stimulation as a therapeutic intervention to treat pain is presented. The following areas are addressed:

- Terminology differences and expectations for analgesia and anesthesia
- Pain reduction versus pain management with the use of electrical stimulation
- General principles of pain management with the use of electrical stimulation
- Treatment rationale and methods for pain reduction and pain management with electrical stimulation
- Treatment expectations and progression for pain reduction and pain management with electrical stimulation
- Appropriate documentation for pain reduction and pain management with electrical stimulation

Physiology Review

Pain sensation occurs as a result of damage to sensory receptors in the skin and internal structures. This damage may be of several different forms, and thus cause the excitation of different sensory receptors. One type of sensory receptor includes the nerve fiber types that are the mediators of and responsible for pain impulses or **noxious** sensation in the central nervous system—the A-delta and C fibers. A-delta fibers provide fast pain sensation, and C fibers provide a deeper, dull or achy pain sensation. A-beta fibers transmit discriminative touch stimuli from the skin.

According to the original work of Melzack and Wall,[1] the sensory pain fibers also have the property of being able to be blocked and to stop their ability to transmit their input to the brain, thus temporarily altering pain perception. This original work sparked the development of a tremendous market for electrical stimulation devices that could be used for this purpose, as described in previous chapters. The devices were termed **transcutaneous** electrical nerve stimulation (TENS) units. TENS has since been used to accomplish pain relief for a multitude of conditions.[7–10]

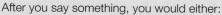

LET'S THINK ABOUT IT...

Instinctively, we already know what to do to reduce the perception of pain. If you accidentally hit your thumb with a hammer, what would you do to make it feel better?

After you say something, you would either:

a. Shake it, which would help make it feel better, or
b. Rub it very quickly, which would make it feel better, or
c. Squeeze it tightly, which would make it feel better, or
d. Run cold water over it, which would also make it feel better.

Each of these options is an example of blocking pain perception by overloading the area with sensory stimulation or mechano-receptive stimulation. That's the goal with electrical stimulation. Keep this in mind as we proceed.

The term TENS actually refers to the application of electrical stimulation across the skin, which applies to most of the electrical stimulation that is applied in physical therapy clinical settings, except for needle insertion for electromyographic (EMG) studies. (For more information, refer to Chapter 2.)

PAIN FIBER TYPES, CENTRAL PATHWAYS

Once a pain receptor is stimulated, the nerve fiber transmits a signal to the dorsal horn of the spinal cord. A few ascending and descending fibers branch off to form Lissauer's tract and communicate with neighboring spinal segments (Fig. 15-1). The main fiber continues in the dorsal horn to make connections with neurons of the lamina I, II, III, IV, and V. Lamina III is also known as the substantia gelatinosa. Synaptic connections are then made with neurons, giving rise to the lateral spinothalamic tract. These neurons cross over to the opposite side of the spinal cord at the ventral white commissure. The fibers of the lateral spinothalamic tract ascend the spinal cord and enter the brainstem (Fig. 15-2).

Electrical stimulation has the ability to block ascending transmission of nerve fibers; therefore, it has the ability to block pain perception. There is a crossing over of information to the opposite side of the spinal cord, so it is also possible in theory to block pain perception on the right side of the body with stimulation on the left side at the same spinal cord level. Pain has both physical and psychological factors associated with it. However, research has indicated that there is a more complex mechanism than just the specificity theory that clinicians have been relying on to explain successes with electrical stimulation.[11]

Analgesia, Anesthesia, and Paresthesia

TERMINOLOGY

The use of appropriate terminology is helpful when discussing the treatment of pain and pain management. To review, **analgesia** is defined as the absence of pain or noxious stimulation; the absence of the sensitivity to pain; or the relief of pain without a loss of consciousness. **Anesthesia** is defined as a loss of sensation, usually by damage to a nerve or receptor, that is, numbness; or the loss of the ability to feel pain caused by the administration of drugs or medical interventions. **Paresthesia** is any abnormal sensation of tingling, pricking, or numbness in the skin without an identifiable cause. **Pain management** involves the patient in the process of providing feedback as to when analgesia (reduction in pain perception) has been accomplished. It may also involve the patient in making decisions concerning when the therapeutic intervention will be used.

These terms are similar but there are important distinctions between them. Electrical stimulation can be used to accomplish analgesia and pain management and it may be the cause for paresthesia but it cannot be used to cause anesthesia. One of the advantages of using electrical stimulation for pain management is that if there is an acute injury in addition to any preexisting condition that is being treated, the patient will feel the discomfort of the new injury. This would not be the case if the patient were anesthetized.

LET'S THINK ABOUT IT

Professional athletes have relatively short careers competing in their sports, in part due to the number of injuries that they have sustained during that professional career. How often have you heard about an athlete receiving an anesthetic injection to permit him or her to continue competing during a critical competitive event? After the competition, the athlete finds out the true extent of the injury. Sometimes, the injury is a career ender.

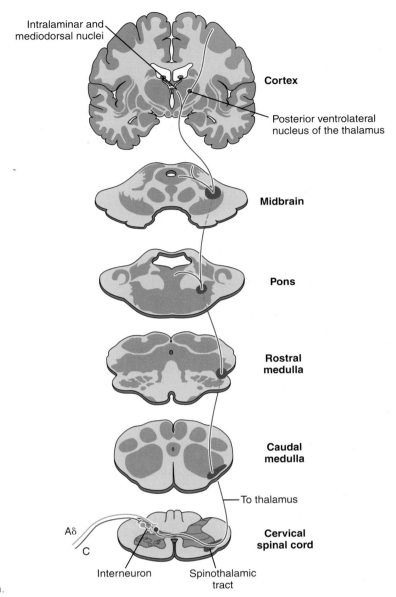

Intralaminar and mediodorsal nuclei

Cortex

Posterior ventrolateral nucleus of the thalamus

Midbrain

Pons

Rostral medulla

Caudal medulla

To thalamus

Cervical spinal cord

Aδ

C

Interneuron

Spinothalamic tract

FIGURE 15-1 Lissauer's tract path of sensation.

If the area were not anesthetized, but instead were provided with analgesia, which is what electrical stimulation is capable of providing, pain from additional injury would break through to warn the individual. Anesthesia removes all sensation from the area.

SENSORY ANALGESIA

Sensory analgesia can be produced by causing a tingling sensation. The stimulation may be activity of A-beta nerve fibers. The sensation produced may affect the gating mechanism at the spinal cord level, so pain impulses are not transmitted to the higher centers.[1] In effect, the patient experiences a tolerable stimulus that blocks pain impulses. Electrode placement sites have several options including surrounding the painful site, along the corresponding dermatome of the area, along the cutaneous nerve distribution of the painful area, or along the area superficial to the nerve trunk supplying the painful site (Fig. 15-3).

The necessary parameters of stimulation include a rate that falls between 50 pulses per second (pps) and 125 pps, a pulse duration of 60 to 100 microseconds, and an amplitude to produce a strong tingling sensation without a muscle contraction.[6] Duration of treatment initially can be up to an hour to assess the therapeutic effect. Although there is no potential harm to stimulation times lasting more than an hour, there have also been no demonstrated benefits to patients. Depending upon its effectiveness, this form of stimulation can be used up to 24 hours per day; however, if a patient is using a home stimulator, he or she is encouraged to turn the stimulator off each hour to determine whether or not it is needed. If the stimulator is left on continuously, the patient may not know what it feels like without it. Pain relief usually occurs during the time the stimulus is applied. This relief then may enable the patient to perform functional activities much sooner than if the TENS had not been used.[4,6,7,12]

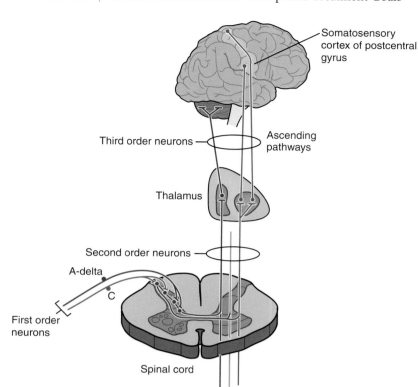

Somatosensory cortex of postcentral gyrus

Third order neurons

Ascending pathways

Thalamus

Second order neurons

A-delta

C

First order neurons

Spinal cord

FIGURE 15-2 The spinothalamic tract, an ascending tract in the spinal column, uses three neurons to convey sensory information from the periphery to conscious level at the cerebral cortex. Neurons ascend one or two vertebral levels via Lissauer's tract and then synapse with secondary neurons in either the substantia gelatinosa or the nucleus proprius.

Endogenous Opiate Liberation

Endogenous refers to something from within or that is developed from internal systems. **Opiates** are drugs containing opium or its derivatives and are used in medicine for inducing sleep and relieving pain. When the terms are used together, it refers to the ability of the body to produce and release strong pain-relieving substances.

Theoretically, stimulation of the endogenous opiate system can also lead to pain relief. Electrical stimulators capable of rates of 1 to 5 pps, a pulse duration greater than 200 microseconds, and an intensity to create a muscle twitch may generate pain relief through this mechanism. The duration of treatment is 30 to 45 minutes. Electrode placement sites may include motor points that may also be acupuncture points or trigger points. (See the Appendix at the end of this chapter for more information regarding electrode placement.)

Stimulation of the A-delta and C fibers by the parameters described may affect the production of endorphins and enkephalin release that mimic the action of narcotic drugs to promote decreased perception of pain. Pain reduction usually lasts longer with this form of electrical stimulation than the application to produce sensory analgesia. This form of electrical stimulation may be used for the treatment of intense or chronic pain.[13,14] Endorphins and enkephalins are examples of endogenous opiates, each of which has a known period of effectiveness. Beta-endorphin has a half-life, or the amount of time when half of the compound is still present and half has decayed, of 4 hours and encephalin has a half-life of 2 minutes.[15]

Selection of specific parameters of stimulation will theoretically result in the liberation of specific endogenous opiates that are either of the longer lasting or shorter lasting variety. In general, high frequency stimulation in the range of approximately 100 Hz with short pulse durations tend to produce shorter lasting pain relief and lower frequency stimulation (less than 10 Hz) with longer pulse durations producing longer lasting relief.[25–27] However, recent investigators have also found that results suggest that there may also be a strong placebo effect with TENS.[28] Since pain is a subjective complaint, the value of the placebo cannot be overlooked and clinicians must be mindful of the power of the placebo in whatever they do in addition to the therapeutic benefits of the therapeutic interventions that they employ.

Other Considerations

When using electrical stimulation for promoting pain reduction, other factors need to be considered. The patient's attitude toward the use of electrical stimulation is important in the successful use of the modality. Explanations of the intended purpose and mechanism of affecting the pain experience need to be presented to the patient in appropriate, understandable terminology. Also, the expected results of treatment need to be discussed. Do not set the patient up for failure by trying to attain unrealistic goals. If a patient has heard of a form of electrical stimulation or has been treated with this modality in the past, find out more details about what the modality was, how it was used, and how effective it was for that patient. If the patient is biased toward

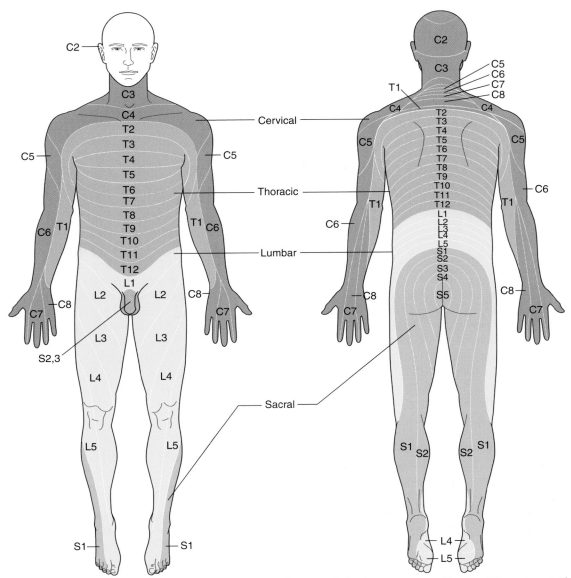

FIGURE 15-3 Dermatome for C7 nerve root distribution shows the area of skin that is innervated by the C7 nerve root. Electrode placement along this distribution would help reduce pain arising from the C7 spinal level.

the success of the treatment, build upon the experience and how the treatment has effectively been used on other patients with similar conditions. If electrical stimulation is used, the patient should be informed that there is a great variety of treatment parameters and electrode placements that can lead to a successful treatment outcome. If the stimulation was used in the past for sensory analgesia, emphasize the effectiveness of endogenous opiate stimulation or vice versa. If the patient indicates a certain type of electrode placement, discuss other options that can be used.

Most important, the practitioner needs to discuss expected results of the use of electrical stimulation by developing realistic goals. If a patient is of the attitude that electrical stimulation does not help or if he or she has had a bad experience with the modality, the practitioner may choose another technique for pain control (see Treatment Expectations later in this chapter).

Narcotic pain medications produce analgesia by decreasing the perception of pain. The release of endogenous opiates by electrical stimulation produces pain relief through the same mechanism. If electrical stimulation is effective in alleviating pain, a decrease in the amount of prescribed medication may be indicated. This must be discussed with the physician who prescribed the medication prior to making a comment to a patient about changing the dosage level.

Alcohol consumption by the patient needs to be considered by the clinician. Alcohol is considered a sedative-hypnotic agent. The effects of dose-dependent central nervous system depression from alcohol produce analgesia. Judgment is also impaired with alcohol consumption; therefore, home use of an electrical stimulator may not be recommended for patients who have a tendency to abuse alcohol by consuming large quantities on a regular basis.

The intensity necessary to elicit the desired response may have to be significantly increased in order to be perceived by the patient. In either case, safety of the patient becomes an even greater concern. The clinician must always be vigilant to maintain patient safety when providing patient instruction that the patient is cognitively capable of receiving what is being presented at that time.

BEFORE YOU BEGIN

Ask yourself the following questions:
- Has the patient already had a bad experience with electrical stimulation that you will have to overcome?
- Does the patient have a fear of electricity?
- Have you thoroughly explained what you are going to do and what the patient should expect?

The use of exercise is also a consideration when using electrical stimulation for pain relief. Patients will be able to detect sharp A-delta pain if an exercise is being done beyond the recommended range of motion (ROM) or at an excessive level that could be causing tissue damage. Protective pain mechanisms remain intact when sensory analgesia is produced via electrical stimulation. Depending on the diagnosis of the patient, the desired response to treatment and the perception of pain, electrical stimulation can be used to facilitate exercise by decreasing pain perception. Specific guidelines need to be reinforced for a home exercise program that is also being done by a patient who is using a portable electrical stimulation device with a home exercise program. (Portable stimulators may be worn during therapeutic exercise; however, that is not the typical application for the devices.)

Potential Treatments and How to Achieve Success

CLINICAL DECISION-MAKING

Many electrical stimulation devices exist that allow several treatment options. These include, but are not limited to, interferential current stimulators (IFC), high-voltage pulsed current muscle stimulators, and low-voltage units. The details of the various types of devices are presented in various chapters in this text. Look at the parameters a given machine is capable of producing to determine if its use is appropriate for the type of treatment for which you want to use it.

The purpose of this section is to develop a process by which the clinician can determine the most appropriate forms of electrical stimulation treatments for a patient. In order to provide effective treatment, the clinician goes through a decision-making process that concludes in treatment alternatives for the patient. Through thorough examination and assessment, the clinician may identify the source of a patient's painful symptoms. Past medical history and the history of the present condition assist the clinician in identifying contraindications and precautions relevant

to the use of electrical stimulation. A summary of contraindications and precautions is presented in Box 15-1. In the presence of contraindications, a different pain-reducing modality that presents fewer risks to the patient should be selected. If precautions are present, the patient should be monitored closely for signs of adverse reactions to treatment. If electrical stimulation is the chosen treatment, parameters are further delineated by identifying the type of pain present, the location of the pain, the characteristics of the pain, and the other rehabilitative needs of the patient. The findings influence treatment parameters, options for electrode placement, and goal setting. A decision-making paradigm is presented in Figure 15-4.

Remember, pain management is only one aspect of the complete care of the patient. Depending upon the additional rehabilitation needs of the individual, other therapeutic interventions will be used.[2-5] Electrical stimulation, as with any other treatment intervention, is to be implemented to help achieve functional goals for a patient. For example, to facilitate greater force gains in a shorter period of time enabling a patient to perform recreational and activities of daily living, a patient may use electrical stimulation for postoperative physical therapy interventions.[5]

BOX 15-1 | Contraindications and Precautions With the Use of Electrical Stimulation for Pain Management

Contraindications
- Demand type cardiac pacemaker
- Carotid sinus, stimulation over the area may result in a hypotensive incident
- Directly over the eye
- Epilepsy
- Malignancies (see below)
- Loss of or decreased sensation

Precautions
- Patients with known cardiac disease or arrhythmias should be closely monitored for signs of adverse effects.
- Directly over an open wound.
- Directly over the lumbar paraspinal muscles and abdominal area during the first trimester of pregnancy electrical stimulation is *contraindicated*.
- During labor and delivery, electrical stimulation may provide relief for lumbar pain if the mother is having an uncomplicated pregnancy. ES devices may interfere with fetal monitors, which is why they need to be used with extreme caution.
- ES may be used for pain control with informed consent of the patient in those instances where there are patients with a diagnosed malignancy that is known to be terminal. ES has been helpful in providing palliative relief.
- Electrical stimulators are for external use only and should be kept out of the reach of children.

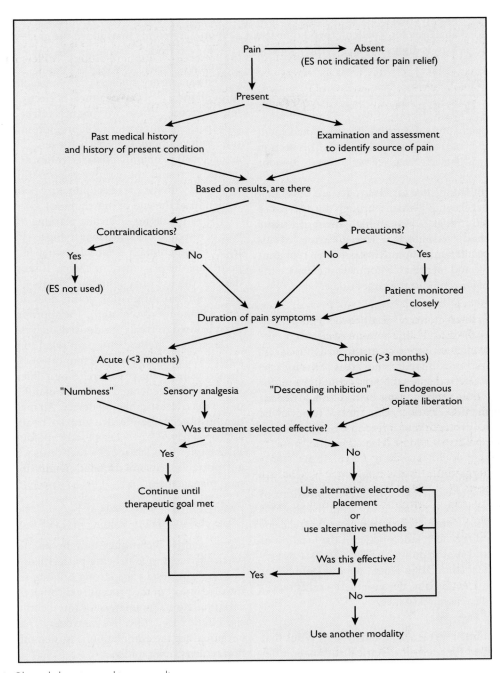

FIGURE 15-4 Clinical decision-making paradigm.

General Principles of Pain Management

Therapeutic intervention with the use of electrical stimulation can provide an analgesic effect. This occurs through a number of postulated neurophysiological mechanisms (see Chapter 2 for this information).

Pain management involves controlling the perception and/or sensation of pain. Management of pain allows the patient to better control his or her discomfort. This can lead to improved function. Electrical stimulation is a physical agent that can be used as one tool for pain management.[6]

Electrical stimulation is believed to produce analgesic effects through the stimulation of the peripheral and central nervous systems. Electrical stimulation devices are available as both clinical and portable models that the patient can use at appropriate times during the day as needed. The portable units are generally the size of a beeper and run on rechargeable batteries. The portability of the electrical stimulators allows the patient greater autonomy in his or her care as well as the option for use of extended periods of stimulation. When the unit and electrodes are used appropriately, side effects are minimal. There is a chance for a chemical burn at the stimulation site, hypersensitivity reactions to the stimulation, or allergic reactions to the self-adhering electrodes. If clinical use of electrical stimulation has provided analgesia for a patient, then home use might be beneficial. This is discussed later in this chapter.

Treatment Methods

RATIONALE FOR ELECTRODE PLACEMENT

Several previous chapters discussed electrode placement sites for a number of treatment applications. This section deals specifically with electrode placement site selection for analgesia.

Optimal stimulation sites for electrodes are those that will facilitate goal accomplishment through the delivery of current. If the skin resistance is too high, the target tissue may not be reached at a comfortable level of current. Motor points, trigger points, and acupuncture points all represent electrically active and identifiable points that enhance the potential flow of current into the target tissue.

Motor Points

Motor points are the anatomical location where the peripheral nerve enters the muscle. The amount of electrical current necessary to elicit a motor response from a muscle will be less over the motor point than other areas of the muscle. Placement of an electrode over this area facilitates a motor response of the underlying muscle belly with a lower intensity setting than other nonspecific sites. Whenever the desired response involves a motor response or muscle contraction, motor points should be selected for use.[17-19]

Trigger Points

Trigger points are those areas that exhibit hypersensitivity to both pressure and electrical stimulation. Palpations of these sites causes pain to radiate away from the site.[17-20] Trigger points have a decreased resistance to electrical energy. There is a direct correlation between the location of trigger points and motor points.[19] Selection of a trigger point for electrical stimulation would tend to yield better results than not selecting one, because these points represent an area of decreased resistance.

Acupuncture Points

Acupuncture points represent another type of point that has been described for use with electrical stimulation devices. These points are located over the entire surface of the body and have been mapped out for centuries. Acupuncture points may lie over muscle or connective tissue. They are also electrically active, exhibiting a decreased resistance to the flow of electrical current.[19] If the desired response to the electrical stimulation is a diffuse sensory analgesia, then acupuncture points may afford the greatest availability of sites for electrode placements. See Table 15-1 for a comparison among all three types of points.

Diffuse sensory analgesia can be readily accomplished through the use of two channels of electrodes for a total of four electrodes. These two channels can be set up in a crisscross pattern. This pattern will promote an increase in sensation throughout the area with less discrimination of actual location of individual electrodes, as long as the electrodes surround the painful region. This setup will be enhanced with the use of acupuncture points. (Refer to the Appendix at the end of this chapter.)

The rationale for electrode placement is based on the type of response the clinician is trying to elicit through electrical stimulation. If a muscle twitch is desired, motor points are the placement of choice. If sensory analgesia is desired, the use of acupuncture points is warranted. The use of optimal stimulation points does not guarantee the desired amount of sensation. The appropriate parameters must be used to create the desired analgesic effect.

Treatment methods for pain relief to be produced by electrical stimulation fall into four categories. Each method theoretically produces pain relief by a different neurophysiological effect generated by the use of different parameters of the electrical stimulation device. All methods have been demonstrated to be effective forms of treatment when used appropriately.[1,2,4-7,9,10] Let's Find Out, found at the end of this chapter, is a lab activity that deals with both clinical and portable electrical stimulation units for the purpose of pain management.

PRODUCING ANALGESIA FOR A PAINFUL PROCEDURE

Some manual techniques may be painful for a patient when the technique is being performed. It is possible to produce analgesia via a strong tingling sensation to ease the discomfort of the procedure through the use of electrical stimulation. Parameters for this technique are summarized in Box 15-2. Effective carryover of pain relief is brief, because once the stimulation is turned off, normal sensation returns very rapidly.

PRODUCING SENSORY-LEVEL ANALGESIA

Sensory analgesia is suggested to activate the gating mechanism in the spinal cord. This reduces pain impulses from reaching the brain to be processed.[1] Appropriate parameters

TABLE 15-1	Comparisons Between Acupuncture, Motor, and Trigger Points		
	EXHIBIT DECREASED RESISTANCE	**CAUSE PAIN TO RADIATE AWAY WHEN PALPATED**	**MAPPED OUT ON CHARTS**
Acupuncture points	X		X
Trigger points	X	X	X
Motor points	X		X

> **BOX 15-2 | Parameters for Producing Analgesia During a Painful Procedure [21,22]**
>
> - Frequency: 150 + pulses per second
> - Pulse duration: Greater than 150 µsec
> - Intensity: A strong tingling sensation to tolerance. *Note:* A non-rhythmical muscle contraction may be produced at this intensity.
> - Electrode placement sites: Along involved dermatome, two points where the nerve is superficial.
> - Treatment time: 5 minutes prior to initiation of the painful technique, 15–30 minutes total time.
> - Indications: Acute pain, pain associated with wound débridement, pain associated with transverse friction massage, pain associated with aggressive stretching techniques, pain associated with aggressive joint mobilization techniques.

> **BOX 15-4 | Parameters for Producing "Hyper-Stimulation Analgesia" [21,22]**
>
> - Frequency: 1–4 pulses per second
> - Pulse duration: ≥1 msec
> - Intensity: Highest tolerable level of noxious stimulation
> - Electrode placement sites: Active electrode is a small diameter probe that is placed over a point with decreased resistance to the flow of current. It may be an acupuncture point, trigger point, or motor point. The dispersive electrode can be held by the patient or placed on the skin at a point distal to the site of stimulation.
> - Treatement time: 30 seconds per point
> - Indications: Acute or chronic pain syndromes

> **BOX 15-5 | Parameters for Endogenous Opiate Liberation [21–23]**
>
> | | |
> |---|---|
> | Frequency: | 1–5 pulses per second |
> | Pulse duration: | 200–300 µsec |
> | Intensity: | Muscle twitch |
> | Electrode placement sites: | Motor points |
> | Treatment time: | 30–45 minutes |
> | Indications: | Chronic pain syndromes |

and treatment indications are described in Box 15-3. Effective carryover is pain relief that persists after the stimulation is no longer present.

NOXIOUS STIMULATION TO PRODUCE ANALGESIA

Electrical stimulation, which is theorized to induce "descending inhibition," uses a noxious form of stimulation to help control pain. The painful stimulus activates the smaller pain fibers, which then make connections in the brainstem reticular formation. Information is then conducted to the midbrain to an area called the periaqueductal gray matter. This area of the brain activates a descending pathway that inhibits pain at the spinal cord level.[1] Analgesia occurs quickly with this form of stimulation and effective carryover can last a few minutes to a few hours. Treatment parameters and indications are presented in Box 15-4. A disadvantage of this form of stimulation is that the patient must experience noxious (painful) stimuli to produce the desired effect.

ENDOGENOUS OPIATE LIBERATION

Low-rate electrical stimulation can potentially produce analgesia through the liberation of endogenous opiates. Parameters for pain relief by this method and indications are summarized in Box 15-5. The onset of pain relief may

> **BOX 15-3 | Parameters for Producing Sensory-Level Analgesia [21,22]**
>
> - Frequency: 75–150 pulses per second
> - Pulse duration: Less than 200 µsec
> - Intensity: Strong, but comfortable tingling sensation
> - Electrode placement sites: Surrounding the site of pain
> - Indications: Acute pain conditions, chronic pain conditions

occur by the end of a treatment session or several hours later with potentially long-term carryover of pain relief.

TREATMENT EXPECTATIONS

When employing electrical stimulation as a tool in a pain management program, realistic goals must be considered. Goal determination is based upon evaluative findings, the nature of the disabling condition, the previous activity level of the patient, the patient's psychosocial condition, and the prognosis of recovery. The goals established will also vary depending on the stage of the healing process and the nature of the pain acute versus chronic. If a patient is not invested in or motivated toward his or her own recovery, the efforts of a clinician may have limited success.

A patient who is experiencing acute pain experiences decreased pain intensity and pain patterns as a result of the resolution of the inflammatory response and the healing process. During the acute phase, patients may experience pain at rest as well as with any movement.[12] The use of electrical stimulation can facilitate the healing process because of physiological responses to the modality. Once pain decreases, the patient may also experience a decrease in the intensity of muscle guarding. The use of electrical stimulation can be used to help break up the pain-muscle guarding-pain cycle. Goals for a patient during the acute phase of the inflammatory response and the healing process include decreasing the intensity of pain at rest and with movement. This response, if elicited by the use of electrical stimulation, may occur within the treatment time of

20 to 30 minutes. The desired response with other patients may be elicited only while the patient is using an electrical stimulation device. In that case, the patient may be a good candidate for a portable device to be used at times outside the clinical setting.

As the healing process enters the subacute phase, pain may be experienced at the end ROM.[12] Pain at rest has usually resolved by this time. This process tends to occur from 7 to 21 days after the onset of injury, but may last up to 6 weeks. Tendons and ligaments may take several weeks to go through this initial healing phase. The severity of injury will also determine the duration of the subacute phase. The use of electrical stimulation may continue to be a treatment option for the patient; however, the underlying purpose for its use will change. The purpose now becomes directed toward controlling the pain that is created as a result of other therapeutic interventions that stress the tissue at end ROM. The patient may have little discomfort prior to treatment, but the gentle therapeutic techniques used to enhance ROM may cause an increase in pain perception. Electrical stimulation may then be used as a post-treatment modality. In this situation, the goal would be to bring the pain level back to a pretreatment level.

When the healing process has reached the maturation and remodeling phase, therapeutic interventions tend to become more aggressive to promote the patient's functional abilities. Progressive stretching, strengthening, and functional activities are commonly the emphasis of treatment. Therapeutic techniques at this phase are intended to stress the immature collagen fibrils laid down in the subacute phase to develop stronger chemical bonds and to orient fibers in a direction that is conducive to function. This process lasts for an additional 8 to 14 weeks after the initial injury. The denser the connective tissue, the longer is the process. During this phase of healing, pain may be experienced at the end ROM when overpressure is applied to shortened or weakened structures. Electrical stimulation can be used for the purpose of treating pain created by the therapeutic intervention with the intent to bring pain levels back to pretreatment levels.

The purpose of the use of electrical stimulation during the normal course of the healing of an acute injury is a transition from managing pain at rest, to post-treatment pain reduction. Each patient's response will vary; therefore, the goals formulated are to be individualized for the patient and adjusted accordingly. If pain is at a tolerable level, not interfering with recovery, or can be controlled by other physical agents effectively, the use of electrical stimulation may be discontinued.

Individuals with chronic pain conditions may also benefit from the use of electrical stimulation. The expectation of eliminating pain symptoms may be unrealistic for the majority of patients; thus, the goal of electrical stimulation is to control pain to allow for better function. Electrical stimulation may be effective for at least three different purposes in treating a chronic pain patient.

1. Electrical stimulation can be used to decrease the intensity of the pain the patient is experiencing at rest.

2. It can decrease the pain associated with the therapeutic techniques used to enhance muscle flexibility and functional activity during and after treatment.

3. Finally, it can also help treat acute flare-ups or exacerbations in pain symptoms.

Treatment goals for the use of electrical stimulation with patients who have chronic pain may emphasize functional ability while keeping pain symptoms at a manageable level. The goal may be an effective reduction in pain that allows the patient to walk for longer periods of time or that provides greater comfort for a person to do work-related tasks. The patient should also be able to use a home electrical stimulation unit effectively to manage his or her pain symptoms.

The complete treatment of a patient with chronic pain is a multifaceted approach involving many medical disciplines and is beyond the scope of this text. Developing relaxation skills; improving coping skills; and increasing flexibility, strength, and endurance will further enhance patient recovery. The use of electrical stimulation is only one tool used to help these patients.

Transcutaneous Electrical Nerve Stimulation (TENS) for Home Use

The portability of some electrical stimulation units allows for home use of the device, thus providing the patient treatment opportunities as needed for pain relief. The patient needs sufficient joint ROM and dexterity to apply electrodes, to plug in wires, and to operate the controls. If the patient is not physically capable of using the machine, the individual may have another person at home that can apply the electrodes and adjust the controls as needed. The patient should also have the ability to understand the appropriate use of the machine. Clinicians should be able to explain the purpose and use of the device in understandable terms. The patient should also be instructed to monitor skin condition and respond accordingly.

Some form of written and/or pictorial home instruction material outlining the safe use of the unit should be provided. All important information concerning the safe and appropriate use of the unit should be included. This form should include, but is not limited to, the following information:

- Purpose of the unit
- Settings of the controls (pulse duration, pulse rate)
- Some form of pain assessment chart to monitor results
- Electrode placement site charts
- Battery insertion instructions
- Electrode care and instructions for use
- The name and telephone number of the clinician or another resource person to answer questions
- A list of dos and don'ts regarding the use of the device
- Potential troubleshooting tips for the unit
- Instructions on appropriate skin care
- A sample form is given in Figure 15-5.

TENS
Home Instruction Form

Your clinician will determine the electrode placement sites and method of stimulation that will provide the most effective degree of pain control with the shortest treatment time. Your cooperation is essential to this process.

Complete the chart below recording your pain ratings as requested. If you have any questions call your clinician.

1	2	3	4	5	6	7	8	9	10
No pain									Maximal pain

pre-TENS rating	Treatment time	post-TENS rating	Relief time	Comments

Setting up the TENS unit . . .

The following descriptions will assist you in setting the controls on the TENS unit. Do not experiment with the settings unless instructed to do so by the clinician.

I Conventional

Pulse Duration: (PD, width)	Preset to the lowest setting
Frequency: (Hz, PPS, rate)	Preset to the highest setting
Amplitude: (intensity)	Increase to a comfortable level of tingling. Increase if it "fades."
Treatment time:	Leave it ON until you do not feel pain. Do not leave it turned ON for more than 60 minutes without turning if OFF to see how it feels.

II Acupuncturelike

Pulse Duration: (PD, width)	Preset to the highest setting
Frequency: (Hz, PPS, rate)	Preset to the lowest setting
Amplitude: (intensity)	Increase until muscle "thumping" occurs
Treatment time:	25 to 30 minutes while resting.

III Brief Intense

Pulse Duration: (width)	Preset to the highest setting
Frequency: (Hz, PPS, rate)	Preset to the highest setting
Amplitude: (intensity)	Increase to the strongest level tolerable.
Treatment time:	5 to 30 minutes as instructed

Electrode Placement Sites

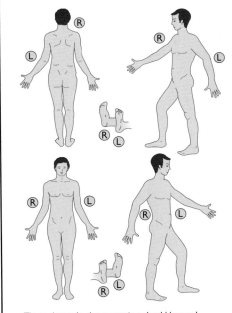

These electrode placement sites should be used. "X's" are one channel, and "O's" are the other channel.

TENS Reminders . . .

1. Do not wear the TENS unit while bathing, showering, or sleeping. Remove the electrodes and replace them after the activity.
2. The TENS unit may be worn at all other times, and turned ON whenever you are experiencing pain. There is no limit to the number of times (treatments) per day.
3. The TENS unit should be turned OFF when not in use, to ensure a longer battery life.
4. If your TENS unit has rechargeable batteries, the extra set should be plugged into the recharger to ensure the availability of charged batteries at all times.
5. Carefully inspect the electrodes before applying them. Make sure that there is no metal or bare rubber showing through the side of the electrode that touches your skin. If the electrodes do break down, replace them.
6. If you need more electrodes, or new lead wires, call the TENS distributor.

Notes:

Important #'s:

Date: _____ Model: _____ Serial # _____

Clinician: _____

TENS Distributor: _____

FIGURE 15-5 Sample written and pictorial home instruction material. (Diagram courtesy of Barbara J. Behrens, PTA, MS.)

Patient Perspective

Remember that this may be the first time that this patient has really been included in his or her own pain management program. This means that the patient has to accept some responsibility for monitoring his or her discomfort and then act appropriately. If the patient is using a TENS unit, then the patient is responsible for making sure that batteries are available as needed to provide uninterrupted stimulation periods. If other methods are being employed, it is important for the patient to accurately report his or her perception of pain and take careful note of the use of pain medications. The approach must be a team effort to be successful.

Patients' Frequently Asked Questions

1. **Can I wear this [a TENS unit] in the shower?**
2. **Can I wear this [a TENS unit] in a thunderstorm?**
3. **If I hurt myself more, will I still be able to feel it?**
4. **What are the side effects of this? It seems too simple.**
5. **Why does that form of electrical stimulation hurt so much and the others do not?**

Although TENS will not provide success for pain relief for all patients, clinicians have successfully used this modality to help in pain management with many patients who seek relief of their symptoms. Combining the appropriate parameters and electrode placements with the principles of the healing process and the appropriate communication approach to the patient provides the treatment that has a high potential for success. Pain may not be eliminated, but it may be controlled sufficiently to facilitate a more comfortable recovery, facilitate other goals of treatment, and restore functional ability as a result of pain control.

Documentation

The documentation of treatment parameters and patient responses are essential to the practice of determining the efficacy of any treatment. The treatment parameters that one clinician uses should be reproducible by another. Documentation is the key for accomplishing consistency in treatment between practitioners. When using the Subjective, Objective, Assessment, Plan (SOAP) note format for documentation, different aspects of the pain management should be noted throughout different headings of documentation.

Objective (O in SOAP) information for the documentation of pain management includes the measurable aspects of the patient's condition and the treatment rendered. Parameters used with electrical stimulation must be indicated. Documentation should include the type of electrical stimulation used, the mode of delivery, pulse duration (PD), frequency (F), rise and fall time (if used), treatment area, electrode placement sites, duration of treatment, and goal of or response to the intensity.

Summary

The use of electrical stimulation as a physical agent for the treatment of pain symptoms is multifaceted. The clinician should have a thorough understanding of the neurophysiological basis of pain modulation and the variety of methods to achieve pain reduction with electrical stimulation. Treatment applications are based on this knowledge as well as the results of a thorough evaluation of the patient. Any modification of parameters is based on treatment outcome. This chapter presented a review of the underlying tenets of pain modulation and a variety of methods to achieve pain reduction. The paradigm of clinical decision-making provides the practitioner with a framework of the process for treatment selection or modification to achieve the desired goals of electrical stimulation as an instrument for pain reduction.

Review Questions

1. What is the difference between pain management and pain relief?
   a. There is no difference
   b. Pain management is what medications do and pain relief is what occurs through the use of physical therapy
   c. Both pain relief and pain management can be accomplished with physical agents but one is managed by the patient with a portable device
   d. Pain management is temporary and pain relief is constant

2. What fiber type would potentially need to be stimulated with electrical stimulation to cause the liberation of the longest lasting endogenous mechanisms for pain management?
   a. A-beta
   b. A-delta
   c. Motor
   d. C fibers

3. What would the rationale be for using a clinical versus portable option for pain management with electrical stimulation?
   a. Clinical electrical stimulation can be used in combination with manual techniques so that the patient feels no discomfort during therapy
   b. Clinical electrical stimulation units are battery operated and offer more power output potential than portable units for sustained benefit
   c. Clinical electrical stimulation units are more expensive than portable units, which means that the reimbursement from insurance carriers would be higher for the same service billed to the patient
   d. Portable electrical stimulators are the most convenient form of electrical stimulation for use in the clinic and would save clinicians money because they would not need to purchase clinical models

4. Electrode placement site selection guidelines for pain management involve the selection of which of the following considerations?
   a. Sites that exhibit an increased resistance to the flow of electrical current
   b. Acupuncture points in the area surrounding the treatment area and referral area of pain
   c. Motor points in the treatment area so that a strong muscle contraction can easily be generated in the painful region
   d. Trigger points in the treatment area

5. Which of the following parameters would *not* be important to document for the use of electrical stimulation to promote analgesia?
   a. The name of the electrical stimulator
   b. The location of the electrodes and general setup
   c. The treatment goal and amount of time for the application
   d. the patient's pre- and post-treatment

CASE STUDY

Carol is a cartoonist who has been referred to physical therapy for pain management techniques subsequent to a cervical strain injury. She was involved in a motor vehicle accident in which she was hit from behind. She now has muscle guarding and marked decreases in her cervical ROM in all directions. Her primary complaint is of occipital headaches. She lives alone and works from a home office. Most of her day is spent at an artist's table that is angled at 45 degrees. Medications to reduce muscle guarding and inflammation caused other complications because they interacted with other medications that she was already taking.

- Would Carol potentially benefit from any form of electrical stimulation to help manage her pain? If yes, what form(s) and where would you place the electrodes?

- If you wanted to use electrical stimulation to attempt to deal with Carol's pain, what parameters would you select and how would you explain what she should expect to feel? Is there more than one potential option? Please support your response.
- Would there be any reason that you might suspect that home use of a TENS unit for Carol could be contraindicated? Why or why not? Please support your response.

DISCUSSION QUESTIONS

1. What forms of electrical stimulation can be used to treat the pain associated with the performance of a painful manual technique such as a deep tissue massage? What parameters would you use and why?

2. Explain the neurophysiological mechanisms of the effects of electrical stimulation in terms that a patient would understand.

3. A patient is diagnosed with phantom limb pain. What information would you need to know about this patient in order to recommend a form of electrical stimulation for treatment of this syndrome?

4. What are the advantages and disadvantages of electrical stimulation for analgesia compared with others that reduce pain perception?

5. Describe three possible forms of electrical stimulation treatments for an individual with a chronic pain syndrome.

REFERENCES

1. Melzack, R: Pain: past, present and future. Can J Exp Psych 47:615–629, 1993.
2. Hurley, DA, Minder, PM, McDonough, SM, et al: Interferential therapy electrode placement technique in acute low back pain: a preliminary investigation. Arch Phys Med Rehabil 82: 485–493, 2001.
3. Draper, V, and Ballard, L: Electrical stimulation versus electromyographic biofeedback in the recovery of quadriceps femoris function following anterior cruciate ligament surgery. Phys Ther 71:455–465, 1991.
4. Gotlin, RS, Hershkowitz, S, Juris, PM, et al: Electrical stimulation effect on extensor lag and length of hospital stay after total knee arthroplasty. Arch Phys Med Rehabil. 75:957–959, 1994.
5. Lewek, M, Steven, J, and Snyder-Mackler, L: The use of electrical stimulation to increase quadriceps femoris muscle force in an elderly patient following total knee arthroplasty. Phys Ther 81:1565–1571, 2001.
6. Jarit, GJ, Mohr, KJ, Waller, R, et al: The effects of home interferential therapy on post-operative pain, edema, and range of motion of the knee. Clin J Sport Med 13:16–20, 2003.
7. Rakel, B, and Frantz, R: Effectiveness of transcutaneous electrical nerve stimulation on postoperative pain with movement. J Pain 4:455–464, 2003.
8. Sluka, KA, and Walsh, D: Transcutaneous electrical nerve stimulation: basic science mechanisms and clinical effectiveness. J Pain 4:109–121, 2003.
9. Chesterton, LS, Foster, NE, Wright, CC, et al: Effects of TENS frequency, intensity and stimulation site parameter manipulation of pressure pain threshold in healthy human subjects. Pain 106:73–80, 2003.
10. Moore, SR, and Shurman, J: Combined neuromuscular electrical stimulation and transcutaneous electrical nerve stimulation for treatment of chronic back pain: a double-blind, repeated measures comparison. Arch Phys Med Rehabil 78:55–60, 1997.
11. Melzack, R, Coderre, TJ, Katz, J, et al: Central neuroplasticity and pathological pain. Ann N Y Acad Sci 933:157–174, 2001.
12. Zizic, TM, Hoffman, KC, Holt, PA, et al: The treatment of osteoarthritis of the knee with pulsed electrical stimulation. J Rheumatol 22:1757–1761, 1995.
13. Wells, PE, Frampton, V, and Bowsher, D: Pain Management by Physical Therapy. Appleton & Lange, Norwalk, CT, 1988.
14. Tollison, CD, Satterthwaite, JR, and Tollison, JW: Handbook of Pain Management, ed 2. Williams & Wilkins, Baltimore, 1994.
15. Bishop, B: Pain: Its physiology and rationale for management. Part II. Analgesic systems of the CNS. Phys Ter 60:21–23, 1980.
16. Lin, JG, and Chen, WL: Acupuncture analgesia: a review of its mechanisms of action. Am J Chin Med 36(4):635–645, 2008.
17. Travell, J, and Rinzler, SH: The myofascial genesis of pain. Postgrad Med 11:425–435, 1952.
18. Melzack, R: Myofascial trigger points: relation to acupuncture and mechanisms of pain. Arch Phys Med Rehabil 62:114, 1981.
19. Melzack, R, Stilwell, DM, and Fox, EJ: Trigger points and acupuncture points for pain: correlations and implications. Pain 3:3, 1977.
20. Baldry, P: Management of myofascial trigger point pain. Acupoint Med 20: 2–10, 2002.
21. American Physical Therapy Association: Electrotherapeutic Terminology in Physical Therapy. Section on Clinical Electrophysiology. Author, Alexandria, VA, 2001.
22. Howson, D: Peripheral neural excitability: implications for transcutaneous electrical nerve stimulation. Phys Ther 58:1467, 1978.
23. Alon, G: High voltage stimulation: effects of electrode size on basic excitatory responses. Phys Ther 66:890, 1985.
24. Han, JS: Acupuncture and endorphins. Neurosci Lett 361(1–3):258–261, 2004.
25. Sabino, GS, Santos, CM, Francischi, JN, and de Resende, MA: Release of endogenout opiods following transcutaneous electric nerve stimulation in an experimental model of acute inflammatory pain. J Pain 9(2):157–163, 2008.
26. Kocyigit, F, Akalin, E, Gezer, NS, et al: Functional magnetic resonance imaging of the effects of low-frequency transcutaneous electrical nerve stimulation on central pain modulation: a double blind, placebo-controlled trial. Clin J Pain 28(7):581–588, 2012.
27. Chen, CC, and Johnson, MI: An investigation into the hypoalgesic effects of high- and low-frequency transcutaneous electrical nerve stimulation (TENS) on experimentally induced blunt pressure pain in health human subjects. J Pain 11(1):53–61, 2010.
28. Vance, CG, Rakel, BA, Blodgett, NP, et al: Effects of transcutaneous electrical nerve stimulation on pain, pain sensitivity, and function in people with knee osteoarthritis: a randomized controlled trial. Phys Ther 92(7):898–910, 2012.

LET'S FIND OUT

Lab Activity: Pain Management With Electrical Stimulation

Purpose

This lab activity is designed to familiarize students/learners with the application of and expected patient responses to transcutaneous electrical nerve stimulation (TENS) for the relief of pain. It will also familiarize students/learners with electrode placement site selection and stimulation parameters for sensory analgesia. Students/learners will have the opportunity to experience various parameters on both portable and clinical stimulation devices.

Equipment

TENS stimulators (clinical and portable)

- lead wires for the stimulators
- electrically conductive gel

OR
self-adhering electrodes
4 equal-sized electrodes
cloth or paper tape to secure electrodes
electrical stimulators with adjustable pulse durations
electrical stimulation unit with an adjustable pulse duration capable of being set in excess of 1 millisecond (msec)

Precautions and Why

PRECAUTIONS	WHY
Unstable fracture	If electrical stimulation is used for a motor response, this is a contraindication. However, if no motor response is elicited, electrical stimulation can be considered safe.
Decreased sensation	If the desired response is dependent on sensation, then electrical stimulation may be useless. However, if the desired response relies on a motor response, then the application may be considered safe.
	If the application involves the transmission of ions through the skin, the patient must be able to report sensation to avoid an adverse response.
Impaired cognitive ability	If the desired response is dependent on sensation, then electrical stimulation may be useless. However, if the desired response relies on a motor response, then the application may be considered safe.
	If the application involves the transmission of ions through the skin, the patient must be able to report sensation to avoid an adverse response.
Pregnancy	If the application is after the first trimester, there is little risk to the fetus or the patient. Electrical stimulation has been safely used for analgesia during labor and delivery, but it may interfere with fetal monitors.
Documented evidence of epilepsy, cerebral vascular accident, or reversible ischemic neurological deficit	Patients should be monitored carefully when electrical stimulation is used in the cervical region. Possible adverse responses may include temporary change in cognitive status, headache, vertigo, and other neurological signs.
Demand pacemaker	Electrical stimulation devices may interfere with the electrical demands of the pacemaker.

Contraindications and Why

CONTRAINDICATIONS	WHY
Pregnancy (first trimester)	There are no data to indicate the level of safety for the fetus with the application of electrical stimulation during the first trimester of pregnancy.
Over the carotid sinus	If the circulation to the brain is altered, there could be adverse effects.
Malignancies	Most application techniques have the potential to produce an increase in circulation to the area. The possibility exists that electrical stimulation over or in proximity to cancerous lesions may enhance the development of metastasis.

Lab Activities

Orientation to TENS Equipment

1. Familiarize yourself with the TENS device that you have selected by reviewing both the controls on the stimulator and the instruction manual for the device. You may use either a clinical or portable stimulator for this exercise. What are the available ranges of parameters?

Frequency:

Pulse duration:

Intensity:

2. Are there any other controls on the device? If yes, what are they and what do they do?

_____

_____

_____

_____

3. Familiarize yourself with electrode placement site charts in your textbooks or recommended readings. See Table 15-2 for optimal stimulation sites for TENS electrode placement.

Orientation to Types of Electrode Placement Sites

1. There are numerous areas on the skin that exhibit decreased resistance to the flow of electrical current. What are the differences among them?

	DESCRIPTIONS	DIFFERENCES
Motor points:		
Trigger points:		
Acupuncture points:		
Dermatomes:		
Spinal nerve roots:		

2. What are some options for electrode placement sites if the patient had been referred to the department for pain management for the lower back?

Observing Patient Responses to Electrode Placement Site Selections

1. Select one of your classmates to act as a patient to receive TENS application for pain management for his or her lower back. Position the patient so that the lower back is exposed and accessible and the patient is comfortable.

2. Prepare the electrodes and the unit to be applied to the patient.

Vertical Placement (Fig. 15-6)

1. Apply one channel of electrodes to the right side and one channel to the left side of the paraspinal musculature using the sites that you identified from the charts.

2. Preset the parameters for sensory analgesia:

Frequency	70–120 Hz (high)
Pulse duration	50 μsec (short)

3. Slowly increase the intensity of the first channel and ask the patient to let you know when he or she first starts to feel something, where he or she feels it, and how it feels, and then to let you know when the intensity is strong but tolerable, and record these observations. Channel 1:

Where?

How does it feel?

Intensity level?

4. Gradually increase the intensity of the second channel and repeat the sequence as above. Assess the area vertically between the electrodes. Channel 2.

Where?

How does it feel?

Intensity level?

What is perceived in between channels?

Was the intensity levels equal on both sides?

- What could explain this?

_____

_____

5. Turn both intensities off. Leave the electrodes in place and disconnect the pin tips from the leads.

Horizontal Placement (Fig. 15-7)

1. Connect the leads to the electrodes so that there is one channel above L4–L5 and one channel below. Repeat the same steps as previously listed.

Does the patient feel anything between the electrodes?

What could explain this?

2. Turn both intensities off. Leave the electrodes in place and disconnect the pin tips from the leads.

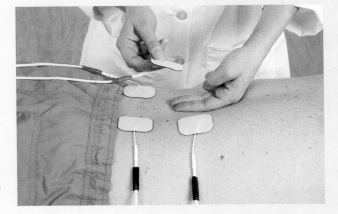

FIGURE 15-6 Two channels of electrodes set up with vertical electrode placements over the paraspinal muscles. A clinical stimulator is depicted; however, a portable device could also have been selected for this exercise.

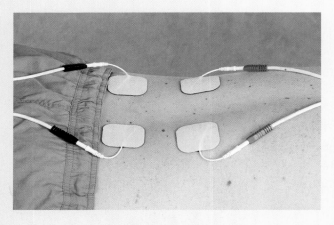

FIGURE 15-7 Two channels of electrodes set up with horizontal electrode placements above and below the area of discomfort. The electrodes are placed on paraspinal muscles but not on unilateral muscles.

Crisscross Placement (Fig. 15-8)

1. Connect the leads to the electrodes so that one channel crosses the other channel.

2. Preset the parameters for sensory analgesia (i.e., frequency, 70–120 Hz; pulse duration, 50 μsec). Slowly increase the intensity of the first channel and ask the patient to let you know when he or she first starts to feel something, where he or she feels it, and how it feels, and then to let you know when the intensity is strong but tolerable, and record these observations.

3. Gradually increase the intensity of the second channel and repeat the sequence as above. Assess the area between the electrodes.

Was the intensity level equal on both sides?

Was it easy for the patient to describe where he or she felt the sensation?

What could explain this?

Does the patient feel anything between the electrodes?

What could explain this?

4. Did any of the setups produce more sensory stimulation than the others? Why or why not?

Problem-Solving Activities
Intensity Adjustment and Patient Instructions for Sensory Analgesia

1. Select one of your classmates to act as the patient and have TENS applied with a portable unit to his or her shoulder. Select electrode placement sites that encompass the entire shoulder and provide sensory analgesia throughout the local area.

2. Set up the electrodes as depicted in Figures 15-9 and 15-10. These represent GB 21 and LI 14 for one channel and SI 10 and SP 20 for the other channel. Why do you think these electrode placement sites were suggested, particularly in this crossed pattern?

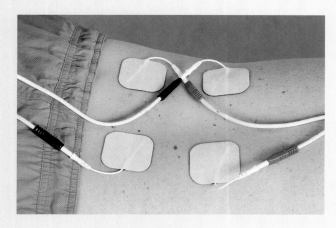

FIGURE 15-8 Two channels of electrodes set up with crossed electrode placements over the paraspinal muscles.

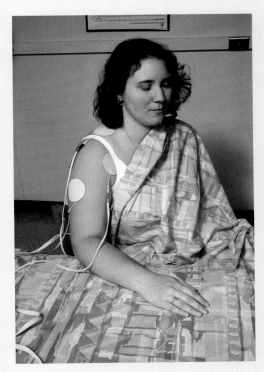

FIGURE 15-9 Anterior electrode placement sites for the shoulder.

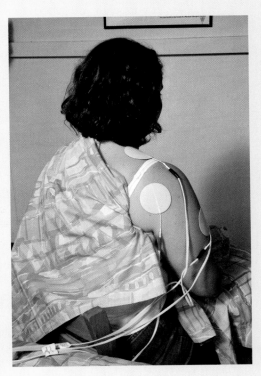

FIGURE 15-10 Posterior electrode placement sites for the shoulder.

3. Preset the parameters on the unit for sensory analgesia.
  • Instruct the patient how and what to adjust to increase the intensity of the stimulation.
    • Also instruct the patient in how and where to apply the electrodes,
    • replace the battery,
    • care for the portable TENS unit and electrodes,
    • self-assess his or her level of discomfort, and
    • record his or her assessment.

4. Give the patient the TENS unit and ask him or her to increase the intensity to a strong but comfortable level.

   a. Instruct him or her to increase the intensity if the sensation "fades" at all.

5. How did the setting of the intensity differ when the patient adjusted it?

   _____

   _____

6. What would be a possible rationale for instructing a patient how to adjust and care for a TENS unit?

   _____

   _____

7. What additional considerations could there be for unit selection for a patient so that he or she could adjust the intensity? (dexterity, cognition)

   _____

   _____

8. Would you expect the intensity for sensory analgesia to change while it was on? Why or why not?

   _____

   _____

9. What would happen if you increased the pulse duration of the stimulation?

   _____

   _____

10. Would this ever be potentially indicated? Why or why not?

    _____

    _____

11. Instruct the patient how to terminate treatment.
    • reassess, and
    • remove his or her electrodes.

12. What instructions did you find most difficult to explain to the patient?

    _____

    _____

Applying and Observing Patient Response to Low Rate Stimulation for Analgesia for Low Back Pain

1. Select one of your classmates to receive application of motor level stimulation to his or her triceps surae bilaterally.

   a. One of the methods to help accomplish long-lasting pain relief is mediated by the release of endogenous opiates from the anterior pituitary deep within the brain. This is facilitated by at least 20 minutes of rhythmic muscle twitching. Selection of muscle groups that are segmentally related to the origin of the discomfort yet distal to the site tend to yield favorable patient responses.

2. Position the patient so that he or she is comfortable and supported with the ankles free to plantarflex and dorsiflex. Consult charts in your books to determine electrode placement sites and apply the electrodes to elicit a motor response from the triceps surae. (If you are consulting an acupuncture chart, BL 57 or BL 58 coupled with BL 60 would work well.)

   a. Preset the TENS unit for motor level stimulation at a low rate.

3. Gradually increase the intensity until a twitch response is visible. Increase the intensity to the highest tolerable level so that joint movement is visible.

4. What are the differences between this level of stimulation and sensory analgesia?

_____

_____

5. How long should it take for a patient to report some decrease in his or her discomfort following this mode of stimulation?

_____

_____

6. What are the patient's subjective responses to this mode of stimulation?

_____

_____

7. Under what circumstances might this mode be considered appropriate for a patient?

_____

_____

8. What is the mechanism for pain relief that this mode is intended to induce?

_____

_____

9. Do you expect the patient to adapt to this mode of stimulation? Why or why not?

_____

_____

10. How long is the carry-over time for relief expected to be for this mode of stimulation?

_____

_____

11. What possible rationale would there be for distally placed electrodes if this setup were recommended for lower back pain?

_____

_____

Experiencing Noxious-Level Stimulation for Analgesia

1. Familiarize yourself with the stimulator. It must be capable of producing pulse durations in excess of 1 millisecond (1 msec).
2. Select one of your classmates to be the patient for hyperstimulation to the web space of the back of his or her hand.
3. Position the patient comfortably and position yourself so that you are at eye level with the patient.
4. There is probably a meter of some form on the stimulator. It may measure conductance or resistance. Familiarize yourself with it by touching the two ends of the leads together and noting what the meter reads. Then hold the larger electrode in your hand and touch yourself with the probe electrode.
5. Compare the meter reading to your first reading. If it was lower, then the meter is reading conductance. If the second meter reading was higher, then it was reading resistance.
6. Preset the following parameters.
   - Frequency: 4 Hz
   - Pulse duration: At least 1 msec
   - On time: 30 sec per activation
7. Give the patient the dispersive/inactive (larger) electrode to hold in his or her other hand. You will not need gel or a conductive interface because the patient will grasp the electrode in the palm of

his or her hand, which usually perspires when grasping something rubber. The perspiration will serve as the contact medium. *(Patients also tend to perspire when they are told that what they are going to experience will be a sensation similar to a hot needle or bee sting.)*

8. Locate the area that is most electrically active within the back of the web space of the back of the patient's hand. This would be the most conductive area (i.e., HoKu or LI 4). See Figure 15-11.

   Once it has been identified, press the on button that activates the stimulation and gradually increase the intensity while watching the patient's eyes. Your observation of the patient's eyes should let you know when the stimulus is as strong as he or she can tolerate. At that point, re-start the timer for 30 seconds. It is intended to be noxious. After the 30-second period is up, remove the probe and ask the patient to describe what he or she felt. Repeat for all members of your group.

9. When would noxious-level stimulation potentially be indicated?

   _____

   _____

10. What would you need to explain to the patient to ensure that your chances of having it work would be enhanced?

    _____

    _____

11. What possible explanations are there for positioning yourself at eye level with the patient?

    _____

    _____

12. Why would this type of stimulator have a conductance/resistance meter?

    _____

    _____

13. How did the sensation of the stimulus differ from sensory analgesia?

    _____

    _____

Patient Scenarios

Read through the patient scenarios and determine the following for each:

- Whether or not electrical stimulation would be indicated for pain relief
- What precautions there might be for the patients described
- What the parameter would be for the patient and your rationale for those parameters
- Where the electrodes should be placed, how many, and why

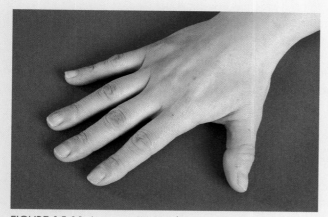 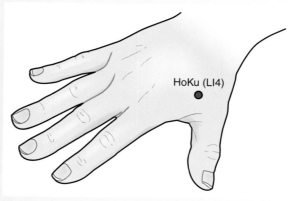

FIGURE 15-11 Locating "HoKu" large intestine 4, which is in the web space of the back of the hand in between the thumb and index finger.

- Whether more than one mode could be indicated for pain relief
- Whether or not the patient might benefit from home use of a portable stimulator, and your rationale
  A. Frank has been referred to the department for pain management. He has been diagnosed with herpes zoster, and on examination there is a large inflamed area on his left side. It starts in the thoracic region in midline posteriorly and extends anteriorly, tracing the last five ribs to the sternum. He is 85 years old, lives alone, and is otherwise healthy aside from an ulcer, which has been controlled successfully by diet and medication for more than 20 years. His primary complaints are hypersensitivity to light touch throughout the inflamed area. It is so sensitive that he guards the area by flexing his trunk so that his clothing does not touch his skin on the left side.
  B. Steve is a maintenance engineer for a retirement community. He has been referred to physical therapy for pain management subsequent to a low back injury he suffered while at work. He is a 42-year-old "workaholic" who has been performing strengthening exercises to stabilize his back. He has also worked through a "work-hardening program," and he is exceedingly anxious to return to his job. His only limitation is chronic low back pain. He is an avid bicyclist, canoeist, and hiker. He is looking for relief that will not interfere with his work with lawnmowers, power tools, and mechanical equipment.
  C. Carol is a cartoonist who has been referred to physical therapy for pain management techniques subsequent to a cervical strain injury. She was involved in a motor vehicle accident in which she was hit from behind. She now has muscle guarding and marked decreases in her cervical ROM in all directions. Her primary complaint is occipital headaches. She lives alone and works from a home office. Most of her day is spent at an artist's table, which is angled at 45 degrees. Medications to reduce muscle guarding and inflammation caused other complications because they interacted with medications she was taking for depression.

Documentation

Electrical stimulation can be used to control or reduce discomfort. Because there are a variety of ways in which this could be accomplished, it is important to document exactly what techniques produced favorable results for a patient. The following parameters must be documented:

- Treatment goal: Sensory analgesia or pain management
- Pretreatment pain assessment: Visual analog or other quantifiable measure
- Post-treatment pain assessment: Same instrument that was applied pretreatment
- Electrode placement sites: Documentation of exact electrode placement sites is not critical if the treatment goal is pain relief and the mode of stimulation is sensory analgesia. However, it can be helpful to the next clinician who treats the patient if alternate sites were used to help eliminate trial and error to achieve a successful result. In, addition, if an alternate mode of stimulation (e.g., hyperstimulation, low rate) was used to accomplish the treatment goal, then the stimulation sites must be documented.
- Specific stimulator used: If the mode of stimulation was sensory analgesia and it was accomplished with a clinical stimulator, then this is not critical to document. However, if the treatment involved home use of a TENS unit, the documentation should include the manufacturer and model of the device.

LAB QUESTIONS

1. What was the most comfortable mode of stimulation for the patients?
2. What was the most uncomfortable mode of stimulation?
3. Which of the parameters would have accomplished A-beta fiber stimulation?
4. What would the necessary parameters be for C fiber stimulation, and when might this be indicated?
5. The patient has increased the intensity to the highest level for a portable TENS unit, and they still do not feel the stimulation. What are the possible remedies, which would you employ first, and why?
6. Discuss the use of ES as a treatment technique in terms of the potential success rate as the sole treatment technique used to treat a patient.
7. Discuss the similarities and differences among the various electrode placement site selection options to accomplish pain relief and provide the rationale for each.

Appendix: Optimal Stimulation Sites for TENS Electrodes

Key				
▼	Acupuncture point		K or K...	Kidney meridian
☐	Motor point		LI or li...	Large intestine
◼	Trigger point		LU or lu...	Lung
gray	Cutaneous nerve		LV or lv...	Liver
black	Peripheral nerve		P or p...	Pericardium
BL. or bl...	Bladder meridian		SI. or si...	Spleen
GB. or gb...	Gallbladder meridian		ST or st...	Stomach
H or h...	Heart meridian		TW or tw...	Triple warmer

*From Mannheimer, JS, and Lampe, GN: Clinical Transcutaneous Electrical Nerve Stimulation. FA Davis, Philadelphia, 1984, pp 301, 306–307, 309–319, 324–325, with permission. Originally researched and developed by Jeffrey S. Mannheimer, RPT, MA, and Barbara J. Behrens, PTA, AAS. © 1980. Repeated on page 413.

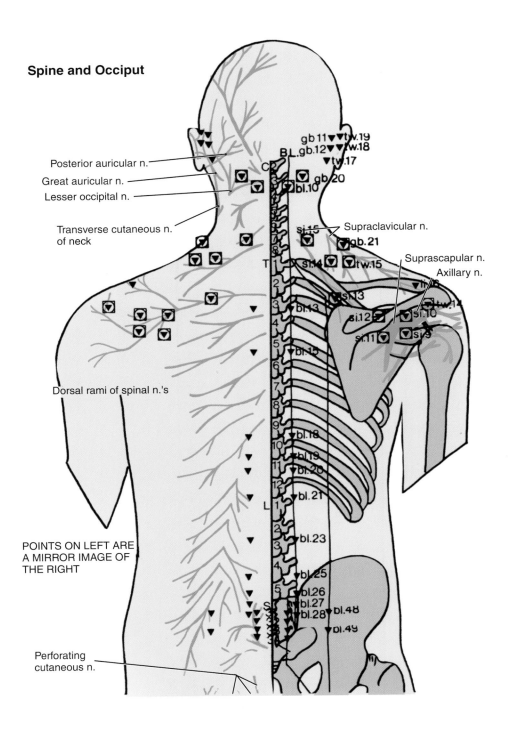

Spine and Occiput

Posterior auricular n.

Great auricular n.

Lesser occipital n.

Transverse cutaneous n. of neck

Dorsal rami of spinal n.'s

POINTS ON LEFT ARE A MIRROR IMAGE OF THE RIGHT

Perforating cutaneous n.

gb 11 ▼▼tw.19
gb.12▼▼tw.18
B.L. ▼tw.17
gb.20
bl.10
si.15
gb.21
si.14 tw.15
si.13
bl.13
si.12
si.11 si.9
bl.15
bl.18
bl.19
bl.20
bl.21
bl.23
bl.25
bl.26
bl.27
bl.28 bl.48
bl.49

Supraclavicular n.

Suprascapular n.
Axillary n.

si.10

TABLE 15-2 | Optimal Stimulation Sites for TENS Electrodes

OCCIPUT

Location	Superficial Nerve Branch	Acupuncture Point	Motor Point	Trigger Point	Segmental Level
Posterior ear upper 3rd (TW 19) same level but slightly more medial on occiput (GB 11)	Great auricular, posterior branch communicates with lesser occipital, auricular branch of vagus, posterior auricular branch of facial. Transverse cutaneous nerve of neck	TW 19 GB 11 is just medial			Cranial C2–C4
Posterior ear middle third (TW 18) same level but slightly more medial on occiput (GB 12)	Same as above	TW 18 GB 12 is just medial			Cranial C2–C4
Behind ear in depression between angle of mandible and mastoid process	Great auricular, posterior branch and lesser occipital	TW 17			C2–C4
Suboccipital depression, between sternocleidomastoid (SCM) and upper trapezius	Greater and lesser occipital nerves	GB 20 BL 10 is nearby, slightly medial and inferior	Splenius capitis (branches from C2–C4) semispinalis capitis	Semispinalis capitis Splenius capitis	C2–C3

The explanation of optimal stimulation sites for the shoulder girdle as seen on this view can be found on the view of posterolateral shoulder and dorsal region of the upper extremity.

TABLE 15-2 | Optimal Stimulation Sites for TENS Electrodes — cont'd

			THE SPINE		
Location	**Superficial Nerve Branch**	**Acupuncture Point**	**Motor Point**	**Trigger Point**	**Segmental Level**
In depression between medial border of posterior superior iliac spine (PSIS) and 1st sacral spinous process	Dorsal ramus of L2	BL 27			L2
2" lateral to spinous process of S2	Dorsal ramus of L2	BL 48	Gluteus maximus (upper motor pt) (inferior gluteal) (L5–S2)	Gluteus maximus	L2 L5–S2
2" lateral to spinous process of S4	Dorsal rami of L2–L3	BL 49	Gluteus maximus (lower motor pt) (piriformis directly below) (inferior gluteal) (L5–S2)	Gluteus maximus (piriformis directly below)	L2–L3 L5–S2
Directly over 1st sacral foramen	Dorsal ramus of S1	BL 31			S1
Directly over 2nd sacral foramen	Dorsal ramus of S2	BL 32			S2
Directly over 3rd sacral foramen	Dorsal ramus of S3	BL 33			S3
Directly over 4th sacral foramen	Dorsal ramus of S4	BL 34			S4

The 12 cutaneous branches of thoracic posterior primary rami become superficial adjacent to the spinous processes. They each have multiple cutaneous twigs. Havelacque considers the dorsal ramus of T2 to be the largest and most diffuse.

The cutaneous distribution of the dorsal ramus of T2 reaches up to the posterior aspect of the acromion, covering the mid-back (to the region of T5–T6) and laterally to the superior region of the posterior axillary fold. A number of optimal stimulation sites are depicted as overlying this nerve.

Cutaneous branches of the dorsal rami of L1–L3 descend as far as the posterior part of the iliac crest, skin of the buttock and almost to the greater trochanter of the femur (see lower extremity, lateral and posterior views). [1(p1033),93]

Continued

Anteromedial Shoulder and Volar Region of Upper Extremity

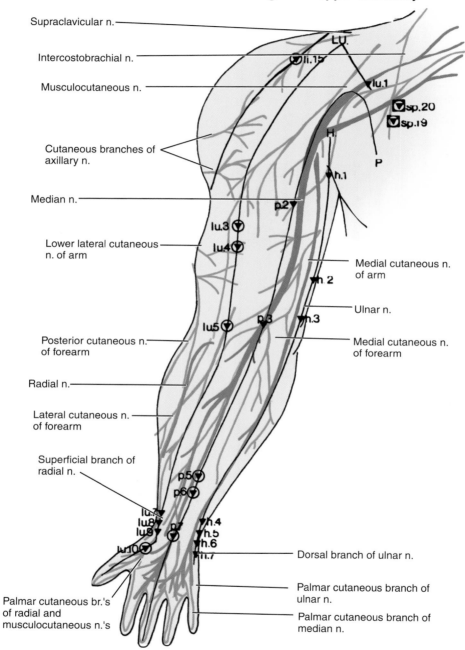

Supraclavicular n.

Intercostobrachial n.

Musculocutaneous n.

Cutaneous branches of axillary n.

Median n.

Lower lateral cutaneous n. of arm

Posterior cutaneous n. of forearm

Radial n.

Lateral cutaneous n. of forearm

Superficial branch of radial n.

Palmar cutaneous br.'s of radial and musculocutaneous n.'s

Medial cutaneous n. of arm

Ulnar n.

Medial cutaneous n. of forearm

Dorsal branch of ulnar n.

Palmar cutaneous branch of ulnar n.

Palmar cutaneous branch of median n.

TABLE 15-2 | Optimal Stimulation Sites for TENS Electrodes—cont'd

ANTEROMEDIAL SHOULDER AND VOLAR REGION OF UPPER EXTREMITY

Location	Superficial Nerve Branch	Acupuncture Point	Motor Point	Trigger Point	Segmental Level
Between first and second ribs, about 4" lateral to sternum, medial to coracoid process	Musculocutaneous nerve	LU 1	Coracobrachialis is nearby (musculocutaneous) (C6)		C5–C7
Radial side of biceps brachii 2" below anterior axillary fold. 3" below anterior axillary fold	Musculocutaneous nerve and its lower lateral cutaneous branch	LU 3 LU 4	Biceps brachii (musculocutaneous) (C5–C6)		C5–C7
In antecubital fossa on crease at radial side of biceps tendon	Lateral cutaneous nerve of arm	LU 5	Brachialis (musculocutaneous) (C5–C6)		C5–C7
Just lateral to radial artery from 1st volar crease to just above radial styloid	Lateral cutaneous nerve of forearm communicating with superficial radial nerve	LU 7–9			C5–C7 C6–C8
Volar surface of hand at midpoint of 1st metacarpal	Superficial branch of radial nerve and palmar cutaneous of median	LU 10	Abductor pollicis brevis (median) (C8–T1)		C6–C8 C5–T1 C5–C7

Continued

TABLE 15-2 | Optimal Stimulation Sites for TENS Electrodes — cont'd

ANTEROMEDIAL SHOULDER AND VOLAR REGION OF UPPER EXTREMITY

Location	Superficial Nerve Branch	Acupuncture Point	Motor Point	Trigger Point	Segmental Level
Between heads of biceps brachii 2" below anterior axillary fold with medial cutaneous	Musculocutaneous and intercostobrachial nerves, may communicate nerve of forearm	P2			T2 C8–T1
Just medial to biceps tendon in antecubital fossa	Median nerve and anterior branch of medial cutaneous nerve of forearm	P3	Pronator teres (median) (C6)		C5–T1 C8–T1
Between tendons of flexor carpi radialis (FCR) and palmaris longus (PL) 2" and 1.5" above volar crease respectively	Median and anterior branch of medial cutaneous nerve of forearm		P5 P6 is 1" below		C5–T1 C8–T1
Between tendons of FCR and PL at midpoint transverse volar wrist crease	Median and anterior branch of medial cutaneous nerve of forearm and palmar cutaneous branch of median	P7			C5–T1 C8–T1
Between ribs 2–3 and 3–4, midway between anterior axillary fold and sternum	Medial and intermedial supraclavicular nerves to 2nd rib, lateral cutaneous nerves of thorax (2–4), the 2nd nerve is the intercostobrachial nerve	SP 19–20	Pectoralis major (medial) and lateral anterior thoracic nerves)	Pectoralis major	C3–C4 T2–T4

TABLE 15-2 | Optimal Stimulation Sites for TENS Electrodes—cont'd

		ANTEROMEDIAL SHOULDER AND VOLAR REGION OF UPPER EXTREMITY			
Location	Superficial Nerve Branch	Acupuncture Point	Motor Point	Trigger Point	Segmental Level
Medial to brachial artery in axilla	Ulnar nerve, intercostobrachial, medial cutaneous nerve of arm and median nerve which is just lateral to artery	H 1			C7–T1 T2 C9–T1 C5–T1
In groove medial to lower third of biceps brachii medial to brachial artery	Median and medial cutaneous nerve of arm		H 2		C5–T1 C8–T1
Just superior to cubital tunnel by medial epicondyle	Medial cutaneous nerve of forearm	H 3			C8–T1
Ulnar aspect of wrist lateral to flexor carpi ulnaris (FCU) tendon from 1.5" above 1st volar wrist crease to pisiform bone	Ulnar nerve and its palmar cutaneous branch	H 4–H 7			C7–T1
In depression anterior and inferior to acromion	Upper lateral cutaneous nerve branch of axillary	LI 15	Anterior deltoid (axillary) (C5–C6)		C5–C6

Continued

Posterolateral Shoulder and Dorsal Region of Upper Extremity

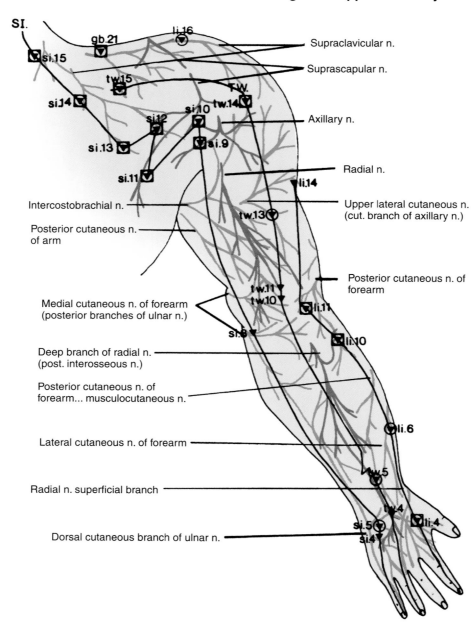

TABLE 15-2 | Optimal Stimulation Sites for TENS Electrodes — cont'd

POSTEROLATERAL SHOULDER AND DORSAL REGION OF UPPER EXTREMITY

Location	Superficial Nerve Branch	Acupuncture Point	Motor Point	Trigger Point	Segmental Level
1.5" lateral to spinous process of C7	Medial branch of supraclavicular	SI 15	Levator scapulae (spinal accessory and dorsal scapular (C3–C4)	Levator scapulae	Cranial C3–C4
1.5" above superior angle of scapula at the level of the spinous process of T1	Lateral (posterior) branch of supraclavicular	SI 14 TW 15 is just lateral	Middle trapezius (spinal accessory) (C3–C4)	Middle trapezius	Cranial C3–C4
Suprascapular fossa (medial end) 3" lateral to spinous process of T2	Lateral (posterior) branch of supraclavicular and dorsal ramus of T2	SI 13	Middle trapezius (spinal accessory) (C3–C4)	Middle trapezius	Cranial C3–C4 T2
At midpoint of suprascapular fossa	Dorsal ramus of T2	SI 12	Supraspinatus (suprascapular) (C5–C6)	Supraspinatus	C5–C6, T2
At midpoint of infrascapular fossa	Dorsal ramus of T2	SI 11	Infraspinatus (suprascapular) (C5–C6)	Infraspinatus	C5–C6, T2

Continued

TABLE 15-2 | Optimal Stimulation Sites for TENS Electrodes—cont'd

POSTEROLATERAL SHOULDER AND DORSAL REGION OF UPPER EXTREMITY					
Location	**Superficial Nerve Branch**	**Acupuncture Point**	**Motor Point**	**Trigger Point**	**Segmental Level**
Directly above posterior axillary fold. Just below spine of scapula	Dorsal ramus of T2 and axillary (posterior branch), which continues as the upper lateral cutaneous nerve of the arm	SI 10 (axillary)	Posterior deltoid (C5–C6)	Posterior deltoid	C5–C6 T2
Directly below SI 10. Just superior to posterior axillary fold	Axillary and dorsal ramus of T2	SI 9	Teres major (subscapular) (C5–C6)	Teres major	C5–C6, T2
In groove between olecranon and medial epicondyle of humerus	Ulnar nerve and its medial cutaneous branches	SI 8			C7–T1
In depression between pisiform bone and ulnar styloid	Dorsal and palmar cutaneous branches of ulnar nerve	SI 5			C7–T1
In depression between fifth metacarpal and triquetral	Dorsal and palmar cutaneous branches of ulnar nerve	SI 4	Palmaris brevis (median) (C8–T1)		C7–T1
On cephalad surface of upper trapezius directly above superior angle of scapula	Supraclavicular	GB 21	Upper trapezius (spinal accessory)	Upper trapezius	Cranial C3–C4

TABLE 15-2 | Optimal Stimulation Sites for TENS Electrodes — cont'd

POSTEROLATERAL SHOULDER AND DORSAL REGION OF UPPER EXTREMITY					
Location	Superficial Nerve Branch	Acupuncture Point	Motor Point	Trigger Point	Segmental Level
In depression posterior and inferior to acromion and above greater tubercle of humerus with arm in anatomical position	Intercostobrachial, upper lateral cutaneous nerve — branch of axillary, and dorsal ramus of T2	TW 14	Posterior deltoid (axillary) (C5–C6)	C5–C6	T2
Just below deltoid insertion by lateral head of triceps	Upper lateral cutaneous nerve branch of axillary	TW 13	Lateral head of triceps (radial) (C7–C8)		C5–C6
In depression 1" above olecranon with the elbow flexed to 90°	Posterior cutaneous of arm (radial) medial cutaneous of forearm (ulnar posterior branches) posterior cutaneous nerve of forearm	TW 10, TW 11 is just above			C5–C8 C8–T1 C5–C8
Between radius and ulna on dorsal surface about 2" proximal to transverse wrist crease	Posterior cutaneous nerve of forearm, branch of radial communications with lateral cutaneous nerve of forearm, branch of musculocutaneous	TW 5	Extensor indicis proprius (radial) (C7)		C5–C8 C5–C6

Continued

Lower Extremity, Anterior View

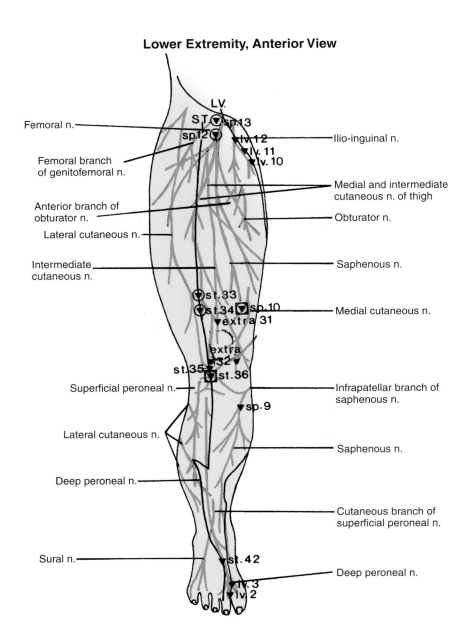

Femoral n.

Femoral branch
of genitofemoral n.

Anterior branch of
obturator n.

Lateral cutaneous n.

Intermediate
cutaneous n.

Superficial peroneal n.

Lateral cutaneous n.

Deep peroneal n.

Sural n.

Ilio-inguinal n.

Medial and intermediate
cutaneous n. of thigh

Obturator n.

Saphenous n.

Medial cutaneous n.

Infrapatellar branch of
saphenous n.

Saphenous n.

Cutaneous branch of
superficial peroneal n.

Deep peroneal n.

LV.
ST. sp.13
sp.12
lv.12
lv. 11
lv. 10

st.33
st.34 sp.10
extra 31
extra 32
st.35 st.36
sp.9
st.42
lv.3
lv.2

TABLE 15-2 | Optimal Stimulation Sites for TENS Electrodes—cont'd

LOWER EXTREMITY, ANTERIOR VIEW

Location	Superficial Nerve Branch	Acupuncture Point	Motor Point	Trigger Point	Segmental Level
2" lateral to superior border of symphysis pubis	Anterior cutaneous branches of iliohypogastric, ilioinguinal, and genitofemoral	LV 10–12	Pectineus (femoral) (L2–L4)		L1 L1 L1–L2
Between 1st and 2nd metatarsals just above web space junction on dorsum of foot	Deep peroneal nerve via its medial terminal and interosseous branches	LV 2–3	1st dorsal interosseus (lateral plantar) (S1–S2)		L4–L5 S1–S2
From inguinal ligament to femoral triangle lateral to femoral artery	Anterior branch of obturator communicating with medial cutaneous. Forms subsartorial plexus.	SP 12 SP 13	Iliopsoas (femoral) (L2–L4)		L2–L4 L2–L4
2" above medial aspect of patellar base	Medial cutaneous nerve of thigh and saphenous nerve (infrapatellar)	SP 10	Vastus medialis (femoral) (L2–L4)	Vastus medialis	L2–L4 L2–L3
Just below medial condyle of tibia, level with tibial tuberosity between sartorius and gracilis	Saphenous nerve	SP 9			L3–L4
Just superior to midpoint of patellar base	Intermediate cutaneous nerve of the thigh	Extra 31			L2–L3
Medial to patellar tendon	Medial cutaneous nerve of thigh	Extra 32 (medial)			L2–L3

Continued

TABLE 15-2 | Optimal Stimulation Sites for TENS Electrodes—cont'd

LOWER EXTREMITY, ANTERIOR VIEW

Location	Superficial Nerve Branch	Acupuncture Point	Motor Point	Trigger Point	Segmental Level
In depression just below patella, lateral to tendon with knee flexed 2"–3" above lateral aspect	Medial and lateral cutaneous nerve of thigh and infrapatellar branch of saphenous which forms a patellar plexus	ST 35 Extra 32 (lateral)			L2–L3 L3–L4
	Intermediate and lateral cutaneous nerve of thigh	ST 33–34	Vastus lateralis (femoral) (L2–L4)		L2–L4
In depression just below patella, lateral to tendon with knee flexed	Medial and lateral cutaneous nerve of thigh and infrapatellar branch of saphenous which form a patellar plexus	ST 35 Extra 32 (lateral)			L2–L3 L3–L4
2" below inferior angle of patella, lateral to tibial crest	Infrapatellar branch of saphenous	ST 36	Superior motor point of anterior tibialis (deep peroneal) (L4–L5)	Anterior tibialis	L3–L4
Below malleoli at center of dorsum of foot, lateral to anterior tibialis tendon	Superficial peroneal	ST 42			L4–S2

Lower Extremity, Posterior View

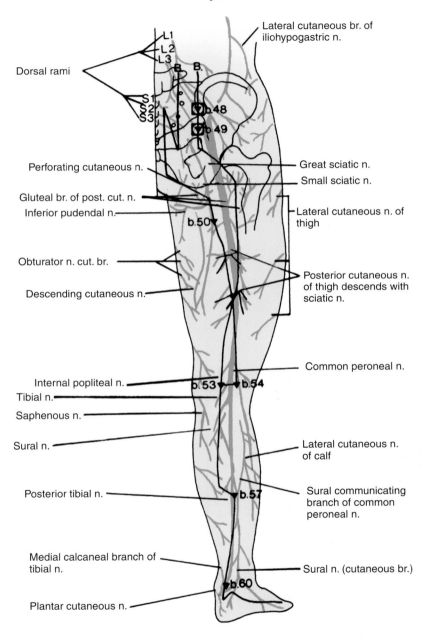

Dorsal rami

L1
L2
L3
B. B.
S1
S2
S3
b.48
b.49

Lateral cutaneous br. of
iliohypogastric n.

Great sciatic n.
Small sciatic n.

Perforating cutaneous n.

Gluteal br. of post. cut. n.
Inferior pudendal n.

b.50

Lateral cutaneous n. of
thigh

Obturator n. cut. br.

Descending cutaneous n.

Posterior cutaneous n.
of thigh descends with
sciatic n.

Common peroneal n.

Internal popliteal n.
Tibial n.
Saphenous n.

Sural n.

b.53 b.54

Lateral cutaneous n.
of calf

Posterior tibial n.

b.57

Sural communicating
branch of common
peroneal n.

Medial calcaneal branch of
tibial n.

Plantar cutaneous n.

b.60

Sural n. (cutaneous br.)

TABLE 15-2 | Optimal Stimulation Sites for TENS Electrodes—cont'd

LOWER EXTREMITY, POSTERIOR VIEW

Location	Superficial Nerve Branch	Acupuncture Point	Motor Point	Trigger Point	Segmental Level
2" lateral to spinous process of S2	Dorsal ramus L2	BL 48	Gluteus maximus (upper motor pt) (inferior gluteal L5–S2)	Gluteus maximus	L2 L5–S2
2" lateral to spinous process of S4	Dorsal rami L2–L3	BL 49	Gluteus maximus (lower motor pt) (piriformis directly below) (inferior gluteal L5–S2)	Gluteus maximus (piriformis directly below)	L2–L3 L5–S2
At midpoint of junction between buttock and posterior thigh	Posterior cutaneous nerve of thigh, medial and lateral branches	BL 50			S1–S3
Popliteal fossa between biceps femoris and semitendinosus tendons	Posterior cutaneous nerve of thigh, medial and lateral branches	*BL 54/40 *BL 53/39 (lateral aspect of popliteal fossa medial to biceps femoris tendon)			S1–S3
Midline of leg below heads of gastrocsoleus at junction of upper 2/3 and lower 1/3 of leg	Sural, communicating branch of lateral cutaneous nerve of calf (common peroneal)	BL 57	Soleus (tibial nerve) S1–S2	Soleus	L5–S2
Between lateral malleolus and heelcord	Dorsal lateral cutaneous nerve-end of sural	BL 60		L4–S2	L4–S2

*Numerical systems differ according to texts, BL 53 & 54 Acupuncture Therapy, BL 39 & 40 An Outline of Chinese Acupuncture

Key			
▼	Acupuncture point	K or K...	Kidney meridian
▯	Motor point	LI or li...	Large intestine
▯	Trigger point	LU or lu...	Lung
gray	Cutaneous nerve	LV or lv...	Liver
black	Peripheral nerve	P or p...	Pericardium
BL. or bl...	Bladder meridian	SI. or si...	Spleen
GB. or gb...	Gallbladder meridian	ST or st...	Stomach
H or h...	Heart meridian	TW or tw...	Triple warmer

*From Mannheimer, JS, and Lampe, GN: Clinical Transcutaneous Electrical Nerve Stimulation. FA Davis, Philadelphia, 1984, pp 301, 306–307, 309–319, 324–325, with permission. Originally researched and developed by Jeffrey S. Mannheimer, RPT, MA, and Barbara J. Behrens, PTA, AAS. © 1980.

CHAPTER 16

Interferential Current Therapy in Clinical Practice

Barbara J. Behrens, PTA, MS

Learning Outcomes

Following the successful completion of this chapter, the learner will be able to:

- Describe the theory behind interferential current therapy (IFC) as a form of electrical stimulation for the accomplishment of therapeutic treatment goals.
- Differentiate between IFC and other forms of electrical stimulation devices citing the potential benefits of IFC versus other forms of electrical stimulation.
- Provide the rationale behind electrode placement site selection for various areas of the body for the accomplishment of pain reduction, edema reduction, and muscle guarding reduction using IFC.
- Problem-solve treatment scenarios that involve the use of IFC as the selected form of electrical stimulation to accomplish the stated treatment goal for a patient.

Key Terms

Interference therapy
Kilohertz

Premodulation
Vector

Wedensky Inhibition

Chapter Outline

Theory Behind Interferential Current Therapy
Setting the Difference
Electrode Placement
The "Third Line" of Current
   Magnets: Here's Why You Learned About Them in
   Kindergarten!

Premodulation and Interferential Current Therapy
Modulation With IFC

"The skin is one of the largest organs on the body and one of its jobs is to prevent electrical current from being able to penetrate it. As clinicians we need to find a way to honor the skin and the patient to accomplish our clinical goals." —B. Behrens

Patient Perspective

"I'm not sure that I can really tell you exactly where I feel that. Is that normal?"

Dr. Hans Nemec was born July 6, 1907 in Vienna and died September 1981. He is credited as being the inventor of **interference therapy,**[1] which is what is now commonly referred to as interferential current therapy (IFC), a form of electrical stimulation that enjoys worldwide use today as a unique form of treatment for a variety of treatment goals including pain reduction, edema reduction, and muscle reeducation.[2]

IFC is most likely one of the most commonly used forms of electrical stimulation in the clinical environment for the reduction of pain, yet very little is published in texts that prepare clinicians in the use of the modality.

The quotes at the beginning of this chapter were selected for two important reasons. First, as clinicians, we must never forget that the patient must be able to tolerate what we are applying to them if we are ever going to be successful with the selected modality, and second, patients must be able to understand what they should be feeling when it is applied correctly. Both of these factors can either lead to the success or failure of any treatment intervention with a modality. IFC is something that has been used clinically since the 1950s, so we should be able to explain it without making it too difficult for our patients to grasp.

Theory Behind Interferential Current Therapy

Chapter 13 dealt with motor responses and electrical stimulation, and one of the greatest limiting factors was always the patient's tolerance of the level of stimulation that might be necessary to elicit a muscle contraction. Chapter 15 dealt with electrical stimulation for pain management. Sometimes patients felt pain at deeper levels than the conventional forms of electrical stimulation was capable of reaching. Both of these types of situations are perfect for IFC, according to those who advocate for it and claim that it's possible to achieve stronger physiological responses that one might desire from lower frequencies without the discomfort.[2] They report that to produce lower frequency effects, or those that would occur at less than 250 pulses per second (pps), the intensity would need to be significantly higher than most patients could bear. This is the result of an inverse relationship that exists between the resistance of the skin and the frequency of the electrical stimulation. The lower the frequency of the electrical stimulation, the higher will be the skin resistance to the passage of current, which means that it will be more uncomfortable for the patient at the skin interface. The skin resistance at 50 pps is approximately 3,200 ohms, and at 4,000 pps it is reduced to approximately 40 ohms.[2] See Figure 16-1 for a graphic representation of the relationship between resistance and frequency.

So, if the resistance at the skin is lower, the electrical energy will pass through more easily and theoretically be able to travel more deeply into the underlying tissues and produce less discomfort for the patient. Please note that this

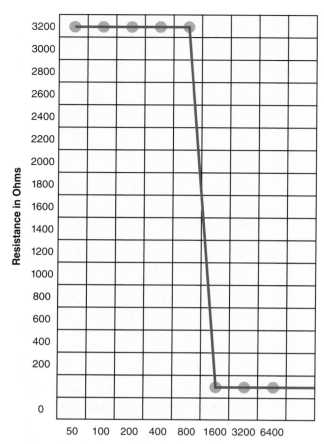

FIGURE 16-1 There is an inverse relationship between the resistance of the skin in ohms and the frequency of electrical stimulation. This figure is for illustrative purposes only and does *not* represent any specific clinical findings.

concept is not supported by all researchers and some believe that frequencies in the thousands are no more comfortable for patients than those delivered at less than 100 pps. There is no scientific evidence to support or refute this theory.[3,4]

IFC is the application of two different and separate sinusoidal currents that are delivered to the same treatment area at the same time at different frequencies with carrier frequencies above 1,000 pps. The difference between the currents produces what is referred to as a beat frequency within the underlying tissue where the current pathways interact with each other (Fig. 16-2).

LET'S THINK ABOUT IT...

Have you ever wondered why you learned how to sing a "round" when you were in kindergarten? Here's your answer! When singing a round such as the song "Row, Row, Row Your Boat," the idea behind it is to have one group start singing the song and then have another group start singing the same song, but start after the first group. This means that the two groups will be out of phase. If you are not taking part in the singing, what you would hear would sometimes be louder and would definitely be different

from either of the original sets of words. You would hear a created third voice that would be analogous to the third line of current created when two channels of IFC are crossed over a treatment area.

Setting the Difference

One of the first questions clinicians ask after hearing the origins of IFC concerns the difference between the frequencies of the two channels. One of the benefits of IFC is that the mechanics of the devices are literally invisible to clinicians. The parameters that one selects for electrical stimulation as a treatment intervention are based upon the treatment goal. This means that you can essentially use it the same way that other electrical stimulation devices have been used. The only difference would be in the selection of electrode placement sites. If the treatment goal is pain relief, then the same frequencies that would have been selected with other forms of electrical stimulation would be selected. The main advantage of IFC is the depth of penetration and that it can cover a larger treatment area than other forms of electrical stimulation (Table 16-1).

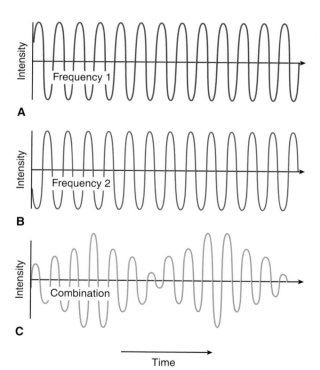

FIGURE 16-2 **(A)** When two sine waves interact with each other and are at the same frequency, they are in phase, meaning the amplitude would double. **(B)** When two sine waves interact with each other and are at the same frequency but 180 degrees out of phase, they would cancel each other out. **(C)** When two sine waves interact with each other and are at different frequencies, they would periodically be in phase and out of phase, which means that the amplitude would double and be canceled out, thus creating a beat frequency.

TABLE 16-1 | Setting the Difference

TREATMENT GOAL	FREQUENCY	BEAT FREQUENCY WITH IFC
Pain reduction (Fast)	70–120 pps	70–120 beats per second (bps)
Edema reduction (muscle pumping with the area elevated)	50 pps	50 bps
Muscle guarding reduction (strong enough to cause a muscle contraction)	80 pps	80 bps

Electrode Placement

The most basic premise behind the application of IFC is that two channels of electrodes must be used and they must be crossed. This will provide the opportunity for the current pathways to interact with each other within the underlying tissue. Current follows the path of least resistance, so it will look for conductive tissues along the way. We know that the body is not uniformly conductive so it would be impossible for the current to travel in a straight line through the underlying tissues; however, we can use the contour of the body to change where the current pathways will most likely interact with each other (Fig. 16-3).

Electrode placement with any form of electrical stimulation is one of the key factors to success in the accomplishment of the therapeutic treatment goal. When using neuromuscular electrical stimulation (NMES), the goal involves eliciting a motor response. This requires that both electrodes be placed on the muscle with one of the electrodes specifically on the motor point of the muscle.

The rationale behind this is simple. The resistance to the flow of electrical energy at the motor point of the muscle is the lowest at the motor end plate, meaning that it will take the least amount of electrical current to accomplish the goal of attaining a muscle contraction. To state this more simply, it means that it's the easiest place to have the current enter the muscle to accomplish the goal and be comfortable for the patient. The motor point of the muscle represents a window into the body, which is much easier to pass through than a "brick wall" of skin resistance. When using IFC, the electrodes come from two channels, not one, so electrode placement is different. However, knowledge of windows in the skin resistance will still be helpful, since it is always easier to pass through them than through "brick walls." This means that knowledge of areas of decreased skin resistance will help in the choice of electrode placement sites. Acupuncture points and trigger points exhibit decreased skin resistance and have been studied and used in the treatment of pain disorders for years. According to Dorsher, they exhibit a clinical correspondence to each other that is likely to be 95% or higher.[5]

The simplest way to think of electrode placement with IFC is "when in doubt, cross it out." The two channels of electrodes need to cross each other over the target treatment area (Fig. 16-4 A,B). This takes into account the use of acupuncture points, found on charts that happen to be located diagonally across from each other on the body.

See the Let's Find Out lab activity at the end of the chapter to guide you through electrode placement and making the sensation of the stimulus with IFC move by changing the position of the joint surrounded by the electrodes.

The "Third Line" of Current

Mention has already been made of two channels of electrodes being crossed over the treatment area. Each of these channels represents one line of current with IFC. The **vector,** or created field—the "third line"—occurs because of the interaction of the two channels inside the

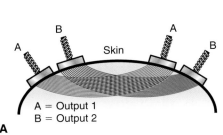

A

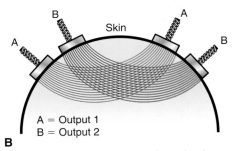

B

FIGURE 16-3 The idea behind IFC is based upon the concept of two sine waves interacting with each other to create a third line of current deep within the tissues. When there is contour between the channels of electrodes, the current must travel through more tissue and is perceived more deeply by the patient. **(A)** There is very little body contour between the electrode channels. **(B)** However, here there is much more contour between the channels of electrodes. The third line occurs deeper within the tissues.

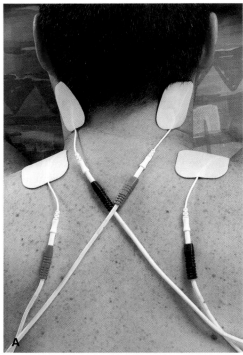

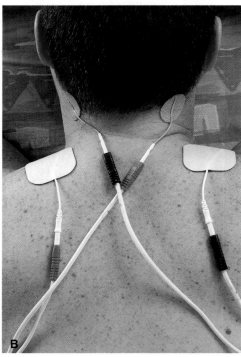

FIGURE 16-4 **(A)** Cervical spine with electrodes placed in a crossed pattern for IFC. The electrodes are equally sized. **(B)** Cervical spine with electrodes placed in a crossed pattern for IFC; however, the electrodes are not the same size. This will result in a shift of the third line of current closer to the smaller electrodes, which is also where the patient will have a greater perception of sensation.

body. This interaction as stated previously is highly dependent upon the conductivity of the underlying tissues in the treatment field. It's also equally dependent upon the relative polarity of the electrodes and the intensity of each of the two channels.

MAGNETS: HERE'S WHY YOU LEARNED ABOUT THEM IN KINDERGARTEN

Virtually everyone learned very early on that a magnet has both a positive and a negative end to it. We also all learned that:

- Opposites attract each other
- Likes repel each other

Now you have the opportunity to learn why you needed to know that!

LET'S THINK ABOUT IT...

If you have two magnets and the positive pole of the two magnets are facing each other, what happens? They repel each other. Think about what a sine wave looks like. It has a positive phase and a negative phase. Now take a look at Figure 16-5.

Clearly, these two channels start out of phase with each other and would be considered opposites. That causes them to repel each other once they encounter each other within the tissue, which is what causes the third line to occur in Figure 16-5. The third line or vector will occur in between the opposite phases of electrodes from separate channels. It will also occur at the beat frequency (Fig. 16.6).

BEFORE YOU BEGIN

1. What is the treatment goal for the IFC?
That prompts the selection of the beat frequency of the device.
2. How deep is what you are attempting to treat? Is there the possibility of placing contour into the field? This will guide you in patient positioning with IFC. A neutral joint position may not be the most optimal position.
3. Are there any acupuncture points or trigger points in the area that could be used?
These have decreased resistance to the flow of electrical current, which will make it easier for the current to cross the skin.
4. What is the direction of the tissues that you are attempting to stimulate?
Current flows most easily parallel to nerves and muscles. Placing your third line parallel to those tissues may enhance the perception of the stimulation for the patient.

Premodulation and Interferential Current Therapy

Many electrical stimulation devices that offer IFC have an additional setting on the device that is referred to as "premod" or premodulated IFC. This phrase is misleading to clinicians as it refers to a beat frequency or pulse trains being delivered from the device from one channel, not two (the basic requirement for interferential). Remember that interferential occurs due to the interference of separate channels within the tissues. If there is just one channel

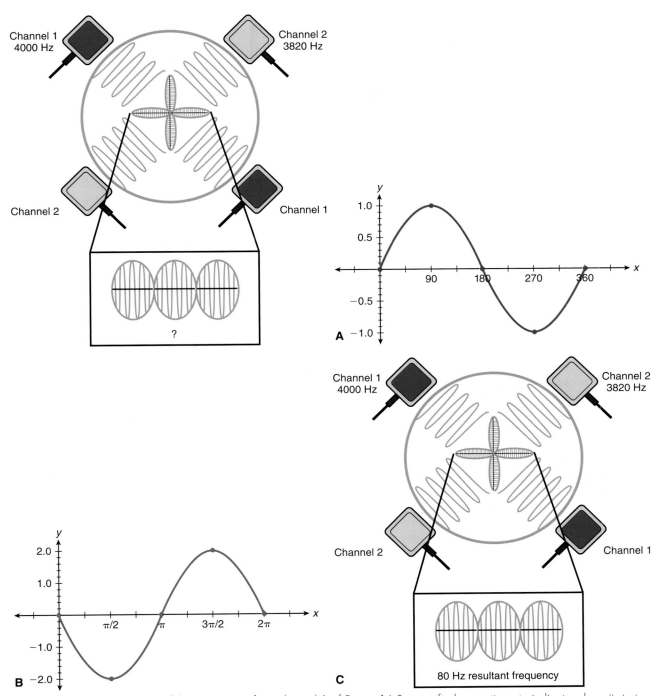

FIGURE 16-5 **(A)** This is one of the sine waves from channel 1 of Figure 16-3 magnified many times to indicate where it starts in terms of polarity. **(B)** This is one of the sine waves from channel 2 of Figure 16-3 magnified many times to indicate where it starts in terms of polarity. A and B sine waves are out of phase with each other. **(C)** The polarities repel each other within the tissue, which is what causes the third line to occur. Notice that the two channels are perpendicular to the treatment field. This would mean that the two electrodes on the top would be the same "phase," either negative or positive.

applied, nothing else is there to "interfere with." **Premodulation** simply means that the device is delivering packets of **kilohertz** frequency (1,000+ pps) that is modulated or interrupted at a lower frequency selected by the clinician as the treatment frequency.

One of the stated advantages of IFC is that of **Wedensky Inhibition,** which, as defined in *Stedman's Medical Dictionary*, is "the damping of muscle response resulting from application of a series of rapidly repeated stimuli to the motor nerve where less frequent stimulation produces muscle response."[6] This means that the stimulations that are provided by the uninterrupted kilohertz frequency under the electrodes of each channel are so rapid that they are incapable of eliciting a specific motor response. However, once two channels interfere with each other and the difference is within a sensory or motor range, the patient

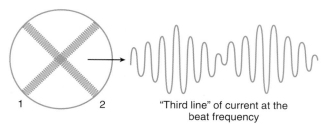

1   2   "Third line" of current at the beat frequency

FIGURE 16-6 A conceptual illustration of IFC. Notice that the two channels are perpendicular to the treatment field, meaning that the two electrodes on the top would be the same phase, either negative or positive.

then perceives the sensation within the tissues rather than under the actual electrodes.

The nerve can only carry impulses at its conduction velocity and must be permitted enough time to repolarize before another impulse can be carried. Until that time, it is in a state of refraction, referred to as its refractory period. Any additional stimulation will not cause a greater response from the nerve or tissues that the clinician is attempting to stimulate. That cannot occur until the nerve repolarizes. When extremely high frequencies such as those in the kilohertz range are administered, these have been described as causing Wedensky Inhibition under the electrodes or altered sensation. There is little to no substantive published literature to support whether or not Wedensky Inhibition for sensory nerves occurs; however, anecdotal evidence from patients supports that sensation under the electrodes is altered. In one study the spread of the IFC into cutaneous, subcutaneous, and muscle tissues was more efficient with true IFC, which used kilohertz frequencies capable of causing the effects described.[7] Another study found that IFC and burst-modulated biphasic pulsed currents yielded greater muscular force than Russian current.[8] Clearly more research is needed before definitive statements can be made; however, Dr. Nemec's early statements should not be completely dismissed regarding a comfortable or altered sensation under the electrodes.

LET'S THINK ABOUT IT...

Suppose you were anxious to purchase tickets to see your favorite performer and knew that the tickets were about to go on sale at a specific time but could only be purchased in person. Most individuals would probably make sure that they were lining up early to purchase the tickets. So, what would happen if there were a revolving door between the entry to the ticket office and the line and everyone in the line started to push the door at the same time, not allowing the door to revolve?

Answer: No one would be able to get through the door.
Why: The only way for anyone to get through the door would be to push the door at the speed that it is capable of revolving to allow someone else to enter.

This model is very similar to the refractory period of a nerve. If a nerve is receiving too much information too quickly, nothing goes through. That's the basic concept behind Wedensky Inhibition.

Modulation with IFC

It is commonly accepted that with alternating current, nerves will accommodate to a constant signal. For this reason, devices are equipped with a variety of options to help prevent this from occurring. The clinical significance of accommodation is that a patient would no longer report the same level of stimulation that he or she originally felt when the device was originally set up for the treatment intervention. If the original goal was to reduce pain, the sensation of the stimulation would need to take place throughout the treatment time. IFC devices have several options to prevent accommodation, each with a different name (Table 16-2).

TABLE 16-2	Modulation and IFC
TYPE OF MODULATION	**MECHANISM TO ACCOMPLISH GOAL**
Sweep	This type of modulation alters the frequency of one of the channels relative to the other channel. The sensation changes slightly so that accommodation is decreased. During setup, the clinician selects a frequency range rather than a set number and also must select a dynamic versus static mode once comfortable intensity levels have been determined. As with all forms of ES, this is determined by patient tolerance.
Amplitude	This type of modulation alters the intensity of one of the channels downward relative to the other channel. The sensation changes slightly so that accommodation is decreased. During setup, the clinician sets the intensity and also must select a dynamic versus static mode once comfortable intensity levels have been determined. As with all forms of ES, this is determined by patient tolerance.
Dynamic	This term refers to whether or not change takes place in the stimulation field. When something is dynamic, it means that it is changing. Changing fields decrease the potential for accommodation to occur.

Summary

Interferential current therapy (IFC) is not a new form of electrical stimulation. Despite that, it has not enjoyed the same level of scientific exploration as other commonly utilized electrical stimulation devices. It is something that can be found in virtually every outpatient physical therapy department and in many facilities is considered the "go-to" form of electrical stimulation for the reduction of acute pain.

IFC produces two independent kilohertz-frequency alternating currents of a constant intensity via two separate channels of electrodes. These channels of electrodes must be set up to cross each other to create interference where they intersect within the treatment field.[4] The effects within the treatment field are based upon the difference between the frequencies of the two channels, which results in a beat frequency in the treatment field that occurs along what is referred to as a vector. That vector can either be stationary or dynamic through the use of settings on the device. The depth of the vector can also be made to be felt more deeply through the use of patient positioning and the contour of his or her body. The literature is sparse regarding specific mechanisms; however, it is also sparse regarding refuting initially proposed mechanisms. It is clear that additional work needs to be done in this area as with other areas in physical medicine and rehabilitation.

Review Questions

1. Which of the following descriptions of the application of electrical stimulation most accurately represents IFC?
   a. Two channels from one stimulator are crossed over the treatment area and the intensity is adjusted to the patient's tolerance
   b. Two channels from separate generators within one stimulator that produces high frequencies in the thousands are crossed over the treatment area and the intensity is adjusted to the patient's tolerance
   c. Two channels from a TENS unit are crossed over the treatment area and the intensity is adjusted to the patient's tolerance
   d. Two channels from one stimulator are crossed over the treatment area and the intensity is adjusted to just above the patient's tolerance

2. What is the main advantage of IFC over other forms of electrical stimulation?
   a. There is no advantage to IFC
   b. IFC is billable at a higher rate than other forms of electrical stimulation
   c. IFC is purported to have a greater depth of penetration than other forms of electrical stimulation
   d. IFC is less comfortable than other forms of electrical stimulation

3. Which of the following treatment goals is inappropriate for IFC due to the crossing of the channels of electrodes that is required?
   a. A motor response
   b. Pain reduction
   c. Muscle guarding reduction
   d. None of the above, since they all could be accomplished with IFC

4. The importance of appropriate electrode placement sites has been discussed in several different chapters. Since IFC relies on the crossing of current pathways within the tissue, which of the following statements is most accurate regarding the type of electrode placement sites that should be considered?
   a. Where the electrodes are placed is irrelevant as long as the channels are crossed over the tissue
   b. As long as areas that have decreased skin resistance are used as electrode placement sites and the channels are crossed, that's all that matters
   c. The electrode placement sites must be motor points for the IFC to be effective
   d. Each channel must be placed over segmentally related electrode placement sites for the stimulation to be effective

5. What does "premodulation" mean when the term is listed on an electrical stimulation unit that is capable of producing IFC?
   a. It means that one channel can be used but there will be no greater depth of the current
   b. It means that two channels are still needed but they do not need to be crossed
   c. It means that the stimulator is an IFC device and nothing more
   d. It means that Wedensky Inhibition can be caused with the selection of a pre-modulated channel

CASE STUDY 1

Steve is a maintenance engineer for a retirement community. He has been referred to physical therapy for an evaluation and treatment for his knee. He has had many, many previous injuries and reconstructions to this knee. Recently, he fell from a second-story scaffolding at work and is now in extreme pain. It is also now necessary for the knee to be replaced. He is a 42-year-old "workaholic" who has been performing strengthening exercises to prepare himself for his impending knee replacement surgery. He is exceedingly anxious to return to his work and leisure activities, which include bicycling, canoeing, and hiking. He's interested in a non–drug-related form of pain relief while he continues to strengthen his vastus medialis oblique (VMO).

CASE STUDY 2

Karen is an analyst for the online education programs provided by a local college, which means that she's essentially working at computers most of the day. She has been complaining of lower back pain that seems to be deeply rooted within her back and often travels down the back of one of her legs. She sought out the assistance of a physical therapist for pain relief who has been helping with IFC and some manual techniques. The PT and PTA are working on her body mechanics and workplace ergonomics and relaxing her paraspinal muscle tightness, which, when inflamed, refers pain along the course of the sciatic nerve. See Figure 16-7 A, B, and C for examples of how IFC was used to handle Karen's pain depending upon where it travels on a given day.

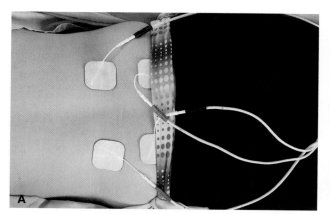
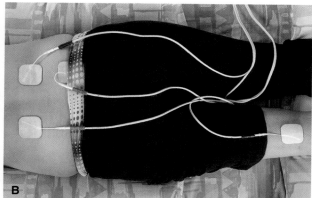
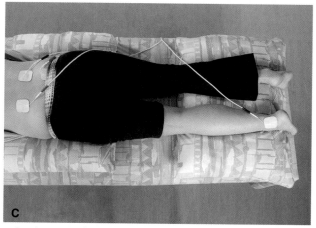

FIGURE 16-7 **(A)** Back with electrode placement for IFC for the lumbar spine. **(B)** Horizontal electrode placement for two channels for lumbar spine with referral down the leg. **(C)** Horizontal electrode placement for two channels for lumbar spine with referral down the leg.

DISCUSSION QUESTIONS

1. You are going to be working with a patient who is complaining of sternal pain following open-heart surgery. Would IFC potentially be indicated to help relieve his discomfort? Why or why not?

2. One of the patients you treated yesterday with IFC for pain reduction following a rotator cuff repair reported that after he returned home, his shoulder actually felt fatigued. He had not yet started a therapeutic exercise program. What could be the possible cause for the fatigue? Could it be related to the IFC? If so, how? Can something be done so that this would not happen again or would IFC need to be discontinued? Please support your responses.

3. One of the patients you will be treating this afternoon has acute chondromalacia of the patella in her left knee, which is edematous and painful. What position would make the most sense for her knee to be placed in for treatment with IFC and what parameters would you use? Please provide support for your response.

4. One of your patients has been diagnosed with piriformis syndrome as the root cause for his sciatica. Would there be any way to potentially use IFC to help provide him with any relief for his discomfort beyond temporary relief? If so, how? How might electrodes be placed and why? What would your parameters be for a treatment setup with him?

5. One of the patients in the department has subscapular pain and irritation. You notice that another therapist is attempting to use IFC to elicit a contraction from the subscapularis by placing the electrodes in a crossed pattern so that they encompass the subscapularis and are parallel to the majority of its muscle fibers. Is this something that you would recommend as a treatment option? Why or why not? Please provide your rationale behind your position.

REFERENCES

1. Dr. Hans Nemec. Web site: http://www.hans-nemec.at/index.php. Accessed July 2012.
2. Watson T. Electrotherapy on the Web. Available at http://www.electrotherapy.org Accessed July 2012.
3. Knight, KL, and Draper, DO: Therapeutic Modalities the Art and Science: Lippincott, Williams & Williams, Philadelphia, 2008, p 159.
4. Ward, AR: Electrical stimulation using kilohertz-frequency alternating current. Phys Ther 89:181–190, 2009.
5. Dorsher, PT: Can classical acupuncture points and trigger points be compared in the treatment of pain disorders? Birch's analysis revisited. J Alternative Complementary Med 14(4):353–359, 2008.
6. Stedman's Medical Dictionary. Lippincott Williams & Wilkins, Philadelphia, 2006.
7. Beati, A, Rayner, A, Chipchase, L, et al: Penetration and spread of interferential current in cutaneous, subcutaneous and muscle tissues. Physiotherapy 97(4):319–326, 2011.
8. Bellew, JW, Beisanger, Z, Freeman, E, et al: Interferential and burst modulated biphasic currents yield greater muscular force than Russian current. Physiother Theory Pract 28(5):384–390, 2012.

LET'S FIND OUT

Lab Activity: Electrode Placement Sites With IFC

Equipment
IFC stimulation unit
Self-adhering electrodes

Lead wires for the stimulator
4 equal-sized electrodes

Precautions and Why

Precautions	Why
Decreased sensation	If the desired response is dependent upon sensation, then ES may be useless. However if the desired response relies on a motor response, then the application may be considered safe.
Febrile conditions	The outcome of the first treatment should be monitored to determine whether or not any increase in circulation is too stressful for the immune system or not.
Epilepsy	This should be treated at the discretion of the physiotherapist in consultation with the appropriate medical practitioner, as adverse responses to IFC have included temporary changes in cognitive status, headache, vertigo, and other neurological signs when used in the cervical region.
Advanced cardiovascular conditions or cardiac arrhythmias	Treatment that involves placement of electrodes over the anterior chest wall may interfere with cardiac rhythm or electrically implanted devices.
Demands pacemakers	Electrical stimulation devices may interfere with the electrical demands of the pacemaker.

Contraindications and Why

Contraindications	Why
Pregnancy (first trimester)	There are no data to indicate the level of safety for the fetus with the application of electrical stimulation during the first trimester of pregnancy.
The anterior aspect of the neck or carotid sinuses	If circulation to the brain is altered, there could be adverse effects.
Malignancy active or suspected except in hospice, palliative, terminal care	Most application techniques have the potential to produce an increase in circulation to the area. The possibility exists that ES over or in proximity to a malignancy may enhance the development of metastasis.
Transthoracically	The heart is a muscle that can be stimulated electrically. IFC must *not* be administered across the contours of the thorax anterior to posterior or laterally where the heart could potentially be in the treatment field.

Interferential Current Electrode Placement Sites and Target Treatment Areas

Interferential current requires the use of two separate generators that produce a frequency greater than 100 Hz. The devices produce 2,000, 4,000, or 5,000 Hz, which is referred to as the *carrier frequency* of the stimulator. Familiarize yourself with the parameters that are available and how you would adjust them.

1. What is the carrier frequency of the device that you are using?

2. Are there any other carrier frequencies available on the device that you are using, and if so what are they?

3. What would be the appropriate pulse burst rate or *beat frequency* for sensory analgesia? _____

4. For a tetanic motor response? _____

Experiencing Interferential Electrical Stimulation and Joint Movement

Select a classmate for electrical stimulation to the knee. You will be applying interferential current (IFC) for generalized pain reduction throughout the knee joint, as if your patient had been diagnosed with chondromalacia of the patella that was producing pain posterior to the patella and inflammation on the superior medial aspect of the knee joint (Fig. 16-8 A,B).

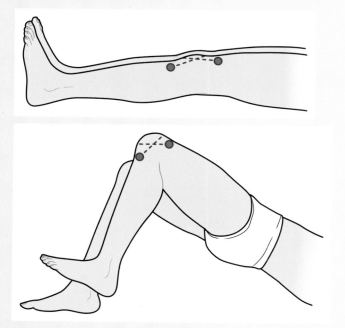

FIGURE 16-8 **(A)** When the knee is extended, the current pathways intersect more superficially. This makes it possible to change the location of the sensation without moving the electrodes but by changing the position of the patient instead. **(B)** When the knee is flexed, the current pathways intersect deeper within the joint.

Position your patient so that the knee is supported in about 20° of knee flexion (Fig. 16-9). Set up the electrodes (four electrodes of equal size) so that they crisscross over the knee on both the medial and the lateral aspects of the knee (Fig. 16-10).

1. Slowly increase the intensity controls on both channels, and ask your patient to describe what he or she is feeling and where he or she is feeling it.
2. What happens to the sensation when your patient increases knee flexion to about 90°?
3. Does the patient still feel the sensation in the same area?

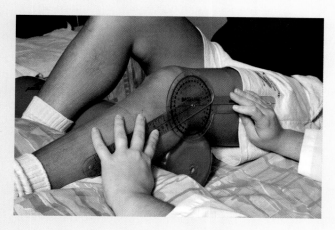

FIGURE 16-9 Appropriate positioning for the knee for placement of electrodes for treatment with IFC. The knee is supported and in an open joint position.

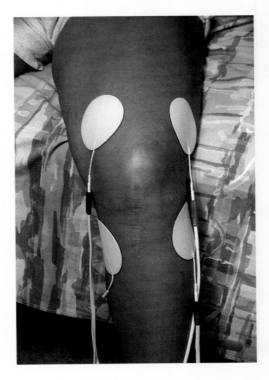

FIGURE 16-10 Application of IFC to knee, with two channels of electrodes that have been crossed.

4. Can the patient tolerate more intensity now? (If yes, increase the intensity.)

5. Locate the control on the device that will make the current move and ask the patient to describe what he or she is feeling now.

6. Is it easier or more difficult for your patient to locate the stimulus than it was before you added the dynamic component to the IFC?

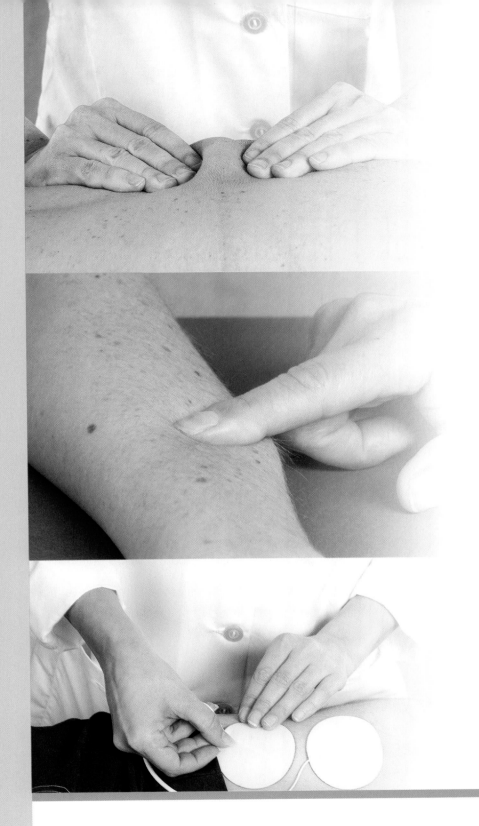

Comprehensive
Approach to Treatment

Integration of Physical Agents: Clinical Decision-Making

Barbara J. Behrens, PTA, MS | *Stacie Larkin, PT, MEd*

Learning Outcomes

Following the successful completion of this chapter, the learner will be able to:

- Describe how clinicians can find evidence to support their choices in treatment interventions for various patient diagnoses.
- Select the best interventions for a given patient based on the patient's goals, treatment goals, patient safety, time constraints, cost effectiveness, and equipment availability.
- Sequence treatment interventions that use modalities to complement and enhance other treatment interventions.
- Describe the essential information to be included when documenting the objective portion of a SOAP note.

Key Terms

Adherence
Assessment
Contraindications
Documentation

Indications
Objective
Plan
Precautions

Reliable
Subjective
Tolerate

Chapter Outline

U.S. Food and Drug Administration (FDA)
Evidence-Based Practice
    Hooked on Evidence
    Other Online Databases
Therapeutic Treatment Goals: Is a Physical Agent
    Appropriate?
Available Treatment Time
Acuity of the Injury

Medical Stability of the Patient
    *The Impact of Patient Adherence to Therapy on
        Recovery*
    Patient Expectations
Available Physical Agents
Integration Principles for Physical Agents: What to
    Choose?
    Indications: Primary and Secondary

> *"Why should I care? What does it mean to me in*
> *my practice?"* —Anonymous

Patient Perspective

"Are you sure that this really works, or is this something that you just dreamed up one night?"

Once again, these perspectives are perhaps seemingly unrelated on the surface, but are critical to the overall success of virtually every treatment intervention in physical therapy. Clinicians must be able to demonstrate to patients that what they plan on doing with them in the clinic is based upon sound physiological research that is supported in the literature. Clinicians must be able to support the approaches that they take with a sound rationale and the requisite patient education to explain what they are planning on doing to help that patient. This will not only help the patient but it will also help to assure that the clinician can demonstrate why the approach was taken to third parties. Those third parties might be individuals who are making reimbursement decisions. So, to answer the question "What does it mean to me in my practice?" it could mean the difference of being paid or not being paid for what one does.

The patient's perspective is also critical to consider and understand. It can be as simple as providing the rationale in simple terms for a patient to understand why you as a clinician have selected the treatment interventions that you have selected. In addition, being able to support those decisions with research articles that bolster your decision-making process should help patients feel more comfortable

in your ability to help them improve. Patients also are interested in having their insurance company pay for their rehabilitation. So, anything that can be done to help a patient understand why clinicians do what they do can help the patients buy into the process as well.

The practice of physical therapy is forever changing. According to the APTA *Guide to Physical Therapist Practice* (2001), a document developed and reviewed by a contingent of more than 600 physical therapists, treatment interventions using electrotherapeutic modalities, physical agents, and mechanical modalities are used for the purpose of (1) reduction of a symptom or (2) promotion of a response. This includes promoting tissue healing,[1-4] increasing blood flow to an injured area,[5,6] muscle strengthening,[7-9] increasing tissue extensibility,[10-12] and promoting pain relief.[13-16] These treatment goals have therapeutic benefits that can be visually observed and manually or mechanically measured.

These goals can often be interdependent. For example, a modality used for the reduction of pain may reduce the level of discomfort enough to decrease the protective muscle guarding in the area. If the guarding subsides, then the potential exists that the blood flow into or from

Continued

the area will no longer be impeded by the muscle guarding, and metabolite retention in the area will have a chance to diminish, resulting in less chemical irritation (from the metabolic retention) and ultimately less pain. Pain can also be considered a protective response, warning the individual not to further stress the injured area. The area is no longer as strong as it once was. Pain perception may intensify because of the muscle guarding and the resulting metabolite retention in the injured tissue.

Many of the individual techniques presented throughout this text address the three sides of the pain triangle—pain, dysfunction, and muscle guarding—but for a discussion of the different degrees refer to Chapter 2. Some techniques primarily target the pain or the muscle guarding and indirectly address the dysfunction. Others specifically target the dysfunction by promoting tissue healing and experience a resultant decrease in pain perception and muscle guarding as the area heals.

One important consideration in the selection of physical agents is the concept of causal factors. The mark of excellence in clinical practice is the attention paid to the cause-and-effect relationship and acknowledgment of the importance of understanding the relationship. Clinicians treat the patient by considering the patient and the normal courses of response to therapeutic interventions. By identifying the cause of the patient's problems, effective treatment interventions can be used, thus decreasing the potential of reoccurrence. Technicians treat the individual symptom without regard for causal factors. Patients treated in this manner are more likely to get frustrated, as their symptom relief is often temporary (Table 17-1).

Skilled clinicians must select the appropriate treatment intervention to fit (1) the diagnosis of the patient, (2) the medical stability of the patient, (3) the anticipated goals of the intervention, (4) the experience of the clinician, and (5) the choices available to the clinician. The influence of each of these factors will vary from individual to individual. Patient safety must remain foremost in this aspect of the decision-making process.

Patient Perspective

Remember that if your patient has previously received physical therapy for an injury, your patient is probably one of your best resources for information regarding what works and what does not.

Your patient must be included in the treatment intervention process. You must be considerate of his or her time as well as your own. Instructions must be stated in terms that your patient or significant other will be able to understand. If you are asking your patient for feedback, make sure that your patient knows how to provide appropriate feedback. Some patients may have the misconception that "no pain means no gain." It is your responsibility to explain what you are doing and why this philosophy does not apply to physical therapy treatment interventions with physical agents.

Patients' Frequently Asked Questions

1. Why can't you just do everything at the same time?
2. Why do I need to have ice after exercise? I really want to leave sooner.
3. Why don't you do the same thing with every patient? That patient seemed to "get more" than I did and our bills were the same.
4. Yesterday when I went to that other place and had the traction with the heat and electrical stimulation then my neck hurt afterward. Why?

This chapter focuses on each of the anticipated outcomes from direct treatment interventions identified within the APTA *Guide to Physical Therapist Practice* resulting from electrotherapeutic modalities, mechanical modalities, and physical agents (Box 17-1). In order to determine whether a goal has been accomplished, the clinician must be able to collect the appropriate information from the patient through tests and measures. The clinician must also recognize that his or her overall approach to the treatment intervention and to the patient will affect the results. The clinician's approach in treating a patient experiencing pain involves the recognition of the pain and assessment of its impact on functional activities and the patient's life in general.[17,18] Determining what factors contributed to the patient's symptoms and how to help the patient limit the potential for the return of

TABLE 17-1	Clinicians Versus Technicians in Their Treatment Approach to Patients	
CLINICIAN	**TECHNICIAN**
Identifies the cause for the problem	Treats symptoms
Treats the cause and educates the patient	No regard for causal factors
Decreases the potential for recurrence, resulting in higher patient satisfaction	Recurrence common and relief is temporary, leading to patient frustration

Electrotherapeutic Modalities
- Biofeedback
- Electrical muscle stimulation
- Functional electrical stimulation (FES)
- Iontophoresis
- Neuromuscular electrical stimulation (NMES)
- Transcutaneous electrical nerve stimulation (TENS)

Anticipated Goals From Electrotherapeutic Modalities
- Ability to perform physical tasks is increased.
- Ventilation, respiration (gas exchange), and circulation are improved.
- Complications are reduced.
- Edema, lymphedema, or effusion is reduced.
- Motor function (motor control and motor learning) is improved.
- Muscle performance is increased.
- Pain is decreased.
- Joint integrity and mobility are improved.
- Risk of secondary impairments is reduced.
- Soft tissue swelling, inflammation, and restriction are reduced.
- Wound and soft tissue healing is enhanced.

Direct Interventions: Physical Agents and Mechanical Modalities

Physical Agents
- Cryotherapy (cold pack, ice massage)
- Deep thermal modalities (ultrasound, phonophoresis)

   From the APTA *Guide to Physical Therapist Practice*, ed 2.
- Superficial thermal modalities (heat, paraffin baths, hot packs, Fluidotherapy)
- Hydrotherapy (aquatic therapy, whirlpool tanks, contrast baths, pulsatile lavage)
- Phototherapy (ultraviolet)

Mechanical Modalities
- Traction (sustained, intermittent, or positional)
- Compression therapies (vasopneumatic compression devices, compression bandaging, compression garments, taping, total contact casting)
- Tilt table or standing table
- Continuous passive motion (CPM)

Anticipated Goals From Physical Agents and Mechanical Modalities
- Ability to perform movement tasks is increased.
- Complications from soft tissue and circulatory disorders are decreased.
- Edema, effusion, or lymphedema is reduced.
- Motor function (motor control and motor learning) is improved.
- Pain is decreased.
- Joint integrity and mobility are improved.
- Risk of secondary impairments is reduced.
- Soft tissue swelling, inflammation, or restriction is reduced.
- Tolerance to positions and activities is increased.
- Independence in airway clearance is increased.

symptoms is essential. The technician who merely applies a modality indicated for the treatment of pain may not have lasting success if the cause of the pain is not addressed. This is where patient education becomes an important component of the treatment plan.

There are several different approaches to treatment interventions that will result in favorable responses from and for the patient. The clinician must be a good observer and know what tests and measures to apply before and after performing any therapeutic treatment intervention to determine whether the chosen intervention had a positive outcome.

U. S. Food and Drug Administration (FDA)

The past has taught us that we can no longer take for granted that something works without asking the basic science questions regarding the "why and how." Before May 1976, medical devices were regulated as a new drug, and because of their use and lack of specific scrutiny within that division, those in existence were grandfathered in as safe and effective. Now they are regulated by the FDA's Center for Devices and Radiological Health, which manages and facilitates a highly structured process for medical devices including regulations, classifications, premarket approvals, investigational device exemptions, and labeling and tracking guidelines. Essentially, these regulations require manufacturers to first prove that a device is not only safe for use on human subjects but is also effective before it is marketed to the clinical community. This process requires that testing take place to determine exactly what results can be expected from the application of the device to a patient.[19]

Very few new devices have gone through this scrutiny, which can take years. An excellent example is the recent introduction and premarket approval of low-level or cold LASER (acronym for "light amplification of stimulated emission of radiation") devices for adjunctive use in the temporary relief of hand and wrist pain associated with carpal tunnel syndrome. Although laser has been commonly used outside the United States for many years, in 2002 only one manufacturer was granted 510(k) approval for this application. Since that time, other manufacturers have received clearance from the FDA by demonstrating that their devices are substantially equivalent to devices on the market. Using a medical device for interventions that are not preapproved by the FDA is not reimbursable by insurance carriers and such uses are termed off-label applications. This policy and procedure was put into place to protect the public from unsafe or unfounded claims being made and equipment from being used in an untested manner and billed to a patient's insurance carrier.

In addition, the FDA has implemented a Medical Device User Fee and Modernization Act of 2002 (MDUFMA), which charges a fee to those companies that apply for premarket approval for a new device. The goal of the MDUFMA is to fund the FDA's medical device directives to "ensure that safe and effective new products get to consumers as quickly as possible."[20]

Evidence-Based Practice

The impact of the FDA on the practice of physical therapy may seem remote to some clinicians but, in reality, it helped spark a movement leading toward evidence-based practice (EBP). Evidence-based practice has been defined as "the conscientious and judicious use of current best evidence in making decisions about the care of individual patients."[21]

When a profession places more value on past practice or previous experience rather than EBP, the potential exists for negative outcomes to be interpreted as a failure of physical therapy when, in reality, the technique and not the profession was at fault. Reliance on EBP to set the standard for care should eliminate potential negative outcomes.[22] Evidence is more than just the experience of a clinician; it is based upon the documented outcomes of multiple clinicians with standardized sets of patient groups, symptoms, and treatment parameters. In addition, the measurement tools for EBP tend to be more objective than personal experience.

HOOKED ON EVIDENCE

The need for evidence has grown considerably stronger through the efforts of the American Physical Therapy Association (APTA), which developed an online searchable database called Hooked on Evidence. This database is a compilation of article extractions related to physical therapy interventions submitted by members of the APTA. Those who submit an extraction use a prescribed detailed template to extract the following information from a published research article: general information, study design, study details, methods, treatment, and outcomes. As of 2012, there were approximately 7,500 article extractions included in the database.[23] Part of the process involves an attempt to take a body of preexisting work and attempt to quantify the results using the same markers, some taken from the APTA *Guide to Physical Therapist Practice*. For example, the following headings are highlighted for each reviewed article:[23]

- Target condition
- Element of patient/client management model
- Practice pattern
- Design type
- Study population
- Population location
- Inclusion criteria
- Exclusion criteria
- How were subjects selected?
- How many subjects were contacted initially?
- How many subjects were eligible to participate?
- How many subjects agreed to participate?
- Nonclinical characteristics of study participants
- Clinical characteristics of study participants
- Blinded clinicians
- Blinded subjects
- Same person providing treatment and testing measures
- Intention-to-treat analysis
- Treatment groups

- Authors' stated purpose interventions
- Study outcomes
- Authors' conclusions
- Reviewers' comments

OTHER ONLINE DATABASES

Databases or online resources vary significantly in the types of information that they search. There are online databases that cover business-related journals to help researchers track business conditions (ABI Inform) through PsycINFO, which contains articles from more than 1,700 journals that deal with psychology-related topics. Although it would seem logical to find all things medical in the MEDLINE database (the National Library of Medicine's electronic database), this is not the case. Each of the databases has its own inclusion and exclusion criteria, which is one of the reasons that it is better to consult more than one online database. It is important to remember that these services are subscription services, unlike Google, which is a nonspecific metasearch engine that is available to everyone and provides all "hits" with the key terms. Items retrieved through a nonsubscription service must be carefully evaluated for their value. Not all articles published on the Internet are reviewed, so it is important when looking at these articles that you consider the source and currency of the information presented. Just because something can be accessed via the Internet does not make it reliable or valuable. *Remember: Articles published in professional journals that are peer reviewed are still the most reliable sources of information regarding patient and treatment intervention information.* Table 17-2 depicts online databases and the types of information that can be accessed through them.

Therapeutic Treatment Goals: Is a Physical Agent Appropriate?

The physical agents that this text addresses are used in the management of numerous soft tissue injuries and some selected neurological conditions. These conditions are associated with symptoms that may include pain, altered sensation, edema, muscle guarding, muscle weakness, decreased soft tissue extensibility, or lack of muscle function. Each of these symptoms may be managed in part through the application of one or several physical agents as components of a physical therapy treatment intervention. Many of the aforementioned signs and symptoms can also be addressed through the use of therapeutic exercise, manual techniques, pharmacological agents (medications), and rest as a part of the total care of the patient. However, physical agent approaches can be used in combination with any or all of the other approaches to help facilitate recovery for the patient. The ultimate question for all clinicians will remain the same: "Am I doing all that I can do to improve the condition of the patient safely, efficiently, and cost effectively?"

The overzealous or inexperienced clinician may use a "shotgun" approach. This involves the use of multiple techniques both manual and mechanical to accomplish a goal.

TABLE 17-2 | Online Databases and the Types of Accessible Information

ONLINE DATABASE	TYPE OF INFORMATION
PubMed	The National Library of Medicine's premier bibliographical database covering the fields of medicine, nursing, dentistry, veterinary medicine, the health care system, and the preclinical sciences. The database contains more than 12 million citations dating back to the mid-1960s. (www.ncbi.nlm.nih.gov/pubmed)
APTA's Hooked on Evidence Web site	APTA's Hooked on Evidence Web site represents a grassroots effort to develop a database containing current research evidence on the effectiveness of physical therapy interventions. This database is available to all APTA members. (www.hookedonevidence/com)
Cumulative Index to Nursing and Allied Health Literature (CINAHL), owned by EBSCO Host	Index with abstracts from 1,200 of the leading journals in nursing and allied health
EBSCO Host—Academic Search	Provides full text for nearly 3,200 scholarly publications covering academic areas of study, including social sciences, humanities, education, computer sciences, engineering, language and linguistics, arts and literature, medical sciences, and ethnic studies
EBSCO Host—Health Source, Consumer Edition	Indexing and many full text for more than 270 health periodicals, more than 1,100 health pamphlets, and 20 health reference books
EBSCO Host—Nursing Academic	Provides more than 520 scholarly full-text journals focusing on many medical disciplines. Also featured are abstracts and indexing for more than 560 journals.
Educational Resource Information Center (ERIC)	Contains citations and abstracts from more than 980 educational and education-related journals, as well as full text of more than 2,200 digests
LexisNexis—Academic Universe: Medical PsycINFO (owned by Reed Elsevier)	Full text and abstracted medical and health information Indexing and abstracts for more than 1 million articles in 1,700 journals dating back to 1887 with some full-text articles available through PsycARTICLES

Some of these databases require subscription fees or are limited access and may be available through college or university libraries.

Unfortunately, the patient may report a negative treatment outcome that then could not be traced back to any individual source, because all of the pieces were administered together. For example, suppose a patient is receiving a therapeutic treatment intervention for a primary complaint of pain, which, upon examination, is thought to be attributed to protective muscle guarding throughout the cervical musculature, limiting the motion and thus protectively guarding the injured area from further trauma. The therapeutic treatment interventions that are used include hot packs, traction, electrical stimulation, ultrasound, massage, joint mobilization, and therapeutic exercises. Several of the chosen treatment techniques address the primary complaint of pain, and several of the techniques might be capable of relieving the cause underlying pain or protective muscle guarding. The combination of treatment techniques may or may not relieve the symptoms. The patient's symptoms may increase if any one of the techniques used is not appropriate for this patient and, with this approach, it will not be possible to determine which technique is at fault.

Clinicians can also get lost in the multitude of symptoms that a patient may offer. Prudent practitioners will identify the primary functional goals and address the impairments that are limiting the patient's ability to perform a given functional activity. When a selected intervention is used, the therapist must assess the patient's response following the individual treatment intervention to determine whether a positive change has occurred. If there are remaining impairments, another physical agent or treatment intervention *might* be indicated. Reduction of the patient's chief complaint may result in reductions of his or her other symptoms, but this will be evident only to the observant clinician. If, for example, pain is worsened by the underlying muscle guarding, reduction of the guarding should reduce the pain. It may or may not be true that relieving the pain will reduce the muscle guarding. This is why it is important to focus treatments on what is causing the pain rather than just trying to treat pain in isolation. Pain is a symptom that may affect a patient's ability to perform functional tasks. It is the ability to perform these tasks that must also be reassessed to determine whether physical therapy was successful.

Available Treatment Time

Patients receive physical therapy in a variety of settings including hospitals, outpatient clinics, skilled nursing facilities, schools, and their own homes when they are well enough to be home but cannot easily commute to an outpatient clinic. The time constraints and support mechanisms will vary significantly among these settings. It is important to consider the patient's needs and goals when designing a treatment program. Patients will not realistically devote every waking hour to their recovery. Time management in the accomplishment of therapeutic treatment goals must be taken into consideration. Treatment sessions that involve physical agents may require approximately 10 to 20 minutes with the remaining treatment time dedicated to manual techniques, patient education, therapeutic exercise, and re-assessment. Although there are exceptions, based upon the diagnosis and other related factors, most treatment sessions usually last approximately 1 hour.

During this time, the goals that have been established and negotiated with the patient need to be addressed. This is the point at which true integration must take place. Many of the techniques will treat the primary patient complaints and indirectly address the other patient problems. It is not necessary or realistic to use every modality that could possibly be used to treat a patient because of this overlapping of responses. Time management and intervention assessment revolve around carefully limited choices to accomplish a goal, assessing the outcome of a given physical agent, and then making modifications when indicated.

Use of every unattended physical agent conceivable for one impairment could involve several hours of time with an end result that is no more significant than if the clinician carefully selected one of the physical agents and used it for 15 to 20 minutes. The general guideline that therapists should follow is to choose the minimum number of treatment interventions that will achieve the maximal response. Whenever possible, treatments should be combined in order to be more efficient. For example, a patient with a painful and edematous knee could receive ice, compression, and elevation at the same time. Another example is combining active range-of-motion (ROM) exercises while receiving a whirlpool treatment. It is important to be judicious in the selection of interventions and conscious of time requirements to use them, as this will directly have an impact on your schedule and ability to treat other scheduled patients. Also, reimbursement can be an issue depending on how a third-party payer reimburses physical therapy treatment sessions. Some carriers may pay for their patients to receive up to three different treatment interventions. Others carriers may pay a flat rate for treatment, regardless of the number of individual treatment interventions used or the amount of time spent with a patient. Remember that patients, too, desire and deserve efficient use of their time. If the treatments become excessively long, the patient may become frustrated and not return for future appointments. Box 17-2 provides the clinician with questions to consider when treating patients with physical agents.

Some treatment interventions that might be indicated for a given patient, based upon their condition, may produce

BEFORE YOU BEGIN

Choose the minimum treatment interventions that will achieve the maximum response.

> **BOX 17-2 | Clinical Considerations When Treating With Physical Agents**
>
> - What is the available treatment time? How much time will it take? (more or less than 1 hour?)
> - How long has it been since the actual injury?
> - What is the medical stability of the patient?
> - What expectations does the patient have about the treatment?
> - What modalities are available to accomplish the treatment goals in the time available for treatment?

comparable results through completely different mechanisms. The approach taken may be more reflective of the individuality of the patient and his or her responses to previous treatment intervention techniques than a specific technique itself. If, for example, a patient had read an article in a magazine that outlined the successes of the use of electrical stimulation for the relief of muscle tension via pain relief, he or she may respond better to electrical stimulation than to traction. Their beliefs may influence the potential benefits of the selected physical agent (see Box 17-2).

Acuity of the Injury

When treating an acute injury, the emphasis of treatment is on maintaining mobility and preventing further injury while the impairments of pain, edema formation, and muscle guarding are addressed.[24] Severely involved patients with multiple trauma and those with neurological impairment will most often be seen for treatment initially in an acute care hospital setting and then be transferred to a rehabilitation facility for a more intensive approach to their recovery. Generally, when there is more tissue destruction, the recovery time will be longer. In these instances, the patient may be seen by a clinician twice daily in an inpatient setting. Even there, the focus on careful selection of treatment intervention techniques should not change. Because these patients have experienced a significant change in their functional ability, they will be involved in a more broad-based therapeutic program. There will be a greater emphasis on therapeutic exercise and adaptive skills for functional independence. Physical agents as treatment interventions will be chosen as an adjunct to their treatment plan to reduce symptoms and to enhance their return to function. Overall, time management and goal optimization in the use of therapeutic agents should remain the same regardless of the treatment setting.

Medical Stability of the Patient

Therapeutic treatment interventions are performed to promote optimal recovery of the patient, not the symptom. Patients with comorbidities might limit your potential choices of physical agents as treatment interventions. Suppose, for example, that a patient sought out physical therapy for the treatment of a cervical strain and sprain, and her primary complaints included pain with limited motion in the cervical spine due to muscle guarding. The patient's medical history reveals that she has osteoporosis. Although cervical traction may be beneficial for the relaxation of the cervical musculature, it would be contraindicated for this patient. The intervention choice may change to one of managing the pain with a portable electrical stimulation device and focusing predominantly on the patient's pain to decrease the muscle guarding rather than the opposite.

Another example of an alteration in treatment intervention selection arising from medical stability issues is the patient who is referred to therapy for lower extremity edema. Upon assessment of the lower extremity, there are no palpable pedal pulses. Although one of the treatment interventions that might have been used for the management of the edema could have been intermittent compression, it would be contraindicated for this patient. The lack of pedal pulses would indicate a decrease in the blood supply to the lower extremity and may be indicative of further medical complications that would need to be evaluated by a physician. It is important to be sure that the cause of the edema is known and that it is appropriate to receive physical therapy interventions. When edema is the result of medical conditions such as congestive heart failure or kidney dysfunction, treating the edema can cause undesirable responses. Box 17-3 depicts indications, contraindications, and precautions and "why."

THE IMPACT OF PATIENT ADHERENCE TO THERAPY ON RECOVERY

Patient **adherence** to a therapy regimen or patient reliability regarding following through with home programs when assigned plays a crucial role in the recovery process. The patient must be able to understand the purpose of the therapeutic interventions so that there is follow-through during the times he or she is not in therapy. Most treatment plans incorporate patient education and/or a home exercise plan so that gains made in therapy can be maintained or further developed at home. Those who are too young or have impaired ability to follow instructions may need to rely on a family member to help with a home program. When progress is slowed or when gains that were made in therapy are not present in the next treatment session, it becomes evident that adherence to therapy is not happening. Patients and their families must understand that the therapy that they receive is only for about 1 hour three times each week. The other 23 hours of those days and the 24 hours of the days without therapy are the responsibility of the patient.

Suppose, for example, that a pediatric patient is with her parents seeking physical therapy to assist in the reduction of the lateral curvature of her scoliosis. The therapist may suggest a trial use of electrical stimulation on the concave side of the curvature to fatigue the musculature and on the convex side for strengthening. The optimal time for the application is at night while the child sleeps. Success with this intervention may obviate the need for surgical correction of the curvature. Unfortunately, the parents feel sorry for their child and use the device every other night rather than the recommended nightly protocol. This course of therapy is unsupported by the parents and deemed a failure, resulting in the child requiring corrective surgery. The intervention may have been appropriate and effective if it had been applied as instructed, but without parental support, it is a failure (Box 17-4).

BOX 17-3 | Know Your Indications, Contraindications, and Precautions!

Why?

- **Indications**: If you do not have a sound physiological rationale for why you are doing something, then you should not be doing it.
- **Contraindications**: Check the patient's medical record for possible contraindications. For example: if treating over the lower back region of a female patient, ask her whether she is pregnant or whether there is any chance that she is pregnant. Pregnancy is a common contraindication for many physical agents. It is better to be safe than sorry. Do not assume someone else asked the patient these questions yet!
- **Precautions**: Be familiar with your patient's medical history and review the medications he or she is taking. Precautions are conditions that need to be closely monitored when providing a specific intervention. If the patient is taking analgesics, he or she may not be able to accurately report painful sensations, so you would need to be more cautious when working with him or her. Another example: if your patient has a pacemaker, the heart rate will not change in the same way that a patient without a pacemaker would respond.

BOX 17-4 | Enhancing Patient Adherence to Therapy

Patient Education

- If you don't know what to expect, how will you know if you are getting it?
- If you don't know what you should be feeling, how will you know if you are feeling it?
- If you don't understand what you shouldn't be feeling, how will you protect yourself?

Significant Others/Family Members

- Do they understand the intent of the intervention and that it is not painful?
- Do they understand that the intervention is not a form of punishment?
- Do they understand the importance of managing the symptoms when the patient is not in the clinic? Do they understand that a break from the activities may cause a patient setback?

PATIENT EXPECTATIONS

Another problem that exists is the perpetuation of the phrase among fitness fanatics and athletes of "no pain, no gain." It is important to realize that when administering a treatment intervention or physical agent, the appropriate responses to the treatment must be explained to the patient as well as the inappropriate responses to treatment.

Let us use the example of an athlete who seeks physical therapy for the treatment of a contusion to the quadriceps. Ultrasound has been recommended for the alteration of the scar tissue that is now limiting the athlete's torque production. During the application of the ultrasound, the patient thinks of the "no pain, no gain" philosophy. The patient begins to feel a prickling sensation leading to a burning sensation, and thinks: "OK, now it's really working, it's really beginning to burn now" without ever making a comment to the clinician delivering the intervention. The patient probably experienced a periosteal burn, which is detrimental to the tissue. The outer lining of bone, the periosteum is highly innervated and rich in collagen. The patient should have been informed about ultrasound and what it should and should not feel like and told to report any perceived sensation to the clinician during the delivery of ultrasound. Instruction needs to be clear prior to applying the physical agent, and the patient's ability to respond appropriately needs to be assessed to determine whether the selected physical agent will be safe for the patient (Box 17-5).

Available Physical Agents

Because there is a wide degree of overlap of many clinical physical agent treatment interventions for the accomplishment of therapeutic goals and because several of the agents address primary complaints as well as secondary complaints, it is important to recognize what tools are available. Patients may plateau with their progress after repeated attempts with a given treatment intervention. It is also

---

BOX 17-6 | Available Physical Agents

- What are the goals that I need to accomplish?
- Which modalities are capable of accomplishing the goals?
- What is not at present in use by someone else?
- Can more than one goal be accomplished with what is available?
- Is there another way to address the goal with the modalities that are available?

---

feasible that when a patient arrives in the department for treatment, the specific physical agent that was used during the last treatment session may not be available. Clinicians need to understand how to accomplish the same treatment goals using alternate methods if their first choice is unavailable (Box 17-6).

Integration Principles for Physical Agents: What to Choose?

INDICATIONS: PRIMARY AND SECONDARY

The first step in determining what physical agent or agents lies in the **indications**. What are the direct effects, and what are the secondary benefits of selecting a given physical agent? Is it primarily used to reduce edema? Will it reduce pain indirectly because of the decreased edema? By establishing a list of the primary and secondary indications of a physical agent and comparing that list with the treatment goals for a patient, you can determine which physical agents might be of benefit for that patient.

SAFETY CONSIDERATIONS: PRECAUTIONS AND CONTRAINDICATIONS

After this initial list is compiled, review each of the physical agents selected and compare them with the medical condition of the patient. Determine whether there are any safety concerns, such as impaired cognition, compromised sensation, or peripheral vascular disease that could eliminate any of the physical agents as potential treatment options. It is the responsibility of the clinician to know the **contraindications** and **precautions** for each specific treatment intervention with or without physical agents and to screen for them. In other words, clinicians must know when it is inappropriate to use a physical agent (contraindication) and when it might be possible to use the physical agent but it must be used judiciously (precaution).

EQUIPMENT AVAILABILITY

Next, look at the availability of the potential physical agents that you have selected. There are usually several

---

BOX 17-5 | Previous Patient Experience With Selected Physical Agents

- Has your patient ever been treated with this physical agent before?
- What was his or her experience with it?
- Was it ever explained to the patient, and did the patient understand what to expect?
- Is your patient willing to try your use of the physical agent again?
- You will explain what the patient should expect.
- Make sure your patient understands normal and adverse responses that he or she needs to report to you.

pieces of equipment in any therapy department that can accomplish a multitude of goals—some better than others. Determine exactly what is available by looking at the necessary parameters for the protocol that you have selected. Do any of the pieces of equipment available meet the parameter requirements?

EQUIPMENT RELIABILITY

Of the pieces of equipment available to you that are not contraindicated for your patient and meet the appropriate parameters for you to accomplish your treatment goals, how many are reliable? When was the last inspection date from the biomedical engineering department? Most electrical equipment should be professionally inspected at minimum once a year and the date of the inspection should be identified with a sticker on the device. If there is no indication that the device has recently been inspected, then there is also no reason for you as a clinician to know whether or not the device is **reliable**, or will work correctly when you need it to operate safely for your patient. The clinician must inspect the equipment and its accessories to determine whether it is complete and operating properly *before* applying it to a patient. Any device that appears faulty should be labeled so and removed from the treatment area. Also, make sure that you are familiar with all of the unit's controls and parameters *before* applying it to a patient.

LET'S THINK ABOUT IT...

When was the last time that you rented a car? If you know how to drive, it is expected that you are responsible enough to know that you will need to find:

- The brakes
- The gas pedal
- The headlights
- The windshield wipers
- The controls to open and close the windows

When you rent a car, no one shows you where any of the above controls are located. That's up to you to find them before you leave the lot! The same thing is true for all of the "boxes" in a physical therapy department. You need to know how to find what you need (in terms of operating controls) *before* you are in front of a patient.

PREVIOUS PATIENT EXPERIENCE WITH THE SELECTED PHYSICAL AGENT

One valuable resource that can easily be overlooked is the patient! Many patients who are receiving therapy have received physical therapy previously. The patient may have had a memorable experience with a physical agent. Ask your patient about his or her previous experiences with therapy and with physical agents. Knowing what has worked well for the patient in the past may help you decide what to use. Likewise, if a patient has a particular aversion to a certain physical agent, as often seen with cryotherapy, then you might want to suggest other appropriate alternatives or find out what the circumstances were behind that application which might not have been appropriate.

What Does the Rest of the Plan of Care Include?

It is important to look at your choices in terms of efficient use of time and expected outcomes. If you selected a physical agent that will address only the primary complaints requiring 20 minutes to apply and you identify that you will also need to use something else to address additional symptoms, can you combine two physical agents and apply them simultaneously? If you do, would this compromise the therapeutic benefit of either one? This is often done with cold packs and electrical stimulation, when the treatment goal is to decrease pain and inflammation.

PREPARATORY TREATMENT

Is your goal for the physical agent one that involves preparation for another activity within the plan of care? For example, heat is often used prior to interventions that focus on increasing the extensibility of connective tissue, such as joint mobilization, soft tissue mobilization, and traction. The heat serves to relax the patient and heat the superficial structures, which can enhance the patient's response to the mobilizing techniques that follow.

FOLLOW-UP TO AN ACTIVITY OR TREATMENT APPROACH

Treatment sessions may involve a wide variety of treatment techniques, some of which may result in some minor levels of discomfort to the patient. Therapeutic exercise may increase the amount of friction in the joint structures, which may result in some localized edema following the activity. Ice may be applied post-exercise to reduce the localized discomfort that was just caused by the increased activity level of the injured area. If the plan involves the application of a physical agent to reduce discomfort after an activity, it is important for the clinician to explain the process to the patient so that the discomfort can be understood and not offset fear of the activity in the future.

Putting It All Together: The Decisions and the Evidence

There is a great deal of decision-making involved when choosing and incorporating a physical agent into a patient's treatment program. As discussed, clinicians must consider many issues when deciding which intervention is best for a particular patient. Part of the decision-making process includes knowing what evidence is credible and available to support a particular intervention with a physical agent. Finding evidence is getting easier and easier as electronic databases are making the search quicker for clinicians to find up-to-date information, but the strength of that information must be carefully evaluated as to the source, reproducibility, and adherence to published guidelines established by licensing agencies where applicable, such as the FDA.

Observation of the initial condition and then reassessment of the patient following any therapeutic intervention will justify their continuation, modification, or the termination of a treatment. Without a carefully constructed process for these assessments, it is difficult to ascertain whether progress is being made (refer to Chapter 2 for assessment techniques). If a patient is beginning to regain strength, experiences a decrease in pain, has less edema, or has less muscle guarding, then he or she will likely resume functional activities. Return to function is the cornerstone of therapeutic interventions (Box 17-7).

Documentation

Documentation is an essential form of communication that serves the needs of the patient, the physical therapist, the physical therapist assistant, third-party payers, and other health care providers involved with the care of the patient including nursing, other therapists, and the physician.[25] It is the legal document that serves to substantiate the treatments provided, and they are often used by third-party payers to determine reimbursement for the interventions. It also provides the details necessary for someone else to reproduce the treatment. For these reasons, it is essential that documentation is clear, concise, and accurate. All pertinent information must be recorded for it to be useful as a record.

BOX 17-7 | Keys to Success With Physical Agents

- Review the published literature.
- Explain treatment techniques to your patients.
- Keep treatment plans simple.
- Observe your patient and record those observations.
- Portray confidence to your patients.
- Reassess after every individual treatment technique and intervention.
- Observe again! And continue to record your observations.

SOAP NOTES

One common documentation format is the SOAP note format. SOAP is an acronym for Subjective, Objective, Assessment, and Plan. A SOAP note is a form of progress note used to document both the treatment and the patient's responses to the treatment. This form of documentation is recorded in the patient's chart and becomes a permanent record of therapy for that patient. It is these progress notes that will answer the basic questions of how a patient responded to a given treatment technique when the chart is reviewed. The chart should present a clear and concise record of exactly what was done and how the patient responded so that anyone reading the chart would understand exactly why the particular course of actions took place upon subsequent patient visits. When documenting a treatment intervention with a physical agent, the details of the treatment must be readily apparent to whoever reads it. This would include the type of physical agent, the parameters chosen (for example, duration, intensity/temperature, frequency), patient positioning (if unusual), and the body part or structure treated. These details are typically found in the objective portion of the treatment note. The patient's response to treatment and suggestions for progressing or modifying the treatment must also be documented, usually in the assessment and plan sections of the progress note. Box 17-8 outlines the components of a SOAP note. Please remember the key to documentation: "If it wasn't documented, it didn't happen."

Summary

Tools are wonderful to have, but without the knowledge of what to do with them they are useless. In physical therapy, as in other areas, this is also true. If we do not stop and take the time to think about what we need to accomplish or the most efficient way to accomplish it, we will fail. This is especially true if we neglect to reassess what we have done and document it. Box 17-9 provides selected key points to keep in mind during the process of providing physical therapy treatment.

Throughout this chapter, we have presented a way to integrate the information from this text and to find credible sources of new information for new tools. We have also provided a systematic approach to documenting what you have done with your patients.

BOX 17-8 | SOAP Notes

- **S = Subjective:** Subjective information refers to the information offered by the patients pertaining to how they feel. Personal biases and emotional background influence subjective information. It may encompass physical complaints and emotional or psychological difficulties. The comments by the patient are entered into the patient record in quotation marks and identified by the phrase "the patient stated that . . ." Asking patients how they feel lets them report their perception of their current state, and can also orient the clinician to pertinent questions that should be asked next.
- **O = Objective:** Objective information, unlike subjective information, is unbiased, impersonal, unprejudiced, factual information. This is the portion of the documentation that includes all relative parameters of the treatment approach so that anyone reading the chart could duplicate the treatment. Examples of objective entries for each modality are listed with the modality to which they pertain:

  Thermal modalities
  Ultrasound
  Hydrotherapy
  CPM
  Intermittent compression
  Electrical stimulation

- **A = Assessment:** The assessment portion of the documentation deals with the patient's response to treatment. The tendency for the use of the phrase "pt. tolerated treatment well" *must* be avoided, because the word "tolerated" provides little information regarding the response to the treatment. To **tolerate** something literally means to bear up under or to endure without injury. It offers no positive or negative comments regarding the treatment effectiveness. The assessment is your professional judgment of how the patient is progressing with the plan of care.
- **P = Plan:** The plan should involve a description of anticipated treatment sessions, based upon the assessment of the present treatment intervention. It also includes information regarding potential discharge or new techniques or exercises for the next session.

BOX 17-9 | Some Key Take-Home Concepts

Following are selected key concepts to which practitioners should be alerted when "putting it all together" for client care:

- **Causes of Pain:** It is important to focus treatments on what is causing the pain rather than just trying to treat pain in isolation. Pain is a symptom that may affect a patient's ability to perform functional tasks. It is the ability to perform these tasks that must also be reassessed to determine whether physical therapy was successful.
- **Functional Goals Versus Impairments:** Prudent practitioners will identify the primary functional goals and address the impairments that are limiting the patient's ability to perform a given functional activity.
- **General Guideline for Treatment:** The general guideline that therapists should follow is to choose the minimum number of treatment interventions that will achieve the maximal response.
- **Evidence-Based Practice:** When searching for EBP-supported treatment methods, keep in mind that articles published in professional journals that are peer reviewed are still the most reliable sources of information regarding patient and treatment intervention information.
- **Patient Education:** Clinicians must be able to support the approaches that they take with a sound rationale and the requisite patient education to explain what they are planning on doing to help that patient.
- **Contraindications and Precautions:** It is the responsibility of the clinician to know the contraindications and precautions for each specific treatment intervention with or without physical agents and to screen for them.
- **Equipment Reliability:** The clinician must inspect the equipment and its accessories to determine whether it is complete and operating properly *before* applying it to a patient.

Finally, the ultimate questions for all clinicians:

- "Am I doing all that I can do to improve the condition of the patient safely, efficiently, and cost effectively?"

CASE STUDY 1

Richard is a 55-year-old retired truck driver who decided to seek out a physical therapist for treatment to relieve pain and stiffness in his right knee. X-rays revealed arthritic changes in both knees. He had a medial meniscectomy in the right knee 2 years ago. His recent complaints of pain and stiffness are related to his present leisure and work activities. Richard is an avid golfer, country-western dancer, and chauffeur.

- Which physical agents could potentially provide sustained relief for Richard if they were used as a part of a comprehensive treatment approach to address his symptoms?

- If you decided to use electrical stimulation for pain relief, which form would you use? Please provide your rationale for your selection.
- Would Richard potentially benefit from the use of a TENS unit at home? If yes, why? If no, why not? Please be sure to support your answer with consideration of his lifestyle and activity level.

CASE STUDY 2

Charlotte is a 50-year-old secretary who went to the outpatient physical therapy department to see if she could receive treatment to relieve symptoms associated with the automobile accident that she was involved in 3 weeks ago. She is having difficulty maintaining an upright posture due to severe headaches, back pain, and intermittent paresthesia in her dominant right hand. She is a frail woman who taught aerobics classes five nights a week. She is unable to teach at all now. Her orthopedist told her that there were no fractures, and she is otherwise healthy.

- Which physical agents could potentially provide sustained relief for Charlotte if they were used as a part of a comprehensive treatment approach to address her symptoms?

- If you decided to use electrical stimulation for pain relief, which form would you use? Please provide your rationale for your selection.
- Would Charlotte potentially benefit from the use of a TENS unit at home? If yes, why? If no, why not? Please be sure to support your answer with consideration of her lifestyle and activity level.
- Would Charlotte potentially benefit from the use of cervical traction to provide relief of her radiculopathies? Please be sure to support your answer.
- Based upon the information that was provided for you, would there be any concerns that you might have regarding proceeding with treatment with Charlotte? If so, what additional information would you want to know? If not, why not?

DISCUSSION QUESTIONS

1. Using an electronic database, find evidence to support the use of electrical stimulation to facilitate wound healing.

2. A patient you are treating presents with edema as a result of a recent ankle sprain. List all the interventions that you could consider for treating the edema. What must you consider when deciding the best intervention to decrease her swelling?

3. As a therapist, how would you monitor patient adherence to a home exercise program?

4. Search the Internet for Web sites that would be helpful to you as a physical therapy student. Your search results should include the address that you visited, how you found the address, the date you visited it, and what you found useful about it. You will also need to consider the validity of the content by identifying the source of information—for example, did the information come from the National Institutes of Health's Web site or from a commercial vendor? And

when was the Web site last updated? The course director will keep all search results in a resource notebook. You may have future access to the sites that each of your classmates found.

5. Your mother is scheduled to see a physical therapist after her recent car accident. She has heard you speak about electrical stimulation and is terrified. How could this affect the results that she is able to attain? What could be done to help alleviate her fears of this modality? (This can be either a written assignment or class discussion.)

6. A colleague has stated that there is no time in the clinic for patient explanations to take place regarding treatment. The colleague stated that he just wants patients to come in, receive treatment, and leave and that this has been successful so far. How would you respond to this and what if anything would you suggest to the colleague? (This can be either a written assignment or class discussion.)

REFERENCES

1. Houghton, PE, Kincaid, CB, Lovel, M, et al: Effect of electrical stimulation on chronic leg ulcer size and appearance. Phys Ther 83:17–28, 2003.
2. Debreceni, L, Gyulai, M, Debreceni, A, et al: Results of transcutaneous electrical stimulation (TES) in cure of lower extremity arterial disease. Angiology 46:613–618, 1995.
3. Karba, R, Semrov, D, Vodovnik, L, et al: DC electrical stimulation for chronic wound healing enhancement. Part 1. Clinical study and determination of electrical field distribution in the numerical wound model. Bioelectrochem Bioenerg 43:265–270, 1997.
4. Gentzkow, G, Pollack, S, Kloth, L, et al: Improved healing of pressure ulcers using Dermapulse, a new electrical stimulation device. Wounds 3:158–170, 1991.
5. Field-Fote, EC, and Tevavac, D: Improving intralimb coordination in people with incomplete spinal cord injury following training with body weight support and electrical stimulation. Phys Ther 82:707–715, 2002.
6. Griffin, JW, et al: Reduction of chronic post-traumatic hand edema: a comparison of high voltage pulsed current, intermittent pneumatic compression, and placebo treatments. Phys Ther 70:279, 1990.
7. Fitzgerald, GK, Piva, SR, and Irrgang, JJ: A modified neuromuscular electrical stimulation protocol for quadriceps strength training following anterior cruciate ligament reconstruction. J Orthop Sports Phys Ther 33:492–501, 2003.
8. Snyder-Mackler, L, Delitto, A, et al: Strength of the quadriceps femoris muscle and functional recovery after reconstruction of the anterior cruciate ligament. A prospective, randomized clinical trial of electrical stimulation. J Bone Joint Surg Am 77:1166–1173, 1995.

9. Lewek, M, Steven, J, Snyder-Mackler, L: The use of electrical stimulation to increase quadriceps femoris muscle force in an elderly patient following a total knee arthroplasty. Phys Ther 81:1565–1571, 2001.

10. Peres, SE, Draper, DO, Knight, KL, et al: Pulsed shortwave diathermy and prolonged long duration stretching increase dorsiflexion range of motion more than identical stretching without diathermy. J Athl Train 37:43–50, 2002.

11. Knight, CA, Rutledge, CR, Cox, ME, et al: Effect of superficial heat, deep heat, and active exercise warm-up on the extensibility of the plantar flexors. Phys Ther 81:1206–1214. 2001.

12. Funk, D, Swank, AM, Adams, KJ, et al: Efficacy of moist heat pack application over static stretching on hamstring flexibility. J Strength Cond Res 15:123–126, 2001.

13. Jarit, GJ, Mohr, KJ, Waller, R, et al: The effects of home interferential therapy on post-operative pain, edema, and range of motion of the knee. Clin J Sport Med 13:16–20, 2003.

14. Hurley, DA, Minder, PM, McDonough, SM, et al: Interferential therapy electrode placement technique in acute low back pain: a preliminary investigation. Arch Phys Med Rehabil 82: 485–493, 2001.

15. Albright, J, Allman, R, Bonfiglio, RB, et al: Philadelphia panel evidence-based clinical practice guidelines on selected rehabilitation interventions for knee pain. Phys Ther 81:1675–1700, 2001.

16. Moore, SR, and Shurman, J: Combined neuromuscular electrical stimulation and transcutaneous electrical nerve stimulation for treatment of chronic pain: a double-blind, repeated measures comparison. Arch Phys Med Rehabil 78:55–60, 1997.

17. Waddell, G, and Richardson, J: Observation of overt pain behavior by physicians during routine clinical examination of patients with low back pain. Psychosom Res 36:77, 1992.

18. Vlayen, JWS, et al: Assessment of the components of observed chronic pain behavior: the Checklist for Interpersonal Pain Behavior (CHIP). Pain 43:337, 1990.

19. Device Advice: Device Advice is CDRH's self-service site for medical device and radiation emitting product information. Device advice is an interactive system obtaining information concerning medical devices. Web site: www.fda.gov/cdrh/deadvice/2004.

20. FDA Talk Paper: FDA Meets with Stakeholders to Address Issues Related to the Implementation of the Medical Device User Fee and Modernization Act of 2002 (MDUFMA). Web site: www.fda.gov/bbs/topics/ANSWERS/2003/ANSO 2004.

21. Sackett, DL, Rosenberg, WM, Gray, JA, et al: Evidence based medicine: what it is and what it isn't. BMJ 312:71–72, 1996.

22. Fritz, JM, and Wainner, RS: Perspective examining diagnostic tests: an evidence-based perspective. Phys Ther 81:1546–1564, 2001.

23. Hooked on Evidence. Web site: http://www.hookedonevidence.com.

24. Soderberg, GL: Skeletal muscle function. In Currier, DP, and Nelson, RM (eds): Dynamics of Human Biologic Tissues. FA Davis, Philadelphia, 1992, pp 92–93.

24. Miller, CR, and Webers, RL: The effects of ice massage on an individual's tolerance level to electrical stimulation. J Orthop Sports Phys Ther 12:105, 1990.

25. Kettenbach, G: Writing SOAP Notes—With Patient/Client Formats, ed 3. FA Davis, Philadelphia, 2004, p 2.

Page numbers followed by "f" denote figures, "t" denote tables, and "b" denote boxes